For my mother, Belle, who always believed in me.

And for Luke. My first, my last, my everything.

MODALITIES

FOR Massage AND Bodywork

MODALITIES
for Massage and Bodywork

Elaine Stillerman, LMT

Founder, MotherMassage®
New York, New York

Foreword by George Peter Kousaleos, BA, LMT

Founder and President, Core Institute School
of Massage Therapy and Structural Bodywork

Tallahassee, Florida

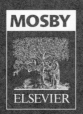

MOSBY

ELSEVIER

11830 Westline Industrial Drive
St. Louis, Missouri 63146

MODALITIES FOR MASSAGE AND BODYWORK ISBN: 978-0-323-05255-9

Notice

Neither the Publisher nor the Authors assume any responsibility for any loss or injury and/or damage to persons or property arising out of or related to any use of the material contained in this book. It is the responsibility of the treating practitioner, relying on independent expertise and knowledge of the patient, to determine the best treatment and method of application for the patient.

The Publisher

ISBN: 978-0-323-05255-9
ISBN 10: 0-323-05255-X

Vice President and Publisher: Linda Duncan
Senior Acquisitions Editor: Kellie White
Associate Developmental Editor: Kelly Milford
Publishing Services Manager: Julie Eddy
Project Manager: Marquita Parker
Designer: Paula Catalano

Printed in Canada

Last digit is the print number: 9 8 7 6 5 4 3

Working together to grow
libraries in developing countries

www.elsevier.com | www.bookaid.org | www.sabre.org

ELSEVIER   BOOK AID International   Sabre Foundation

CONTRIBUTORS

Sandra K. Anderson, BA, LMT, NCTMB
Massage and Bodywork Educator and Freelance
    Writer
Practitioner, Massage Therapy, Shiatsu, Thai Massage
Co-Founder, Tucson Touch Therapies
Tucson, Arizona

**Jack Blackburn, LMP, Masters in
    Theological Studies**
Registered Counselor, Spiritual Director
Trager Practitioner, Focusing Trainer, Reiki Master
Seattle, Washington

Beverly Byers, EdD, RN, LMT, MTI
Associate Professor, MSN Coordinator – Nursing
Lubbock Christian University
Founder, Owner, Director, Oceans Massage
    Therapy Center
Lubbock, Texas

R. Makana Risser Chai, LMT, JD
Author of two books on Lomilomi
CEO, Hawaiian Insights, Inc.
Kailua, Oahu, Hawaii

Judith DeLany, LMT
Director and International Instructor
NMT Center
Saint Petersburg, Florida

Sharon Desjarlais, CC
Certified Business Coach and Communications
    Consultant for CranioSacral Therapists
Owner, Your True-Calling Coach
Developer, CranioSacral Success™ Marketing System
Jupiter, Florida

Sandy Fritz, BS, MS, NCTMB
Owner and Head Instructor
Health Enrichment Center School of
    Therapeutic Massage
Lapeer, Michigan

Richard M. Gold, PhD, LAc
Professor, Body Therapy and Somatics
Pacific College of Oriental Medicine
International Professional School of Bodywork
San Diego, California

Keith Eric Grant, PhD, MS, BS
Senior Instructor, Sports &
    Deep Tissue
McKinnon Institute
Freelance Physicist & Writer
Ramblemuse Associates
Oakland/Pleasanton, California

Robert Harris, HND, RMT, CLT-LANA
Director and Senior Instructor
Dr. Vodder School – International
Victoria, British Columbia

Leslie Korn, PhD, MPH, RPP, NCBTMB
Director, Health Alternatives, LLC
Center for Traditional Medicine
Olympia, Washington

Whitney Lowe, LMT
Director
OMERI
Sisters, Oregon

Sonia Elisa Masocco, MT, LDT, CAy
Senior Instructor, The Ayurvedic Institute
Private Practice, Ayurveda and
    Phytotherapy
Albuquerque, New Mexico

Diana Moore, BS, MS, LMT, CIMI®
Certified Infant and Toddler Mental
Health Specialist
President and Founder, Loving Touch®
Certified Infant Massage Instructor Training Program
International Loving Touch Foundation, Inc.
Portland, Oregon

Joseph E. Muscolino, DC
Instructor
The Connecticut Center for Massage Therapy
Newington, Connecticut

Laura Norman, BS, MS, LMT, ARCB
Internationally Certified Reflexologist
Certified Inspired Life Coach
Founder, Owner, Director
Laura Norman Wellness Centers
Delray Beach, Florida

Terry Norman, BME, LMT
Exam Review Committee Member, NCBTMB
Certified Practitioner, ALBTA
Instructor, University Texas–Arlington and Mountain
    View Community College–Dallas
Private Practitioner
Mansfield, Texas

Art Riggs, CMT
Certified Advanced Rolfer
Private Practice
Instructor/Director, Deep Tissue Massage Program
San Francisco School of Massage
Oakland, California

Susan G. Salvo, BEd, LMT, NTS, CI, NCTMB
Co-Director and Instructor
Louisiana Institute of Massage Therapy
Lake Charles, Louisiana

Peter Schwind, PhD
Director/Founder, Munich Group
Instructor Barral Institute
West Palm Beach, Florida
Certified Advanced Rolfer
Advanced Rolfing Instructor
Munich, Germany

Dane Kaohelani Silva, DC, LMT
Center for Spirituality & Healing
Faculty, University of Minnesota
Minneapolis, Minnesota

Elaine Stillerman, LMT
Founder, MotherMassage®: Massage During
    Pregnancy Training Course
Contributor, Massage Today
Writer/Consultant, "Real Moms, Real Stories,
    Real Savvy"
New York, New York

John E. Upledger, DO, OMM
President and Founder, The Upledger Institute, Inc.
Medical Director, The Upledger Clinic
Certified Specialist of Osteopathic Manipulative
    Medicine
Palm Beach Gardens, Florida

REVIEWERS

Don Ash, PT, CST-D
Physical Therapist
Alliance Physical Therapy
Rochester, New Hampshire

Susan G. Beck, BS, CIMI, NCTMB
Coordinator/Instructor, Massage Therapy Program
Dept. of Health Occupations, College of Technology
Idaho State University
Pocatello, Idaho

Cheryl Chapman, RN, HNC, NCTMB, NJSC
Oncology and Mastectomy Massage Specialist
Continuing Education Educator
Certified Holistic Nurse Practitioner
Private Practice
Millburn, New Jersey

Giovanni Felicioni

Alexandra Hamer, MA, LMBT
Orthopedic Massage Therapist
KMI Structural Integrator
Durham, North Carolina

Michaela Johnson, BA,LMT
Tucson, Arizona

Deane Juhan
Bodyworker
Instructor, Trager Institute
Orinda, California

Don Kelley, LMT
Hohenwald, Tennessessee

Eleanora Lipton, BA, RPE
Registered Polarity Educator, American Polarity
   Therapy Association
Founding Director, Atlanta Polarity Center
Atlanta, GA

Janet Markovits, LMT
AMTA
New York, New York

Stefan Matte, LMT
AIS Practitioner
Stretching Boston
Boston, Massachusetts

Tamara Mondragon
Hawaiian Lomilomi Instructor
Hawaiian Healing Arts
Honolulu, Hawaii

Thomas W. Myers, LMT, NCTMB, ARP
Director
Kinesis, Inc.
Walpole, Maine

Dianne Polseno
President
Cortiva Institute
Boston, Massachusetts

Sharon Puszko, PhD, LMT
Owner, Director, Educator
Day-Break Geriatric Massage Institute
Indianapolis, Indiana

Joseph F. Recknagel, BS, ATC
Assistant Athletic Trainer
Detroit Lions, Inc.
Allen Park, Michigan

Sande Rosen, LMT, NCR
Boynton Beach, Florida

Maureen Stott, LMT
Therapeutic Massage Center Vernon
Vernon, Connecticut

Stewart Wild, LMT, CNMT
AMTA, NCBTMB
Holliston, Massachusetts

Hildegard Wittlinger
Professor
Dr. Vodder Schule/Wittlinger Therapy Center
Walchsee, Austria

Qianzhi Wu, BS, MS (China), LAc
Professor, Preceptor, and
    Vice President of Faculty
The Academy of Oriental
    Medicine at Austin
Austin, Texas

FOREWORD

Each of us has benefited greatly from the creation and advancement of practical knowledge. We understand that sharing pertinent information is both a professional and personal mandate, especially when that knowledge has a far-reaching positive effect on the health and well-being of humanity. There have also been important professional and educational experiences in our lives when we immediately realized that the knowledge gleaned from these precious moments would have a great impact on who we could become, on what we could then do for others, and on how we could live a more fulfilling life. The publication of *Modalities for Massage and Bodywork* feels to me like one of those moments. The valuable information contained in these pages, representing the most popular modalities of therapeutic massage and bodywork, comes at a critical time for the massage and bodywork profession as it integrates more fully with the cultures of health and wellness, medicine and rehabilitation, and sports and fitness. This project has pulled together an impressive body of theoretic and clinical information, incorporating the history, theory, science, art, skill, and competency of each modality with insightful clarity. This publication has manifested an expansion of the profession's ever-expanding knowledge base.

Modalities for Massage and Bodywork is unique because it was written by a dedicated group of educational leaders with vast clinical experience, clearly representing the broadest knowledge base of therapeutic massage and bodywork available in the world today. These authors have dedicated their lives to the health of their clients and patients and have invested many years of profound study to master and teach their particular form of somatic therapy. Their personal and professional qualifications engender trust and respect from their colleagues and from tens of thousands of massage therapists and bodywork practitioners who have previously gained from their wisdom and clarity. Indeed, they are the stewards of a living tradition that reaches into the past, while defining our present, and preparing us for the future.

Many practitioners have sought to educate themselves about the diversity in the profession by reading general textbooks, professional magazine and journal articles, and other educational resources. Their desire to gain an understanding about the width and breadth of these modern and centuries-old traditions has grown exponentially with the growing acceptance of the profession by the general public. While reading the chapters of this book you may find yourself marveling again and again at the complexities and diversities in each modality of touch therapy. The editing of this valuable book by Elaine Stillerman has brought together valuable knowledge for everyone who seeks to understand the practical nature and intricate characteristics of each system. Her guidance and support for the contributors and their somatic modalities were evident in the development of each chapter. Her respect and passion for this profession served as a guiding beacon that kept everyone focused on this important compilation.

Whether you are a student of massage therapy who is searching for a fuller understanding of the art and science of this field, or you are a new practitioner who is contemplating how to choose a modality to specialize in, this book will offer you a wealth of information from disciplines that cover the broad spectrum of Asian, traditional European, contemporary western, energetic, medical, sports, and structural forms of somatic therapy. For seasoned practitioners this book is an incredible source of detailed information that will add substance to the modalities that you have been practicing, while inspiring you to learn more about those modalities that have escaped your past training.

As a founder, executive director, and faculty member of a leading school of massage therapy, I am delighted to add this book and DVD to our curriculum's resource list. Most massage therapy schools teach introductory courses on many of the modalities in the following chapters. This book will help massage and bodywork instructors refine their class curriculum through expansion of the content areas in each learning objective. For those who offer continuing education and advanced certification training, this book will improve the confidence that teachers and students must have in resource material that supports the foundation of each program. This book will also benefit the general public as they search for practical information about the massage and bodywork modalities that are practiced in their local communities. I can see this book being strategically placed in school libraries and in the waiting rooms of massage therapy clinics, bodywork centers, rehabilitation facilities, and multidisciplined wellness centers.

For the visual learner *Modalities for Massage and Bodywork* has a companion DVD that highlights seven of the most popular modalities. This amazing video allows the learner to witness the clinical techniques and treatment protocols that are essential for safe and effective practice. You will watch the hands of these gifted practitioners as they explain their strategies and hopeful outcomes. This DVD is a unique resource that brings both clarity and practical reality to the written content of the book.

For 30 years I have engaged in both the clinical practice and teaching of somatic therapies, specializing in structural integration, myofascial therapy, and athletic performance strategies. I have been fortunate to have practiced and taught in several countries with unique sociocultural heritages. In some of those cultures massage therapy was a primary medical component and fully integrated into wellness-oriented care and education. My perspective of the diversity of massage and bodywork was further enhanced by my early involvement in state regulatory and licensure issues, national certification standards, massage-related research, educational scholarship, and international approval of massage therapy as a medical service at Olympic and world championship events. I have attended hundreds of state, regional, national, and international conventions and conferences and met with thousands of massage therapists, bodywork practitioners, educators, scientists, and other allied health professionals. Each of these experiences added layers of understanding and appreciation for the vast territorial expanse that covers this amazing field. Through all of these professional and personal encounters I was inspired to appreciate the uniqueness of each form of manual therapy. I sought to understand the differences and similarities, the unique histories and philosophies, and the primary clinical procedures and accepted treatment standards. It wasn't until I had this book in my hands that I knew that here was a resource that I had always been hoping for — a textbook that brought together the most vibrant notes and clearest voices of this amazing symphony of somatic therapy.

Modalities for Massage and Bodywork has had an immediate impact on my expanding professional awareness, and reading it reminded me of an event that happened eighteen years ago. I was one of the organizers of the 1990 International Congress of Massage and Bodywork, where over 100 practitioners and teachers from eight countries gathered in the Canary Islands for 1 week to share their knowledge and skills. During that week, people from different cultures who spoke different languages shared the embodiment of their disciplines through lecture, demonstration, and discussion. Like this book, we shared the critical information on modalities and clinical systems that we had learned and developed. We sought a common language that described the true essence of our approaches, while singling out the special terminology that exemplified the unique character of each modality. We also recognized how similar our life's path had been and how many were pioneers in their respected fields. We were uplifted by the common forces that drove our professional lives and from the somatic forces that gave us the energy to look for the singular truth in the healing modality that we practiced. And we all agreed that no matter what system we practiced, no matter what culture and history we embraced, and no matter how we interpreted the human body, we deeply knew that the essence of our work was in restoring balance to the human condition. We understood that we were personally transformed by this ability to provide somatic homeostasis that benefits the human condition.

I believe that the special wisdom of these modalities, expressed by an incredibly gifted group of authors and healers, will provide a foundation for understanding the myriad of possibilities that rest in our fingertips. This book, under the expert guidance of Elaine Stillerman, represents a remarkable undertaking that has seamlessly integrated the highest qualities and standards of our professional traditions and will serve as a landmark resource for many years to come.

George Peter Kousaleos, BA, LMT
CORE Institute
Tallahassee, Florida

PREFACE

Modalities for Massage and Bodywork introduces readers to 21 different bodywork techniques written by the pre-eminent leaders in their respective fields. No other text offers instruction from such a prestigious listing of innovative and renowned practitioners. The modalities that are included in this book are the most sought after classes in advanced training and continuing education seminars at massage schools across the country.

Students and practitioners of the somatic arts and massage schools are the primary audiences for this book. Although this book is not a substitute for appropriate on-site training, students and practitioners can reaffirm their knowledge of techniques they have already studied and can also learn about different bodywork modalities they may want to pursue. This is especially important if your massage school does not offer some of these modalities. The chapters can help you decide if it is a subject you want to study in more depth. In addition, massage schools can adapt their continuing education program based upon the teachings of these highly regarded professionals. Instructors who are proficient with a particular modality may use that chapter to create a syllabus for their own introductory classes.

Modalities for Massage and Bodywork is arranged alphabetically for ease in reading. Each chapter starts with Student Objectives and lists the Key Terms that are unique to that particular modality. These terms will be defined within the text when they initially appear for greater explanation.

A brief description of the modality is followed by its historical development. The body of the chapter describes the modality in greater detail and includes its benefits, contraindications, and specific techniques for basic training.

Case Histories serve to illustrate the effects of each modality within a therapeutic context. These experts also provide personal insights about specific techniques. Each chapter includes Multiple Choice Test Questions to help measure your understanding of the modality, a list of resources for more information, and a suggested readings list.

Modalities for Massage and Bodywork also offers readers an opportunity to witness seven of these experts teaching their modality. The DVD that is included offers lectures from our experts in these fields: Dr. Lisa Upledger in CranioSacral Therapy, Judith DeLany in Myofascial Release and Neuromuscular Therapy, Kathleen Crawford in Reflexology, Sandy Anderson in Shiatsu, Richard Gold in Thai Massage, and Elaine Stillerman in Prenatal Massage.

For massage schools and instructors, *Modalities for Massage and Bodywork* provides the appropriate context for you to teach each bodywork technique. The curriculum for each subject is offered, and a test with an answer bank and explanations helps determine your students' comprehension of key points. The DVD helps those students who are visual learners while the text provides essential elements for those students who prefer to read the material.

It is important to reiterate that no bodywork technique can be learned from a book or a video. It is irresponsible for anyone, student or instructor, to read this book and assume authority on its subjects. Hands-on training can only be learned in a classroom setting with a qualified instructor.

This compilation of bodywork techniques is unique in its scope and contributors. I hope you will use it to further your knowledge and interest in a variety of subjects that enrich your practices and provide appropriate care for your clients.

Elaine Stillerman

ACKNOWLEDGMENTS

A book of this scope and depth could not have been possible without the help from all the dedicated and talented contributors. I want to pay my respects for their innovative work and thank Joe Muscolino, Sonia Elisa Masocco, Bev Byers, John Upledger, Sharon Desjarlais, Susan Salvo, Diana Moore, Makana Risser Chai, Dane Silva, Robert Harris, Keith Eric Grant, Art Riggs, Whitney Lowe, Leslie Korn, Laura Norman, Sandra Anderson, Sandy Fritz, Peter Schwind, Richard Gold, Jack Blackburn, Judith DeLany, and Terry Norman for their inspirational contributions.

A big thank you goes out to Stefan Matte, Laura Humphreys, Cheryl Chapman, Don Ash, Sharon Puszko, Susan Beck, Tamara Mondragon, Hildegard Wittlinger, Tom Myers, Alexandra Hamer, Eleanora Lipton, Janet Markovits, Sande Rosen, Michaela Johnson, Joe Recknegal, Giovanni Felicioni, Deane Juhan, Don Kelley, Stewart Wild, Maureen Stott, and Qianzhi Wu for their careful reviews. Dianne Polseno oversaw and reviewed the cohesiveness and the educational content of this textbook. Her dedication to this project was admirable, and her careful scrutiny helped develop and realize this book's fullest potential.

Not every author can sing the praises of their editorial and publishing team, but I reach high C's for this group of professionals: Kellie White, Kelly Milford (the 2 K's), and April Falast in the editorial department; Julie Eddy and Marquita Parker on the production side; Anita Lott in marketing; and the design coordinator, Paula Catalano.

Working on this project also requires personal support. Once again, I thank Olga Debord, Alice Apolinaris, and Augusta Green for affording me the time to work while they loved and attended to my beautiful, special boy.

I also want to acknowledge and recognize the numerous leaders in the field of bodywork whose innovative work continues to enrich our profession.

INTRODUCTION

As readers continue their quest for increased knowledge and their exploration of various bodywork techniques, it becomes clear that a textbook that provides substantive information on advanced training is needed. *Modalities for Massage and Bodywork* is that book. This text provides students and practitioners of the somatic arts with the fundamental understanding of 21 different and popular modalities to enhance their palpation and treatment skills and enrich their practices.

This text also provides massage schools with the resources they need to formulate their own advanced studies curricula. Experienced, trained faculty members can refer to the appropriate chapter and create their syllabi based upon the teachings of our experts.

A word of caution is necessary from the onset, however: no one can learn hands-on techniques from a book, home study program, or video regardless of how detailed they are or who is providing the instruction. In order to truly assimilate the theories and techniques of any modality, and to act responsibly, readers are advised to take professional certification classes where the on-site supervision of skilled instructors personally guides you through the practicum and ensures your complete understanding of the concepts and techniques. One goal of this book is to stimulate your thirst and desire for this necessary advanced instruction and to encourage you to seek out appropriate training in areas that are of interest to you.

The publishers and I reviewed the most popular continuing education courses being offered at massage schools around the country to arrive at this prestigious list of modalities. Choosing who would write each chapter was easy. Each contributor is a recognized leader and expert in their respective fields. They bring years of wisdom and experience to each chapter and share with readers the history, far-reaching benefits, and values of their techniques. Many of our contributors have become adept and thoroughly proficient in time-honored modalities. Others have been the originators or leading proponents of certain bodyworks. But all of them share their expertise and years of dedicated work.

The modalities in this textbook are varied. Ayurvedic therapies, Lomilomi, Polarity therapy, Reflexology, Shiatsu, Thai Massage, and Tuina are based on cultural and time-honored traditions that have been passed down over many millennia. Active isolated stretching, CranioSacral Therapy, Manual Lymphatic Drainage, Myofascial Release, Structural Integration, and Trager are evidence-based, innovative modalities that address specific biologic and physiologic systems. Cancer Massage, Geriatric Massage, Infant and Pediatric Massage, Neuromuscular therapy, Orthopedic massage, Prenatal Massage, Sports and Fitness Massage, and Trigger point release are all forms of bodywork that are adapted to suit certain physiologic needs and medical or therapeutic conditions.

Although the origins of these modalities may be different, two things are constant: all of them recognize and respect the intimate and indivisible relationship among the body/mind/spirit, and all of them produce profound physiologic, emotional, and spiritual changes in the person receiving them. The common thread is that human touch stimulates sensory receptors in the skin and deeper tissues. These signals are transmitted to the spinal cord and brain stem, which, in turn, send the messages to the entire body. When we are touched by another person, our pituitary gland secretes the hormone oxytocin, which combines with dopamine to lower blood pressure, stress, and make us feel good. So regardless of the nature or form of therapeutic touch, the effects are universal and health-affirming.

Over 100 years ago, the English researcher Sir Henry Dale identified a substance in the pituitary gland that speeded up childbirth. He also learned that this same hormone promoted milk let-down. He coined the name oxytocin from the Greek words for "rapid birth." Years later, the role of oxytocin was recognized to play a major physiologic role in calming, soothing, and influencing many vital systems in the body, including encouraging maternal and baby bonding and love.[1]

Touch is the principal trigger for the release of oxytocin. Since our skin is the largest sensory organ in our body, touch stimulates the secretion of neurochemicals that influence the blood, muscles, tissues, nerves, organs and systems. These advantages also affect the provider of touch — massage practitioners and bodyworkers. Many of the contributors to this book describe the peaceful state of mind they enjoy while doing their work. Physiologically, bodyworkers also benefit from

---

[1] Cohen S: *The magic of touch*, New York, 1987, Harper & Row.

the secretion of oxytocin. As a result, your stress hormone levels and blood pressure decline and your sense of well-being is enhanced.[2]

Since all forms of bodywork release oxytocin and boast numerous health benefits, the choice of which modalities to learn and incorporate into your work is your personal decision. *Modalities for Massage and Bodywork* affords you a unique opportunity to fine tune those techniques you already use or introduce you to other forms of bodywork perhaps for the first time.

This book has been one of the best educational experiences I have ever had. Reading and editing each chapter written by the preeminent, acknowledged leaders in their respective fields have been the equivalent of private tutorials with each of them. I am astounded by their vast knowledge and experience, as well as the dedication and passion with which they offer their unique modalities.

It is my hope that the readers will also benefit from the teachings of these renowned professionals and that their curiosity will be piqued and stimulated to pursue further education.

Elaine Stillerman

---

[2] Moberg K: *The oxytocin factor*, Cambridge, MA, 2003, De Capo Press.

CONTENTS

Active Isolated Stretching

Joseph E. Muscolino

1

INTRODUCTION

Active isolated stretching (**AIS**) is a stretching technique that employs the neurologic reflex known as **reciprocal inhibition** (Box 1-1),[1] as well as a specific protocol for how each of the 200+ stretches is done. It is a powerful treatment tool that can be applied to suit most every population, whether the individual is young, old, male, female, athletic, active, or sedentary.[2,3] Because it is a stretching technique, its primary focus is on stretching taut and/or contracted soft tissues, thereby increasing flexibility of the body.[1,4,5] Because it also involves active movements by the client, it has the added benefit of increasing the client's strength and stability.[4,6] AIS can be done by the client at home or with the assistance of a therapist.[1,7]

HISTORY OF AIS

AIS was developed by Aaron Mattes, both as a result of his professional relationship working with college athletes and his personal experience of having suffered a severe low back injury. Mattes began developing the AIS technique in 1972, when he was a clinical supervisor

BOX 1-1 Reciprocal Inhibition

Reciprocal inhibition is a neurologic reflex that causes the antagonists to a joint action to relax, by inhibiting them from contracting, when a mover of that joint action is directed to contract.[4,6] This is a necessary reflex for the body because when a mover on one side of a joint is directed by the central nervous system to contract and shorten, the antagonists on the other side must lengthen. For this reason, whenever the nervous system desires a joint action to occur, it sends both facilitory signals to the motor neurons that control the mover muscles of that joint action and inhibitory signals to the motor neurons that control the antagonist muscles of that joint action.

The mechanisms of this reflex can be exploited to increase the effectiveness of a stretch. Instead of receiving a passive stretch from the therapist, the client actively contracts mover muscles during a stretching maneuver. This will cause a reflex reciprocal inhibition to the antagonist muscles on the other side of the joint; these antagonist muscles are the target muscles that we desire to stretch.[4,6] Now that these target muscles have been reflexively inhibited to relax, stretching them can be performed with greater effectiveness. Figure 1-1 illustrates the neurologic mechanism of reciprocal inhibition.

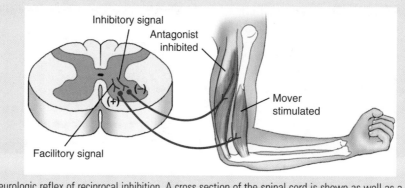

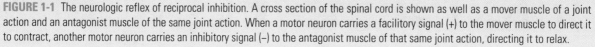

FIGURE 1-1 The neurologic reflex of reciprocal inhibition. A cross section of the spinal cord is shown as well as a mover muscle of a joint action and an antagonist muscle of the same joint action. When a motor neuron carries a facilitory signal (+) to the mover muscle to direct it to contract, another motor neuron carries an inhibitory signal (–) to the antagonist muscle of that same joint action, directing it to relax.

and coach in the sports department at the University of Illinois at the Champaign-Urbana campus. In working with athletes, he noticed how inflexible his athletes were, some of whom were world class, even though a stretching program was part of their regimen. Working from the assumption that flexible athletes would experience fewer injuries and perform better, Mattes began to investigate how to develop a more effective stretching regimen. Given his background in athletics, it was natural for his stretching technique to be geared more toward an active and dynamic approach. Personally, he also leaned toward shorter durations of holding each stretch because he had always felt that longer-duration stretches tended to irritate his muscles. Implementing these techniques into the training program at his university yielded positive results, so he expanded the development of his approach, introducing it to other universities as well as high school sports programs in the area.

In 1976, Mattes transferred to the University of Toledo, where he was able to create a large clinical

program and a sports training center. He continued to develop new stretches for the athletes and found excellent results working on all athletes, including those who had experienced injuries and those recovering from surgeries as a result of severe injuries. Mattes has described this period as a "golden era" because he had the support of the entire sports department at the University of Toledo. All the coaches promoted his stretching technique, and from 1976 to 1979 there were no athletic surgeries at the school.

Mattes' own severe back injury, which eventually required surgery, was only a further impetus for him to research and develop his technique. He increased his own readings and studies, including cadaver lab research, in his quest to improve and perfect his technique.[8]

Thirty-five years later, the Mattes technique of AIS has gained world-wide recognition and acceptance as a premier approach to stretching. Mattes now resides in Florida, where hundreds of students of his technique have come to assist him at his clinic, working on clients who come from all over, presenting with a wide variety of conditions. AIS has proven to be beneficial for most everyone, ranging from the average person, who through a sedentary lifestyle has become increasingly less flexible, to athletes, for whom the technique originated, to people suffering the effects of more devastating injuries such as Parkinson's disease, Lou Gehrig's disease, and incomplete spinal cord lesions.

STRETCHING DEFINED

A **stretch** is a type of movement exercise wherein a force is directed into the soft tissues of the body that creates a line of tension (i.e., a line of pulling) that elongates all the soft tissues located along that line.[4,9,10] The term **target tissue** is used to describe the soft tissue (or tissues) that is to be stretched.[9] (If the target tissue is a muscle, it may be called the **target muscle**; if the target tissue is a ligament, it may be called the target ligament, etc.) These soft tissues are muscles and their tendons, ligaments, joint capsules, other fascial tissues, and skin.[1,6,9,11] By elongating soft tissues that are taut, stretching increases the body's flexibility.

Variety of Stretching Techniques

Before exploring the exact protocol of AIS, it will be helpful to define and explain the vast array of stretching techniques that exist, some of which are part of the AIS technique and some of which are not. While stretching techniques may be classified in a number of ways, they may be subdivided into two broad categories: static and dynamic stretching.[4,9,11]

AIS employs dynamic stretching within its protocol. To better understand dynamic stretching and AIS technique, it is helpful to first discuss static stretching.

Static Stretching, Passive and Active

A **static stretch** is one where a body part is brought into a specific position and held without moving (statically) for a period of time (like a yoga pose).[1] The recommended period of time to hold the stretch has usually been between 10 and 30 seconds, although some sources recommend holding the stretch for as long as 60 seconds.[1] This is how stretching has been done for decades.[9] The manner in which the client's body is brought to the position of stretch can be either passive or active.

A **passive stretch** is defined as one in which the muscles of the joint being stretched are relaxed. This can be accomplished with the assistance of a therapist or by the client alone.[4] (For example, a client can stretch his neck extensors by using a hand to passively move the head and neck into flexion; even though the client performed the stretch on himself, he did not contract his neck muscles.) An **active stretch** is defined as one where the muscles of the joint being stretched create the movement. The definitions of passive and active stretches have often been misinterpreted.[5,7]

Dynamic Stretching, Passive and Active

In contrast to static stretching, **dynamic stretching** (often called **mobilization stretching**) involves more movement of the client's body. But like static stretching, it can be performed passively and/or actively. With dynamic stretching the client or therapist brings the body to the position of the stretch but this position is not held very long, usually only 1 to 3 seconds.[1,4,10] Dynamic stretching emphasizes the *movement* that brings the body into the stretch, not the end position. AIS employs active dynamic stretching.

Static and Dynamic Stretching Compared

In recent years, static stretching has lost favor in some circles, and dynamic stretching has been recommended instead.[4,10] The pros and cons of each type have been debated extensively. Proponents of static stretching state that for a soft tissue to stretch and stay stretched, it needs to be statically held in a stretched position for a longer period of time.[3,5,12] Proponents of dynamic stretching point to the benefits of more stretching repetitions involving active movement, each one held for a shorter period of time. on the part of the client.[1,4]

Advanced Stretching Techniques

Beyond static and dynamic stretching, more **advanced stretching techniques** can be done. These stretching techniques are considered advanced because they employ a neurologic reflex to increase the efficiency of the stretch. There are two types of advanced stretching techniques. The first is **proprioceptive neuromuscular facilitation** (**PNF**), also known as **contract relax** (**CR**) or **postisometric relaxation** (**PIR**) stretching, which utilizes the golgi tendon organ reflex (Box 1-2).[4,7] The second is **agonist contract** (**AC**), which utilizes reciprocal inhibition.[4,7,9,10] AIS is a type of AC stretching.[4]

When to Stretch

Stretching is a method of body conditioning that can either stand alone or be done in conjunction with strengthening exercise.

BOX 1-2 The Golgi Tendon Organ Reflex

The Golgi tendon organ (GTO) reflex (also known as the tendon reflex) is a proprioceptive neurologic reflex that inhibits a muscle from contracting in response to an excessive contraction of that muscle.[4] This reflex prevents the muscle's contraction from tearing its tendons. GTOs, which are located within tendons, are sensitive to stretch. When a muscle belly contracts excessively, it pulls forcefully upon its tendons, causing the GTOs to stretch. This sends a signal into the spinal cord along a sensory neuron, which synapses with an interneuron, which in turn inhibits the lower motor neurons (LMNs) that control the muscle fibers. Inhibition of a muscle's LMNs results in relaxation of the muscle (Figure 1-2). A GTO reflex can be utilized to help relax a muscle, thereby allowing a greater stretch of the muscle than otherwise would have been possible. Proprioceptive neuromuscular facilitation (PNF) stretching, and not AIS, utilizes the GTO reflex.

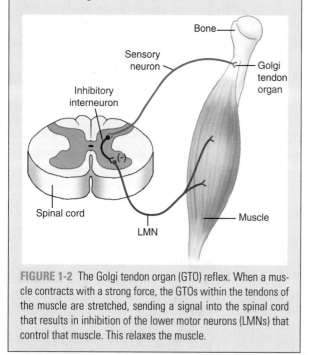

FIGURE 1-2 The Golgi tendon organ (GTO) reflex. When a muscle contracts with a strong force, the GTOs within the tendons of the muscle are stretched, sending a signal into the spinal cord that results in inhibition of the lower motor neurons (LMNs) that control that muscle. This relaxes the muscle.

When done in conjunction with strengthening exercise, stretching has traditionally been performed first.[4] The premise has been that stretching and loosening the musculature of the body decrease the risk of injury to a person performing strengthening exercises. However, that belief is now in doubt, at least with regard to classic static stretching.[10] The reason is that stretching tends to be effective only if soft tissues are first warmed up.[4] Therefore, stretching before exercising is not as effective because the tissues are cold. Proponents are now advocating that static stretching should be done after the strengthening exercise, when the tissues are already warmed up.[10]

However, this does not mean that no stretching should be done before the strengthening phase of a workout. Because most sources believe that being flexible before initiating strength exercises lessens the risk of injury, they continue to recommend some type of stretching motions. Instead of static stretching, however, dynamic stretching is becoming more accepted as the appropriate method of warming up and making the body flexible before strengthening exercise.[4,10] Dynamic stretching has the advantage of warming the tissues, lubricating the joints, facilitating neuromuscular pathways, and also stretching soft tissues. In short, it appears to be the ideal method of stretching before strengthening is done. Because of the active joint motions involved, AIS is a method of active dynamic stretching and is therefore a well-suited preface to strengthening exercise.

Of course, stretching does not have to be linked to strengthening exercise; it can also be done as a stand-alone method of body conditioning. However, given the fact that warm tissues stretch better than cold ones,[1] it is useful to engage in some type of activity that warms the tissues before beginning the stretching routine. Walking, jogging, or cycling for a few moments may all be effective. Alternately, the tissue may be warmed up by means of a hot shower, bath, heating pad, or a massage. Regardless of the means used, warming the tissues before beginning the stretching routine will facilitate the efficiency of the stretching. This rule is less critical when the type of stretching done is active dynamic because it involves muscle contractions, which will serve to warm the tissues in addition to stretching them. Being a type of active dynamic stretching, AIS requires little or no warm-up before being done.

AIS TECHNIQUE PROTOCOL

There is a specific protocol to performing AIS. An active isolated stretch can be **assisted** or **unassisted**. If an active isolated stretch is assisted, a therapist aids or assists the client in performing the stretch. If it is unassisted, the client performs the stretch alone; no therapist is involved in the stretching activity. The following steps illustrate how an assisted active isolated stretch is performed.

1. Identify the target muscles and other adjacent target soft tissues that are to be stretched.
2. Have the client stretch the target muscles (or other target tissues) by actively contracting the muscles on the opposite side of the joint (i.e., the muscles that are antagonistic to the target muscles). This motion should be gentle.

3. At the end of the client's range of motion, the therapist increases the intensity of the stretch by adding a gentle force that further stretches the target muscles. The added stretch force by the therapist should always be gentle (less than 1 pound of force) so that the target muscles are not excessively irritated; otherwise a muscle spindle reflex may be triggered (Box 1-3). Note:

Steps 2 and 3 are called the **stretch phase;** the entire duration of the stretch phase should be no more than 2 seconds.

4. The client is now supported and guided back to the starting position. This step is called the **recovery phase** (Note: The client should always be brought back to the original starting position at the end of each repetition.)

BOX 1-3 Muscle Spindle Reflex

Whenever a target muscle is stretched excessively or too quickly, a **muscle spindle reflex** (also known as the **stretch reflex** or **myotatic reflex**) is triggered that causes the muscle to contract.[1,4,7,10] Given that the purpose of stretching is to stretch and elongate the target muscle, having it contract defeats this purpose. For this reason, stretching should never be done too vigorously. In other words, stretching can never be forced; instead, target muscles must be gently coaxed to stretch.

A muscle spindle reflex is a neurologic reflex of proprioception. **Proprioception** is defined as the ability to determine our body's position in space and our body's movement through space.[4] By responding to the length of a muscle, muscle spindles help to give us proprioceptive awareness because knowing the length of musculature gives us information about the static and dynamic position of our joints.

A major purpose of a muscle spindle reflex is to protect the muscle belly from being overstretched and torn.[4] The reflex is initiated by a specialized cell called a muscle spindle cell, hence the name of the reflex. Muscle spindle cells are specialized muscle cells located within the muscle belly, parallel to the fibers of the muscle. When a muscle is stretched, the muscle spindle cells located within the muscle are also stretched. These muscle spindles are sensitive to being stretched, and if the stretch is beyond the threshold of the muscle spindles, they send a signal into the spinal cord via a sensory neuron. This sensory neuron then synapses with a lower motor neuron, which then exits the spinal cord and returns to the muscle being stretched, ordering it to contract and thus preventing it from being overstretched and torn (Figure 1-3).

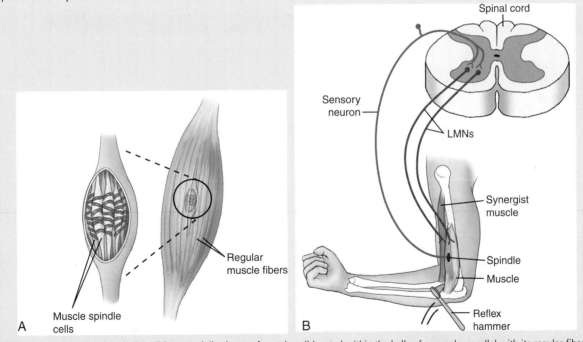

FIGURE 1-3 **A,** A muscle spindle cell is a specialized type of muscle cell located within the belly of a muscle, parallel with its regular fibers. When a muscle is stretched either too far or too quickly, a muscle spindle reflex is triggered. **B,** This figure demonstrates the tendon of a muscle being tapped with a reflex hammer that momentarily elongates it, thereby creating a pulling force on the muscle belly. This reflex consists of a sensory neuron entering the spinal cord and synapsing with lower motor neurons (LMNs), which then exit the cord, carrying a signal telling the muscle and its synergists to contract.

Continued

BOX 1-3 Muscle Spindle Reflex—cont'd

Muscle spindles also maintain resting muscle tone.[16] Because a muscle spindle cell is a specialized type of muscle cell, it can contract and shorten or relax and lengthen. This contraction/relaxation is controlled by a functional region of the brain known as the **gamma nervous system**.[16] When the gamma nervous system directs the contraction of the muscle spindles within a muscle, they become tighter and shorter and therefore more sensitive to being stretched. If the muscle is then stretched even slightly beyond that shortened length, the muscle spindle reflex is triggered, which causes the entire muscle to contract to that shortened length. In this manner, whatever tension level the gamma nervous system sets for the muscle spindles will eventually be followed by the entire muscle. There are many factors that determine the tension level that the gamma motor system sets for the muscle spindles of a muscle. These factors include chronic tension levels of that muscle due to use and postures assumed, previous traumas, and general psychologic and emotional stress levels. Note: When the term **muscle memory** is used to describe the tendency of a muscle to have a certain resting tone, this muscle memory does not reside in the muscle itself; rather it resides in the brain's gamma nervous system control of the muscle spindles of the muscle.[4]

The protocol of the stretch and recovery phases is repeated approximately 8 to 10 times.[1,7] Each successive repetition usually allows for an incremental gain of a few degrees of motion of the stretch. The client should breathe out during the stretch phase and breathe in during the recovery phase (Box 1-4).[1] These steps are shown in Figure 1-4, where the target muscles being stretched are the right lateral flexor muscles of the neck.

BOX 1-4 Stretching and Breathing

When stretching, the typical protocol for breathing is to breathe out (exhale).[14] This is especially true when exerting; think *e* for exertion; *e* for *exhale*. Because AIS requires that the client actively contract to move the body part during the stretch phase, it is the stretch phase that involves exertion, making it the phase during which the client should exhale. Exhalation requires a contraction of the diaphragm and abdominal wall muscles that helps stabilize the spine (protecting it when performing contractions that require exertion) and increase the strength of the muscles that are contracting (which increases the degree of the reciprocal inhibition reflex).[4,14,15]

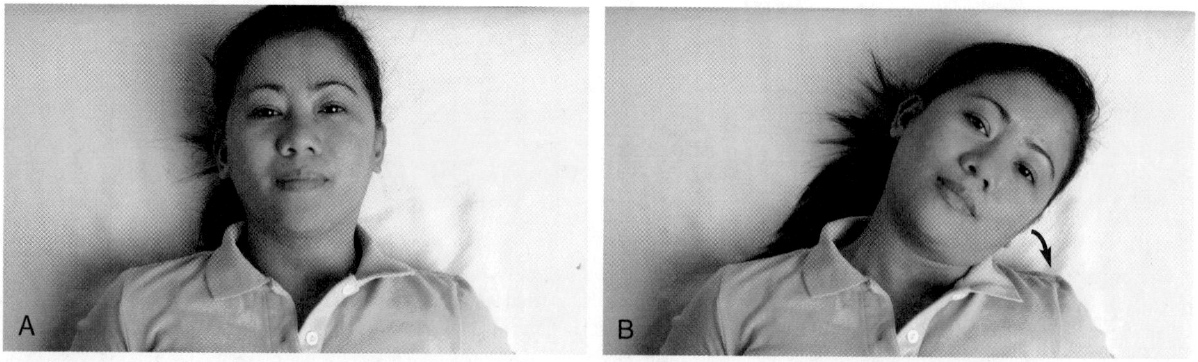

FIGURE 1-4 A, An active isolated stretch of the right lateral flexor muscles of the neck, with the client supine. **B,** The protocol begins with the client contracting her left lateral flexor musculature, actively bringing her neck into left lateral flexion at the spinal joints, thereby beginning the stretch of the right lateral flexors of the neck. (Photo by Yanik Chauvin.)

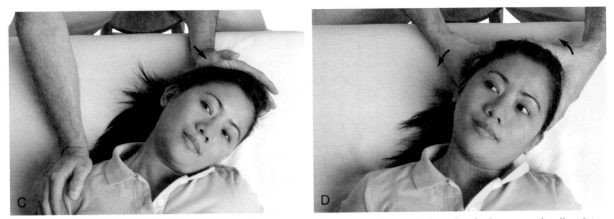

FIGURE 1-4 cont'd C, At the end of the client's active motion, the therapist adds a gentle force that further moves the client into left lateral flexion, further stretching the right lateral flexors (*B* and *C* comprise the stretch phase.) **D,** The client is then supported and guided back to the original starting position for the next repetition; this is the recovery phase. Eight to ten reps are usually performed. (Photo by Yanik Chauvin.)

AIS, ANATOMIC, PHYSIOLOGIC, AND CLINICAL FOUNDATIONS

The rationale for the AIS method is clear and involves many anatomic, physiologic, and clinical principles.

Each active isolated stretch begins by choosing the target musculature that is to be stretched. Aaron Mattes has developed more than 200 stretches, each one designed to isolate a specific muscle or muscle group. Isolating a target muscle or muscle group allows for specific and precise stretching, which is especially important when working clinically to rehabilitate a region of the client's body.[1,13]

The first part of the stretch begins by having the client contract the target muscle's antagonistic muscles (i.e., located on the other side of the joint). When these antagonist muscles contract, the client's body part moves in the opposite direction from where the target muscles are located. This causes the target muscles and other target soft tissues to stretch. Because the antagonist muscles are actively contracted, the target muscles are also reciprocally inhibited, allowing them to be manually stretched further by the therapist at the end of the range of motion.

Other benefits also occur when the client contracts the antagonist muscles and actively moves during the first part of the stretch. For example, the contraction strengthens the antagonist muscles and facilitates the neural connections between the nervous system and the antagonist muscles.[1] Active movement on the part of the client also increases blood and lymph circulation to the area, bringing in needed nutrients and draining away waste products of metabolism.[1,12] It also causes a circulation of the synovial fluid, lubricating the joints and aiding nutrient supply to the intraarticular joint structures. Movement by the client also warms all the soft tissues and hydrates the connective tissue fascia.[1,6] This increases the pliability of the connective tissue fascia, allowing soft tissues to stretch more easily.

The second and more important part of the stretch is done by the therapist (when assisted AIS is being performed). Taking advantage of the reciprocal inhibition reflex and the fact that the target tissues are warmed and hydrated, the therapist can add a gentle further stretch that will be more effective than it otherwise would have been. It is important that this additional stretch not be excessive; otherwise the muscle spindle stretch reflex might be triggered, which would result in a tightening of the target muscles.[1,10,13] Given that AIS involves multiple repetitions, usually 8 to 10, each successive repetition allows the therapist to increase the degree of the stretch. Even though each rep adds only a few degrees of stretch, multiplying this by 8 to 10 repetitions allows for an excellent overall stretch. Aaron Mattes is fond of saying that he is patient. He does not feel the need to force the stretch because he will have the opportunity to repeat the stretch and build upon it so many times. Only a few degrees of additional stretch are needed each time to make for a successful overall stretch.

When performing AIS stretching, clients never hold their breath. The protocol is to breathe out during the exertion of actively contracting (the antagonist muscles) and moving; and to then breathe in during the recovery phase when the therapist supports and guides the client back to the starting position, so as to be ready for the next rep. It is important that the client keep breathing to ensure that the body is constantly being supplied with oxygen, a needed nutrient for the tissues to burn glucose to supply energy for the body.[1] Furthermore, breathing out during the exertion phase of the stretch helps to increase the stabilization of the body, protecting the joints of the body and facilitating a more efficient active movement.

◼◼◼ IN MY EXPERIENCE

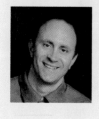

In my experience, AIS can be successfully practiced not only by practitioners looking to perform entire hour-long sessions on a client, but also those practitioners who desire to integrate AIS into the practice of other types of bodywork, including massage therapy. In fact, stretching, and AIS in particular, is a perfect adjunct to massage, adding another tool to loosen and relax the client. AIS can be performed for a specific muscle or muscle group, requiring less than one minute; it can be used to stretch all the muscles around a specific joint, requiring approximately 5 minutes or so; or it can be used to stretch an entire region of the body, requiring perhaps 10 to 20 minutes or more. How it is integrated into a massage session is flexible and can vary depending upon the needs of the client and the time available.

INTEGRATING AIS INTO A MASSAGE SESSION

An added advantage of AIS to massage therapists is that it is very time efficient. It allows for many repetitions because each rep requires only 2 to 3 seconds. Therefore, it is easy to integrate AIS into a massage session without subtracting much time from the massage itself. An entire AIS protocol for a target muscle requires only 20 to 30 seconds. An ideal way to include AIS stretching into a massage session is to first massage the area, helping to warm up and relax the tissues. Then AIS can be done to the muscle groups of this region, capitalizing upon the effects of the massage. If, for example, the neck has been massaged, it would take only 3 to 4 minutes to stretch all six major muscle groups of the neck (flexors, extensors, lateral flexors to both sides, and rotators to both sides).

UNASSISTED AIS

AIS can also be done without the assistance of a therapist. In Mattes' book, *Active Isolated Stretching: The Mattes Method,* both assisted and unassisted active isolated stretches are shown for every muscle and muscle group.

The protocol for an unassisted active isolated stretch is similar to that of assisted AIS. The only difference is that the client must perform the second part of the stretch alone. This usually requires using a hand to bring the body part further into the stretch. Because the client cannot always easily reach the body part to be stretched, the AIS method makes use of a rope that the client can hold and use to pull on the body part being stretched.[1,2] Figure 1-5 demonstrates an unassisted active isolated stretch in which the client uses her hand to further the stretch; Figure 1-6 demonstrates an unassisted active isolated stretch in which a rope is used instead.

STABILIZATION

A crucial but often overlooked aspect of any stretching maneuver is stabilization of the rest of the client's body. Whenever a stretch is done, the idea is to create a line of tension that pulls on the target tissues. However, this force often pulls on the rest of the body. If the rest of the body is moved by this force, the stretch to the target tissues will be diminished or lost. In cases such as these, it is important that the rest of the body be **stabilized**. Aaron Mattes has paid close attention to the stabilization necessary to effectively perform each of the active isolated stretching maneuvers. For each stretch, it is important to note the position of the therapist's other hand, which is acting to stabilize another part of the client's body.[1,9] This hand is called the **stabilization hand**.

While important for every stretch, stabilization is especially important for stretching the muscles that cross the hip joint. These muscles are stretched by moving the thigh at the hip joint while the pelvis is stabilized. To facilitate this stretch, AIS therapists use a seat belt that wraps around the client's pelvis. For client comfort, a piece of foam rubber is used to cushion and spread out the restraining force of the seat belt upon the client.[1] An example of using a seat belt for stabilization is shown in Figure 1-7. The client is prone

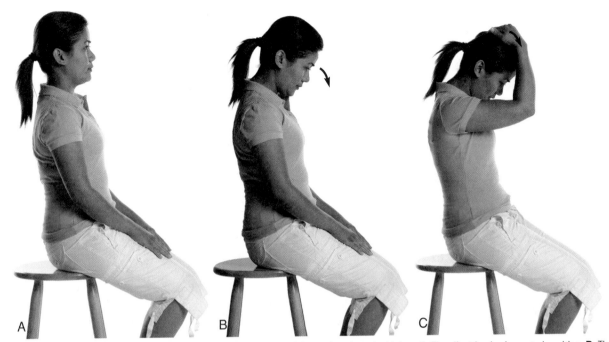

FIGURE 1-5 An unassisted active isolated stretch of the extensors of the neck at the spinal joints. **A,** The client begins in neutral position. **B,** The client actively contracts the flexors (antagonists to the extensors) and moves the neck into flexion, thereby beginning the stretch of the extensors (and reciprocally inhibiting the extensors). **C,** The client now uses her hands to move her neck further into flexion, thereby increasing the stretch of the extensors of the neck. (Photo by Yanik Chauvin.)

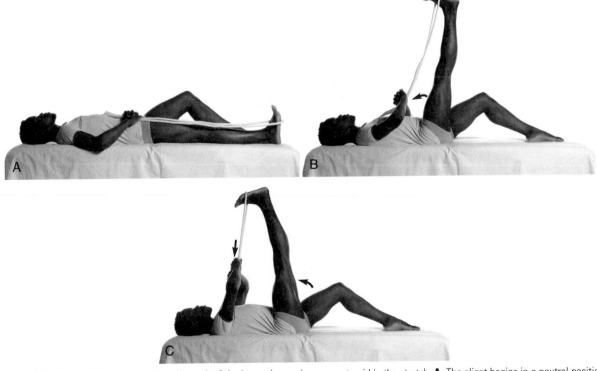

FIGURE 1-6 An unassisted active isolated stretch of the hamstrings using a rope to aid in the stretch. **A,** The client begins in a neutral position. **B,** The client actively contracts the flexors of the hip joint and extensors of the knee joint (antagonists to the hamstrings), beginning the stretch of (and reciprocally inhibiting) the hamstrings. **C,** The client now uses the rope to pull the thigh into further flexion at the hip joint, thereby increasing the stretch of the hamstrings. (Photo by Yanik Chauvin.)

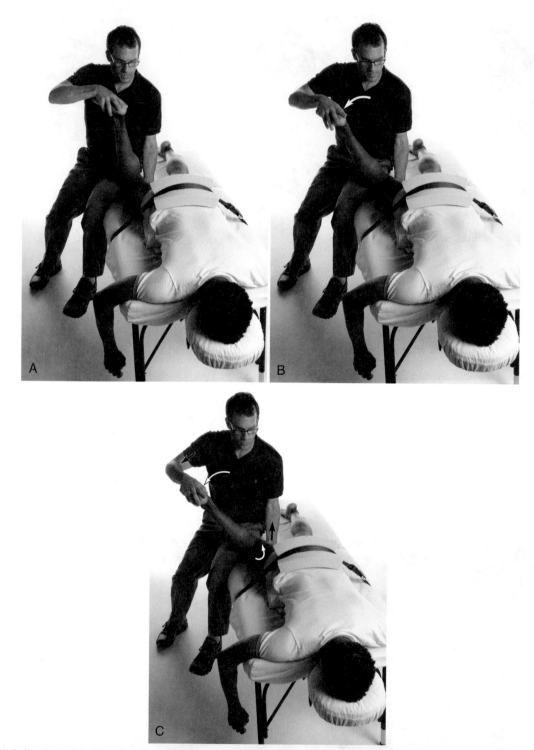

FIGURE 1-7 A stretch of the lateral rotators of the thigh at the hip joint with the client prone. A seat belt is used to stabilize the pelvis (with foam rubber placed between the seat belt and client for cushioning) so that when the thigh is medially rotated stretching the lateral rotators, the pelvis does not move. Keeping the pelvis stabilized in this manner allows for a better stretch of the target muscles across the hip joint. (Photo by Yanik Chauvin.)

with a seat belt wrapped around the pelvis, cushioned by foam rubber. The client can now medially rotate the thigh at the hip joint (as well as have the therapist add in further medial rotation motion), stretching the lateral rotators at the hip joint, without having the stretching force lost because of pelvic motion (i.e., instability).

CONTRAINDICATIONS

There are not many contraindications to AIS. The contraindications that do exist depend upon the particular body part that is being stretched. If the tissues being stretched have sufficient integrity to be able to accept this stretch, then AIS may be done. In other words, if the client is healthy enough to be able to move a certain amount in a certain direction without causing actual tissue damage, then the client is healthy enough to have tissues stretched within that range of motion. If, however, the tissues of a region have recently been torn due to trauma (e.g., a fractured bone, moderate or marked sprain or strain, or bleeding in the region), then AIS is contraindicated until the tissue damage has been healed. If the tissues have been markedly overused and are irritated or swollen, AIS may also be contraindicated until the irritation or swelling has abated.[3,6] Additionally, if the stretching involves the spine, then the presence of a moderate/marked disc pathologic condition (a bulge or herniation) and/or marked spinal **degenerative joint disease (DJD)** may contraindicate certain active isolated stretches (Box 1-5). If there is ever doubt as to the safety of carrying out any stretch, obtain the client's permission to consult with the client's physician.

CERTIFICATION

While Aaron Mattes is currently investigating the possibility of creating a certification program for his AIS technique, no formal certification currently exists. For the most up-to-date information regarding AIS certification, contact Aaron Mattes' organization at www.stretchingusa.com. Even though there is no formal certification, Aaron Mattes does provide a list on his website of "preferred" qualified AIS practitioners who have distinguished themselves by taking at least two AIS seminars and/or by studying and working at his clinic in Florida.

BOX 1-5 Degenerative Joint Disease

Degenerative joint disease (DJD) is a condition that involves degeneration of the articular cartilage of a joint and excessive calcium formation along the bony margins of the joint. DJD is primarily caused by physical stress upon the joint; hence, DJD is a natural result of aging. However, when a person has either excessive degeneration that interferes with normal functioning of the joint, or has a greater degree of this condition than would be expected at the person's age, it is deemed to be a pathologic condition of the joint. DJD is also known as **osteoarthritis (OA)**. When present in the spine, it is also referred to as spondylosis.

ACTIVE ISOLATED STRETCHING EXAMPLES

While it is not the purpose of this chapter to exhaustively cover all of the 200+ stretches within the technique of AIS, it is helpful to present a number of examples so that the principles discussed can be better understood. To that end, additional examples of active isolated stretches are given in Figures 1-8 through 1-12.

CHAPTER SUMMARY

AIS is an advanced method of dynamic stretching developed by Aaron Mattes that utilizes the neurologic reflex reciprocal inhibition, as well as a specific protocol for how to carry out the stretching technique. It may be done either unassisted or assisted by a therapist. Within the AIS technique, Mattes has developed over 200 specific stretches that address all of the major muscles and muscle groups of the body. Compared to classic static stretching, AIS more efficiently stretches the target tissues, increases local circulation and warms the local tissues, improves the neural connection between the central nervous system and the musculature, strengthens the musculature, and increases joint fluid motion, thereby increasing joint lubrication as well as nutrient flow to the intraarticular structures of the joint. In short, AIS is an extremely effective technique that can easily be added to your massage therapy practice.

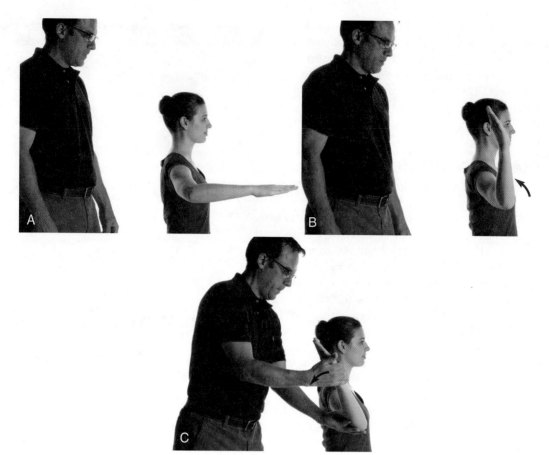

FIGURE 1-8 An assisted active isolated stretch of the medial rotators of the right arm at the shoulder joint. **A,** The client is in the neutral starting position. **B,** The client actively moves the right arm into lateral rotation at the shoulder joint, beginning the stretch of the medial rotators. **C,** The therapist adds a gentle force that moves the right arm into further lateral rotation, thereby further stretching the medial rotators. (Photo by Yanik Chauvin.)

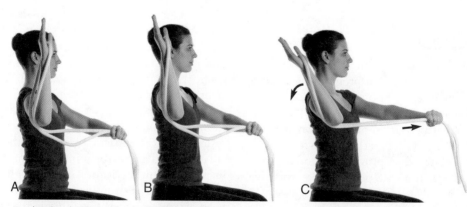

FIGURE 1-9 An unassisted active isolated stretch of the medial rotators of the right arm at the shoulder joint. **A,** The client is in the neutral starting position. **B,** The client actively moves the right arm into lateral rotation at the shoulder joint, beginning the stretch of the medial rotators. **C,** The client gently pulls on the rope with her left hand, bringing the right arm into further lateral rotation, thereby further stretching the medial rotators. (Photo by Yanik Chauvin.)

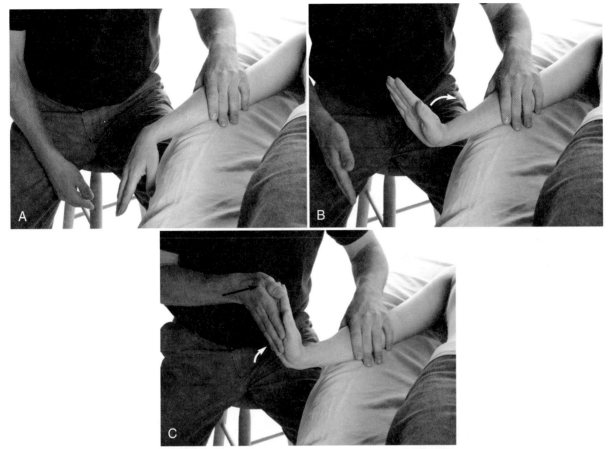

FIGURE 1-10 An assisted active isolated stretch of the flexors of the right hand at the wrist joint. **A,** The client is in the neutral starting position. The client is lying supine on a massage table. **B,** The client actively moves the right hand into extension at the wrist joint, beginning the stretch of the flexors. **C,** The therapist gently moves the client's right hand into further extension, thereby further stretching the flexors. (Photo by Yanik Chauvin.)

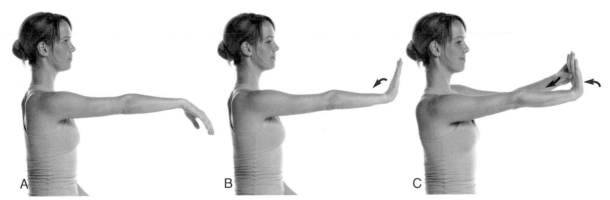

FIGURE 1-11 An unassisted active isolated stretch of the flexors of the right hand at the wrist joint. **A,** The client is in the neutral starting position. **B,** The client actively moves the right hand into extension at the wrist joint, beginning the stretch of the flexors. **C,** The client uses her left hand to gently move the right hand into further extension, thereby further stretching the flexors. (Photo by Yanik Chauvin.)

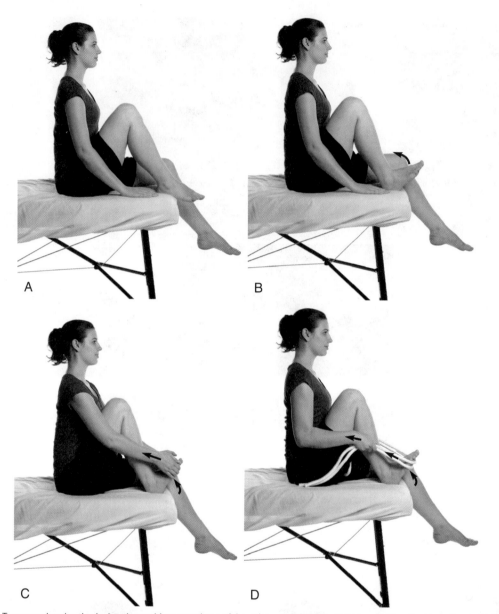

FIGURE 1-12 Two unassisted active isolated stretching procedures of the soleus muscle of the right leg. **A,** The client is in the neutral starting position. **B,** The client actively moves the right foot into dorsiflexion at the ankle joint, beginning the stretch of the soleus. **C,** The client uses her hands to add the further stretch of the soleus. **D,** The client uses a rope to add the further stretch of the soleus. (Photo by Yanik Chauvin.)

CASE HISTORIES

■ Case history 1

This case history involves a middle-aged, right-hand-dominant male. He is a bodyworker who does approximately 10 to 15 hours of massage per week. He had previously played tennis regularly to stay strong and flexible. However, due to a knee meniscus tear, he had stopped playing tennis and had not replaced it with another physical activity for approximately one year. At the same time, he began spending a greater amount of time at a desk, working on a computer keyboard and using a mouse.

The effects of a sedentary lifestyle are not as dramatic as a trauma because they build up insidiously, imperceptibly increasing with each passing day, week, and month. But they can be just as disastrous. Without his noticing, the client's right shoulder had become painful to use and its joint motion restricted. He remained unaware of this condition until one day when he attempted to do a pushup. As soon as he placed body weight on his shoulder joints, he realized that he could barely perform one pushup, and that was with a great deal of pain in his right shoulder. Assuming that the problem was simply tight musculature, he had two 1-hour massages, with a concentration at the musculature of the right shoulder. However, to his disappointment, he received little if any relief.

Coincidentally, a month later he was scheduled to attend an Active Isolated Stretching (AIS) technique seminar being given by Aaron Mattes. While his reason for attending was to learn the technique for the benefit of his clients, he was curious to see what effect the AIS technique would have upon his right shoulder. In the weekend seminar every major muscle of the body was covered, including all muscles of the shoulder joint and shoulder girdle. The stretches to his right shoulder did not cause any pain, but they were certainly challenging and felt effective.

The day after the seminar he decided to test whatever benefit he might have derived from the weekend's stretching by trying to do a pushup. To his amazement, not only was he able to easily perform five to ten pushups in a row, but he did so without any pain. While he had always had confidence in what stretching can do for the body, and he had heard excellent things about the AIS technique in particular, that day sold him on its effectiveness. He now regularly employs AIS as a part of his practice.

■ Case history 2

In this second case history the client, once again, is a bodyworker. She is a middle-aged female bodyworker who is an AIS practitioner, a licensed massage therapist, and a certified Pilates instructor. She recently began to experience carpal tunnel syndrome (CTS) in both of her hands. The cause of her CTS was overuse of her hands from doing massage, AIS, and Pilates; she works approximately 60 hours a week on clients. As she admitted, she forgot about the damage that can happen to her hands by working long hours and not taking care of herself.

Her symptoms included tingling, numbness, and pain in both hands, the left hand being more severe. The pain was so severe that it made it difficult for her to perform many activities of daily life, such as holding a steering wheel when driving or picking up heavy objects. It also often kept her awake at night. These symptoms progressed to the point that it became difficult for her to work on her clients, not only threatening her livelihood, but also potentially leaving her clients without the benefit of her work.

Because her clients had achieved excellent results from the AIS work that she did, she decided to try treating her own CTS with AIS. She began a regular routine using Aaron Mattes' active isolated stretches, as well as Aaron Mattes' active isolated strengthening. She also adjunctively added in massage therapy. Six months later,

her hands were not only free from pain; they were stronger than they had been before. Now healthy and strong, she is able to continue her work, enjoying a full and satisfying practice with her clients.

SUGGESTED READINGS

Mattes AL: *Active isolated strengthening*, Sarasota, Fla, 2006, Aaron Mattes Publishing.

Mattes AL: *Active isolated stretching: The Mattes method*, Sarasota, Fla, 2000, Aaron Mattes Publishing.

Mattes A: *Specific stretching for everyone*, Sarasota, Fla, 2000, Aaron Mattes Publishing.

RESOURCES

www.stretchingusa.com

REFERENCES

1. Mattes AL: *Active isolated stretching: The Mattes method*, Sarasota, Fla, 2004, Aaron Mattes Publishing.
2. Mattes AL: *Specific stretching for everyone*, Sarasota, Fla, 2000, Aaron Mattes Publishing.
3. Anderson B: *Stretching*, 20th Anniversary rev. ed, Bolinas, Calif, 2000, Shelter Publications.
4. Muscolino JE: *Kinesiology: The skeletal system and muscle function*, St. Louis, 2006, Elsevier.
5. Nelson A, Kokkonen J: *Stretching anatomy*, Champaign, Ill, 2007, Human Kinetics.
6. Liebensen C: *Rehabilitation of the spine: A practitioner's manual*, Baltimore, 1996, Lippincott Williams & Wilkins.
7. McAtee R, Charland J: *Facilitated stretching: Assisted and unassisted PNF stretching made easy*, ed 2, Champaign, Ill, 1999, Human Kinetics.
8. Mattes A: Personal communication with the author, 2007.
9. Muscolino JE: Stretch your way to better health, *MTJ* 45:167-171, 2006.
10. Beam J et al: The stretching debate, *Journal of Bodywork and Movement Therapies* 7:80-96, 2003.
11. Chaitow L, DeLany J: *Clinical application of neuromuscular techniques: The upper body*, vol 1, Edinburgh, 2000, Churchill Livingstone of Elsevier.
12. Kraftsow G: *Yoga for wellness*, New York, 1999, Penguin.
13. Wharton J, Wharton P: *The Whartons' stretch book, featuring the breakthrough method of active-isolated stretching*, New York, 1996, Three Rivers Press.
14. Alter M: *Science of flexibility*, ed 3, Champaign, Ill, 2004, Human Kinetics.
15. Muscolino JE, Cipriani S: Pilates and the "powerhouse"—1, *Journal of Bodywork and Movement Therapies* 8:15-24, 2004.
16. Lowe W: *Orthopedic massage*, Edinburgh, 2003, Mosby.

MULTIPLE CHOICE TEST QUESTIONS

1) Who developed AIS?
   a) John Barnes
   b) Andrew Still
   c) Aaron Mattes
   d) Robert King

2) What is the primary purpose of AIS?
   a) increase strength of the body
   b) increase flexibility of the body
   c) decrease range of motion of the body
   d) decrease strength of the body

3) What term is used to describe the tissue that is to be stretched?
   a) target tissue
   b) focus structure
   c) prime muscle
   d) taut band

4) What term describes the stretch in which the person remains in the position of stretch for 10 seconds or more?
   a) dynamic stretch
   b) active isolated stretch
   c) active stretch
   d) static stretch

5) For how long are dynamic stretches usually held?
   a) 1 to 3 seconds
   b) 5 to 10 seconds
   c) 10 to 30 seconds
   d) 60 seconds or longer

6) What is another term for dynamic stretching?
   a) static stretching
   b) contract relax stretching
   c) mobilization stretching
   d) all the above

7) What is the definition of an active stretch?
   a) any stretch in which the client moves his body into the stretch
   b) any stretch in which the therapist moves the client's body into the stretch
   c) a stretch in which the muscles of the joint (where the stretch is occurring) bring the body part to the position of the stretch
   d) a stretch in which the client does multiple reps and holds each one for 3 seconds or less

8) Which of the following statements is true regarding a passive stretch?
   a) It always requires the presence of a therapist.
   b) It never requires the presence of a therapist.
   c) The client cannot perform a passive stretch without assistance from a therapist.
   d) The client may be able to perform a passive stretch without assistance from a therapist.

9) Which of the following are two different types of advanced stretching?
   a) classic static stretching and dynamic stretching
   b) contract relax (CR) and active stretching
   c) mobilization stretching and AIS
   d) proprioceptive neuromuscular facilitation (PNF) and agonist contract (AC) stretching

10) What neurologic reflex is employed with contract relax (CR) stretching?
    a) muscle spindle
    b) Golgi tendon organ
    c) reciprocal inhibition
    d) stretch

11) What neurologic reflex is employed with active isolated stretching (AIS)?
    a) muscle spindle
    b) Golgi tendon organ
    c) reciprocal inhibition
    d) stretch

12) What are the two phases of an active isolated stretch called?
    a) initial and terminal
    b) active and passive
    c) stretch and recovery
    d) static and dynamic

13) During the AIS protocol, when does the client exhale?
    a) when actively moving the body part
    b) when the therapist adds additional stretch
    c) when being returned to the starting position
    d) during the recovery phase

14) How many reps are usually done with AIS protocol?
    a) 1 to 3
    b) 3 to 5
    c) 8 to 10
    d) 20 or more

15) Approximately how much force should be added to the stretch by the therapist after the client has actively moved the body part?
    a) 1 pound or less
    b) 3 to 5 pounds
    c) 5 to 10 pounds
    d) more than 10 pounds

16) If a muscle is either stretched too far or stretched too quickly, what reflex is triggered?
    a) muscle spindle
    b) Golgi tendon organ
    c) reciprocal inhibition
    d) none of the above

17) What muscles of the client are actively contracted during the AIS protocol?
    a) target muscles
    b) agonists to the target muscles
    c) antagonists to the target muscles
    d) all the above

18) Which of the following are benefits of AIS?
    a) increased flexibility of the target muscles and increased strength of the antagonists of the target muscles
    b) increased local circulation and increased warming of the local tissues
    c) increased strengthening of the actively contracted muscles and facilitation of the neural pathways to the contracted muscles
    d) all the above

19) Which of the following describes the stabilization hand?
    a) the therapist's hand that performs the stretch
    b) the client's hand that passively moves the body part into the stretch
    c) the hand that holds the rest of the body still during the stretch
    d) a and b

20) Which of the following may be a contraindication to AIS of the spine?
    a) marked osteoarthritis (OA)
    b) bulging disc
    c) advanced degenerative joint disease (DJD)
    d) all the above

Ayurvedic Therapies

Sonia Elisa Masocco

2

AYURVEDIC FUNDAMENTALS: BASIC PRINCIPLES KEY TO THE UNDERSTANDING OF AYURVEDA

Ayurveda is an eastern Indian system of holistic therapies and medicine that integrates the body, mind, and spirit not only as a means to heal, but also as a way of life. The name Ayurveda comes from two Sanskrit words: *veda* and *ayus,* which combined mean "the science of life." It is believed that healthy people are those who keep a balance between body, mind, and spirit.

HISTORY

Before written history, this ancient wisdom is believed to have come from divine origins, which were communicated directly to the sages through meditation. This wisdom was passed from one generation to the next through oral history and traditions. About 3,000 years ago, an invading nomadic tribe from Central Asia called the Aryans compiled the knowledge into four books called the four Vedas: *Rg, Yajur, Sama,* and *Atharva*. It took thousands of years to finish all four books.

The foundation of Ayurveda comes from the last book, *Atharva*. The first text of Ayurveda, the *Samhita,* dates from 1000 BC.[2] Later versions were written at the turn of the first millennium and embrace the concurrent philosophical teachings of yoga, Buddhism, and other philosophies.[2,4]

Ayurveda flourished through the invasions of nomadic tribes (between 2000 and 600 BC), Alexander the Great (356-323 BC), and the rise of Buddhism in India in the third century BC.

The third Mauryan emperor, Ashoka (ca. 273-232 BC), who converted to Buddhism while ruling India, developed hospitals for humans and animals. He sent emissaries to Sri Lanka, Nepal, and Tibet creating embassies and establishing monasteries to spread the teachings of Buddhism. During his rule, Ayurveda grew in popularity.

When India became a British colony in 1858, Ayurveda was replaced by European knowledge in all areas governed by the East India Company. However, when India regained its independence in 1947, Ayurveda was gradually reestablished and is currently one of the six medical systems officially recognized by the Indian government. Today there are schools throughout the world that teach Ayurvedic therapies.[3]

AYURVEDIC THERAPIES

To understand the basic principles of **Ayurvedic therapies,** it is important to understand the Sanskrit terms used by the three main authors of Ayurvedic ancient texts: Caraka, Susruta, and Vagbhata (Box 2-1). Two of the most important terms are **dosha** and **prakruti**.

The term *dosha* refers to the three psychophysiologic principles of the body, also known as bodily humors, and references the five elements of ether (or space), air, fire, water, and earth.[1] The three doshas are **vata, pitta,** and **kapha.** Each dosha has recognizable qualities that can be observed as characteristics related to the body or personality traits. When functioning normally and present in normal quantities, the doshas maintain all healthy bodily processes. When they are out of balance, disease results.

At the time of conception and then birth we resonate to a specific combination of the doshas. These combinations are known in Ayurveda as *prakruti* and make up our original balanced constitutions.[1,7] For example, a prakruti can have pitta dosha as primary with vata dosha secondary and kapha dosha tertiary. There can also be dual doshic prakruti, where two of the doshas are predominant and the third secondary, or a total balance between the three, called *tridoshic*.[3,7]

It is the prakruti's individual ratio of the three doshas and the blending of the respective dosha's qualities that give each of us our unique constitution (nature) with distinctive strengths and vulnerabilities. When the prakruti's balance becomes disturbed because of poor dietary choices and an unhealthy lifestyle, prakruti becomes **vikruti,** meaning "out of balance."[3,10]

The Doshas
Vata: Space and Air

Vata is responsible for space, movement, breathing, natural urges, and sensory functions and is associated with an astringent taste. **Prana,** the Sanskrit term for "life force," is found in vata.[1]

Characteristics of vata include: cold, dry, light, rough, movement, subtlety, and clarity.[1] People with more vata in their prakruti may have skin that is cool to the touch or may give others a "cold shoulder." Their skin may be dry and flaky, they may suffer from constipation, or they may have a dry sense of humor. They often have a slender frame and are light sleepers. They may have rough calluses on their heels or may speak in a rough tone. They may have trouble focusing their attention or have a hard time sitting still and need to move about. The subtle quality gives this type the ability to perceive and understand the nontangible or metaphysical. The clear quality allows for an open mind. According to the ancient texts, many of the diseases that occur when vata is out of balance involve pain, tingling, numbness, dryness, and stiffness.[2]

Pitta: Fire and Water

Pitta is responsible for metabolic processes, body temperature, digestion, and understanding. It is associated with a pungent taste.[2,7] **Agni,** the digestive fire, and **tejas,** the spark of cellular intelligence, are found in pitta.

Characteristics of pitta include: hot, sharp, penetrating, light, slightly oily, liquid, and foul smelling.[2,7] If someone has pitta dominant, their body temperature tends to be higher than normal and they are uncomfortable with hot temperatures or when overexposed to the sun in the summer. They may be hot tempered. They may have sharp and penetrating facial feature or may be mentally sharp or have a "sharp tongue." They may be sensitive to light or

BOX 2-1	**Ayurvedic Major Classic Ancient Texts**
Author	**Ancient Text Titles**
Caraka	*Caraka Samhita*
Susruta	*Susruta Samhita*
Vagbhata	*Astanga Hrydayam*
	Astanga Samgraha

have a light body frame. They may have slightly oily skin or loose bowel movements. The liquid characteristic can be seen as excessive sweating or urination, while foul odors can come from various body parts.

Many of the diseases that occur when pitta is out of balance involve inflammation, burning, and bleeding.[2]

Kapha: Earth and Water

Kapha is responsible for growth, stability, and energy reserve and is associated with a sweet taste. **Ojas,** the principle of immunity, is found in kapha[7,8] (Box 2-2).

Characteristics of kapha include: heavy and dense, slow, cool, oily, smooth, sticky, and earthlike. People whose prakruti is primarily kapha often have a heavy build with dense bones and muscles. These people are slow in their speech and move slowly. Because they have slower digestion and metabolism, they tend to gain weight easily. Their temperature is often cool, and they have a laid-back temperament that is "calm, cool, and collected." Their skin and hair are considered oily. Their joints are well lubricated and move smoothly. They may have smooth, calming voices. The sticky quality relates to endurance, to an ability to stay in relationships, and to the body's ability to bind and create growths. Being associated with the element earth, they have strength and stamina. Heaviness, excess moisture,

and growths are believed to be responsible for many of the diseases that occur when kapha is out of balance.[2]

Each dosha is associated with a primary site in the body as well as secondary sites (Table 2-1), with certain feelings and emotions (Table 2-2), and with times of day, seasons, and biologic ages (Table 2-3).[2,7]

According to Ayurveda, there are six stages in the development of "dis-ease" or **samprapti.**[7] They are accumulation, provocation, spread, deposition, manifestation, and secondary complications. The first three stages are easily treated with diet and lifestyle modifications. Although the latter three can be modified by diet and lifestyle changes, they require additional measures for management and the intervention of an Ayurvedic physician.[1A]

Another fundamental concept is that of **ama,** or toxicity.[2] Ama manifests as heavy, cold, dull, and sticky qualities. Its opposites are light, hot, sharp, and clear. Ama is a profound concept because it is the undigested

---

[1A] In India the basic training for an Ayurvedic Physician is 4 years, similar to U.S. medical training. Then there are specializations for eight branches: ENT, geriatrics, toxicology, internal medicine, pediatrics, psychiatry, surgery, and virilization (sexual rejuvenation). In the United States, Ayurveda is not a licensed profession, but there are a few schools offering various degrees of training in Ayurveda with an aim to preserve and promote the philosophy, knowledge, and practice of Ayurveda.

BOX 2-2 Ayurvedic 20 Qualities also Known as "The 10 Pairs of Opposites"

Sanskrit	English	Variant	Action
Guru	Heavy	Weight	Nourishing, anabolic
Laghu	Light	Weight	Depleting, catabolic
Manda	Slow/Dull	Intensity	Pacifies
Tikshna	Sharp	Intensity	Cleanses
Ushna	Hot	Temperature	Increases activity
Shita	Cold	Temperature	Condenses
Snigdha	Oily	Emollient	Produces moisture and lubricates
Ruksha	Dry	Emollient	Drying
Shlaksna	Smooth	Texture	Stimulates growth
Khara	Rough	Texture	Depletes
Sandra	Dense	Viscosity	Nourishes
Drava	Liquid	Viscosity	Dissolves
Mrdu	Soft	Compression	Relaxes
Kathina	Hard	Compression	Solidifies
Sthira	Static/Stable	Fluidity and movement	Supports
Cala	Mobile	Fluidity and movement	Excites
Sukshma	Subtle	Density	Penetrating
Sthula	Gross	Density	Protecting
Avila/Picchila	Cloudy/Sticky	Adhesion	Coating
Visada	Clear	Adhesion	Dispersing

TABLE 2-1 Doshas: Primary and Secondary Sites		
Dosha	**Primary Site**	**Secondary Sites**
Vata	Colon	Lower abdomen, pelvic girdle, thighs, bones, ears, and skin
Pitta	Small intestine	Liver, spleen, gallbladder, blood, eyes, gray matter of the brain
Kapha	Stomach	Lung, pancreas, synovial fluid, plasma, lymph nodes, mastic tissue, sinus, and white matter of the brain

TABLE 2-2 Doshas: Feelings and Emotions		
Dosha	**Positive Feeling**	**Emotions**
Vata	Clear insights	Fear, anxiety, and emptiness
Pitta	Wisdom	Anger, hate, and jealousy
Kapha	Compassion	Attachment, accumulation, and possessiveness

byproduct of ingestion and it relates to all spheres: the physical, mental, emotional, and spiritual. Toxicity can also be caused by exogenous factors such as environmental pollutants, or worms and parasites.[12] The agni, or the digestive fire contained within pitta, must be sufficiently fanned and appropriately fed in order to prevent toxicity. Symptoms of toxicity may be low energy, a sense of heaviness, restlessness, lethargy, indigestion, abdominal distention, constipation, congestion, accumulation of urine or sweat, loss of taste, and sexual debility.

It may also manifest as lack of luster, lack of brilliance, lack of appetite, and a coating on the tongue. All of these signs and symptoms of ama can be increased by any food, activity, thought, or relationship that is

heavy, cold, dull, sticky, occurring between 6 to 10 AM or PM, or on a cloudy day. Because poor digestion of food, thoughts, emotions, or experiences is directly related to the health of the digestive fire, agni plays the most significant role. Many Ayurvedic therapies cannot be done if there is ama. Alternative measures have to be used to increase the agni and eliminate the ama.

Physically, digestion can be increased by using herbs that kindle the digestive fire **(dipana)** and toxicity can be eliminated with herbs **(pachana).**[1] In addition to herbs, the practitioner may use yogic techniques[2A] to deal with spiritual toxicity or candle gazing to deal with emotional toxicity. Many Ayurvedic therapies are not effective until the ama is eliminated.

AYURVEDIC THERAPIES

Ayurvedic therapies are performed in conjunction with other protocols. These often involve recommendations for diet and lifestyle changes and herbs. The treatments are tailored to the agni, ama, and health of the person being treated [2A,3A] (Figure 2-1).

[2A]Ayurveda is rooted in seven systems of Indian philosophy. Logical thinking and principles of valid knowledge are derived from *Nyaya*. The concept of reality, category of qualities, and substances stems from *Vaisesika*. From *Samkhya* we get the theory of cause and effect, and evolution of the universe. The concept of duty, rituals, and use of mantras comes from *Mimamsa*. The concept of the soul and the universe stems from *Vedanta*. The eight limbs (i.e., the five restraints, five observances, posture, breathing, withdrawal of the senses, concentration, meditation, and spiritual absorption) originate in *Yoga*, and the four noble truths (suffering exists, there is a cause of suffering, there is cessation of suffering, and there is a mean to cease suffering) are derived from *Buddhism*.

[3A]In Ayurveda there is a strong emphasis on the concept of *bala*, strength. Strength is measured in terms of the dosha as compared with other doshas, the agni, the individual's physical capacity to endure therapy, the mental strength of the client, the strength of the therapy itself, the strength of the medicine used in therapy, and the strength of the person administering the therapy.

TABLE 2-3 Doshas: Time of Day, Seasonal, and Age Associations			
Dosha	**Time (AM and PM)**	**Season**	**Ages**
Vata	Between 2 and 6	Increases in the fall and decreases in the winter	55 to 100
Pitta	Between 10 and 2	Increases in the summer and decreases in the fall	14 to 50
Kapha	Between 6 and 10	Increases in the winter and decreases in the spring	Birth to 12

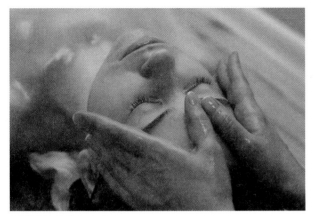

FIGURE 2-1 Use of oil.

The Ayurvedic ancient texts refer to massage as a necessity. The author Caraka states:

"As a pitcher, dry skin, and an axis of a cart become strong and resistant by the application of oil, so by massage of oil the human body becomes strong and smooth skinned, it is not susceptible to the diseases due to vata, it is resistant to exhaustion and exertion."
(*Caraka Samhita*, Ch 5, vs 85-86)

Giving a massage is considered to be a **seva,** or service, and service is considered one of the noble actions (dharma). The Ayurvedic ancient texts make it clear that massage is necessary to achieve and maintain good health.

The importance of massage is further supported in Vagbhata's treatise *Asthanga Hrdayam.* He states that in order to enjoy good health and happiness it is important to receive a massage with oils specifically prepared for one's constitution and according to the season.[14]

There are two types of therapeutic massage: **udvartana,** which is a dry massage using light oil and dry powders, and **abhyanga** or **snehana** (self-massage), which is a massage using only oils.

Udvartana: Dry Massage

Udvartana is the sankrit term that literally means "grinding," "pounding," "rubbing," or "kneading" the body.[1] It also refers to the fragrant oils used in this treatment or in the relief of pain in the limbs.[1]

Dry massage is used to decrease the absorption and crystallization of toxins in the body. Only after these wastes are broken down and the metabolic fire is increased through exercise, applying warmth and moisture, or eating a specialized diet is a person healthy enough to receive abhyanga or snehana massage.

The skin is the most external pathway to the body's innate capacity to heal. With direct contact with the skin, using strokes that are brisk or rubs that create friction, udvartana helps eliminate accumulated kapha or ama.

Benefits of Udvartana

Dry massage aids in digestion and increases metabolism, which can help in weight loss. It reduces toxicity and softens the body tissues, conveys a sense of lightness, and generates clearer perceptions.

Indications for Udvartana

Dry massage should be used for disorders associated with kapha—such as oily, thick hair; clammy skin; sluggishness; excess weight; drooling; sinus or bronchial congestion; lack of energy or motivation; excess ama; or when kapha is prevalent in prakruti or vikruti.

Contraindications to Udvartana

Udvartana is never used at night, regardless of the receiver's state of health. There are also specific conditions where dry massage techniques should not be used—for example, when a person is weak or incapacitated; frail and elderly; worried, anxious, or in an extreme emotional state; has an eating disorder and is emaciated; has a tendency to bleed easily; or has thin or frail skin. Udvartana should be avoided if vata is dominant in either prakruti or vikruti, or if pitta is dominant in the vikruti.

The protocol for the udvartana is the same as that for abhyanga. The main difference is that a segment of the body is effleuraged with a light coat of oil before that segment is sprinkled with powder to encourage venous and lymphatic return. The powder is applied with a combination of palm pressing, kneading and friction strokes, long strokes on long bones and muscles, and circular strokes on all joints and buttocks. This treatment lasts approximately 45 minutes.

After udvartana, the client will have improved digestion, a sense of lightness, be more alert, feel stronger and more energized, and have more color in his or her complexion. If done incompetently, udvartana may leave the client feeling heavy, drowsy, congested, and lethargic. If the treatment is too aggressive, the client may have insomnia, ringing in the ears, feel more stressed, become more emotional or anxious, experience spontaneous bleeding (such as in the gums or nose), feel thirstier, and/or have a burning sensation or a skin rash.

Abyhyanga: Oil Massage

The purpose of abhyanga or snehana is to balance and realign the dosha. The oil sedates the doshas so that toxins can be released more easily. **Panchakarma,** the Ayurvedic purification program, may begin after the body is ready to release toxins (Box 2-3). The daily practice of localized oil massage can be used to treat insomnia; lack of muscle tone; fatigue; dry skin; lack of skin luster and texture; ailments caused by vata in the joints, muscles, and nerve; or to provide postnatal support.

The daily practice of full body oil massage increases vitality, improves circulation and cardiovascular health, and stimulates the release of waste and toxins. According to Ayurveda, when the massage is done at a faster pace, the body becomes more flexible, is better able to prevent the effects of aging, and increases muscle tone.[1A] Abhyanga or snehana is considered to be either nourishing and building, or lubricating treatments.[2]

Nourishing therapy is done if someone is weak or incapacitated; is frail and elderly; is worried, anxious, or in an extreme emotional state; has an eating disorder and is emaciated; has a tendency to bleed easily; or has thin or frail skin.

Due to their intrinsic qualities, Ayurvedic oils lubricate and soften the tissues. The oils are absorbed through the skin and enter the capillaries, where they liquefy and push toxins back to the GI tract for elimination. The application of oil nourishes the body and grounds and calms individual. Oils can also soothe irritation or rekindle the localized metabolic fire.[8,14] A tenet of Ayurveda is that we carry memories of past experiences, feelings, and emotions within our tissues. Through massage, we can release any negative feelings and lighten our emotional load.

During abhyanga specific oils are used to balance and pacify each dosha. When the predominant dosha is vata, sesame oil is used. When the predominant dosha is pitta, oils like coconut or sunflower are used. For kapha predominance, oils such as sunflower, mustard, or corn are typically used.[2,3]

Benefits of Abhyanga

Massaging with oils increases the positive energy of kapha; eliminates toxins, thus calming vata; balances endocrine secretions; improves the tone of tissue and skin, which results in a healthy complexion; brings nourishment to tissue; slows the aging process, which leads to a longer life span; alleviates pain; and eliminates stress, resulting in relaxation and a feeling of harmony. The receiver is happier and healthier with more vitality and vigor.

Indications for Abhyanga

Abhyanga is used as a preparation for panchakarma—for treating disorders associated with vata qualities. It is used when someone is worried, anxious, or stressed; has weak or no muscle tone; has cracking or popping joints; is afflicted with Bell's palsy, stroke, or paralysis; has an eating disorder leading to emaciation; has dry skin; has aches and pains from physical labor; or is elderly and frail.

Contraindications of Abhyanga

Abhyanga is not used on a cold and cloudy day, regardless of the receiver's state of health. There are also specific conditions where oil massage techniques should be avoided. Abhyanga should not be used if someone has very low agni and high ama; is obese; has edema; is nauseous or vomiting; is jaundiced or has hepatitis A; has a fever; has drug or alcohol abuse issues; is severely dehydrated; is menstruating or pregnant; has acute hypoglycemia or insulin-dependent diabetes; has recently taken a laxative or had an enema; or has an abscess or bleeding disorder.

During abhyanga, the client is undressed, covered by a sheet, and lies supine on a massage table. This treatment can be performed by one therapist or by two

---

> **BOX 2-3 Panchakarma – The Ayurvedic Science of Rejuvination[4A]**
>
> Panchakarma: [Sanskrit] a fivefold purification treatment used in *Ayurveda*, usually including a purgative to eliminate *kapha*, a laxative to eliminate *pitta*, an enema to eliminate *vata*, inhalation treatment to clear *doshas* from the head, and bloodletting to purify the blood.

From *Dorland's illustrated medical dictionary*, ed 31, Philadelphia, 2007, Saunders.

[4A]Panchakarma is a process of elimination and rejuvenation and can be literally translated as "five actions." This process is generally overseen by an Ayurvedic physician. The five actions are basti (medicated enema) for vata primary or vata vikruti, virechana (purgation therapy) for pitta primary or pitta vikruti, vamana (emesis therapy) for kapha primary or kapha vikruti, rakta moksa (bloodletting) for vitiation of the blood disorders, nasya (nasal administrations) for any residual dosha. These five actions are preceded by internal intake of oil, external application of oil, and sudation.

therapists massaging with synchronized strokes. Two therapists often massage one client to provide more balance and to save time.[9] The pressure of the strokes used during abhyanga depends upon the predominant dosha. A vata constitution requires soft pressure, pitta requires medium pressure, and kapha needs strong or rough pressure. A chant usually precedes the massage to clear the space and allow for healing. Different schools teach different chants. The chants can be as short as a single "Hari Om" or as long as 108 verses.

The practitioner starts the session by applying oil to the feet, which grounds the client. The lower extremities are then oiled and massaged using long, fluid strokes on long bones, circular strokes on the joints, working distal to proximal, or toward the center of the body. The upper extremities are oiled and massaged in the same manner. The abdomen is then oiled and massaged by following an imaginary spiral stemming from the umbilicus (nabhi), which is considered the seat of the maternal prana. The umbilicus is filled with oil.

The client turns prone and the treatment begins again at the client's feet, followed by the long, fluid strokes on the legs. The buttocks are oiled and massaged with circular movements. The back is then oiled and massaged with a mixture of upward long strokes for the lateral portion and circular strokes medial at the spine.

The client turns face up again as the upper torso gets oiled and massaged with long lateral movements. The sequence concludes with massage of the face. The session comes to an end with a salutation to the divine temple of the soul, the body (Box 2-4).

Depending on the condition of the client, this treatment can last from 40 to 90 minutes. Moderation in diet and lifestyle is usually recommended after an abhyanga.

After the treatment, the client will feel slightly tender, have improved digestion and a soft bowel movement the next day, experience pain relief, have clearer perceptions, have a sense of lightness, be in a better mood, have more energy, and enjoy deeper sleep. If done incompetently, abhyanga can cause hard and dry stools, poor digestion, and adversely affect the movement of prana within the body, creating breathlessness, dizziness, loss of strength and sleep, and sensory dysfunctions. Excessive abhyanga can create paleness, heaviness, stiffness, puffiness, drowsiness, anorexia, nausea, burning pain in the liver area, and indigestion.

When abhyanga is done only to the feet, it is called **padhabhyanga** (*padha* in Sanskrit). When abhyanga is done only to the hands, it is called **hastabhyanga** (*hasta* in Sanskrit). Because feet and hands mirror the body, these treatments can affect the entire body.

It is believed that prana, or life force, and divine energy flow from the fingertips and hands of the therapist to the receiver.[2] Traditionally, therapists begin their day by intoning a specific, personalized chant to increase their energy and the prana in their hands. The chant can also be used before beginning the day's sessions. Because it is believed that there is transference of energy, it is important that therapists work only when they are physically and mentally healthy. And, the therapist must be totally present and focused on the client.[2A]

TECHNIQUES OF AYURVEDIC MASSAGE

Several different techniques are used for Ayurvedic massage.[2,7] In general, for clients with vata types of constitution lesser pressure is used because they are light and slight. For pitta types, who have a small to medium build, a medium pressure is adequate, and for kapha types, with their larger frames, more pressure can be used.

Tapping

Tapping is considered the introduction to massage. It is used to wake up the body and signals the beginning of the massage. It is done by gently patting the person from the feet to the hips, and from the hands to the shoulders (Figure 2-2).

BOX 2-4 Salutation to the Devine in Everyone

According to Vedic tradition the body is the temple of the soul, and therapists are traditionally taught to view a client as a divine being. *Namaste* is a traditional, and common, salutation. *Namas* in Sanskrit means "bow," "reverential salutation," "adoration," and "homage"; *te* in Sanskrit means "to you"; so *namaste* means "I bow" (or "salute" or "pay homage") "to you." This is usually accompanied by a slight bow with hands pressed together in prayer at the chest, chin, nose, or above the head. The right hand signifies the higher self and the left hand represents the worldly self; the merger represents the union of divine and devotee. The gesture can also be performed wordlessly and will carry the same meaning.

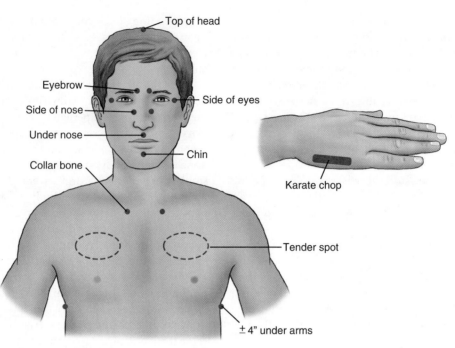

FIGURE 2-2 Tapping points.

Flowing

Flowing consists of soft stroking, which is soothing and gentle and done with one or both hands in a constant motion. This technique is used both as beginning and ending strokes for long bones and muscles and when working on the neck, soles of the feet, and palms of the hands. Using full palmar contact, the therapist works so that the movement and pressure are toward the heart.

Kneading

Kneading is used on larger muscles or anywhere on the body that requires increased tone and vitality. This technique is tridoshic, but excessive pressure may aggravate vata-type individuals.

Rubbing

Rubbing creates friction and is commonly used to encourage circulation, release waste, decrease muscle stiffness, and alleviate fatigue. Rubbing aggravates vata, but, if done rhythmically, it soothes pitta and kapha.

Pinching

In pinching, the tissue is grasped between the forefinger and thumb and pulled away from the bone. Pinches are short, rapid, and rhythmic and are used only on arms, legs, and back.

Squeezing

Similar to pinching, squeezing is used for releasing tension and energy from the extremities, like the toes of the feet and the fingers of the hand. Each squeeze starts at the base of the toe or finger and goes to the tip. It is usually followed by flicking the end of the toe or the fingertip.

Pulling

Similar to pinching but requiring a better grasp, pulling lifts the skin and must always be done gently. A common use is to gently pull the hair when working on the scalp. This technique is used to release stress, suppressed emotions, and blocked energy.

Pressing

Pressing is used to stimulate tissues and regulate vata and the flow of energy. Pressing can be done on hard body surfaces with flat hands moving in a circular manner. On softer tissue, compression is done with a wave-like pressure moving toward the heart. Pressing can also be done on specific points using the thumb or more than one finger.

Circular

Circular, clockwise, and counterclockwise massage movements are generally done on joints and on the abdomen. These movements encourage energy to flow, lubricate the joints, and dispel any tension, ache, or strain.

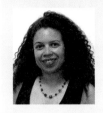
AYURVEDIC TREATMENTS

Netra Basti: Eye Cleansing

Netra basti is the process of cleansing the eyes and improving vision by applying clarified butter (ghee) to the eyes. This treatment lubricates and nourishes the optic nerve and eye tissue. Traditionally, this treatment is done in the evening, one eye each day, to improve eyesight[2,9,17,20] (Figure 2-3).

Nasya: Nasal Clearing

Nasya is the process of administering medications through the nasal passages to improve breathing and memory and to balance the endocrine system. According to Ayurveda, the nose is a direct pathway to the brain where prana, the life force, controls the mind and all neurologic functions. Caraka stated that torticollis, headaches, facial paralysis, lock jaw, irritation and inflammation of the nose, and head tremors can be successfully treated with nasya therapy.[2]

Karna Purana: Ear Cleaning

Karna Purana (from the Sanskrit words *karna,* meaning "ear," and *purana,* meaning "filling") literally means filling the ear with oil. It is a procedure in which warm or medicated oil is poured into the ears.[1] In Ayurveda the ear represents the entire body as an inverted fetus. It is believed that the effect of massaging the ear reach all parts of the body. Karna purana is used to alleviate ringing in the ear, to improve hearing, to loosen ear wax, reduce teeth grinding, and calm the mind.

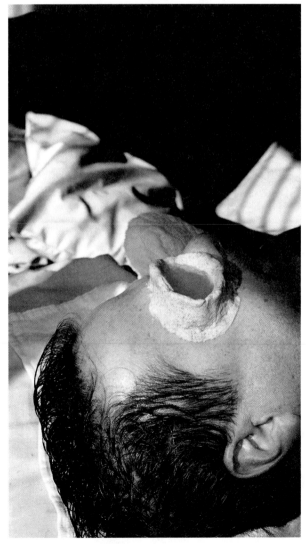

FIGURE 2-3 Netra basti.

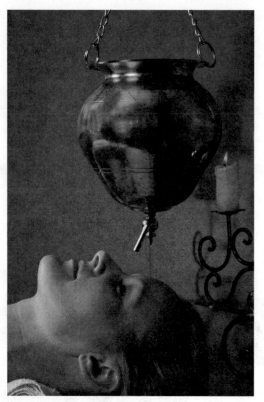

FIGURE 2-4 Shirodhara.

Shirodhara: Continuous Flow of Oil to the Third Eye

Shirodhara comes from the Sanskrit words *shiro,* meaning "head" and *dhaara,*[5A] meaning "coming down in a stream." This treatment balances the central nervous system, quiets the mind, and restores functional integrity within the mind and body, leading to an inner peace (Figure 2-4). It also heals injuries to **marma points**[6A] (Figure 2-5), which are energy points believed to be related to internal organs, doshas, or tissues.[7A] Shirodhara has gained popularity because of its relative simplicity. With the client supine and with protective covering over the eyes, a steady stream of oil drips on the area of the

> **BOX 2-5 Salutation to the Devine in Everyone**
>
> Susruta, author of the Ayurvedic ancient text *Susruta Samhita* and the father of surgery, was the first to mention marma points. The marmas constituted the primary seat of prana (life force), tejas (spark of intelligence), and ojas (principle of immunity) as well as the three fundamental qualities of sattva (purity), rajas (movement), and tamas (stillness). He stated that for those who have an injury to any of the marmas, suffering will be severe. It is thought that the marmas were originally identified and grouped as points to be avoided during surgery.

third eye. Traditionally, this treatment is done in the morning and in complete silence.

If a person needs shirodhara but it is unavailable, pichu can be substituted. **Pichu** is a treatment where a piece of cotton, saturated with the appropriate oil, is pressed across the forehead. (See Box 2-5.)

Kati Basti: Pool of Oil to the Lumbosacral Area

In Sanskrit *kati* means hip and *basti* or *vasti* refers to dwelling of oil. **Kati basti** is the process of loosing tight lower back muscles and relieving lower back tension or pain by pouring oil into a flour and water doughnut that has been placed on the lumbosacral area. This treatment relieves all afflictions of the hip area, such as sciatica and lumbago. The treatment rarely lasts more than 45 minutes (Figure 2-6).

Prustha Basti: Spinal Pool of Oil

Prustha basti is the process of improving mobility and releasing tension in the spine by placing a series of doughnuts consecutively along the spine and filling them with warm or medicated oil. This treatment lubricates the vertebral disks and nourishes the nerve ganglions.

Lepana: Application of Herbal Paste

In a **lepana** treatment session, the therapist applies an herbal paste to an area of the body to reduce swelling, pain, or localized inflammation of tissues. The pastes, called lepas, are usually made from a mixture of different herbs but can also be made with clay, depending on the condition, and are generally applied opposite to the direction of hairs. Traditionally, the herbs are mixed in a bowl with water and a bit of oil

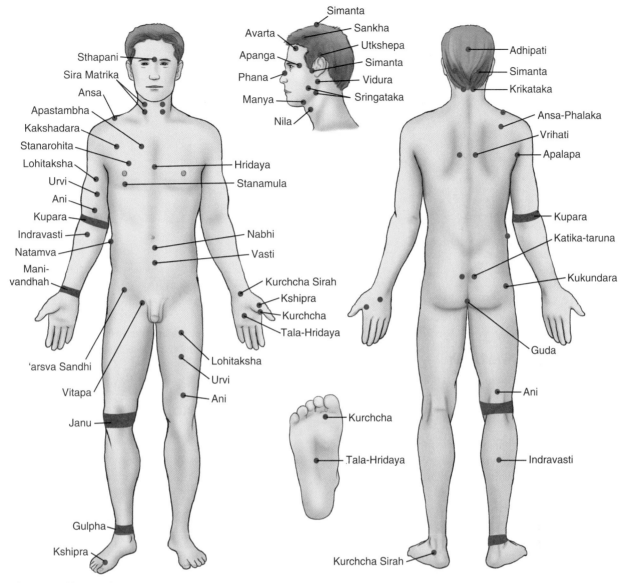

FIGURE 2-5 Marma points.

while singing a mantra.[8A] There are three types of lepas: thin, medium, and thick. Sometimes clients are given thin paste to apply as home care.

Pinda Svedana: Poultice-Pounding Therapy

From the Sanskrit words *pinda*, meaning "round mass" or "heap" and *svedana*, meaning "perspiring," **pinda svedana** is the process of detoxifying and loosing the tissues, and increasing healthy metabolism by wrapping a wet or dry poultice in a cloth and then rubbing or pounding it on the person's body to increase the rate of perspiration.[8,17] Movements for the dry bolus (the mass in the

---

[8A]Mantras are sacred sounds sometimes expressed in chant form to convey the intention to the object of desire.

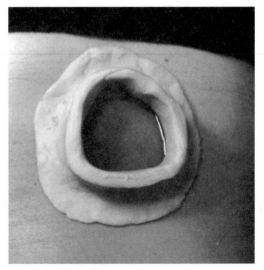

FIGURE 2-6 Omveda.

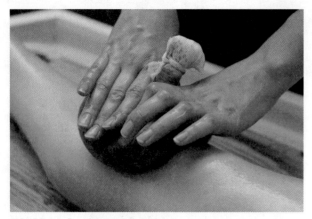

FIGURE 2-7 Poultice pounding therapy.

cloth) are quick and pounding while movements for the wet bolus are usually slower and rubbing (Figure 2-7).

CHAPTER SUMMARY

Ayurvedic therapies are powerful tools to heal the body, mind, and spirit. Ayurveda recognizes each person as a unique, multidimensional being and tailors each session to the needs of that person. However, the treatment goal is always the same: a balanced state for that individual.

Repeated applications of therapies allow the substances to work deeper in the body and promote greater self-awareness and self-understanding. According to Ayurveda, the body is the house of the soul and we must restore and strengthen the body to allow our souls to flourish.

The main focus of the protocol of abhyanga is the rythmic application of 6-8 oz of oil to the body in the one session, this is meant to lubricate and loosen the tissues which allows the doshas which have spread to the peripheral tissues to go back to their original sites at the core of the body.

There are few schools in the United States that offer training in Ayurvedic therapies, so many practicing practitioners were tutored by Ayurvedic physicians or therapists in India. For a current listing of schools offering Ayurvedic training in the United States, contact the National Ayurvedic Medical Association or log on to their website at http://www.ayurveda-nama.org/".

CASE HISTORY

In 2003, an elderly woman came to see me on a recommendation by a massage therapist. She was 80 years of age, frail, and had heart issues. Her pitta nature made her a fighter, though her skin and body were not too strong. After an initial intake and review of her numerous medications and supplements, I decided that light abhyanga would be helpful. Given that she was in a vata stage of life, I recommended medicated oil in a base of sesame and the Ayurvedic herb ashwaghanda *(Withania somnifera)* and to use rose attar at the heart. I taught her the strokes and how to apply the oil. She was to do one complete abhyanga daily preferably in the morning using approximately 4 oz of oil in each application. If the self-massage was too much, I suggested foot massage as an alternative. We met weekly, sometimes bi-monthly to review general progress and make any necessary changes or additions to base oil.

We both noticed that her energy was stronger and her skin looked younger and was less fragile. She is currently 84 years young and continues to apply the oil twice a day since she says her body "wants it and needs it." Very interested in Ayurveda, she meditates and does breathing exercises regularly and is a role model for many of my clients and others who have come to know her.

SUGGESTED READINGS

Johari H: *Ancient Indian massage*, Delhi, 2003, Munshiram Mancharlal.

Lad V: *Ayurveda, textbook of fundamental principles*, Albuquerque, 2002, TAP.

Lad V: *Ayurveda, the science of self healing*, Santa Fe, NM, 1985, Lotus Press.

Svoboda R: *Life, health & longevity*, Albuquerque, 2004, TAP.

Tiwari M: *Secrets of healing*, Twin Lakes, Wis., 1995, Lotus Press.

REFERENCES

1. Williams M: *Sanksrit english dictionary*, New Delhi, 1994, Munshiram Manoharlal Publishers.
2. Sharma D: *Caraka samhita*, Varanasi, 1997, Chowkhambha Series.
3. Svoboda R: *Life, health & longevity*, Albuquerque, 2004, TAP.
4. Radhakrishan M: *A Sourcebook of Indian philosophy*, Princeton, NJ, 1957, Princeton University Press.
5. Tigunait R: *Seven systems of Indian philosophy*, Honesdale, Pa, 1983, Himalayan Institute.
6. Bhishagrantna KK: *Susruta samhita*, Varanasi, 1998, Chowkhamba Sansrit Series.
7. Lad V: *Ayurveda, Textbook of fundamental principles*, Albuquerque, 2002, TAP.
8. Lad V: *Ayurvedic studies program notes, 2000*, 2001, New Mexico
9. Murthy KR: *Vagbhata's asthanga hrydayam*, Varanasi, 1999, Krisnadas Academy

10. Lad V: *Ayurveda, the science of self healing*, Santa Fe, NM, 1985, Lotus Press.

11. Svoboda R: *Prakruti, your ayurvedic constitution*, Twin Lakes, Wis, 1989, Lotus Press.

12 Lad V: *Ayurveda, the complete book of clinical assessment*, Albuquerque, 2006, TAP.

13. Murthy KR: *Bhavaprakasa*, Varanasi, 2000, Krisnadas Academy.

14. Murthy KR: *Sarangadhara samhita*, Varanasi, 1995, Chaukhambha Orientalia.

15. Nadkarni AK: *Indian materia medica*, Bombay, 2000, Popular Prakasham; Paranjpe P: *Indian medicinal plants forgotten healers*, Delhi, 2005, Chaukhamba Sanskrit Pratishthan.

16. Tiwari M: *Secrets of healing*, Twin Lakes, Wis, 1995, Lotus Press; Sala A: *Indian medicinal plants*, Calcutta, 1997, Oriental Longman.

17. Tewari PV: *Kasyapa samhita*, Varanasi, 1996, Chaukhambha Visvabharati.

18. Joshi S: *Ayurveda & panchakarma*, Twin Lakes, Wis, 1996, Lotus Press.

19. Gogte. VM: *Ayurvedic pharmacology & therapeutic uses of medicinal plants*, Mumbai, India, 2000, Bhavan's Book University.

20. Kulkarni, P.H.Dr, *Ayurveda therapy*, Pune, India, 1996, Ayurveda Rasashala.

21. Lad V: *Secrets of the pulse*, Albuquerque, 1996, TAP.

MULTIPLE CHOICE TEST QUESTIONS

1) Which country is considered the homeland of Ayurveda?
   a) China
   b) US
   c) Mexico
   d) India

2) How old is the body of knowledge of Ayurveda?
   a) 20 years old
   b) 100 years old
   c) 500 years old
   d) over 3000 years old

3) The term *dosha* means
   a) two
   b) element
   c) bodily humor
   d) union

4) The qualities of vata are
   a) dry, light, cold, subtle, mobile, clear with astringent taste
   b) hot, sharp, penetrating, slightly oily with pungent taste
   c) heavy, slow, cool, oily, smooth, earthlike with sweet taste
   d) dry, heavy, hot, mobile, penetrating with a salty taste

5) One of the fundamental principles of Ayurveda is
   a) like cures like
   b) like increases like
   c) like does not affect like
   d) none of the above

6) Adulthood is considered to be
   a) a vata stage of life
   b) a kapha stage of life
   c) a pitta stage of life
   d) a combination of all

7) In Ayurveda toxicity shares some qualities with
   a) vata
   b) pitta
   c) kapha
   d) all of the above

8) In Ayurveda most toxicity is
   a) physical
   b) mental
   c) emotional
   d) all of the above

9) Abhyanga, oil massage, is contraindicated in
   a) diseases of vata
   b) panchakarma
   c) low agni, high ama
   d) chronic lower back pain

10) Oils that are light, cooling, and sweet are most suitable for
    a) pitta predominance
    b) vata predominance
    c) kapha predominance
    d) all of the above

11) Udvartana is typically
    a) gentle
    b) slow
    c) rough
    d) oily

12) Udvartana is indicated for
    a) lethargy and lack of motivation
    b) sinus and bronchial congestion
    c) excess kapha
    d) all of the above

13) Which of the following statements is false?
    a) Ayurvedic massage wards off the effects of aging.
    b) Ayurvedic massage stimulates the release of waste and toxins.
    c) Ayurvedic massage is indicated for lack of muscle tone.
    d) Ayurvedic massage can be done when the client has a fever.

14) Which one of the following massage techniques should be avoided if a client has high vata and thin skin?
    a) tapping
    b) rubbing
    c) kneading
    d) pressing

15) Which of the following massage technique helps release suppressed emotions?
   a) kneading
   b) pinching
   c) pulling
   d) circular

16) After treatments such as abhyanga and karna purana one should
   a) take a cold shower to stimulate the system
   b) eat a full meal to further nourish the system
   c) take a walk in the wind to oxygenate
   d) none of the above

17) Pooling of warm oil in the lumbar-sacral area can be useful for
   a) relieving lower back pain and tension
   b) reducing growth of tumors
   c) reducing obesity
   d) improving sexual stamina

18) Lepana is used for
   a) localized swelling
   b) inflammation
   c) generalized heat
   d) all of the above

19) Pinda svedana is used to:
   a) encourage sudation and elimination of toxins
   b) encourage vitality
   c) rejuvenate the tissue
   d) all of the above

20) What is considered to be the pitta time of day?
   a) 6 AM to 10 AM
   b) 10 AM to 2 PM
   c) 2 PM to 4 PM
   d) 6 PM to10 PM

Cancer Massage

Beverly Byers

3

INTRODUCTION

More people are surviving **cancer** than ever before. This is due in part to the awareness of symptoms and early detection as well as the availability of treatment options. Of the more than 10 million **cancer survivors** in the United States, three fourths will develop long-term effects from the cancer and the treatments for cancer.[1] When faced with the diagnosis of cancer, many people seek information about cancer and the treatment options, including complementary and alternative medicine (CAM). With this information they are better able to make informed decisions and have some input into their health care. One complementary therapeutic choice for people with cancer is **massage therapy**. While massage should never replace conventional treatments, it certainly can be integrated into any health care plan (Figure 3-1).

Oncology is the study of cancer and its treatment. Each oncology client has unique circumstances surrounding the disease and its treatment. A client's needs depend on many issues, including age, socioeconomic status, general health, and family support, as well as the phase and the severity of the illness. Cancers are different, treatments for cancer are different, and the side effects of treatments are different. Cancer is not static—it goes through changes and the people with cancer go through changes. Reactions of the body, mind, and emotions differ from person to person. Additionally, changes occur week to week for oncology clients in the way they feel and the way their bodies respond to the disease and the treatments. The **pain** that arises from having cancer and/or the cancer treatment varies depending on location, extent, and side effects. If any vital organs are compromised, this could contribute to pain experienced by clients.

The diagnosis of cancer can be devastating and may seem like a hopeless situation. When people feel hopeless, they are often willing to try numerous approaches to recover and get well. A significant number of people with cancer use complementary and alternative medicine to relieve symptoms and reduce treatment side effects.[2,3]

Massage is a welcome invitation for most people, while cancer is neither welcome nor invited. When cancer has sabotaged a person's life, massage is one method of soothing the body, mind, and spirit. Massage is now

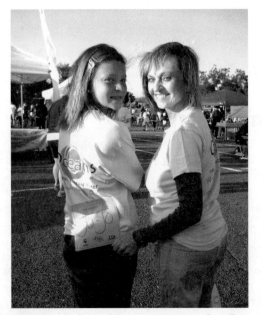

FIGURE 3-1 Beverly Byers and her granddaughter, Race Terry, walk with Oceans Massage Therapy Center's *Hands for the cure,* team in the Susan G. Komen race.

valued in the treatment of cancer and has synergistic effects on the body's healing response.

On the cover of the August 1997 issue of *Life Magazine* is a beautiful photograph of a woman's bare shoulder being touched by massaging hands.[4] The words accompanying the photograph read "Massage feels good. It also reduces stress, eases back pain, fights anorexia, lifts depression and saves lives—the Healing Power of Touch." The article inside the magazine described the research being conducted at the time and how touch made a difference in the growth and development of infants. Additionally, the research revealed the reciprocal effects of relaxation and decreased stress for the givers of massage. This article was instrumental in increasing awareness about the benefits of massage. In addition, it brought increased respectability to massage as a therapeutic modality.

HISTORY OF CANCER MASSAGE

For years, Swedish-based massage was contraindicated for people living with cancer because it was believed massage could spread cancer through the lymphatic and circulatory systems.[6-8] This myth was challenged in the 1990s with the publication of *Massage Therapy and Cancer* by Debra Curties and *Medicine Hands: Massage Therapy for People Living with Cancer* by Gayle MacDonald.[5,6] Thanks to the research, it is now known massage therapy will not cause cancer to **metastasize** or spread. The lymphatic and circulatory systems both constantly move fluids with or without massage. If cancer is going to metastasize, it will do so whether massage is administered or not.[8]

About the same time, certain hospitals began to embrace massage therapy for cancer patients and therapists were hired or contracted in the interested hospitals. It took massage schools and training programs longer to let go of the myth that massage could spread cancer. Even today, some massage schools do not teach that massage is indicated for oncology patients.

UNDERSTANDING CANCER

Much of the success of **cancer massage** rests in the hands and the hearts of therapists. Therefore, it is imperative for therapists to know what cancer is, how it spreads, and where it tends to migrate in the body.

The word *cancer* refers not to just one disease, but many (Box 3-1). The World Health Organization identifies cancer as "a generic term for a group of more than 100 diseases that can affect any part of the body.... One defining feature of cancer is the rapid creation of abnormal cells which grow beyond their usual boundaries, and

BOX 3-1 What is Cancer?

- Cancer begins when cells divide and grow out of control until they form a mass of tissue, known as a **tumor** or **neoplasm.**
- Cancer spreads when the rapidly growing cells break off from the tumor and enter the lymphatic system or the bloodstream.
- **Liquid tumors** are those which are not solid but rather they circulate through the blood stream such as **leukemia** or in the lymphatic system such as **lymphoma.**
- Cancer migrates from the primary site through the lymphatic system or bloodstream to form new tumors in other places such as organs and bones.
- Metastasis is the spread of cancer. For example, cancer that begins in a person's lung may spread to the brain. Cancer that has metastasized to the brain continues to be called by the name of the primary site, lung cancer.

which can invade adjoining parts of the body and spread to other organs, a process referred to as metastasis."[9]

Oncology is the branch of medicine dealing with tumors, and an oncologist is a physician specializing in oncology. An **oncogene** is the gene that can cause a cell to become **malignant**; antioncogenes, on the other hand, suppress tumors.[10] When the cells begin to grow out of control, they create cancers that behave in different ways, grow at different rates, and respond to different treatments. The four characteristics that define cancer are site, stage, grade, and type.

- *Site* is where the cancer occurs in the body. Primary site is where cancer originates (Table 3-1).
- *Stage* refers to how much of the body has been invaded and if the cancer has spread to lymph nodes or other tissues. The stages of cancer

represent the severity and are labeled stage 0, stage I, stage II, stage III, or stage IV with higher numbers indicating greater tissue invasion. Stage 0 is defined as carcinoma **in situ,** or self-contained. Stage I, II, and III indicate the extent of the cancer, the size of the tumor, and the spread to lymph nodes and/or organs bordering the primary tumor. Stage IV means the cancer has metastasized to another organ(s). The common elements considered in most staging systems are the location of the primary tumor, the size and number of tumors, lymph node involvement, cell type and cell grade, and whether or not metastasis has occurred.

Staging is determined by physical exams, imaging procedures, laboratory tests, pathology reports, and surgical reports. Imaging procedures include x-rays, computed tomography (CT) scans, positron emission tomography (PET) scans, and magnetic resonance imaging (MRI) scans. Laboratory tests are studies of fluids and tissues, such as blood, urine, liver function, and tumor markers. Pathology information is derived from tissue and cellular findings in the biopsy and cytology reports. Surgical reports describe the findings during surgery such as tumor size and appearance and the state of nearby tissues.

- *Grade* is determined with a microscopic view of the cancer cells. The cells are classified according to how abnormal they look as well as their growth pattern and likelihood of spreading. A pathologist can determine the grade and whether a tumor is benign or malignant by studying the cells under a microscope. Tumor grades are commonly described as 1, 2, 3, and 4 with the lowest number being the least aggressive. Cancer cells with grades 3 and 4 indicate more rapid growth with the chance to spread faster than grades 1 and 2. Grading systems vary according to the type of cancer and may be seen in different numberings. Tumor grade, along with other factors, determines the treatment plan for the patient.
- There are several main *types* of cancer:
  - **Carcinoma** begins in the skin or in tissues that line or cover internal organs; it arises from the epithelial tissue.
  - **Melanoma** is a malignant tumor originating in melanocytes (the cells that produce the pigment melanin, which colors skin, hair, and eyes).
  - **Sarcoma** begins in bone, cartilage, fat, muscles, blood vessels, or other connective or supportive tissue.

TABLE 3-1 Leading Primary Cancer Sites in United States for All Races in Order of Prevalence

	Men	Women	Children
1.	Prostate	Breast	Leukemia
2.	Lung	Lung*	Brain tumors
3.	Colorectal	Colorectal*	Lymphoma
4.	Bladder	Uterus	

U.S. Cancer Statistics Working Group: *Incidence and mortality web-based report*, Atlanta: U.S. Department of Health and Human Services, Centers for Disease Control and Prevention and National Cancer Institute, 2007 (website): www.cdc.gov/uscs.
*Reversed among black and Asian/Pacific Island women.

- **Leukemia** starts in blood-forming tissue such as bone marrow; it is characterized by rapid growth of abnormal white blood cells.
- **Central nervous system cancers** begin in the brain and spinal cord.
- **Lymphomas** and **multiple myelomas** begin in the cells of the immune system and are cancers of lymphatic tissue.[6,11]
- All of these characteristics—site, stage, grade, and type—will influence the treatment for the person who is diagnosed with cancer.[12]

TREATMENTS

Conventional medical treatments include **surgery, radiation,** and **chemotherapy.** The treatments may be used alone or in conjunction with one or both of the others depending on the type, site, and stage of the cancer. The objective is to destroy the cancerous cells.

Surgery

When the cancer can be surgically removed, surgery often becomes the first treatment of choice. Once the tumor is removed, it is sent to pathology for the initial report which indicates whether the borders of the tissue are free of cancer cells. If there are cancer cells at the borders, then additional tissue will be removed in an attempt to remove all cancer cells without compromising surrounding tissues and organs.

Radiation

Radiation therapy uses energy to kill cancer cells and shrink tumors by damaging their genetic material, thus rendering them incapable of growing and dividing. Unfortunately radiation is unable to target just cancer cells; therefore, normal cells as well as cancer cells are damaged. Most normal cells survive the effects of radiation and continue to function properly.

About half of all oncology patients receive radiation, which may be used alone or along with chemotherapy and/or surgery. It is used to shrink a tumor, to relieve symptoms, or to completely destroy a tumor. Radiation can be used to treat most solid tumors, as well as leukemia and lymphoma. The dose of radiation depends in part on the normal tissues and organs in the region of the cancer so healthy tissue in the area can be spared if possible. When surgery is performed to excise a tumor, radiation may again be utilized to incapacitate any remaining cancer cells. Radiation is done

at timed intervals. It may be performed several days in a row, after which time off is scheduled for the patient to gain strength.[14]

Prophylactic radiation therapy may be given in areas where there is no evidence of cancer in order to prevent cancer cells from growing in that area. *Palliative* radiation therapy is used to reduce symptoms such as the pain from metastatic cancer in the bones or other parts of the body.

The type of radiation given depends on a number of factors, including the health of the patient, the location and type of cancer, and whether the patient will be undergoing other types of cancer treatment. Radiation can be delivered externally, internally, or systemically.

Most cancer patients who need radiation will receive it externally, meaning it is delivered from a machine outside the body. Generally, this is given on an outpatient basis. Internal radiation is performed inside the body and systemic radiation therapy consists of unsealed radioactive materials that go throughout the body.

Patients receiving external radiation present no radioactive danger to others. It is safe for massage therapists to do bodywork on these patients. For patients receiving internal or systemic radiation, no bodywork should be done by massage therapists until the medical staff determines the radiation has been cleared.

Chemotherapy

Chemotherapy is a form of treatment that uses drugs to destroy cancer cells. Unfortunately, the drugs do not recognize the difference between cancerous and noncancerous cells; therefore healthy tissues and organs are also damaged causing side effects for the patient. Chemotherapy may be given into the bloodstream through a central line, which may be an implanted **port** in the arm or upper chest (Figure 3-2). It may also be prescribed for the patient to take orally. Frequently the patient has side effects that present in the gastrointestinal tract in the form of nausea, vomiting, diarrhea, and constipation. The mucus membrane lining the gastrointestinal tract becomes inflamed and sensitive making it painful to take in nourishment. White blood cells, red blood cells, and platelets fall below normal and patients feel fatigued and lethargic and too tired to do much beyond the basics. They may experience mood swings and not think as clearly as usual. Hair loss and changes in the skin may be noticeable.

CONVENTIONAL TREATMENTS AND MASSAGE

So how does massage affect various conventional treatments? When the cancer patient is in the treatment phase, the massage is adjusted based on the type of treatment and the side effects the patient may be experiencing. For example, when surgery is a treatment choice, the incisions will be healing for several weeks. Once the patient has been released by the physician to have massage, it is important for the therapist to know where the incisions are so they can be avoided until healed. In addition, the patient may have ports for chemotherapy to enter the blood vessels and/or **drains** for excess fluid to exit the body (Figures 3-2 and 3-3).

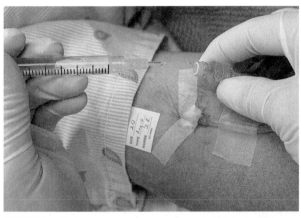

FIGURE 3-2 Port.

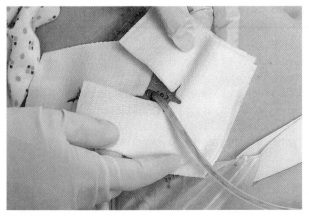

FIGURE 3-3 Drain.

Knowledge of the location of ports and drains, as well as how they appear, will help the therapist avoid these areas.

Generally, a 6-week period is allowed for surgical wounds to heal; however, a physician may allow the patient to have massage before the end of the 6-week period. A gentle massage, lasting 20 to 30 minutes and using less pressure, is a good introductory massage following surgery. Subsequent massages on the same patient are based upon how well the person tolerated the previous massage. Therapists should obtain feedback from clients regarding how the massage made them feel, including the length of the massage, the pressure, and firmness. A record of their progress should be kept and their responses should be documented.

STRESS OF CANCER

Being diagnosed with cancer often changes the direction of a person's life forever. Changes may occur in family dynamics, roles, finances, and employment. Not the least, changes occur within the individual with cancer, including body image and self-esteem. Goals are displaced by the immediate desire to fix the thing that has just hijacked personal plans. **Stress** is placed on the person diagnosed with cancer and all those involved.

Psychologist Dr. Hans Selye described stress as a change in one's life that elicits a response; the change can come from external or internal sources. While stress can be a positive motivating force known as eustress, it can also be a negative debilitating force known as distress. One response, known as "fight or flight," elevates heart rate, blood pressure, and respiration as the circulatory system shunts blood to the vital organs. The diagnosis of cancer creates stress that affects the whole being emotionally, mentally, spiritually, and physically. The response to the stress of cancer diagnosis depends on internal factors such as self-concept, personality, self-esteem, and role; it also depends on external factors such as life events, experiences, environment, and social support.[15]

One nurturing way oncology patients can deal with the emotional and physical stresses of their disease is through massage therapy. Massage to encourage relaxation is an effective way to manage the stress, even if the client is unaware of its numerous scientific benefits (see Box 3-3). As awareness increases among the population, more people with cancer may seek massage as a way to cope and deal with the side effects of treatment (Figures 3-4 to 3-8).

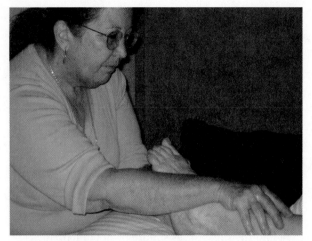

FIGURE 3-4 Massage therapist, Elizabeth Harper, applies a gliding stroke to a client's leg.

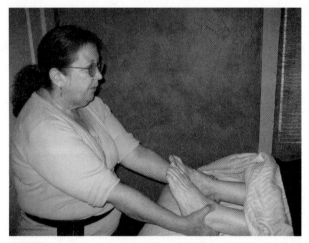

FIGURE 3-5 Massage therapist, Elizabeth Harper, massaging the feet.

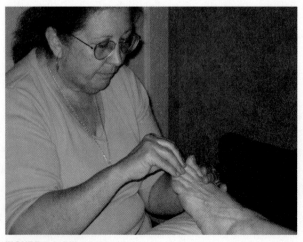

FIGURE 3-6 Effleurage on the toes.

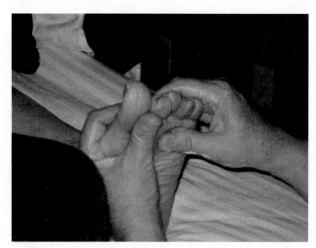

FIGURE 3-7 Kneading the underside of the foot.

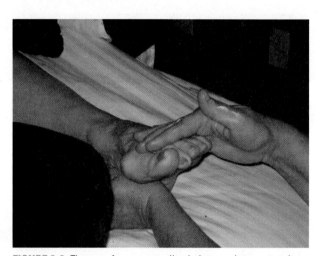

FIGURE 3-8 The use of a massage oil or lotion can decrease unpleasant friction for the client.

PHASES OF CANCER

An oncology patient will go through several phases of the disease. The experience is personal and is not the same for everyone. How people cope with the diagnosis and the phases of cancer will be unique for each person. The transitions of life with cancer are neither constant nor predictable. These phases include diagnosis, pretreatment, treatment, posttreatment, and remission. People are also faced with the possibility of relapse, more treatments, palliative care, and end of life. The phases are not linear, that is, they do not go in order and they are not predictable. Nor do people with cancer enter every phase: only the first, the diagnosis, is a phase every person with cancer experiences.

BOX 3-2 Dynamics and Emotions of Cancer Phases

- Diagnosis—Shock, fear, disbelief, and anger
- Treatment—Loss of control begins; side effects of treatments such as nausea, pain, and fatigue may be exhibited
- Posttreatment—Reality and acceptance; return to normal life and order, but with underlying concerns of relapse
- Possible relapse—Anxiety and anger of return of disease and more treatment
- Palliative Care—No further treatment; comfort measures

The client may experience a wide range of emotions during the phases (Box 3-2). Emotion, fear, and stress may be present at every stage. There are many unknowns that affect emotions, and the toll on the body makes coping with the changes more difficult.

Following the diagnosis, patients are faced with decisions related to the inevitable struggles brought on by cancer. These might include various treatment options for the cancer, financial burdens, and even daily diet and exercise. Kris Carr, in her eloquent documentary describing her personal journey with cancer, states "Cancer becomes a job."[16] Said Carr, "People often ask me why I named the film *Crazy Sexy Cancer*. The answer is simple: to challenge the perceptions, to poke fun, and bring humanity to a disease that is still so misperceived and feared. No matter what happened, I refused to be saddled with the isolating stigma associated with cancer. Just because it had changed my life forever, didn't mean that I had changed."[16]

COMPLEMENTARY, ALTERNATIVE, AND INTEGRATIVE THERAPIES

In addition to the conventional treatments of surgery, radiation, and chemotherapy, oncology patients may seek complementary, alternative, and integrative therapies. While these terms are often used interchangeably, a closer look reveals they are not quite the same. The best explanations come from the National Center for **Complementary** and **Alternative Medicine** (NCCAM).

- Complementary medicine is used *together with* **conventional medicine.**
- Alternative medicine is used *in place of* conventional medicine.
- Integrative medicine combines treatments from conventional medicine and CAM for which there is some high-quality evidence of safety and effectiveness. It is also called integrated medicine.[3]

Dr. David Eisenberg, medical doctor at Harvard, opened the door for the exploration of unconventional therapies when he published his survey results in 1993. He found 10% of the respondents indicated they sought complementary or alternative therapy for medical reasons. Eisenberg conducted a follow-up survey in 1998 and discovered a much greater number of people were adding complementary and alternative therapies as health care. His landmark studies helped bridge conventional and complementary care.[17]

In 1999, the National Institutes of Health, created NCCAM to explore practices that were outside the conventional medical realm. They support research for complementary and alternative health care.

The American Hospital Association (AHA) in 2003 sponsored a study of hospitals and their use of CAM and found 82% of the hospitals offering CAM included massage therapy and more than 70% were using massage for pain management. The patients most often requesting massage therapy included people with cancer, pregnant women, and people seeking general pain management.[18]

Massage has been a complementary therapy for decades and is now part of integrative medicine as research supports its safety and efficacy. Massage may be combined with other complementary therapies to enhance the overall effectiveness of the treatments. These modalities may include light touch, reflexology, acupuncture, craniosacral therapy, and energy work among other types of bodywork. The plan of treatment takes into consideration the type of cancer and the stage of the cancer as well as how the person feels physically and mentally. The benefits of massage for cancer patients are included in Box 3-3.

BOX 3-3 Benefits of Massage for Cancer Patients

Physical Benefits
- Restores **homeostasis**
- Relieves pain
- Releases oxytocin
- Strengthens **immune system**
- Lowers stress levels
- Improves blood circulation
- Improves appetite and quality of sleep

Emotional Benefits
- Decreases anger
- Decreases depression
- Increases energy

MASSAGE FOR CANCER

Cancer massage is a type of massage given to a person with cancer. Oncology massage therapy is a combination of many styles of massage incorporated into the massage sessions.[19] The massage is customized for the client depending on specific variables. These include the site and stage of the cancer, treatments for the cancer, and side effects of the disease or the treatments. The age of the client must be considered since cancer affects all ages from infants to elderly clients. All factors must be considered for the customized massage to promote optimal results. Each massage session for a person with cancer requires the therapist to modify the technique. For example, if a client is undergoing radiation treatment, the radiated area is not to be massaged or rubbed. These patients are instructed after showering or bathing, not to rub, but to pat dry. Even if the area does not appear to be inflamed, the tissue is sensitive to touch. For skin tenderness and inflammation from the radiation, prescription ointments and creams may be effective. For minor inflammation, one-third strength hydrogen peroxide and water may be helpful.

For chemotherapy patients, the massage therapist should be aware of the physical, mental, and emotional highs and lows the clients experience on a day-to-day basis. The massage session is modified according to the patient's needs on that particular day. The intent for the massage should be to increase circulation, not to detoxify. The powerful drugs used to treat the cancer are challenging to the physical body, and the body needs to detoxify at its own rate.[20]

For clients receiving chemotherapy, each element of the massage should be "dialed down."[21] This includes the time, pressure, and speed of the massage. Massage strokes must be gentler to avoid further taxing the body physically and emotionally.

If the patient is feeling nauseated from chemotherapy, therapists should avoid vigorous motion and rocking movements, which tend to exacerbate the nausea. To help with nausea, the patient can be taught to apply pressure to Pericardium 6, the acupressure point that is proximal to the wrist between the flexor ligaments. Visual imagery of a peaceful, still setting with a cool breeze may also be calming for the person experiencing nausea.

Guidelines for Cancer Massage

There is no definitive massage routine because cancer patients respond individually to cancer and their treatments. The basic Swedish massage should be modified based on good clinical judgment, common sense, basic principles in massage, and knowledge of cancer and the treatments as well as the effects on the body.[21,22]

The phrase "less is best" applies to the first massage given to a person with cancer in terms of length of time and amount of pressure. It may take several massages to get the most appropriate timing and pressure for the greatest result. The massage begins with the basic relaxation Swedish massage. Variations to the massage depend on phases of the cancer and the treatment. The first massage for a particular client should be gentle but firm touch that can be felt by the client but is more than nerve or feather strokes. As a general rule, a 15- to 30-minute massage achieves positive results.

A typical massage may not be appropriate for someone recovering from cancer treatment, yet there is still some form of safe, skilled touch for every phase of the cancer experience.[6,23] It is best to limit the session to one or two areas of the body such as the fingers and hands, the neck and shoulders, the low back and sacrum, the hand and forearm, or the back (Figures 3-9 to 3-12). If the therapist determines the client should not receive a traditional massage, the following suggestions are ways to be present with the client and still touch:

- Easy touch is generally welcomed.
- Touch with intention of making the client feel better.
- Be present and focused.
- Assist the client with visual imagery, such as colors, flowers, sky, or ocean views.

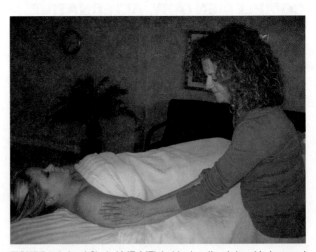

FIGURE 3-9 Lorri Clark, LMT, MTI, holds the client's hand in hers and assists in stretching the muscles to facilitate better movement.

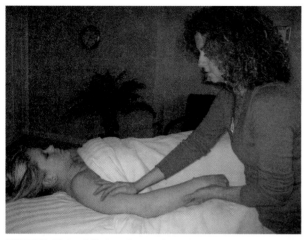

FIGURE 3-10 Lorri Clark performs a kneading stroke on upper arm.

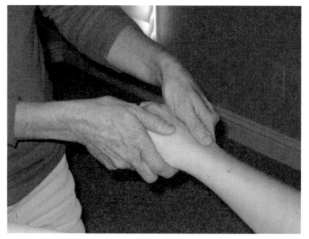

FIGURE 3-12 A close-up of stretching of the arm.

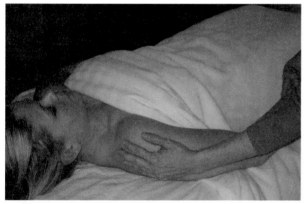

FIGURE 3-11 Gliding stroke along shoulder.

- Encourage the client to breath rhythmically
  - Inhale to a count of four,
  - Hold for a count of seven,
  - Exhale to a count of eight,
  - Repea t up to four cycles of these patterns.[24]
- Hold the head by placing hands on temporal lobes with fingers spread around the ears.
- Pétrissage the ears.
- Rub the base of the occiput.
- Massage the forehead by gently sliding fingers from between the brows to the top of the forehead using one hand then the other for six times (see Figure 3-13)
- Hold the client's hand and rub the palm with your thumbs
- Massage each finger by gently rolling the skin, then pulling each finger distally
- Friction across the wrist
- Hold one hand on the upper chest just inferior to the clavicles and the other hand on the solar plexus

for one or two minutes. Avoid this method if the client has had a mastectomy as it may be too invasive.
- Squeeze the trapezius muscles[6]

Cancer Patients in the Spa Setting

Many people who enjoy spa settings are cancer survivors. Spa clients with a history of cancer provide special opportunities for the therapists to be part of the healing process.[25] The treatments for cancer—including surgery, radiation, and chemotherapy—have long-term and short-term side effects. It is important for therapists to recognize that cancer clients who are able to enjoy spa settings may also be dealing with the aftereffects of the cancer and the treatments. For example, fatigue may linger for months, and people who have had one or more lymph nodes removed are always at risk for **lymphedema,** or swelling in the extremities. Chemotherapy and radiation may cause permanent damage to tissues and vital organs. Healing may be ongoing for months and therapists must understand that the tissues beneath the surface may still be healing and in need of tender, loving care.

There are special considerations for treating people with cancer in a spa setting where many choices of massage and body treatments are part of the menu services. However, not every service is appropriate for the person with cancer, whether in treatment or weeks out of treatment. The therapist trained in massage for cancer helps the client choose the treatment that will provide the best outcome for the client. A detoxifying massage should be avoided within 12 months of treatment. MacDonald[25] suggests using a less-demanding approach in a spa setting in the following ways:

- Use less pressure and slower movements to soothe the body, mind, and spirit.
- Shorten the time of the massage.
- Use less heat; think of warmth rather than hot applications to the skin. For instance, use a warm rock for 5 minutes on the abdomen rather than a hot rock for 30 minutes.
- Use products that are calming rather than stimulating, such as essential oils and exfoliates that are less coarse.
- Assist client in choosing less-demanding services such as energy work or a foot massage.
- Nurture the client.

Therapists generally have a caring nature that includes compassion and dedication. As massage for people with cancer has become a specialty, the desire to work with cancer survivors has surfaced in many areas. Yet, it takes much more than trained-in-massage hands to work with those who have cancer. It takes an understanding of the physical, mental, and emotional challenges as well as the life and role changes being faced by people with person. Therapists who seek training, information, instruction, and supervision in the field of cancer and people with cancer will make better assessments and decisions for their clients.[26] Just as the word "cancer" describes many disorders, so does the phrase "massage for cancer" describe many types of bodywork. While there is not one massage technique or routine for the person with cancer, there are many types, variations, and considerations so that the massage can be tailored to fit the individual.

Perhaps most important, professional massage therapists must be informed and educated on what cancer is and what it is not. Additionally, discernment and critical thinking help to make an accurate assessment of the client and incorporate the variables involved. Knowledge brings about the best-informed decisions in working with cancer clients. In brief, some of what massage therapists need to know includes:

- Condition of the person with cancer
- The phase of the cancer
- The treatments the person is undergoing
- The stage of the treatment
- How the person feels physically, mentally, and emotionally
- Palliative care/comfort measures
- Goals or reasons for seeking massage

With the client's input, the massage therapist determines areas of the body that can be massaged as well as the length of time for the massage. While much of the cancer massage is orchestrated by the therapist, the client's wishes should be honored. Massage therapy is one area of treatment where clients have a large measure of control.

Setting the Stage for the Massage

The massage therapist and the cancer client both play active roles in the massage session. By working as a team, they increase the benefits of the massage. Before beginning the massage, the therapist makes an assessment of the client's mental and emotional state and then tailors the massage session to the client's physical needs and emotional fragility.

The client and the massage therapist have a unique relationship. The client with cancer deals with intrusive and painful procedures and treatments. The massage therapist provides a caring touch that can help a client feel whole. The more knowledge the therapist has about cancer and the treatments, the greater the understanding of the client's journey through the illness, the treatments, and the possible side effects. "This underlying empathy that is inseparable from the actual technique is what makes it a truly special experience for both client and therapist."[27]

To ensure a successful outcome, here are some suggestions to set the stage:

1. A written health history (Box 3-4) will help the therapist assess the health status of the client.
2. The massage should be planned based on the health history and verbal communications with the client.
3. Each subsequent massage session should be documented with changes that have occurred since the previous massage. Documentation should include how the client physically tolerated the massage session, changes in cancer treatment, level of fatigue, and emotional state. In addition to listening to the client, the therapist should observe the client as well, noting factors such as appearance and tone of voice.
4. Lubricants should not contain chemically enhanced scents. Sesame oil is preferred by some therapists.[22] Lubricants containing zinc should not be used for those in radiation therapy since it can interfere with the treatment.[21]
5. The therapist should be present with the client. Massage therapists should be focused on the healing intent for the session and for the client.
6. The client should be positioned for personal comfort. For example, a breast cancer patient should be massaged in a supine or side-lying position until she is able to sleep on her stomach. When a woman has undergone a mastectomy, she should

BOX 3-4 Health History for The Cancer Client

Name _____ Date _____ Gender _____

Date of birth _____

Describe any stressors you have

_____

What do you do to relieve stress?

_____

_____

When were you diagnosed with cancer   Month _____ Year _____

What is the medical name of the cancer _____

What month & year did you begin treatment _____

What month & year did you complete treatment _____

Which treatments have you received or are currently receiving?

Surgery _____ Date _____

Radiation _____ Date _____

Chemotherapy _____ Date _____

Medications _____ Date _____

_____

_____

How did the treatments make you feel? _____

How do you feel now (most of the time)? _____

Do you have any ports, tubes, or drains at this time? _____ Where are they _____

Have you had any problems with blood clots? _____

Have you had problems with bleeding? _____

Have you had lymph nodes removed? _____

Date _____ How many _____

What area(s) of your body were they taken from? _____

What side effects did you have? _____

Have you ever had a professional massage? _____ Date _____

Have you tried other complementary therapies? Circle all that apply.

Acupuncture

Craniosacral Therapy

Energy work

Polarity

Reflexology

Reiki

Therapeutic Touch

Others

_____

_____

_____

position her own arm on the affected side to her own comfort. The therapist can add a pillow under her elbow, arm, and hand. For the patient who has recently had the reconstruction surgery known as "transverse rectus abdominis muscle flap" (in which extra tissues and muscle from the lower abdominal wall are brought to the breast area), the therapist needs to keep the patient supine with knees flexed and bolstered to reduce abdominal stress.[27]

7. Maintaining cleanliness, including hand washing, is of utmost importance because of compromised **immunity** in clients, especially those receiving treatment. To prevent the spread of infection, hands and arms to the elbow should be washed thoroughly prior to the massage. The therapist who has recently had a viral or bacterial infection should consider wearing a mask or postponing the massage session to decrease the risks to the client.[28]

8. Verbal and nonverbal communication play a role in developing and maintaining a trusting relationship.

The therapist begins the session by encouraging the client to let go of stress. This may be achieved by starting with a visual image and/or instructing the client to breathe in a rhythmical pattern. Dr. Andrew Weil, director of the Integrative Medicine Program at the University of Arizona, has developed an effective breathing routine: rhythmically count to four while inhaling through your nose, count to seven while holding the breath, count to eight while exhaling out your mouth (keep tip of tongue at the ridge behind front teeth), then repeat the sequence for a total of four cycles.[24]

Dr. Weil believes massage therapy is a great benefit to people with cancer. "The idea that it can encourage cancer to spread has no scientific basis. Obviously, unhealed incisions should be avoided, and those with metastatic disease in bones should be handled gently."[29]

Massage helps restore **homeostasis,** or balance, by allowing the parasympathetic nervous system to do its work and calm the body, mind, and spirit. The relaxation response occurs, heart rate slows, blood pressure decreases, and breathing becomes more rhythmical. Massage is a valuable therapy for managing both chronic and acute pain.[18] Massage releases **endorphins,** the body's natural pain relievers.[30]

Dr. Mehmet Oz, a well-respected heart surgeon and believer in complementary therapies, reported, "Massage has also been shown to have profound effects on the hormonal and immunologic systems. . . . Rats undergoing belly massage will release oxytocin, an important hormone from the brain. In addition, AIDs

patients will elevate their natural killer cells in the **immune system** after several massage sessions." Dr. Oz further states that the findings "point to a potential immunologic effect of massage."[31]

Physiologically, therapeutic massage improves blood circulation. When muscles are stretched and kneaded, blood return to the heart is increased and toxins are carried out of the muscle tissue. Improved circulation brings oxygen to tissues and vital organs. Improved perfusion and oxygenation of tissues and organs leads to better functioning: the brain thinks more clearly, digestion and elimination improve, and wounds heal more quickly.

One study conducted by the Touch Research Institute revealed that cancer pain was diminished after massage. The women in the study had breast cancer. After receiving three 30-minute massages each week for 5 weeks, the women reported feeling less angry, less depressed, and more energetic. In addition, their pain levels decreased. The results began with the first massage and continued through the final session.[32]

Massage has been found to lower the levels of the stress hormones, cortisol, and norepinephrines. Massage stimulates the vagus nerve, one of the 12 cranial nerves that influence heart rate, causing the heart to beat at a slower pace.[4] Massage affects cancer by increasing immunity and strengthening other body systems. Chemicals, such as **serotonin** and beta-endorphins are released that boost immunity (Figures 3-13 to 3-15).[33,34]

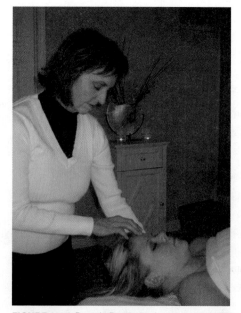

FIGURE 3-13 Beverly Byers gently massages forehead.

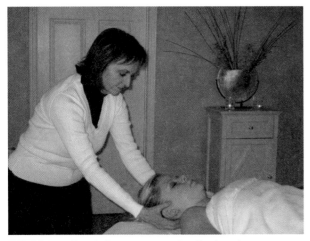

FIGURE 3-14 Beverly Byers massages the client's neck.

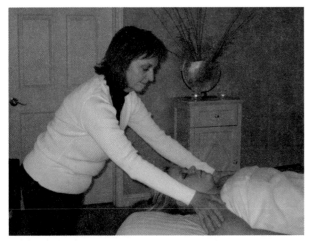

FIGURE 3-15 Beverly Byers finishes the massage with light, gliding strokes.

CONTRAINDICATIONS

Although the benefits of massage far outweigh the risks, there are still cautions and contraindications that must be followed when working with people living with cancer. Surgical incisions should be avoided while they are in the healing stage. Port and drain sites should be avoided in the massage session and caution should be used not to dislodge tubes and ports that enter or exit the client's body. Reducing germs and bacteria by careful hand washing and wearing clean clothing is essential. Tumor sites and radiated tender skin areas are contraindicated for massage.

Patients who have had lymph nodes removed are at risk for lymphedema or swelling of the limb distal to the site where lymph nodes were removed. When lymphedema develops, there are methods including lymphatic drainage massage that help control swelling. Unfortunately lymphedema is a lifelong condition. Because lymphedema can be adversely affected by aggressive massage, it is important that massage therapists receive specialized training in lymphatic drainage when the client's lymph nodes have been removed.

Two major considerations for massage with clients recovering from surgery are the effect of immunosuppressant drugs and **blood clots.** Immunosuppressant drugs are sometimes prescribed for patients following cancer surgery. The drugs do just that—suppress immunity—leaving the patient more susceptible to pathogens and at increased risk for infection. Blood clots, thrombophlebitis, or deep vein thrombosis (DVT), are risks for anyone following major surgery, especially surgery involving the leg, hip, or pelvis.[30] Therefore a client's legs are not to be massaged since surgical patients are more at risk for blood clots (deep vein thrombosis). Gentle massage on hands, arms, back, neck, and face is appropriate.

Blood clots pose a risk of detaching from the walls of veins and floating freely within the circulatory system. The clot can lodge in a vessel resulting in a blockage—this can become a life-threatening situation. Massage therapists must be aware of the risks of DVT, as any pressure or movement could detach a clot from the veins of an extremity, resulting in an embolism. Patients taking anticoagulant drugs to help prevent blood clots may receive gentle massage. Deep or vigorous massage is never advised for patients with low platelet counts or on anticoagulant drug therapy as it may cause bleeding, bruising, and hepatic overload. Massage is contraindicated directly over known tumors, blood clots, or prosthetic body devices.[10]

MASSAGE FOR THE PERSON WITH METASTATIC CANCER

When cancer spreads, or metastasizes, it does so through the blood circulation, the lymphatic system, or through body spaces such as the bronchi. The most common way for cancer to spread is through the lymphatic system. When cancer has spread, the goals of treatment are to relieve symptoms and decrease the side effects of treatment.[28]

Should the metastasis occur in the bone, the therapist must use caution with pressure since the client will be more fragile, bones more brittle, and more susceptible to fractures. Cancer in bones can cause pain; therefore, the massage should be very gentle. [21,29]

SPECIAL POPULATIONS

Touch for the Very Ill or Frail Client

If the client appears too fragile for a massage, certain forms of touch can still be effective. The therapist should consider the client's sensitivity to touch. See the suggestions listed under Guidelines for Cancer Massage (p. 42).

Pain can be a constant reminder that a person is not well. One of the most comforting measures is a foot massage. The foot (or hand) routine can relax the entire body. The therapist can begin by spreading soothing lotion on the entire foot including toes. With the thumb, sliding effleurage can then be applied between the metatarsals proximally and then distally. Each metatarsal-phalangeal joint can be mobilized with circles or figure eights, then each toe petrissaged by gentle squeezing along the sides, then gently squeezing top and bottom sliding proximal to distal. Next, broad pressure can be applied to the sole of the foot with a closed fist. This resembles an ironing motion with one fist while the other hand holds the dorsum with mild resistance. Pressing specific points on the bottom of the feet may improve energy flow in other parts of the body. [35]

Hospice

Patients in hospice care, as well as others who may be terminally ill and nearing end-of-life, are faced with fears, grief, and losses. They have lost certain freedoms and are faced with the end of relationships. They may feel isolated with fear of being alone or fear of pain and death. The touch of massage may bring comfort and care in the last days. Massage may help with physical problems such as breathing difficulties, digestion, elimination, or insomnia. Massage sessions may be whatever the patient wants them to be. Generally, the sessions are softer, gentler, and shorter. [36]

Massage for Children with Cancer

Camp TLC at Lake Tahoe is a wellness center for children ages 6 to 18 with life-shortening illnesses. The camp accepts children with any condition including multiple sclerosis, muscular dystrophy, HIV, and cancer. Camp TLC intends to add quality to the children's lives and to decrease the stress brought on by their conditions. Massage is integral to the healing process of the children. Physically, massage is therapeutic and provides greater range of motion; mentally, it provides comfort and relaxation.

In addition to receiving massages at Camp TLC, the children also learn how to give massages. The camp's massage therapists teach the children specific techniques for massaging and stretching a person's hand. Buford reports while the children liked receiving the massages, they also enjoyed performing them on others. [37]

When children are diagnosed with cancer, their lives change in the same ways as those of adults with cancer. They are faced with uncomfortable treatments, changes in everyday life and diet, multiple hospitalizations, and social adjustments, all of which place stress on the children. When these children receive massages, their stress levels decrease.

Massage for Hospitalized Patients

Massage in the hospital is not a brand-new concept. Not too many years ago, nurses gave backrubs to their patients. However, backrubs are no longer a routine part of nursing care, although some institutions are teaching massage techniques to nurses (Box 3-5).

BOX 3-5 Teaching Massage to Nurses

Developing and teaching the course, *Complementary Therapies*, at a private liberal arts university in west Texas provided me with the opportunity to blend massage and nursing. Students in the class were registered nurses (RN) enrolled in an RN-BSN program. The nurses were introduced to massage therapy techniques and were taught how to perform a simple hand, foot, and back massage. Licensed massage therapists taught the RNs these specific massage techniques. The RNs were given an assignment using the massage techniques they had learned. The assignment was to find out whether massage therapy made a difference in blood pressure, heart rate, and breathing rates (vital signs) of hospitalized patients. The students were to administer one of the learned massage techniques to five patients who agreed to the massage. The RNs and the patients determined whether the 15- to 20-minute massage would be on the back, hands, or feet. The patients who agreed to receive the massages were monitored prior to the massage for blood pressure, heart rate, and respiration and again after the massage. Twenty-four of the twenty-five patients had a decrease in blood pressure, heart rate, and respiration following the massage. In addition, they verbally stated it was a pleasant experience. The five RNs conducting the assignment reported they too felt better following the massage. They were uplifted as they ministered to the patients through their hands.

Today, more hospitals are adding complementary or integrative medicine programs that give patients the opportunity to receive massage from professional massage therapists. In the event massage is not offered by the hospital program, patients or their family members may elect to hire a specially trained massage therapist. In this case, the physician will determine whether or not the patient can medically receive massage and must write the order for the patient to receive massage.

In the hospital setting, the massage therapist must adapt to the situation and often improvise. For example, the patient is generally in a hospital bed which makes it necessary to adapt body mechanics to suit the height of the bed and work around the equipment that is supporting the patient's care.

Cautions

As a massage therapist, you cannot really know what patients' tolerance to the massage might be—the patients may not even know. They may get lost in the "feel good moment" not realizing the amount of toxins being stirred up. Later, they may experience the "aftershock" or the effects that filter out of a relaxing massage which may cause flulike symptoms. It is best to err on the side of caution and use the "less is best" approach in the beginning. This includes less time for the massage, less pressure, and less work for the therapist.

The therapist should be informed about any ongoing symptoms such as fatigue, pain, and anxiety the client may be experiencing. Therapists should also be aware of the types of treatment the client has had and how they were tolerated. Finally, the therapist should listen for verbal and nonverbal cues such as words, tones, and expressions.

WHY CANCER MASSAGE IS RECOGNIZED

As physicians and scientists have accepted and embraced the benefits of massage, they have increased the awareness among the public through their voices and their writings. This fact, coupled with the desire of people to seek out complementary and alternative therapies as a means to contribute to their own health and healing, has helped create widespread acceptance of the benefits of massage therapy. Bodyworkers are seeking more information and training in massage for medical conditions, including cancer. Massage schools are reexamining and dismissing the notion that massage causes cancer to spread and are now teaching the benefits of massage for people with cancer, as well as pointing out

the career path to working on patients in a cancer clinic or hospital.[39] In addition, information about massage for cancer is available on internet has had an enormous impact on the education of the public.

As clinical trials are now proving the scientific basis for massage for people with cancer, it is becoming more credible among the scientific community. The Touch Research Institute (TRI) at the University of Miami announced research results that pointed to increases in dopamine levels and the immune system's natural killer cells or lymphocytes known to destroy cancer cells in women with breast cancer, which would increase patient immune function.[34]

TRAINING AND EDUCATION

Educating massage therapists in the art of cancer massage includes the study of cancer and its treatments, considerations for the client's current condition, as well as contraindications and cautions. Benefits for people living with cancer when the massage is provided by a properly educated and trained oncology massage therapist. Dr. Barrie Cassileth of Memorial Sloan-Kettering Cancer Center, New York City, advocates that cancer patients should only visit a certified, licensed therapist who knows how to care for cancer patients, many of whom may need a lighter touch.[40]

Training and educational resources include, but are not limited to, those listed in the Resources section at the end of this chapter.

CHAPTER SUMMARY

Techniques for massage for cancer clients depend on many variables, each of which can affect the others. In essence, the techniques are based on three variables, the first of which is the cancer itself (including site, type, grade, and stage). Second, techniques are also adapted according to variables surrounding cancer treatments, including surgery, radiation, and chemotherapy. Third, techniques for the massage are tailored to the uniqueness of the client, including age, mobility, physical feelings of health, and emotional well-being. Massage therapists use knowledge, training, and discretion to administer the most appropriate massage for the specific client.

People diagnosed with cancer experience dramatic life changes. A journey of endurance begins; it becomes emotionally, socially, and physically painful and frightening. Cancer is a diagnosis no one chooses—yet treatments are available in both conventional medicine and complementary medicine. A holistic approach in caring for the client yields the greatest benefit.

▪▫▫▫ IN MY EXPERIENCE

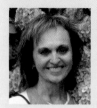

While a student of Medical Massage at Memorial Sloan Kettering Cancer Center (MSKCC) in New York, one of the best experiences I had was following and observing the MSKCC therapists as they gave massages to patients in the hospital. One young mother sat in her hospital bed surrounded by pictures of her young son and husband. With a turban covering the cancer treatment evidence, she spoke briefly about herself and the cancer that had recently returned. She spoke softly, "Massage is the only thing I look forward to." She positioned herself for the massage in her hospital bed as she relaxed with her eyes closed. As the therapist gave compression and rubbed her feet gently, the room became quiet and slow as we were engulfed in the peacefulness that blanketed us. After about 10 minutes, we watched as the therapist moved toward the patient's head and asked her to get comfortable on her side. The therapist began slow effleurage strokes to her back for about 10 minutes. At the close of the massage session, we quietly exited the room while the patient remained in a quiet, relaxed state.

Research studies have been conducted since the early 1990s, and the evidence continues to support the benefits of massage for cancer patients. Massages for people with cancer are generally relaxing, gentle, and often shorter in length (20 to 30 minutes). The clients' condition determines the length and type of massage they will receive. Testimonials of the clients indicate they feel better following the massages, and the research indicates massages enhance the immune system. Just as there is not one cancer, but many, so there are many variations of massage for cancer. The outcome of massage for the person with cancer may not be fully understood; yet a caring attitude and gentle touch toward the cancer client may allow healing to take place.

Working with cancer patients is a rewarding experience. Because massage for people living with cancer differs from general massage, it is imperative for therapists to have an adequate understanding of people with cancer, cancer as a disease, and the treatments for cancer. The skillful hands and the caring hearts of the massage therapist are paramount; but without proper education and knowledge of the concepts, massage therapists cannot effectively fulfill their role.

CASE HISTORY

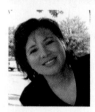

In December 2005, the client noticed an increase in the size of her breasts which she attributed to a new work-out exercise routine. After a while, and following the persistence of her husband that something wasn't normal, it became evident the increase in breast size was not due to the exercise and she made an appointment with her doctor. The diagnosis was breast cancer. After further testing, the client underwent a bilateral mastectomy.

While no cancer had been discovered in the right breast prior to surgery, the oncology surgeon said it was likely it would become cancerous too. Following the surgery, the pathology report revealed the right breast also had cancer cells.

The client began chemotherapy and was focused on getting rid of any cancer that might remain in her body. As the harsh chemicals fought the cancer cells, she endured the side effects. When her hair fell out, she wore a baseball cap—"I never wore a wig."

She came for her first massage in the spring 2007, about 16 months after her diagnosis weekly sessions of half-hour massages began. The client beamed as she described her massages. "She (the massage therapist) takes me away. I am transported into a different body—I am normal again." She said, "I feel like Franken boobie—I'm not normal. I get in a valley once in a while. Liz relieves me of those feelings. It's like fuel—I get gassed up and I am ready to go for the next few days or the week."

The treatments were weekly hour-long massages. The therapist began the session at the feet with the client in supine position. The client turned to each side to make her back accessible. She was unable to be prone because of the recent reconstructive breast surgery. Soothing effleurage strokes were applied to her extremities and her back. Gentle petrissage and friction were used on leg and back. The client experienced mild lymphedema in her left arm; therefore, the only strokes used on both arms were centripetal light effleurage. The massages were tolerated well.

When the client was asked if she saw a change after the massage, she said "It makes everything flow better. The therapist has given me back that flexibility—I walk better. When I don't go for massage, I start feeling unsteady." Then she was diagnosed with metastatic cancer—"the hot spots showed up on my liver and my lumbar spine." She was beautiful and appeared youthful. She currently is on oral medications, both of which are known to increase blood pressure. With a smile she reported, "There has not been an increase in my blood pressure with massage." The

▐▐▐▌ IN MY EXPERIENCE

For several weeks, I went to Cora's house three to four times each week to give her a hand and foot massage while she reclined in her favorite chair just before bedtime. Her pain was in her left pelvis, where the colon cancer had metastasized months earlier. For the 30 to 40 minutes I was there, Cora seemed to relax as she closed her eyes while I talked to her of pleasant visual scenarios; then I gently massaged each hand/forearm and each foot/leg.

I took it personally when she died. I had believed that somehow I could make a difference. I could not—at least in her prognosis. You have to accept that you can't cure the patient; hopefully, you can ease the burden of pain and offer comfort through touch, holding, and massage. And in the end, the recovery came for Cora—when she was released from the bone pain in her pelvis and the limitations of cancer were lifted as she passed from this life. Did I ease some of the anxiety, pain, and stress brought on by the disease of cancer? I have to believe I lessened some of them.

client continues with the massages on a weekly basis and each session is adjusted based on how she feels and what she believes her needs are. For example, when she feels very low energy and is unable to do her daily activities, she will request a massage to help elevate her energy level.

SUGGESTED READINGS

Chapman C: Training manuals for cancer and mastectomy massage; (website) www.cherylchapman.com.

Curties D: *Breast massage*, New Brunswick, Canada, 1999, Curties-Overzet Publications.

Curties D: *Massage therapy and cancer*, New Brunswick, Canada, 1999, Curties-Overzet Publications.

MacDonald G: *Medicine hands: massage for people with cancer*, Findhorn, Scotland, 2007, Findhorn.

MacDonald G: *Massage for the hospital patient and medically frail client*, Philadelphia, 2005, Lippincott Williams & Wilkins.S.

RESOURCES

Memorial Sloan Kettering Cancer Center
New York City
www.mskcc.org

M.D. Anderson Cancer Center
Houston, TX
www.mdanderson.org

REFERENCES

1. Haylock P et al: The cancer survivor's prescription for living, *Am J Nurs* 107:58-70, 2007.
2. MD Anderson Cancer Center (website): retrieved from http://mdanderson.org.
3. NCCAM: (website) http://nccam.nih.gov/health/cam-cancer/. Accessed Sept 21, 2007.
4. Colt G: The magic of touch, *Life*, August 1997.
5. Curties D: *Massage therapy and cancer*, Toronto, 1991, Curties-Overzet.
6. MacDonald G: *Medicine hands: massage therapy for people with cancer*, Forres, Morayshire, UK, 1999, Findhorn Press.
7. Walton T: Developments in oncology massage, *Massage Today* 6: 2006.
8. Williams D: Touching cancer patients: guidelines for massage therapists, *Massage* 84:74-79, 2000.
9. World Health Organization: *WHO traditional medicine strategy: 2002-2005* (website): http://www.who.int/medicines/organization/trm/orgtrmmair.html.
10. *Tabers cyclopedic medical dictionary*, ed 18, Philadelphia, 1997, F.A. Davis.
11. Salvo S: *Massage therapy: principles and practice*, ed 3, St. Louis, 2003, Saunders.
12. National Cancer Institute: *Tumor grade: questions and answers* (website): http://www.cancer.gov/cancertopics/factsheet/Detection/tumor-grade.
13. U.S. Cancer Statistics Working Group: *Incidence and mortality web-based report*, Atlanta: U.S. Department of Health and Human Services, Centers for Disease Control and Prevention and National Cancer Institute, 2007 (website): www.cdc.gov/uscs.
14. Curties D: Cancer therapies, *MTJ* 39:80-89, 2001.
15. Selye H: *Stress without distress*, New York, 1974, Lippincott.
16. Carr K: *My crazy, sexy cancer*, documentary aired on TLC, Sept. 2007. http://tlc.discovery.com/tv/specials/crazy-sexy-cancer/crazy-sexy-cancer.html
17. Eisenberg DM : Trends in alternative medicine use in the United States, 1990-1997: results of a follow-up national survey, *JAMA* 280:1569-1575, 1998.
18. Milivojevic J: Massage and pain relief, *MTJ*, Spring 2004, 48.
19. Handley WC: Massage for cancer patients: indicated or contraindicated? *Massage Today* 7: 2007.
20. MacDonald G: Oncology bodywork for cancer patients: the need for a less demanding approach, *Massage and Bodywork*, 7:16-26, 2005.
21. Walton T: Cancer massage therapy: essential contraindications, *MTJ*, Summer 2006.

22. Howard L: Oriental therapies, *Massage and Bodywork*, August/September 2000.

23. Walton T: Massage therapy for people with cancer: fear, healing, and changes in the field (serial online): http://amtamassage.org/journal/pdf/CE-Cancer-MT.pdf.

24. Weil A: *Spontaneous healing*, New York, 1995, Ballantine.

25. MacDonald G: A vacation from cancer, *Massage and Bodywork*, April/May 2007.

26. Vanderbilt S: Oncology: Cancer and human connection—the making of an oncology massage therapist, *Massage and Bodywork*, June/July 2005.

27. Thiagarajan K: Post-mastectomy massage, *Massage*, Oct. 2006, p. 84.

28. Malloy J: Do the benefits of massage outweigh the risks? *MTJ* 39:60-73, 2001.

29. Weil A: Personal email correspondence, Sept. 2007.

30. Werner R: *A massage therapist's guide to pathology*, ed 3, New York, 2003, Lippincott Williams & Wilkens.

31. Oz M: *Healing from the heart*, New York, 1998, Penguin Group.

32. Touch Research Institute (TRI) (website): retrieved from http://www6.miami.edu/touch-research/Massage.htm July 13, 2007.

33. *Nurses's handbook of alternative & complementary therapies*, ed 2, New York, 2003, Lippincott Williams & Wilkins.

34. Memorial Sloan Kettering Cancer Center (MSKCC) (website): retrieved from http://library.mskcc.org/scripts/portal/index.pl July 13, 2007.

35. Vanderbilt S: Easing cancer pain and anxiety—the value of a good foot rub, *Massage and Bodywork*, June/July 2001.

36. Tappan F, Benjamin P: *Healing massage techniques*, Connecticut, 1998, Appleton & Lange.

37. Buford, D: Camp TLC for terminally ill children: tender, loving care, *Massage and Bodywork*, June/July 2001.

38. Vanderbilt S: Children and massage—a powerful combination, *Body Sense*, Spring 2003.

39. McConnellogue K: Massage and the cancer patient: the courage of touch, *Massage and Bodywork*, December/January 2000.

40. Cassileth B, Deng G: Complementary and alternative therapies for cancer, *The Oncologist* 9:80-89, 2004.

MULTIPLE CHOICE TEST QUESTIONS

1) Rapid creation of abnormal cells which grow beyond their usual boundaries are known as:
   a) healthy cell growth
   b) depression
   c) cancer
   d) lymphedema

2) Massage for people living with cancer
   a) is applied using deep tissue massage
   b) enhances the immune system
   c) has never been contraindicated
   d) is one cause for cancer metastasis

3) Five common side effects from cancer treatments are:
   a) nausea, pain, anxiety, fatigue, and depression.
   b) Hunger, pain, anxiety, fatigue, and rashes
   c) Nausea, hunger, fatigue, energy, and pain
   d) Depression, infection, hernia, rashes, and fatigue

4) Massage has many benefits for cancer patients. Some of these are
   a) relieves pain
   b) improved immune system
   c) improved appetite and quality of sleep
   d) all of the above

5) When lymph nodes are removed from areas of the body, swelling can occur. This condition is known as
   a) lypossage
   b) lymphedema
   c) deep vein thrombosis (DVT)
   d) vital organ dysfunction

6) One common type of treatment for cancer uses a beam externally delivered to a specific area of the body. In some cases it is internally implanted. This is known as
   a) chemotherapy
   b) immunotherapy
   c) radiation therapy
   d) surgery

7) Chemotherapy is a very strong medicine used to destroy tumors. This type of treatment mandates that all elements of massage—pressure, speed, circulatory intent, etc. be which of the following?
   a) lessened or dialed down
   b) increased
   c) contraindicated
   d) deeper

8) When working with a client experiencing nausea you should forego
   a) jostling
   b) joint movements
   c) scented lubricants
   d) all of the above

9) Patients undergoing surgery as a cancer treatment are at risk for
   a) deep vein thrombosis (DVT)
   b) hernias
   c) muscle strains
   d) rashes

10) In cancer treatment, massage therapy is considered to be
   a) contraindicated
   b) complementary therapy
   c) cure
   d) conventional medicine

11) When cancerous cells grow and spread to other sites in the body, it is known as
   a) grade of cancer
   b) an oncogene
   c) metastasis
   d) deep vein thrombosis

12) Some cancers such as lymphoma or leukemia develop and live in the blood or lymph systems. These are referred to as
   a) solid tumors
   b) lymphedema
   c) radiation
   d) liquid tumors

13) Frequent sites of primary cancers include
   a) breast, prostate, lung
   b) kidney, liver, intestines
   c) gall bladder, pancreas, colon
   d) lung, heart, diaphragm

14) A _____ is a device used to transport chemotherapy drugs into the body
   a) shunt
   b) drain
   c) port
   d) all the above

15) Palliative care refers to the
   a) pretreatment care
   b) care given to ease a client's suffering
   c) care given to those undergoing radiation
   d) home care for clients

16) Massage for people with cancer must be adapted for the individual due to the _____ involved
   a) detoxification
   b) variables
   c) plan of action
   d) palliative care

17) Which variables will affect the techniques for cancer massage?
   a) type and phase of cancer they have
   b) type and stage of treatment they are in
   c) side effects and conditions currently being experienced by the client
   d) all of the above

18) For an oncology client who has just completed treatment, a deep tissue massage
   a) is highly recommended for its detoxifying effects
   b) is contraindicated
   c) can cause the client to have flulike symptoms
   d) both b and c

19) A thorough health history can reveal whether an oncology client is experiencing
   a) pain
   b) lymphedema
   c) fatigue
   d) all of the above

20) There are many phases that a person with cancer may or may not go through but the one phase all have in common is
   a) diagnosis
   b) lymphedema
   c) posttreatment
   d) survivor

CranioSacral Therapy

John E. Upledger and Sharon Desjarlais

4

DEFINITION OF CRANIOSACRAL THERAPY

CranioSacral Therapy (CST) is a light-touch method of releasing tensions in and around the central nervous system to relieve pain and dysfunction and improve whole-body health and performance. Applying a gentle, knowing touch along with a healing intention helps stimulate the rhythmical flow of cerebrospinal fluid within the membranes and ventricles of the **craniosacral system** that surrounds the brain and spinal cord. These waves of fluid keep the brain and spinal cord healthy so they can send balanced electrical impulses to the body's tissues, organs, and systems.

By mobilizing the fluid and soft tissues throughout the body, CranioSacral Therapy triggers each individual's natural self-healing mechanisms to improve health all the way down to the cells. Whether you use it as a primary modality or as a complement to other approaches, it can produce significant results with a full spectrum of medical conditions.

History

My personal journey with CranioSacral Therapy began in 1970 when I was assisting a spinal surgery on a man named Delbert. Inside the spinal canal there is a membrane that surrounds and protects the spinal cord. All I had to do was hold that membrane still while the operating surgeon removed a calcium deposit from its outer surface.

It may sound simple, but I just couldn't do it. The membrane kept moving no matter how carefully I tried to hold it still. What was even stranger was that it was pulsing at a rate of about eight beats per minute. That particular rhythm didn't correspond to either Delbert's breathing or heart rate, which we were monitoring.

After Delbert made it through surgery, I discovered that the odd pulsing rhythm of the membrane inside his

To better understand concepts in this chapter, watch *CranioSacral Therapy* video on the **DVD** found at the back of this book.

55

spinal canal was new to all the doctors in the operating room. We didn't know it at the time, but what we were seeing was the rhythm of cerebrospinal fluid pumping through the craniosacral system.

A year or so later I attended a short course on cranial osteopathy, a field developed by Dr. William Sutherland. The course focused mainly on the bones of the skull and the fact that they weren't fused at the sutures as doctors had been taught in medical schools. Sutherland's material demonstrated how skull bones had the potential to continue to move ever so minutely throughout a person's life.

As I was in this seminar palpating the motion of the bones, people started asking about the pulsing rhythm they were feeling. That's when I realized I had seen the driving force behind those moving skull bones during Delbert's surgery. I put the two episodes together—what I saw in surgery and what I was feeling now with my own hands. They seemed linked, yet no one knew how.

That lack of information enticed me to refine my **palpation** skills. I began experimenting with a variety of methods of connecting with the mysterious rhythm of the craniosacral system. Yet instead of focusing on the skull bones as Sutherland and other cranial osteopaths had, I was continually drawn to work with the membranes and fluid. I could clearly see the potential of this new approach to release restrictions in the central nervous system to help disorders like headaches and migraines, TMJ syndrome, chronic fatigue, fibromyalgia, and a multitude of other challenges.

Over time news of my work began to spread. In 1975 I was invited by Michigan State University to help uncover a scientific basis for Sutherland's theories about the movable nature of the cranium. From 1975 through 1983 I worked as a professor of biomechanics at MSU's College of Osteopathic Medicine. It was an exhilarating time. While I was there I led a team of anatomists, physiologists, biophysicists, and bioengineers, all working together to test and document the influence of the craniosacral system on the body.

Out of those years of research and clinical trials, we were finally able to explain the function of the craniosacral system. Then we went on to demonstrate how the system could be used to evaluate and treat numerous health problems involving the brain and spinal cord. I refined and named this new approach CranioSacral Therapy.

MECHANISM OF CRANIOSACRAL THERAPY

CranioSacral Therapy focuses on normalizing the craniosacral system. This core body system extends from the skull, face, and mouth down to the sacrum

and coccyx (Figure 4-1). It consists of a compartment formed by the dura mater membrane, the cerebrospinal fluid contained within the dura mater, the systems that regulate fluid flow, the bones that attach to the

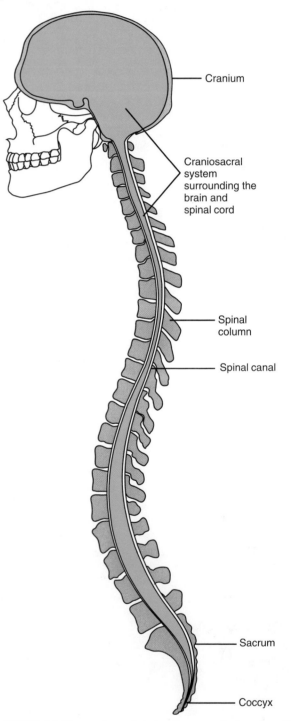

FIGURE 4-1 The craniosacral system is a core body system that extends from the skull, face, and mouth down to the sacrum and coccyx. (Drawing courtesy of Tad Wanveer.)

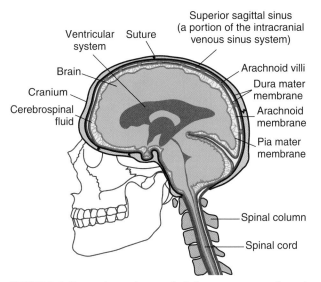

FIGURE 4-2 The craniosacral system includes a compartment formed by the dura mater membrane and cerebrospinal fluid in the dura mater, the bones that attach to the membranes, and joints and sutures interconnecting these bones. (Drawing courtesy of Tad Wanveer.)

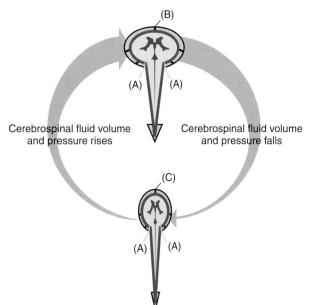

FIGURE 4-3 Changes in the dura mater tensions induce movements in the bones attached to the dura mater compartment. (Drawing courtesy of Tad Wanveer.)

membranes, and the joints and sutures that interconnect these bones (Figure 4-2).

In its most basic sense, the craniosacral system functions as a semiclosed hydraulic system that bathes the brain and spinal cord and their cells in cerebrospinal fluid pumped rhythmically at a rate of 6 to 12 cycles per minute. In order to accommodate these pressure changes, the bones of the cranium and sacrum must remain somewhat mobile throughout life, as Dr. Sutherland first noted in the 1930s.

The research and clinical trials that we conducted at MSU supported Sutherland's conclusion. Studying bone specimens from live surgical patients 7 to 57 years old, our team was able to demonstrate definitive potential for movement between the cranial sutures.[1-5] Our findings also supported those published in *Anatomica Humanica* by Italian professor Guiseppi Sperino,[6] who noted that cranial sutures fuse before death only under pathologic circumstances.

Several other studies of ours then laid the foundation for developing what we called the **Pressurstat Model**, which explains the mechanism of the craniosacral system. Essentially, as cerebrospinal fluid volume and pressure rise and fall within the craniosacral system, corresponding changes occur in the dura mater membrane tensions. These changes in turn induce movements in the bones that attach to the dura mater compartment (Figure 4-3).

When the natural mobility of the dura mater or any of its attached bones is impaired, the function of the craniosacral system may be impaired as well. And because of the contents of the craniosacral system—the brain, the spinal cord, and all its related structures—tissue restrictions or imbalances there can directly affect any or all aspects of central nervous system performance (Figure 4-4).

Fortunately these problems can be detected and corrected by a skilled therapist using simple methods of palpation. Starting with a very light touch—about 5 grams, or roughly the weight of a nickel—you can evaluate the system by testing for the ease of motion and the rhythm of cerebrospinal fluid as it flows within the membranes. Then you can use specific hands-on techniques to release restrictions in the membranes, the fascia, and any other tissues that influence the craniosacral system. The result is an improved internal environment that frees the central nervous system to return to its greatest levels of health and performance.

Encouraging the Body to Self-Correct

CranioSacral Therapy is based on the idea that each person's body contains all the necessary information to uncover the underlying cause of any health problem. As the therapist, you simply open your line of communication with the client's body to obtain this information and facilitate the client's self-healing processes.

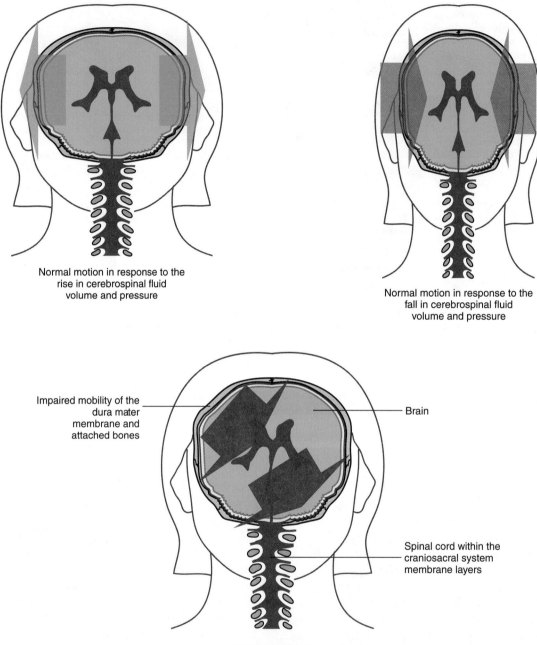

Normal motion in response to the
rise in cerebrospinal fluid
volume and pressure

Normal motion in response to the
fall in cerebrospinal fluid
volume and pressure

Impaired mobility of the
dura mater
membrane and
attached bones

Brain

Spinal cord within the
craniosacral system
membrane layers

Impaired mobility

FIGURE 4-4 Tissue imbalances can directly affect any or all aspects of central nervous system performance. (Drawing courtesy of Tad Wanveer.)

Because of this direct approach of listening to the client's body, the usual intake process carried out in conventional medicine is generally reversed when it comes to CST. Rather than taking a verbal medical history, you may choose to begin with gentle palpation. If you become familiar with the client's history beforehand, you may find only what you expect to find rather than sensing the subtle clues offered by the client's body, energy, and psyche. For that reason, CST clients are usually asked to write their medical histories and bring them in for their files. You can then review the history later, after you complete your hands-on evaluation and you feel safe from the issue of suggestibility.

CranioSacral Therapy also diverges from conventional medicine in its approach to symptoms. Rather than trying to simply relieve them, your goal is to resolve the primary dysfunction underlying the presenting symptom complex. For instance, consider strabismus, which is a lack of coordination between the eyes. Rather than seeing this as a condition to be corrected by surgery, you might use CranioSacral Therapy to search for a cause within the intracranial membrane system and the motor control system of the eyes.

In the case of strabismus, the cause is often an abnormal tension pattern in the tentorium cerebelli. These tension patterns are frequently referred from the occiput or the low back and pelvis, which makes sense when you understand that the craniosacral system runs from the cranium all the way to the tailbone (sacrum). That's how a trauma, strain, or torsion type of injury at one end of the system can affect the other end of the system.

So imagine that your CST evaluation indicates intracranial membrane strain of the tentorium cerebelli due to occipital or low back and pelvic dysfunctions resulting in secondary motor dysfunction of the eyes. Clearly, you would focus first on the sacrum, the pelvis, and the occiput, and then on the tentorium cerebelli. A "spontaneous correction" of the strabismus would indicate an accurate CST evaluation and resolution.

You can use a similar approach for almost any problem, from TMJ disorders to spastic colitis. The nature of the presenting problem is usually of secondary importance unless fast relief of symptoms is critical, or if the client doesn't understand CranioSacral Therapy. In these cases you may want to attend to the immediate complaints while the client's full understanding of CST evolves.

Palpating the CranioSacral Rhythm

With CranioSacral Therapy, you use gentle palpation to meld with the body so you can discern a wide spectrum of internal changes. While heavy palpation can evoke a defensive reaction, gentle and intentioned touch allows you to explore the full range of internal structures, tissue motion, and energies.

Just as you can use touch to distinguish the cardiac and respiratory pulses, you can feel the **craniosacral rhythm** throughout the body. This rhythm has a distinctive character at different body locations. When you're able to fully evaluate the rhythm, you can get specific information as to how well the craniosacral system is functioning. You can also use it to tell whether your efforts at reestablishing normal function have been successful.

To use the craniosacral motion as an evaluation tool, you'll want to palpate the rhythm throughout the body to determine where the fascia is restricted and where it's moving efficiently. There are certain **listening stations** that can quickly give you a general evaluation of the craniosacral motion (Box 4-1).

Learning to palpate the craniosacral rhythm is the foundation for successful CranioSacral Therapy. The more you practice, the more your hands will develop skills and wisdom all their own. Eventually you can free your hands to play a beautiful concerto while you listen for the melody and communicate with the intelligence of the body.

Tracing Tensions Through the Fascial System

An integral aspect of CranioSacral Therapy involves the **fascial system.** Fascia runs like a continuous web of tissue throughout the body. It covers every structure, organ, and cavity, from the top of the head to the tip of the toes. Everything from the tiniest nerve to the largest bone has its own fascial sheath or envelope. Indeed, you can travel from any one place in the body to any other place without ever leaving the fascia. You can begin in the falx cerebri, move into the tentorium cerebelli, travel down the lining of the internal aspect of the occiput, and end up at the carotid foramen in the temporal bone. At this juncture you can continue your journey down the carotid sheath that becomes the pericardium in the thorax. You can then travel down the fascial fibers of the pericardium, which pierce the respiratory diaphragm. Once through the diaphragm you can continue down its inferior fascial covering to the fascia of the psoas muscle. You can then follow the psoas fascia into the pelvis and the leg. From this point it's a straight shot to the bottom of the foot (Figure 4-6).

Because you can make this journey to anywhere in the body using fascia as the vehicle, you can see how fascia interconnects the entire body. That means that abnormal tension patterns in the fascia can be transmitted from one body part to another in what can appear to be bizarre ways unless you understand the unity of the entire fascial system.

It's critical to note that fascia should remain somewhat mobile under normal physiologic conditions. The tissue is tough yet flexible, allowing for movement from the subtle, like those that allow your heart to beat, to the gross, like those that allow you to throw a ball.

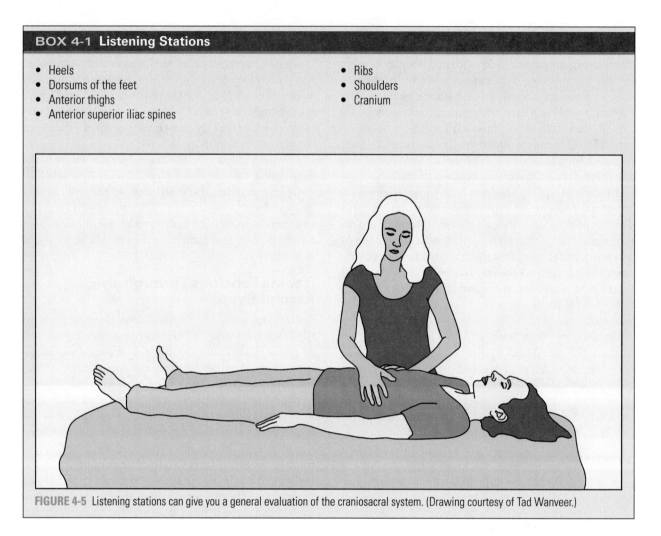

BOX 4-1 Listening Stations

- Heels
- Dorsums of the feet
- Anterior thighs
- Anterior superior iliac spines

- Ribs
- Shoulders
- Cranium

FIGURE 4-5 Listening stations can give you a general evaluation of the craniosacral system. (Drawing courtesy of Tad Wanveer.)

From a therapeutic perspective, applying gentle traction techniques to the fascia in arbitrary directions from various positions can help localize restricted areas. You can then interpret those areas of restricted mobility as either sites of current problems or residue from previous lesions.

Arcing for Active Lesions

A lesion can be classified as any type of tissue or organ abnormality resulting from disease or injury. In CranioSacral Therapy, active lesions are differentiated from inactive residual effects by **arcing** (pronounced 'är-king), a technique I developed along with biophysicist Zvi Karni at Michigan State University. By using a process of mechano-electrical monitoring, we discovered that skilled therapists are able to palpate energies inside and off the body.[7]

Arcing requires you to sense the energetic waves of interference produced by an active lesion. These waves

of energy tend to be superimposed over the normal subtle motions of the body and its organs, tissues, and energies. You can then trace the waves to their source by manually sensing the arcs that they form.[7-9] The source of the waves is considered to be the core site of the underlying lesion. It may even be distant from the location of your client's symptoms. Usually an active lesion disrupts gross physiologic activities, as well as more subtle energy functions and patterns such as acupuncture meridians (Figure 4-7).

As you arc and discover sites of dysfunction and disruption, you can attempt to restore mobility to the involved tissues and energy fields. More often than not, your attempts will be partially if not completely successful. In either case, you'll often discover a deeper lesion that the dysfunction you just addressed was actually adapting to. You can then follow the clues layer by layer until you discover the primary problem. You might get there in the first CST evaluation, or it may require more

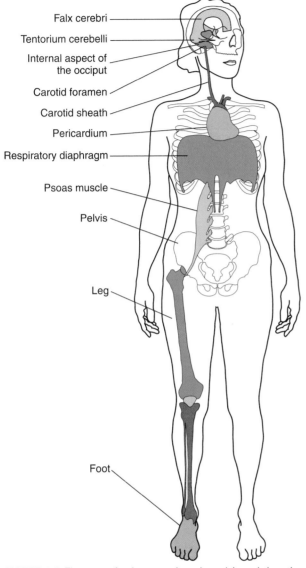

Falx cerebri
Tentorium cerebelli
Internal aspect of the occiput
Carotid foramen
Carotid sheath
Pericardium
Respiratory diaphragm
Psoas muscle
Pelvis
Leg
Foot

FIGURE 4-6 The psoas fascia moves into the pelvis and then the leg and from this point is a straight shot to the bottom of the foot. (Drawing courtesy of Tad Wanveer.)

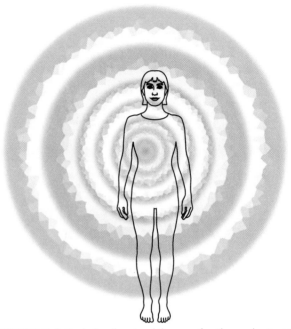

FIGURE 4-7 Active lesion disrupts subtle energy functions and patterns such as acupuncture meridians. (Drawing courtesy of Tad Wanveer.)

than one session to bring the deepest underlying problem to the surface.

Inducing the Still Point

In CranioSacral Therapy, a **still point** occurs when the cerebrospinal fluid gently, gradually, and naturally comes to a rest in what can best be described as an extended pause. A still point can occur spontaneously or you can induce it intentionally to help facilitate the release of restrictions in the membranes around the brain and spinal cord.

It works quite simply. By delicately interrupting the fluid flow, you can cause a momentary buildup of fluid in the system. When you subsequently release the tissues and the fluid begins to flow again, it gently flushes the system, causing the membranes to stretch a tiny bit and release tissue restrictions or adhesions.

The results, which include increased blood flow to the brain, can have a therapeutic effect on the central nervous system and the entire body. Some highly beneficial effects include the relief of headache and muscle pain, a reduced state of stress and ready response, a deep state of relaxation, and an overall sense of well-being.

A still point represents one of the few times a therapist actually alters the functioning of the craniosacral system. To illustrate how this occurs, it is important to understand how the terms "flexion" and "extension" apply to CranioSacral Therapy. In the flexion phase of the craniosacral rhythm, the whole body externally rotates. The head actually widens and the base of the sacrum moves posteriorly. In contrast, the body rotates internally in the extension phase (Figure 4-8).

We theorize that the flexion phase of the rhythmical cycle is created when the inflow of cerebrospinal fluid (CSF) into the semiclosed hydraulic system formed by the dura mater membrane exceeds the outflow. During the extension phase of the rhythm, the inflow of CSF

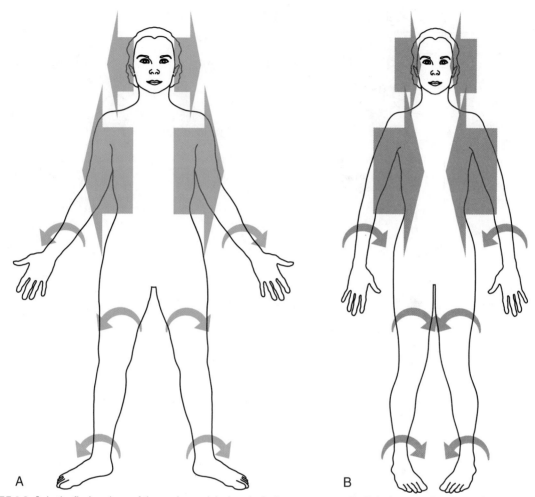

FIGURE 4-8 A, In the flexion phase of the craniosacral rhythm, the body rotates externally. **B,** In the extension phase of the craniosacral rhythm, the body rotates internally. (Drawing courtesy of Tad Wanveer.)

is either completely shut down or significantly less than the outflow. Thus, we might say that the flexion phase is one of filling and the extension phase is one of emptying.

You can induce a still point by using manual techniques to resist either the flexion or the extension phase. Generally, it is easier and more efficient to resist the filling (flexion) than the emptying (extension).

Releasing the Energy Cyst

Have you ever had a client whose injury continued to cause problems long after the site had healed? That's not all that unusual. Research I conducted in the 1970s along with Dr. Karni led us to discover that the body can retain the imprint of physical trauma in the tissues.[10] These imprints, which can include the intense emotions that occurred at the time of injury, actually leave a residue embedded in the body. I call these areas of restricted or disorganized energy "**energy cysts**."

The idea goes something like this: When an accident occurs, the energy of the trauma enters the body. This fits with the laws of thermodynamics which tell us that energy cannot be created or destroyed. They also tell us that the natural tendency of atoms, molecules, and energy is toward disorganization.

When this external, disorganized energy—the "energy of injury"—is forced into the body, it penetrates into the tissues to a depth determined by the amount of force versus the density of the tissues it's trying to penetrate. For instance, the energy from a blow to the foot might penetrate through the leg all the way up to the pelvis. When it reaches the depth of maximum penetration, it stops and forms a localized ball of energy that doesn't belong there.

If your body is vital and able, the energy of injury can dissipate and normal healing can occur. But if your body is compromised or in any way unable to dissipate this energy, it's compacted into a smaller and smaller ball in order to minimize the area of tissue-function disruption. As it becomes more and more compressed and localized, the disorganization within this compressed energy increases until it becomes an energy cyst.

Although the body can adapt to energy cysts, over time it needs extra energy to continue to accommodate them while still performing its day-to-day functions. As years pass and the body becomes more stressed, it can lose its ability to adapt altogether. That's when symptoms and dysfunctions begin to appear and become difficult to suppress or ignore.

In CranioSacral Therapy we use a technique called energy cyst release that can help you deal with these particular challenges. Often that process is as simple as allowing your client's body to spontaneously return to the same position it was in when the injury was first sustained. When that happens, through gentle palpation you can feel the tissues of the body relax as the energy cyst is expelled. Then the body is free to return to its optimal levels of functioning.

Relieving the Facilitated Segment

Peripheral body problems often refer into segments of the spinal cord via the nerve root connections. This greatly affects the dura mater membrane, which is key to the functioning of the craniosacral system.

According to the CranioSacral Therapy model, the dura mater within the vertebral canal (dural tube) has the freedom to glide up and down for a range of 0.5 to 2 cm. This movement is allowed by the slackness and direction of the dural sleeves as they depart the dural tube and attach to the intertransverse foramina of the spinal column.

When nerve roots refer increased impulse activity into the spinal cord from their peripheral locations, it creates a facilitated condition of the related spinal cord segment. Hyperactivity in the **facilitated segment** sends out impulses to the related dural tube and dural sleeves. The result is a tightening and loss of mobility of the dural tube related to the involved segment.

Our clinical observations suggest that CST is effective in releasing dural tube restrictions to normalize the activity of facilitated spinal cord segments. To locate these areas of restricted mobility, you test the mobility of the dural tube and release restrictions as you find them using gentle traction techniques. These releases are necessary. If a peripheral restriction is released but the dural tube restriction and facilitated spinal cord segment aren't released, the peripheral problem usually reoccurs.

Once the peripheral body and the dural tube have been released of restrictions, you can then focus on the cranium and sacrum. This is where you help gently release tissue tensions to allow the self-correction of primary and secondary dysfunctions of the skull bones, facial bones, hard palate, and sacrococcygeal complex.

By working with the dural membranes inside the skull and spinal canal, you very gently mobilize all the related sutures and joints. After the bony restrictions are mobilized, you can then focus on correcting abnormal dural membrane restrictions, irregularities in cerebrospinal fluid activities, and dysfunctional energy patterns and fluctuations related to the craniosacral system.

At this point your client may be shifting from a stage of having obstacles removed to one of self-healing as you simply help facilitate the process. In essence, it's no longer about "fighting disease" as much as enhancing health. That's why CST is such an effective preventive-health modality. It mobilizes the body's natural defenses rather than focusing on the causal agents of diseases.

■□■ IN MY EXPERIENCE

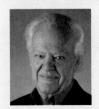

One element shared by all effective healing methods is the process of leading the client on a journey to authentic self-discovery. This "golden thread" is necessary for the initiation and continuation of self-healing, because it is only through self-healing that any human being can experience both permanent recovery and spiritual growth.

Using the Craniosacral Rhythm as a Significance Detector

In CranioSacral Therapy, the craniosacral rhythm is a key indicator you use to locate and release tissue restrictions. One important way you can use this rhythm is to gauge the significance of different types of internal physiologic events.

When a client's body is involved in an important process, the craniosacral rhythm will often come to a sudden stop. This abrupt halt of the rhythm is called the **significance detector.** Unlike the still point in which the cerebrospinal fluid seems to gently and naturally come to a rest, the significance detector feels like the fluid has run into a solid wall.

The sensation generally indicates that your client's body is going through some type of important underlying event. Often, when the craniosacral rhythm comes to an abrupt stop, it indicates that the client is in the same body position in which a physical trauma originally occurred. Again, this may be a point at which an energy cyst can be naturally expelled.

Using Gentle Forces

To evaluate and release restrictions in the craniosacral system, you generally use very gentle traction or lifting forces directed along the natural pathways of cranial bone movement in the flexion or extension phases of the craniosacral cycle. If this gentle traction reveals that the cranial bones are moving freely and smoothly through their normal range of motion, then no underlying restriction exists. However, you will often encounter some resistance to these delicate forces. When you do, it indicates there is an underlying restriction in the craniosacral system.

Restrictions, which are simply barriers to the free and natural motion of the craniosacral system, can occur between cranial bones or within the dura mater membrane system. In this way you can distinguish between osseous and membranous restriction, which each provide you with a different palpation sensation.

Osseous restrictions feel rigid. They lack mobility at the cranial sutures, often resulting from sutural jamming. It feels as if the cranial bones are cemented at the junctions of the sutures. Membranous restrictions are elastic. When you're using gentle traction on a membranous restriction, it feels like a rubber band that's been pulled and is ready to snap back.

Distinguishing between osseous and membranous restrictions is a critical component of evaluating and addressing the craniosacral system. While osseous restrictions inhibit normal cranial bone motion, the primary target of CranioSacral Therapy is the craniosacral membrane system. These underlying membranous restrictions interfere with the natural functioning of the craniosacral system and often serve to hold the osseous restrictions in place.

Sensing the Tissue Release

Tissue release, also called simply "release," is the palpable sense of softening and relaxation that we feel in the tissues when a CranioSacral Therapy technique has come to a successful completion. It doesn't necessarily mean that the whole session is over, only that one phase has finished.

A release generally feels like the tissues loosen and move laterally in a reasonably symmetric manner. Other common signs include softening, lengthening, increased fluid flow, increased energy flow, heat, a sense of energetic repelling (like two opposing magnets), and the client taking a deep breath. To put it simply, any change in the tissue can be considered a sign of release.

BENEFITS AND CLINICAL APPLICATIONS OF CRANIOSACRAL THERAPY

CranioSacral Therapy is well known for its multiple applications and positive results in thousands of cases. By facilitating and enhancing the body's self-corrective mechanisms, it has proven useful as both a primary and complementary modality for a wide variety of dysfunctions, from coronary insufficiency to Crohn's disease.

The number of sessions required to achieve positive results depends on a number of factors, including how complex the client's defense mechanisms are. After you conduct an initial hands-on evaluation, you can make a recommendation. In general, if there is no change in your client's condition after five or six sessions, CST may not be effective for that individual.

Following is a partial list of conditions that have responded well to CST in clinical applications. While research conducted at MSU proved the existence of the craniosacral system and its effect on health and disease, this information is based primarily on more than three decades of clinical observations.

Pain Syndromes

These include all types, including myofascial, neuromusculoskeletal, and radicular pain syndromes. Because of its effects on the autonomic nervous system,

CST desensitizes facilitated segments and strengthens fluid exchange throughout the body. It also addresses many of the psychoemotional factors that may be contributing to chronic neck and back pain.

Headache Syndromes

These include migraine, tension cephalalgia, fluid congestion, and hormonally related syndromes. CST is excellent at helping you identify and relieve the underlying causes of headaches. The immobility of cranial sutures seems to be a contributing factor in migraines for many clients. CST addresses this problem along with autonomic and neuromusculoskeletal dysfunctions, both of which may contribute to headache syndromes.

Temporomandibular Joint (TMJ) Syndrome

This painful problem arises when the joints of the lower jaw become dysfunctional. Surprisingly, the problem can originate from a craniosacral system restriction that results in an imbalance between the temporal bones on each side of the head. Other causes include nervous tension resulting in tooth grinding or jaw clenching, whiplash to the neck, and malocclusion of the teeth. CST is highly effective at locating and relieving the underlying problems and mobilizing the temporal bones.

Spinal Dysfunctions

This includes scoliosis, low-back (lumbar and lumbosacral) instability, disc compression, postoperative complications, and other dysfunctions. Once you determine the underlying cause, CST is effective at solving biomechanical, neurogenic, and facilitated segment problems.

Traumatic Injuries

With CST you can work with a multitude of traumatic brain and spinal cord injuries, including closed head injuries, spinal cord injuries, whiplash and other spinal ligament strains, and nervous system conditions due to injuries. Your success will vary depending on the severity of the injury.

While many therapists usually do well with clients who suffer seizures subsequent to head injuries, we've seen moderate improvement in the movement of paralyzed limbs due to head injuries. The greatest progress usually appears in the area of intellect and social responsiveness.

We've also seen remarkable improvement in vision, hearing, smell, and taste, and in secondary autonomic dysfunction such as disequilibrium, cardiac pulmonary function, bowel function, urinary tract function, sexual function, and related conditions. The positive results are probably due to the effect of CST on the autonomic and related spinal cord segments, as well as its ability to reduce stress and anxiety.

Degenerative Diseases of the Central Nervous System

Until a few years ago it was thought that CSF simply bathed the surface of the brain. All that changed with the use of radioactive tracers that flow with the fluid. Now it's understood that when tracers are injected into the ventricular system of the brain, they're distributed throughout the brain within minutes.

Since CSF carries all sorts of messenger molecules that facilitate communication between cells of different systems, it stands to reason that improving this fluid circulation may explain the success we've seen using CST to treat degenerative diseases. People who struggle with these types of diseases respond to CST in a variety of ways depending on the severity and the systems affected.

A colleague and good friend of mine, Don Ash, PT, CST-D, recently worked with an elderly man who was extremely agitated due to chronic back pain. He had Parkinson's disease with the classically rigid, forward-flexed spine, and the small shuffling step gait.

Don treated him with CranioSacral Therapy every 2 weeks for nearly 2 years with surprising results. His patient became more relaxed and the muscle tone in his spine decreased, which also decreased his pain. With the absence of pain he was less agitated and more congenial with his family, which greatly lifted the mood and social interaction.

Unfortunately, this relaxed state only lasted about 10 to 12 days before another CST session was needed. After 2 years the effects of the disease could no longer be handled by CST alone. But you can clearly see that it's a solid adjunctive therapy. With medications and other interventions, it can be very beneficial in adding months and even years of improved quality of life.

Another recent discovery that may help explain the effectiveness of CST in cases of degenerative diseases of the central nervous system is that CSF contains molecules that attach to metallic atoms that are deposited in the brain. These atoms are then carried away and excreted from the body in a process known as chelation. Metal atoms deposited in the brain tissue are thought to be contributing factors to problems such as Alzheimer's disease and senility. Because of that, improving CSF circulation through CST may be considered preventive therapy.

In the case of Alzheimer's, CST can temporarily improve mental function if it's capable of being recovered. As with other degenerative diseases of the nervous system, this depends on the severity of each individual's case. I've seen Alzheimer's patients have a brighter affect with more ability to comprehend and communicate. Physical effects of the disease such as tremors, clonus, and pill-rolling movements can be diminished.

I've also had great success improving the mental alertness and brain function of elderly clients who were having trouble concentrating and putting words together. I'm sure that by improving the circulation of blood, CSF, interstitial, and intracellular fluid, we're helping clear toxic waste accumulated in the brain cells and tissues.

Once again, the positive effects of CST may be temporary. But it can provide windows of good quality of life in an otherwise very dark place for many patients and their families.

Postsurgery Rehabilitation

CST is an excellent addition to any postoperative rehab program. It restores the movement of body fluids to areas traumatized by surgical procedures. In this way it enhances the healing process and can potentially reduce the formation of adhesions and scar tissue. CST also helps remove toxic residue from anesthetics and pain medications.

In the early 1970s I treated several postoperative neurologic clients as early as the first day after surgery with very good results. The neurosurgeon felt his clients demonstrated a decreased number of complications, lowered morbidity rates, and shortened recovery times. In general, we found that the sooner we began therapy, the more it helped prevent complications.

Autism

CST has shown great promise in cases of autism, which is actually a complex set of symptoms with no known origin. (At least 30% of known cases of autism are caused by the genetic disorder Fragile X.) While it's not clear precisely which mechanisms are at work in either causing or "curing" the condition, it has been widely noted that after CST, these particular clients generally inflict much less pain on themselves. They also tend to display more affection toward others and improved social behavior.

In my experience, autism has several unique qualitative effects on the craniosacral system. First, there seems to be a universal hypertonicity of the dura mater in the circumference of the cranial vault. It's global and feels like the membrane is rigid, unyielding, and lacking the subtle quality that is common in fascial tissue. Having said that, it also seems to respond very well to repeated still points and the directing of energy into the cranial vault from the hands on each side of the head.

Additionally, areas of specific motor and sensory control and cognition can sometimes be beneficially influenced. If the client has learning delays, a frontal lift technique aids the frontal cortex. Clients who exhibit hyperactivity and extreme emotions can sometimes become very quiet with techniques on the temporal bones that help alleviate restrictions in the limbic system. Therapy on the cranial base and occiput also tends to be very useful for those with tactile defensiveness, hyper- or hypoactivity, or developmental delay in gait, balance, and hand dexterity.

The important point in working with autism is gaining the client's confidence and trust through the use of still points, which encourages the patient to relax and the body to recognize the benefit of light touch. This creates an element of trust leading to subtle yet progressively positive changes to a nervous system that has been overwhelmed by the difficult problem of autism.

Cerebral Palsy

This is basically a catchall term that means the brain isn't working properly. Because CST often has a positive impact on the motor control system, including the relief of muscle spasticity, it works well with most cerebral palsy clients. While sometimes there appears to be little or no change, occasionally there is remarkable improvement.

Either way, the rule holds true—the younger the clients are when you work with them, the better they usually do. By the time they're adolescents you may be able to correct the underlying problem, but the nerve pathways necessary for proper functioning may not be there because they never had a chance to form in the first place.

Learning Disabilities

In 1978 I conducted a standardized craniosacral examination on a mixed sample of 203 children in the Michigan school system. I found a positive relationship between elevated craniosacral system motion scores and children the school authorities said had learning disabilities, behavioral problems, and/or poor motor coordination.[11]

Since then CranioSacral Therapy has been used with thousands of learning-disabled children. I suspect more than half of them had problems with their craniosacral systems. When these problems are resolved, the kids have up to a 90 percent chance of overcoming these disabilities. This is especially true in cases of dyslexia and hyperkinesis. Often the disability simply disappears as the children grow and develop without the presence of restrictions.

Motor System Problems

CST can almost always improve motor and speech problems. Even in the case of eye-motor problems, a skilled practitioner can tell in a matter of minutes whether the problem is caused by tension in the membranes that the nerves pass through to get to the eyes. When this is the case, especially in children, the problem is often permanently correctable in two or three sessions. Clients have also reported great success in cases of olfactory dysfunction and vertigo, though we've seen only moderate success with tinnitus.

Endocrine Disorders

Many of these problems, including premenstrual tension, pituitary dysfunction, pineal gland problems, and related emotional problems, often respond favorably to CST. It helps mobilize fluids, balance the autonomic nervous system, improve endocrine control, and relieve neuromusculoskeletal and psychoemotional symptoms. Releasing the dural sleeves that may be restricting nerve outflow to the adrenals, thyroid, spleen, liver, thymus and reproductive glands is also very helpful.

Endocrine disorders can occur as the developing brain evolves. In addition, they can happen following physical trauma such as shaken baby syndrome, or viral or bacterial infection like meningitis. As hormonal changes occur in the maturing bodies of women, CST can be exceptionally useful in returning balance to the client, whether in the premenopausal, postmenopausal or perimenopausal stage.

CST is just as effective for men in the throes of aging. The aging spine responds to fascial release techniques of the dural tube. Hormone-producing organs like the pituitary gland and thyroid respond to increasing CSF production. The governing organ in the brain, the nerve pathways (both efferent and afferent), and the end organ or structure can be returned to optimal function by liberating fascial restrictions in the spine and promoting the circulation of CSF, both of which are facilitated by CST. Combining CranioSacral Therapy with allopathic approaches can only maximize the potential for healing in almost every instance.

Other Conditions

CranioSacral Therapy can successfully address a wide range of pain, dysfunction, and disease. The most important thing to remember is that it's extremely gentle and often resolves conditions in a shorter timeframe than many other approaches. It can almost always help in some fashion, even if simply to improve the success of other therapies.

CONTRAINDICATIONS OF CRANIOSACRAL THERAPY

Even in the most critical cases, CranioSacral Therapy has wide applications. However, it is contraindicated anytime you have a concern about changing a client's intracranial pressure. Such conditions include but are not limited to:

Acute brain hemorrhage or stroke—CST is contraindicated when any bleeding or interruption of blood flow in the brain has occurred.

Recent spinal tap or puncture in the craniosacral system—Do not proceed with CST unless the client's physician says there is no more leaking of spinal fluid and it's safe to use light-touch therapy that may alter intracranial fluid-pressure dynamics.

Recent fracture of skull bones, vertebral column, or ribs—Take a very careful approach here in case an increase in cranial bone motion leads to bleeding or a membranous tear. Proceed cautiously and refer to an advanced therapist if you have any concern. You can find one by visiting the online directory at www.iahp.com.

Intracranial aneurysm—It is contraindicated to change intracranial fluid pressure when it could potentially precipitate a leak or rupture of a dangerous intracranial aneurysm.

Herniation of the medulla oblongata—A herniation of the medulla oblongata through the foramen magnum is a life-threatening situation. You would not want to alter fluid pressures within the craniosacral system by any means.

Arnold Chiari malformation—This is an incomplete foramen magnum in which the inferior poles of the cerebellar hemispheres and the medulla protrude and may herniate through the foramen magnum. Don't do anything that places more strain—or shifts the fluid pressure to place more strain—on the foramen magnum, brain stem, or dural tube.

Whenever you come across any of these contraindicated conditions, it's critical that you consult the client's physician. Proceed only after you get the green light confirming that there's no problem altering intracranial pressure at this stage of recovery. If you're still uncomfortable, refer the client to an advanced CranioSacral Therapist.

THE 10-STEP PROTOCOL

If you're just starting to use CST, one of the most helpful approaches is the 10-step protocol (Figure 4-9). It consists of a series of basic steps that enhance the client's overall craniosacral system function. Each step acts as both an evaluation and correction. The techniques are so gentle and noninvasive that they're virtually risk-free.

The steps for the 10-step protocol are generally broken down as follows (Figure 4-9):

1. Still point (CV-4)
2. Diaphragm releases: pelvic, respiratory, thoracic inlet, hyoid, cranial base
3. Traction release (L5-S1), medical compression asis
4. Dural tube rock and glide
5. Frontal lift
6. Parietal lift
7. Sphenoid compression and decompression
8. Temporal techniques: temporal wobble, finger in ear, temporal compression
9. TMJ compression and decompression
10. Still point (CV-4)

As you become skilled in these 10 basic steps, you can alter the order to better suit your professional style. After all, it's not the precise order that's important but the exact procedures and their applications. Once you understand what you're doing with the techniques and why, you can let the creativity of your spirit and hands guide you through the process.

CHAPTER SUMMARY

Few body structures have more influence over health than the central nervous system. And few body systems have more impact on the central nervous system than the soft tissues and fluid that protect the brain and spinal cord—the craniosacral system.

Every day we endure stresses and strains and our bodies absorb them. But the body can only handle so much before it finally reaches the tipping point. Then tissues can tighten and compromise the function of the craniosacral system and nearly every other system in the body.

CranioSacral Therapy is a very gentle approach that releases these tensions in and around the central nervous system so the body can relax and self-correct. Using a gentle touch—starting at about the weight of a nickel—you can effectively evaluate the internal environment for any restrictions that may be affecting the craniosacral system. Then you can use distinctive light-touch techniques to release any tensions you find.

By freeing the central nervous system to perform at its best, CranioSacral Therapy naturally eliminates pain and stress, strengthens resistance to disease, and enhances general health and well-being. It's deeply relaxing, performed with the client fully clothed on a comfortable massage table. And because it's so gentle, it's effective for all ages, from newborns to elders.

"Many people have a belief that life is difficult and healing is painful. CranioSacral Therapy helps them let go of that belief. The healing process can be much more gentle and subtle."

- Scott, Abbeville, LA

CASE HISTORIES

■ Case history 1: Mighty Joe defies the odds

By most doctors' accounts, this is a little boy who shouldn't be here. He was born on October 15, 1998, with arthrogryposis, an extreme case of congenital joint contractures. His condition had been diagnosed through a level-two ultrasound while he was still in the womb. "Doctors first told me he had trisomy 18," said his mother, a longtime critical care nurse and lactation consultant. Trisomy 18 indicates the presence of an extra chromosome, which creates a condition normally incompatible with life. Doctors advised her and her husband to immediately terminate the pregnancy. Instead they decided to fall back on their faith, a choice they believed had served them well in the prior births of four healthy children. She simply refused further prenatal testing.

It turned out the doctors were wrong about much of the child's diagnosis. This was the first of many ways they would underestimate the spirited little boy who became known as Mighty Joe. As expected, Joe was born with severely contracted, hardened limbs. "He looked like a pretzel," his mother said. "His arms were straight and hard. His elbows weren't discernible. His wrists were bent in full flexion and his fingers were completely crippled. On top of that his feet were flipped up."

Fortunately, he didn't have the trisomy 18 doctors had diagnosed, and his other vital signs were all healthy. He cried heartily, sucked strongly, and scored high on both Apgar tests. Yet all those positive signs barely softened the blow of the overwhelming obstacles now facing Joe and his family. "Right away doctors told me his arms were paralyzed and he'd need at least seven surgeries," his mother

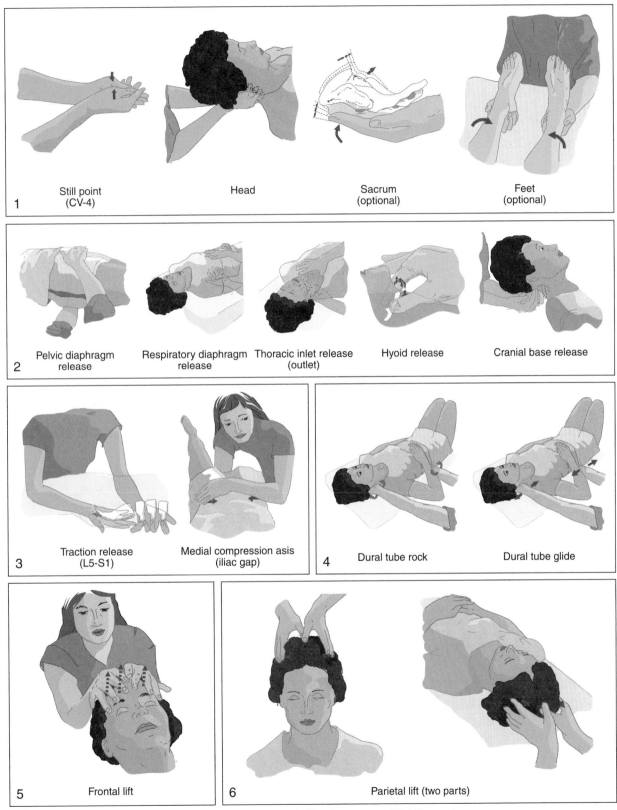

1 Still point (CV-4) Head Sacrum (optional) Feet (optional)

2 Pelvic diaphragm release Respiratory diaphragm release Thoracic inlet release (outlet) Hyoid release Cranial base release

3 Traction release (L5-S1) Medial compression asis (iliac gap)

4 Dural tube rock Dural tube glide

5 Frontal lift

6 Parietal lift (two parts)

FIGURE 4-9 10-step protocol. (Drawing courtesy of Tad Wanveer.)

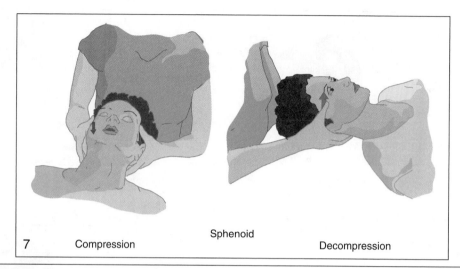

7   Compression   Sphenoid   Decompression

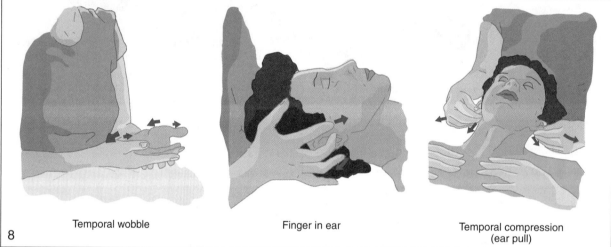

8   Temporal wobble   Finger in ear   Temporal compression (ear pull)

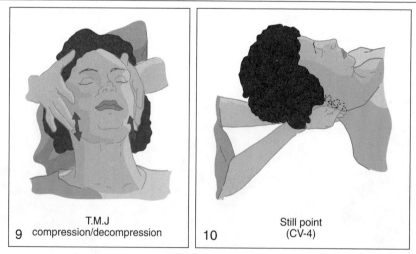

9   T.M.J compression/decompression   10   Still point (CV-4)

FIGURE 4-9 cont'd

said. "They even suggested a drastic move that would fix one arm in a state of flexion so he could feed himself. Then they wanted to permanently place his other arm down to accommodate his toiletry."

Two leading Chicago specialists confirmed this course of treatment, acknowledging it would leave Joe severely handicapped. While both parents agreed to foot surgery for Joe to avoid long-term use of leg braces, they were reluctant to take such radical steps with his arms and hands. That's when his mother got the idea to pursue another form of therapy she had heard about.

"I had taken a board-certified lactation course before Joe was born," she said. "The instructor mentioned something called CranioSacral Therapy for suck disorders. I had no idea if it would help in Joe's case, but I read up on it and thought it couldn't hurt." So when Joe was 5 months old, she took him to a CranioSacral Therapist in their Wisconsin hometown. "After the first session he started moving his fingers and his arm muscles softened a bit," she said.

Encouraged, she then brought Joe to see me when I was in their area teaching a symposium. After examining Joe, I told her that I felt he would regain full use of his arms and hands. How did Joe's surgeon react to the news? "He just laughed," his mother said.

Refusing to be discouraged, she brought Joe to The Upledger Clinic in Palm Beach Gardens, Florida. He received 3 days of concentrated CranioSacral Therapy from staff clinicians Roy Desjarlais, LMT, CST-D, and Rebecca Flowers, OTR, BCP, CST-D. "We did a lot of dural tube mobilization to free up the spinal cord segmentally as well as globally," Roy said of his sessions with Mighty Joe. "His nerve roots were then able to relax and work more efficiently, which in turn facilitated releases in the contractures in his hips and elbows.

"We also balanced his reticular alarm and autonomic nervous systems to help free up the cranial membranes. And there were significant sessions releasing the maxilla and vomer that helped with Joe's cranial base, brain stem, and again, his alarm system. Of course all the work helped facilitate fluid exchange between Joe's central nervous system and the rest of his body, which did a great deal to increase body efficiency overall."

"The change was dramatic," his mother said. "Joe's whole body posture and physical appearance changed. His face filled out. He started obtaining more range of motion in his wrist joints and elbows, and he was moving all his fingers." Back home a week later Joe began bringing his arms and hands to his face to play peekaboo, and he was finally using a sippy cup on his own. "Our whole family celebrated," she said.

Since his first visit, Joe has been to The Upledger Clinic once again and has seen other therapists for ongoing CST. His mother said Joe can now feed himself, color with crayons, and cut with scissors. And the doctors no longer suggest surgery. Indeed, Joe has already gone far beyond what anyone had predicted. "He's an incredible little child," she said. "He's very intelligent with an extensive vocabulary. He's also loving and kind and very, very sensitive. He's just a wonderful person."

Yet his mother concurs Mighty Joe's biggest strength may well be his will to fight. "Despite all the odds, he's pulled through," she said. And what lesson has she taken from all this? "No matter what body or mind we are given," she said, "that soul is precious and vital. You can't devalue that perfectness in any person, any living being. That's what I've learned that's profound."[12]

■ Case history 2: 21-year-old enters adulthood pain-free

The smile on the client's face spoke volumes beyond her simple words: "I've had pain for 12 years and now it's gone." With that one look, the tall, soft-spoken 21-year-old conveyed all the hope of someone given a new chance in life—the first, really, for her.

Since the age of 8, the client had lived at the mercy of reflexive sympathetic dystrophy (RSD), a neurologic syndrome brought on, in her case, from a simple fall while roller skating. Little explanation can be offered as to why she developed a life-altering condition from such a common childhood mishap. Little beyond "the right set of circumstances all colliding together," as she put it.

The pain began in her left foot about 2 days after the accident. A deep, persistent, on-fire kind of pain. The orthopedic doctor her parents took her to thought it was a sprain and put her in an air cast for 6 weeks. "The worst thing you can do," she said. Casting and immobilization can actually worsen the symptoms of RSD. "My skin got a silvery sheen and was blue and purple."

A family friend who was a nurse practitioner recognized her problem for what it was and recommended a doctor in the pain-management clinic where she worked. Tests there and at Shand's Children's Hospital finally brought the correct diagnosis of RSD—a condition that, unfortunately, has no known remedy.

She found some relief during her teen years. "I was able to be in the marching band and on the swim team," she said. Then she started college, where she tried to do too much. The RSD flared up with a vengeance, spreading for the first time up to her left hand. In a 4-month span she went through seven lumbar punctures, two rhizotomies (where they severed the sympathetic ganglion nerves), and an epidural catheter that left her paralyzed from the waist down for 11 days. That's when a friend of her mom's recommended CranioSacral Therapy at The Upledger Clinic. It had helped her with her TMJ problem, so she thought she might find some relief as well.

In a 2 week intensive program, she was found to have severe restrictions of her intracranial membrane system and dural tube, a compromised craniosacral system, and severe imbalances in her autonomic nervous system and myofascia. During the course of therapy, "I knew something was going on inside me," she said. "There were times I forgot my methadone. And methadone is a drug that's really hard to forget to take because of the withdrawal symptoms and the pain that comes right back." By the end of the program her pain had improved enough that she was able to go back to school.

Then in January 2002 she faced another setback when she contracted encephalitis. Once again the correct diagnosis was slow in coming. A neurologist, an infectious disease specialist, and a rheumatologist all concluded that her condition was a complication of the RSD and medication. "They automatically assumed it was the RSD and was psychosomatic," she recalled. In April another neurologist finally confirmed the problem was encephalitis. She stepped up her appointments at The Upledger Clinic, coming at least twice a week and going through another week-long intensive program. Finally, in December, "everything started to get better," she said. Though she readily admitted it was a tough process.

"There were times when I got very discouraged, wondering if this was even working. It took a good year to recover from the encephalitis, and I'm still feeling some of the effects. Especially when I'm under stress, I get very tired and the pain in my foot comes back. But I'm pain-free most days of the week now, which actually is a weird feeling. I honestly didn't remember life without pain."

Tad Wanveer, LMBT, CST-D, worked on the client for her official last appointment. "What a difference," he observed. "She shows a high level of improvement and balance of the areas in which she initially presented. It's wonderful to see this extremely courageous, intelligent, and sensitive young woman able to go back and live her life."

Living her life is exactly what she began doing. "I have a lot more focus, and I'm more sure about what I want to do," she said. "One of my goals is to run a triathlon, which I would never have been able to do. I've never been able to run even a quarter of a mile. I'm also graduating from community college and going to college in Ft. Myers for their premed program." From there she wants to go to Kirksville College of Osteopathy.

Laughing, she said, "I have a twin sister and we've always been very competitive. Right now she's up in Tennessee going to school. She's a chemistry major with a biology minor and I'll be a biology major with a chemistry minor. During the summers she works for a big pharmaceutical company, and she's been gearing all her research toward finding a cure for pain. I keep telling her, "It's right in front of your eyes!'"

The sparkle in her own eyes revealed that she's anxious for the chance to prove her point. "A year ago I didn't even know if I'd get this far. I didn't even know if I'd graduate with my AA degree," she recounted. "I look at everything as a gift. I have my life back now. And it's a lot better life than I had before."[13]

SUGGESTED READINGS

Ash D: *Lessons from the sessions: reflections of journeys in CranioSacral Therapy*, Rochester, NH, 2005.

Leskowitz E, ed: *Complementary and alternative medicine in rehabilitation*, Oxford, 2002, Churchill Livingstone.

Upledger JE: *A brain is born: exploring the birth and development of the central nervous system*, Berkeley, Calif, 1996, North Atlantic Books.

Upledger JE: *Cell talk*, Berkeley, Calif, 2003, North Atlantic Books.

Upledger JE: *CranioSacral Therapy: touchstone for natural healing*, Berkeley, Calif, 2001, North Atlantic Books.

Upledger JE: *CranioSacral Therapy II: beyond the dura*, Vista, Calif, 1990, Eastland Press.

Upledger JE: *SomatoEmotional release and beyond*, Palm Beach Gardens, Fla, 1990, UI Publishing.

Upledger JE: *SomatoEmotional release: deciphering the language of life*, Berkeley, Calif, 2002, North Atlantic Books.

Upledger JE: *Working wonders: changing lives with CranioSacral Therapy*, Berkeley, Calif, 2005, North Atlantic Books.

Upledger JE: *Your inner physician and you*, Berkeley, Calif, 1997, North Atlantic Books.

Upledger JE, Vredevoogd JD: *CranioSacral Therapy*, Vista, Calif, 1983, Eastland Press.

RESOURCES

The Upledger Institute
www.upledger.com
1-800-233-5880
561-622-4334
11211 Prosperity Farms Rd., D-325
Palm Beach Gardens, FL 33418

The Upledger Clinic
www.upledgerclinic.com
561-622-4706
11211 Prosperity Farms Rd., D-223
Palm Beach Gardens, FL 33418

Your True-Calling Coach™
Supporting CranioSacral Therapists who want full and prosperous practices.
www.craniosacralsuccess.com
561-746-2273

REFERENCES

1. Retzlaff EW et al: Nerve fibers and endings in cranial sutures research report, *J Am Osteopath Assoc* 77:474-5, 1978.
2. Retzlaff EW et al: *Possible functional significance of cranial bone sutures*, report, 88th Session American Association of Anatomists, 1975.
3. Retzlaff EW et al: Structure of cranial bone sutures, research report, *J Am Osteopath Assoc* 75:607-8, 1976.
4. Retzlaff EW et al: Sutural collagenous and their innervation in saimiri sciurus, *Ana Rec* 187:692, 1977.
5. Retzlaff EW, Mitchell FL Jr: *The cranium and its sutures*, Berlin, 1987, Springer-Verlag.
6. Sperino G: *Anatomica Humana* 1:202-203, 1931.
7. Upledger JE, Vredevoogd J: *CranioSacral Therapy*, Seattle, Calif, 1983, Eastland Press.
8. Upledger, JE: *Craniosacral Therapy II: beyond the dura*, Seattle, Calif, 1987, Eastland Press.
9. Upledger, JE: *SomatoEmotional release and beyond*, Palm Beach Gardens, Fla, 1990, UI Publishing.
10. Upledger JE: Releasing the energy cyst, *Massage Today* 3 (serial online): www.massagetoday.com.
11. Upledger JE: The relationship of craniosacral examination findings in grade school children with developmental problems, *J Am Osteopath Assoc* 77:760-769, 1978.
12. Upledger JE: Mighty Joe defies the odds, *Massage Today* 2 (serial online): www.massagetoday.com.
13. Upledger JE: 21-Year-Old looks forward to pain-free adulthood, *Massage Today* 4 (serial online): www.massage today.com.

MULTIPLE CHOICE TEST QUESTIONS

1) Describe the basic anatomy of the craniosacral system:
   a) the skull, face, and mouth down to the sternum
   b) the skull, face, and mouth down to the dorsum of the feet
   c) the skull, face, and mouth down to the sacrum and coccyx, and the brain and spinal cord contained within
   d) the skull, face, and mouth down to the sacroiliac joints

2) What is the core intent behind releasing or mobilizing the craniosacral system?
   a) to relieve the symptoms associated with pain and dysfunction
   b) to trigger/facilitate self-healing
   c) to help the client feel taller and less tense
   d) to help the cranium widen and soften

3) What is fascia?
   a) the outermost tissue of the craniosacral system
   b) the outermost tissue of the viscera
   c) the membrane just under the dura mater
   d) one piece of continuous connective tissue in the body that covers and connects every structure in the body

4) What is the Pressurestat Model based on?
   a) cerebrospinal fluid pressure and volume rising and falling
   b) lymph fluid pressure and volume rising and falling
   c) blood fluid pressure and volume rising and falling
   d) general circulation patterns throughout the body

5) What is directly affected if the craniosacral system is imbalanced?
   a) hormone level
   b) muscle tension
   c) all aspects of the central nervous system
   d) metabolism

6) How is CST different from most conventional medicine?
   a) CST is cause-focused while most conventional medicine is symptom-focused.
   b) CST always involves more than one practitioner at a time.
   c) CST practitioners take a more thorough medical history before an initial session.
   d) CST is symptom-focused while most conventional medicine is cause-focused.

7) Why is gentle palpation more effective than heavy palpation when evaluating the body?
   a) It allows you to tune in to one body system at a time.
   b) It's easier on the hands, enabling you to spend more time on each client.
   c) It helps you find areas on the skin that indicate a lesion deeper in the body.
   d) It allows you to explore the full range of structures without eliciting a defensive reaction from the client or the client's body.

8) What benefit do you get by evaluating the CSR throughout the body?
   a) You can get specific information on how well the lymph fluid is circulating.
   b) You can get specific information as to how well the body is functioning.
   c) You can get specific information on how well the blood is circulating.
   d) You can get specific information on how well the upper extremities are functioning.

9) What are listening stations and why are they helpful?
   a) The ears. They allow you to hear what's going on deep in the body.
   b) The viscera. They allow you to tune into the effects of the craniosacral motion on organ function.
   c) The heels, dorsums of the feet, anterior thighs, anterior superior iliac spines, ribs, shoulders, and the cranium. These areas can quickly give you a general evaluation of the CS motion.
   d) The cranium. This is the most direct route into the craniosacral system.

10) What is an active lesion?
   a) an open wound
   b) waves of interference energy superimposed over normal subtle motions in the body commonly caused by trauma or injury
   c) any area of the body that is hot to the touch
   d) any tissue change that occurs as the client is undergoing a still point

11) What are the benefits of a still point?
   a) It has an overall therapeutic effect on the central nervous system and the entire body. Some benefits are relief from headache and muscle pain, reduced stress, a deep state of relaxation, and an overall sense of well-being.
   b) It helps reduce congestion.
   c) It assists with hormonal imbalances.
   d) It helps reduce inflammation.

12) Describe the motion of CranioSacral flexion and extension in the body and cranium.
   a) Flexion in the body: internal rotation. Flexion in the cranium: narrowing. Extension in the body: external rotation. Extension in the cranium: widening.
   b) Flexion in the body: external rotation. Flexion in the cranium: widening. Extension in the body: internal rotation. Extension in the cranium: narrowing.
   c) Flexion in the body: tightening of the muscles. Flexion in the cranium: tightening of the sutures. Extension in the body: releasing of the muscles. Extension in the cranium: releasing of the sutures.
   d) Flexion in the body: lengthening of the extremities. Flexion in the cranium: narrowing. Extension in the body: tightening of the extremities. Extension in the cranium: widening.

13) How would a practitioner induce a still point?
   a) by holding the client's heels very still
   b) by holding the client's head very still
   c) by pressing gently on the sternum
   d) by resisting either the flexion or extension phase of body movement until the CSR stops

14) What are the potential long-term effects of an energy cyst?
   a) The soft tissues will become fibrotic around the energy cyst, making it impossible to remove.
   b) The cyst could erupt, causing an open wound that doesn't heal easily.
   c) The body will need extra energy to continue to accommodate the energy cyst, which ultimately creates a "drag" on overall function.
   d) Memory will decrease.

15) What is a facilitated segment?
   a) any segment of the musculoskeletal system involved in inflammation
   b) hyperactivity/hyperirritability of a spinal cord segment
   c) a segment of the body that has reached a still point
   d) an area of soft tissue that has experienced a release

16) How is the significance detector useful therapeutically?
   a) to determine nutritional deficiencies
   b) to understand when a CranioSacral Therapy session is complete
   c) to help you decide where to start working on the client's body
   d) to indicate when the client's body is involved in an important process (the CSR stops, suddenly indicating a thought or position that's important to explore)

17) How might body positioning be important in a CST session?
   a) Sometimes a client's body needs to recreate the position it was in when a trauma occurred in order to release the energy and/or restrictions.
   b) The client needs to feel fully relaxed in order for a session to proceed.
   c) When a client can maintain a tense position, the potential for release is greater.
   d) Body position has no significance in a CranioSacral session.

18) What is a tissue release?
    a) The muscles contract before softening and lengthening.
    b) The dura mater unwinds.
    c) Generally, any change in the tissue is a release. Commonly there is softening, lengthening, heat, and other subtle indications of release.
    d) The tissue remains the same.

19) Name some common conditions that can be helped by CST.
    a) emphysema and other lung-related issues
    b) pain syndromes, headaches and migraines, TMJ dysfunction, and central nervous system disorders
    c) genetic anomalies
    d) broken bones and open wounds

20) What is the overall contraindication for CST?
    a) children under the age of 7 and adults over the age of 80
    b) smoking and drinking alcoholic beverages
    c) anytime there is a concern about changing a client's intracranial pressure: for instance, in cases of hemorrhage, stroke, or recent skull fracture
    d) interleukin-2 hypersensitivity

Geriatric Massage

Susan G. Salvo

5

INTRODUCTION

The elderly are the fastest growing population in the country.[1-4] Worldwide, the number of people 65 or older is increasing faster than ever before.[4] Most of this increase is occurring in developed countries.[4] In the United States the percentage of people 65 or older increased from 3% in 1900 to about 34% in the late 1990s. Population experts estimate that more than 50 million Americans, about 17% of the population, will be 65 or older in 2020[5] (Box 5-1) (Figure 5-1).

The elderly present massage therapists with some unique challenges. There are the obvious physical changes such as thinning skin, reduced muscle mass, and vision and hearing impairments.[6] Sensorineural deficits and the effects of illness predispose the elderly to accidental injury.[5-7] In 2005 90% of the elderly reported having at least one chronic medical condition, most often managed with medications, so a thorough intake is crucial. This population faces many lifestyle and emotional changes such as retirement, reduced income, and the loss of loved ones.[6,8] To meet the challenges of this population segment, the therapist needs to cultivate patience, tolerance, caution, thoroughness, kindness, and attentiveness.[9]

Geriatric massage is a form of massage designed to meet the specific needs of the elderly population. The main consideration is the client's current health status and limitations, which determine adaptation measures such as avoidance of an area or elevation of the client's upper body to promote proper breathing.[10] By definition, **geriatrics** is the branch of medicine concerned with the diagnosis and treatment of old age.[5] Although massage therapists do not diagnose a prudent therapist takes into consideration all aspects of a client's health to arrive at an appropriate treatment plan.

At present, there are two main geriatric massage techniques: one taught by the Day-Break Geriatric Massage Institute and one taught by Comfort Touch. The original technique was developed by Dietrich Miesler, who founded the Day-Break Geriatric Massage Institute in 1986.

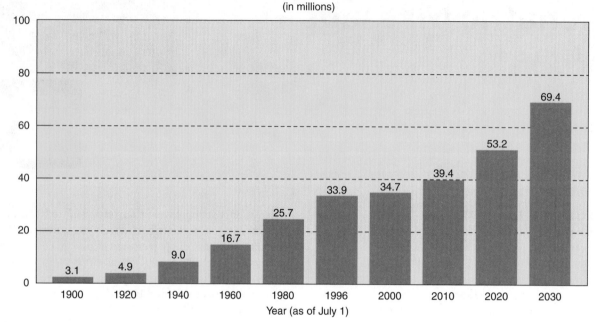

FIGURE 5-1 Population trends of persons 65 and older. (Courtesy AARP.)

According to data collected from the 2000 census, approximately half of the people 65 and older live in nine states. In order of size, they are California, Florida, New York, Texas, Pennsylvania, Ohio, Illinois, Michigan, and New Jersey. When looking at the number of elderly per capita, Florida leads the nation with 18% of its population over 65.[5]

Reported illness increases with age. In 2005, 90% of older persons reported having at least one chronic condition and the majority had multiple conditions. Among the most frequently occurring conditions were hypertension (48%), arthritis (47%), all types of heart disease (29%), cancer (20%), diabetes (16%), and sinusitis (14%).[5]

Reported disability increases with age. In 2002, 52% of older persons reported that they had some type of disability (sensory, physical, or mental). Some disabilities were minor while others required assistance to meet important personal needs. Almost 37% of older persons reported severe disabilities and 16% reported that they needed some type of assistance as a result. 57% of persons over 80 reported severe disabilities and 30% of the over-80 population reported that they needed assistance.

Data releases from the web sites of the National Center for Health Statistics: http://www.cdc.gov/nchs/ (including the Data Warehouse on Trends in Health and Aging: http://www.cdc.gov/nchs/datawh.htm); the Agency for Healthcare Research and Quality: http://www.ahrq.gov/; and the Bureau of Labor Statistics: http://www.bls.gov/.

It is essentially traditional massage adapted to the aging population. There are a few unique techniques, such as fluffing, which takes into account the thinning skin of the senior and circulatory issues. After retirement in 1996, Miesler passed his ownership to Sharon Puszko, who worked and studied with him for a number of years and remains the Institute's owner director. Dietrich Miesler died in May 2006.

The second technique, Comfort Touch, was developed by Mary Kathleen Rose. After graduating from massage school in 1985, she began working with HospiceCare. By 1991, she was teaching her form of massage and coined the phrase Comfort Touch. This nurturing form of acupressure, which avoids conventional massage in favor of broad perpendicular pressure, was consistent with hospice's philosophy of palliative care.

Another technique, called Compassionate Touch, is very similar in theory and practice to Comfort Touch. Dawn Nelson, its founder, started her outreach program in San Mateo in 1991, the same year Comfort Touch was introduced. In this modality, verbal interaction is not necessary. Nelson published a book in 2001 titled *From the Heart Through the Hands: The Power of Touch in Caregiving.*

In this chapter, we will explore both the challenges and the many rewards of working with the elderly. All references to massage will be to that of adapted traditional Swedish, as it is the most widely used method.

Comparing Geriatric Massage to Swedish Massage

Geriatric massage takes into account the needs and challenges of the aging. Swedish strokes are adapted to reduce damage to the skin, so pressure and shearing is reduced.

The client position is adapted to the needs of the elderly as well, favoring seated, supine, or side lying. Many conditions, such as advanced osteoporosis or breathing difficulties, make the prone position unsuitable for the elderly.

Treatment time is generally shorter, usually no longer than 30 minutes, as treatments longer in length may fatigue the elderly. However, the elderly frequently need more time to get on and off the table, get undressed and redressed, or go to the toilet. The shorter treatment time reduces the cost of a massage, making it more affordable for elderly clients.Additionally, many massage therapists offer discounts to elderly clients because most are living on fixed incomes.

WHAT IS OLD AGE?

Old age is regarded as nearing the end of the average life span of human beings. Today, average life expectancy is around 77.[5] The longest documented human life span is 122 years (Jeanne Calment, Arles, France, 1875-1997).

The baby boomers are those persons born after WWII, between 1946 and 1964.[11] This group constitutes approximately one third of the American population today.[5] Because of its size, this groups has had and will continue to have a big influence on our society. The oldest baby boomers are now in their 60s.[11]

Senescence refers to the period of life from old age to death.[12] When is someone old? Webster defines old as "having lived or existed for a long time."[5] Although chronological age, the number of years lived, is the easiest to identify and measure, it is the least meaningful measurement of aging.[5] Just as there are no typical 30-year-olds, there are no typical 70-year-olds. An elderly person can be quite active and independent, living without assistance with their activities of daily living (Figure 5-2). Some require assistance accomplishing various daily activities and may live at home or in an assisted living facility. Others can be frail and cannot function without skilled help; most of the latter are found in long-term care facilities, and the rest are often at home with family or caregivers.[13]

So how do the elderly view themselves? Bernard Baruch, on his 85th birthday said that "Old age is fifteen

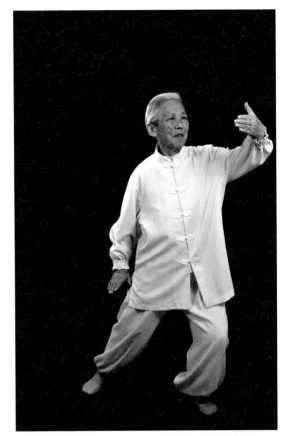

FIGURE 5-2 An elderly person can be quite active and independent, living without assistance with activities of daily living. (Courtesy David L. Frazier, 1999.)

years older than I am." That quote is very true, especially when you consider a recent study that revealed people younger than 30 view people 63 as getting older. People 65 and older do not think people are getting older until they are 75.[5]

Even though membership with American Association of Retired Persons (AARP) is open to persons 50 years of age and older, most Americans consider 65 to be the beginning of old age.[14] This is most likely because United States workers become eligible to retire with full Social Security benefits at age 65. When the New Deal politicians established the Social Security program in the 1930s, they set the age at which benefits could be collected at 65. Life expectancy at that time was 63.[5] If the same standards were applied today, retirement age would be 79.

People in the 65-and-over age group are often called **senior citizens.** The age at which a person becomes eligible for full Social Security benefits will increase gradually until it reaches age 67 in 2027. In Western societies, everybody is declared to be "old" when they reach the age of 65 and secure their pension entitlement.

How does this relate to massage? Sixty-five years old is the age at which the massage therapist begins to take into account the aging process and how it might have affected a client's body. Although each client is assessed individually, there are most often physical changes that might affect massage treatment. Next, we will look at the aging process.

THE AGING PROCESS

The branch of study concerned with normal aging is **gerontology.** Although aging is poorly understood, the differences between a younger person and an older person are easily noted. Aging is a physiologic process that is universal, progressive, inevitable, irreversible, and decremental. There is no single factor responsible for the aging; the process is unique to each person.

There are many theories as to why we age, but two gerontologic hypotheses predominate: the *wear and tear theory* and the *genetic theory*.[15] Because cells are the basic units of life, it is believed that cellular aging is the beginning of the decline and is the result of gradual wear and tear.[16] Changes (or atrophy) in our skin, our nervous system, and our organs are the result of dysfunctions at the cellular level.[17] This is the basis of the wear and tear theory. However, not all people wrinkle at the same age. This is the basis of the genetic theory. One can see how they both have value.

One perspective gaining in popularity is the *free radical theory*. It states that free radicals (byproducts of metabolism) accumulate and damage cell membranes, which decreases their efficiency. When free radicals kill or damage enough cells in an organism, the organism ages.[4] The body also contains antioxidants, which scavenge free radicals, slowing or reducing cell damage. Antioxidant production increases with physical activity and with the consumption of certain nutrients (vitamins C and E and coenzyme Q_{10}), and its supply is reduced by disease and environmental pollutants.

It is important to separate the irreversible process of aging from the often reversible processes of disease. Many physiologic and structural changes are a normal part of aging, such as those seen in joints, blood vessel walls, and the brain. When these normal aging processes become significant enough to cause a health disability, we regard them as diseases (e.g., arthritis, atherosclerosis, or Alzheimer's disease). Some disease processes accelerate aging and aging predisposes a person to some diseases because older people have limited regenerative abilities. Even with the absence of disease, a person's fragility increases with age, leaving a person vulnerable to falls (Box 5-2).[5,18]

BOX 5-2 Fall Risk Factors for Elders

Anxiety
Area rugs
Confusion, dementia
Decreased vision or hearing
Depression
Disability in lower extremities
Electrical cords
Foot problems
General clutter
Glossy, waxed floors
High massage tables
Hip or knee replacements
Inadequate lighting
Inadequate or missing safely rails
Mobility devices
Problems with balance and gait
Recent illness
Sedatives and antidepressants
Severe chronic illness
Skeletal and neuromuscular changes that predispose to weakness and postural instability
Unsteadiness, dizziness
Women 75+

From, Ebersole P, Hess P, Schmidt Luggen A: *Toward healthy aging, human needs and nursing response,* ed 7, St Louis, 2008, Mosby.

Some of the diseases that occur more frequently in the elderly are arthritis and hypertension.[17] Both are seen in almost 50% of elderly. The therapist must be aware of the possibility and frequency of **orthostatic hypotension** (OH, or **postural hypotension**) related to medications taken for these health concerns.[13] OH is addressed in the section on Treatment Guidelines. Changes in the skeletal and urinary systems predispose many elderly women to osteoporosis and to urinary incontinence (Box 5-3). Cerebral changes increase the likelihood of Alzheimer's disease.[14] In fact, from 65 to 85, incidences double about every 5 years.[4] Roughly 9% of seniors reported having problems with balance and coordination.[4] Cataracts, glaucoma, macular degeneration, and diabetic retinopathy are the most common problems of aging eyes, and hearing impairment increases with age as 1 in 3 people older than 60, and half of all people older than 85, have significant hearing loss[14] (Box 5-4). However, as common as some disease is with the elderly, old age is not synonymous with disease.[4]

BOX 5-3 Risk Factors for Urinary Incontinence

Age
Dementia
Diabetes
Environmental barriers
Estrogen deficiency
High caffeine intake
High-impact physical exercise
Hysterectomy in older women
Immobility
Low fluid intake
Medications such as sedatives and diuretics
Obesity
Past pregnancy
Pelvic muscle weakness
Smoking
Stroke

From, Ebersole P, Hess P, Schmidt Luggen A: *Toward healthy aging, human needs and nursing response,* ed 7, St Louis, 2008, Mosby.

BOX 5-4 Suggestions for Working with Elders Who Are Visually or Hearing Impaired

- Keep in mind that there are many degrees of impairment.
- Access your position in relation to the individual. One eye or ear may be better than the other.
- When in the presence of a visually impaired person, speak promptly and clearly, identify yourself and others with you. State when you are leaving to make sure the person is aware of your departure.
- Make sure you have the individual's attention before you start talking.
- Listen attentively and avoid interrupting or finishing his or her sentences.
- If you are having difficulty understanding the client, repeat what you understood, and allow him or her time to respond.
- Speak descriptively of your surroundings and state the position of the people in the room.
- Speak normally but not from a distance; do not raise or lower your voice, and continue to use gestures if that is natural to your communication. Do not alter your vocabulary; words such as see, hear, blind, and deaf are part of normal speech. When others are present, address the client by prefacing remarks with his or her name or a light touch on the arm.
- Try to minimize the number of distractions.

(Continued)

- Use the analogy of a clock face to help a visually impaired person locate objects.
- Check to see that the best possible lighting is available.
- Try to keep the individual between you and the window; you will appear as a dark shadow. This makes lip reading difficult.
- Speak and gesture before handing a visually or hearing impaired person an object.
- When walking with a visually impaired person, offer your arm. Pause before stairs or curbs; mention them. In seating, place the person's hand on the back of the chair.
- Visually impaired people like to know the beauty around them. Describe flowers, scenery, colors, and textures. Elderly people most frequently have been sighted and can enjoy memories of beauty stimulated by descriptive conversations.
- Be careful about labeling an impaired person as confused.
- Assist client with intake form.
- Replace eye wear that is removed for massage.
- Avoid scheduling evening sessions if visually impaired client is driving himself or herself.

Adapted from Ebersole P, Hess P, Touhy T, Jett K: *Gerontological nursing and healthy aging,* ed 2, St Louis, 2005, Mosby; Smith S, Gove J: Physical changes of aging, available online at http://www.edis.ifas.ufl.edu/HE019.

Elderly make up the largest consumers of prescription and over-the-counter medications[7,19] (Box 5-5). According to the Food and Drug Administration (FDA), senior citizens purchase 30% of prescription drugs and 40% of over-the-counter drugs.

Table 5-1 lists many of the body systems' physiologic changes associated with aging, the functional effects of those change, and their implications for the therapist. Use Table 5-1 to cross-reference treatment guidelines for the elderly featured later in the chapter.

BOX 5-5 Most Commonly Used Medications by the Elderly: In Order of Use

Cardiovascular agents
Antihypertensives
Analgesics
Antiarthritic agents
Sedatives
Tranquilizers
Laxatives
Antacids

Adapted from Eliopoulos C: *Manual of gerontologic nursing,* ed 2, Mosby, 1999, St Louis.

TABLE 5-1 Body Systems and Massage Implications

Body System	Physiologic Change	Functional Effect	Massage Implications
Integumentary	Skin loses elasticity and becomes thinner and more frail; wrinkling and sagging are evident	Tears easily, heals more slowly than when younger; bedridden clients are more prone to pressure sores	Reduce pressure and shearing, avoid lesions; bring any sores to attention of client or caregiver
	Decreased subcutaneous fat	Reduced temperature regulation; increased risk of injuries and bruising from weakened support of blood vessels	Keep clients warm with blankets
	Reduced glandular activity (sudoriferous and sebaceous)	Rough, dry, flaky, and itchy skin (xerosis), reduced temperature regulation	Use quality lubricants, keep clients warm with blankets or use a cool washcloth on the forehead or back of neck
	Increased pigmentation	Presence of irregular moles, precancerous and cancerous lesions, keratosis, and liver spots on sun-exposed areas such as arms and face	Avoid suspicious areas and open lesions
	Reduced number of hair follicles	Hair thins and grays	Nonapplicable
	Nails grow slowly	Nails may be thick, rough, splitting; increased fungal infections	Avoid unhealthy nails
Respiratory	Rigidity of chest wall (ribs calcify and muscle tone is reduced) as seen in clients with kyphosis and osteoporosis	Reduced thoracic movement (chest expansion); reduced respiratory function and resultant decreased endurance	Use semireclining position; shorter treatment time
	Loss of lung tissue elasticity	Reduced lung capacity (17% between the ages of 50 and 70) and resultant decreased endurance	Use semireclining position; shorter treatment time
Cardiovascular	Thickening and narrowing of vascular lumen due to accumulation of cholesterol and fats	Decreased circulation, increased blood pressure, increased fatigue and instances of orthostatic hypotension	Shorter treatment time; elevate lower limbs; reduce times client changes positions and assist during the process
	Loss of vessel elasticity	Superficial capillaries break more easily	Reduce pressure and shearing
	Heart enlarged (cardiomyopathy)	Reduces cardiac output (increased CHF*) and increased instances of orthostatic hypotension	Reduce times client changes positions and assist during the process; avoid areas of pitting edema
	Decreased efficiently of venous return	Increased varicosities and blood clot formation in legs, especially in sedentary clients	Elevate legs; and avoid vigorous massage on legs reduce pressure
Gastrointestinal	Decreased saliva production	Dry mouth (xerostomia); medications may contribute to this	Offer water before and after massage
	Decreased gastric secretions and peristalsis	Slowed digestion and increased constipation	Use semireclining position; gently massage abdomen
	Decreased tone of sphincter muscles	Increased esophageal reflux and heartburn and fecal incontinence	Use semireclining position; allow client to remain clothed; adult diapers

TABLE 5-1   Body Systems and Massage Implications—cont'd

Body System	Physiologic Change	Functional Effect	Massage Implications
Musculoskeletal	Bone mass decreased	Bones become more porous, brittle, and fragile (after 60, women lose about 8% bone mass each decade; men lose about 3%); increased instances of osteoporosis and fractures (common fracture sites are the hip, ribs, clavicle, and arm)	Reduce pressure; ROM* and stretches should be avoided or cautiously applied
	Muscle mass decreased (correlated directly to decreased activity)	Decreased strength and altered gait	Reduce pressure; provide unobstructed passage; allow more time for client activities
	Glycogen (fuel) stores in muscles are reduced	Decreased endurance and increased fatigue	Reduce treatment time; allow more time for client activities
	Changes in joint structures	Articular cartilage erodes and synovial fluid becomes fibrotic; decreased mobility; altered gait	Reduce pressure; ROM* and stretches should be avoided or cautiously applied; provide unobstructed passage; allow more time for client activities
	Intervertebral discs dehydrate and narrow	Creates spinal changes such as decreased height and flexed position of kyphosis (osteoporosis may be a cause of this deformity); altered gait	Use semireclining position; ROM* and stretches should be avoided or cautiously applied; provide unobstructed passage; allow more time for client activities
	Elastic fibers in connective tissue degenerate (correlated directly to decreased activity)	Reduced flexibility	Use gentle joint rocking
Neurologic	Nerve cell degeneration and decrease in cerebral blood flow (about 20% between 50-80)	Reduced response time and decreased reflexes; loss or increased sensitivity to pain, which increases injury risk; decreased tolerance to heat or cold; decreased balance and coordination; altered gait	Reduce pressure; shorter treatment time; provide unobstructed passage; allow more time for client activities; provide a warm blanket or cool washcloth on forehead and back of neck
	Decrease in neurotransmitter production	Increased potential for dementing processes and other neurologic diseases	Reduce pressure; shorter treatment time; be tolerant of client's behavior which might change abrupty
Endocrine	Decreased T3* and T4* production	Decreased metabolic rate	Provide a warm blanket; shorter treatment time
	Female ovaries cease to respond to FSH* and LH* from the pituitary	Menopause; symptoms include hot flashes and periodic sweating	Non applicable
	Cessation of female ovulation	Reduces hormones levels of estrogen, which affects bone density	Reduce pressure; ROM* and stretches should be avoided or cautiously applied

Continued

TABLE 5-1	Body Systems and Massage Implications—cont'd		
Body System	**Physiologic Change**	**Functional Effect**	**Massage Implications**
Urinary	Decreased bladder capacity and incomplete bladder emptying	Urinary urgency and frequency	Suggest client use toilet before and after massage
	Decreased tone in sphincter muscles	Urinary (and fecal) incontinence	Suggest client use toilet before and after massage
Sensory	Pupils decreased in size and less light enters eyes	Decreased accommodations to near/far and to light/dark; impaired vision	See adaptive measures outlined in Box 5-4
	Walls of auditory canals thin, ear wax accumulates, and eardrums thicken	Impaired hearing	See adaptive measures outlined in Box 5-4

Data from Wold GH: *Basic geriatric nursing*, ed 4, St Louis, 2008, Mosby; Ebersole P, Hess P, Touhy T, Jett K: *Gerontological nursing and healthy aging*, ed 2, St Louis, 2005, Mosby; Ebersole P, Hess P, Schmidt Luggen A: *Toward healthy aging, human needs & nursing response*, ed 7, St Louis, 2008, Mosby; Gould BE: *Pathophysiology for the health professionals*, ed 3, Philadelphia, 2006, Saunders; Diego MA, Field T, Sanders C, Hernandez-Reif, M: Massage therapy of moderate and light pressure and vibrator effects on EEG and heart rate, *Int J Neurosci* 114:31-44, 2004; Beera MH, Berfow R: *Merck manual of geriatrics*, ed 3, Whitehouse Station, NJ, 2000, Merck Research Laboratories; Worfolk JB: Keep frail elders warm! *Geriatr Nurs* 1:7-11, 1997.

BENEFITS OF GERIATRIC MASSAGE

The following is a brief summary of the benefits of geriatric massage.[5,12,25,26]

- *Blood circulation*—Increases blood circulation, thus speeds healing of injury and illness
- *Lymph circulation*—Increases lymphatic circulation, thus reduces the edema of inactivity
- *Blood pressure*—Decreases blood pressure with increased relaxation
- *Depression*—Reduces depression with increased relaxation and reduced anxiety
- *Gastrointestinal*—Stimulates bowel activity and reduces constipation
- *Mobility*—Partially restores loss of mobility due to inactivity
- *Skin condition*—Improves condition of dry or cracked skin with lubricant use
- *Pain*—Reduces pain by stimulating touch and pressure receptors
- *Sleep*—Improves the quantity and quality of sleep by increasing relaxation and reducing anxiety
- *Vitality*—Increases vitality with reduced pain, increased mobility, and improved sleep
- *Relaxation*—Promotes mental and physical relaxation; deepens breathing; decreases fear and anxiety
- *Increased self-esteem*—Improves client's quality of life, self-esteem, and sense of well-being
- *Reduced isolation*—Decreases feelings of isolation as massage involves contact with another

We often view the elderly in our society as the untouchables. In a study by Barnett published in the *International Journal of Nursing Studies*, the age group touched the least in medical settings was 66 to 100 years of age.[27] However, "The use of touch and physical closeness may be the most important way to communicate to ill and aged persons that they are important as human beings," says Ashley Montagu, author of *Touching: The Human Significance of the Skin.*[28]

Research indicates that social connection is a key component to health and happiness in the elderly when receiving regular massage.[25] An ongoing relationship with a massage therapist can be a significant part of an elderly client's life as he or she knows that he or she will receive focused attention from a caring person.

TREATMENT GUIDELINES FOR THE ELDERLY

The following are simple guidelines to help the therapist provide pleasant and safe massage experiences for the elderly.

Thorough Intake

The purpose of older adult intake procedure is to evaluate the client's health status, both strengths and limitations, so that effective and appropriate massage can be delivered (Figure 5-3).[29] A thorough intake process creates a session that is both age-appropriate and condition-appropriate. Instruction in how to conduct an intake interview or devise a treatment plan is beyond the scope of this chapter, but the therapist should be mindful of a few important principles and items that need special consideration.

The first principle is to listen to the client. What the client has to say is more important than what the therapist

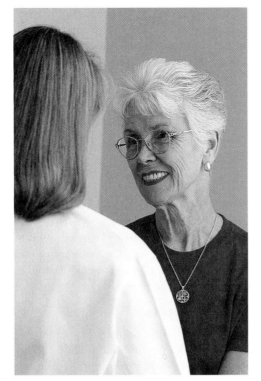

FIGURE 5-3 The purpose of a thorough intake is to evaluate the client's health status, both strengths and limitations.

has to say. Focus on the client's special needs and concerns. Use the interview to get acquainted with your client. This not only provides valuable information, but also eases client tension and anxiety and builds trust and rapport. Be sure you understand what the client is saying, and allow time for asking and answering questions. Most treatment decisions are determined by the needs of the client first and by his or her health status second (Box 5-6).[30]

Next, do not rush through the intake process. Seniors typically need more time to perform tasks, and there is often more medical information to document (see Box 5-1 and 5-5). While there are many elderly people who are in excellent health, approximately 90% of older people have a chronic illness[7] or medical condition that must be taken into consideration when performing the massage. Ask about surgeries that have occurred within the last five years. If applicable, ask why the surgery was needed, if it brought the desired results, and if there are any current problems associated with the past surgery.

Inquire about medications, both what kind and why they are prescribed. The therapist might wish to reference any unfamiliar medications to ascertain any side effects that might affect treatment, such as dizziness, drowsiness, and increased bruising. Additionally, many medications cause dry mouth. If this is the case, drinking water should be offered before and after massage and should be available throughout the massage.

Be sure you have the name and contact number of a family member or friend, in case of an emergency, as well as the client's primary care physician's name and contact number. Consult with the client's physician if questions arise about the client's condition.

Robust and Frail Seniors

Assess the client's vitality and vigor during the intake interview. Decide, based on the client's health status and activity level, if the client is more robust or frail.[31] Use Box 5-7 to help you in making these assessments. Active, robust seniors still experience body changes that accompany the aging process (see

---

BOX 5-6 The Lived Experience: Listen to the Aged

Listen to the aged for they will tell you about living and dying.

Listen to the aged for they will enlighten you about problem-solving, sexuality, grief, sensory deprivation, and survival.

Listen to the aged for they will teach you how to be courageous, loving, and generous.

They are a distinguished faculty without formal classrooms, tenure, sabbaticals. They teach not from books but from long experience in living.

Burnside IM: Listen to the aged, *Am J Nurs* 75:1801, 1975.

BOX 5-7 The CSHA* Clinical Fragility Scale

1) Very fit—robust, active, energetic, well motivated and fit; these people commonly exercise regularly and are in the most fit group for their age
2) Well—without active disease, but less fit than people in category 1
3) Well, with treated comorbid disease—disease symptoms are well-controlled compared with those in category 4
4) Apparently vulnerable—although not frankly dependent, these people commonly complain of being "slowed up" or having disease symptoms
5) Mildly frail—with limited dependence on others for instrumental activities of daily living
6) Moderately frail—help is needed with both instrumental and noninstrumental activities of daily living
7) Severely frail—completely dependent on others for the activities of daily living, or terminally ill

*Canadian Study of Health and Aging.

Table 5-1), but can benefit from a more traditional Swedish massage. Dry skin responds well to highly emollient creams, and the therapist has the opportunity to observe any skin changes while the client is draped on a massage table.

If the client is frail, he or she would benefit more from seated, side-lying, or supine positions while clothed (Figure 5-4). Traditional Swedish massage should be avoided in favor of broad, perpendicular acupressure (taught by Comfort Touch) and rocking and fluffing techniques (taught by Day-Break Institute). The purpose of the latter is to provide some mild form of exercise by gently moving the limbs. However, geriatric massage should not be used as a replacement for exercise. More than 70% of elderly are sedentary.[13,32]

Reducing Pressure

Because of the changes in aging skin, such as reduced elasticity and decreased subcutaneous fat, the elderly are more easily injured (Figure 5-5, *A* to *C*).[17] This necessitates reducing both downward pressure and shearing force of the hands sliding over the skin. Reduced pressure does not translate into a light massage. Maria Mathias, massage instructor and author, uses the phrase "gentle strength" when describing the reduced pressure.[33] Even with reduced pressure, strokes should still be firm and broad; use the entire palm surface of the hand.

Honor the client's request regarding deeper pressure by making immediate modifications, but return to a more appropriate and safer pressure. Puszko offers advice for working with the elderly who insist on deeper pressure. She recommends initially applying more pressure and asking, "Like this?" When you arrive at the depth the client accepts, continue for a few moments, and then return to the previous pressure. Most often, the client will state, "Now, that's more like it!"[34]

Stretching and Joint Movements

Include gentle stretching and joint movements such as rocking if the client feels up to it (Figure 5-6). Constantly monitor the client as these movements can be tiring for him or her. Avoid extreme spinal mobilizations (including the neck), which may harm the client in cases of increased bone porosity.

Shorter Sessions

To reduce the possibility of fatigue treatment time for elderly clients should be limited to about 30 minutes. Day-Break recommends a 5-minute introduction of unhurried effleurage, deep breathing, and gentle rocking; then, 20 minutes of focused work on the feet, legs, shoulder, or neck (client determined). This is followed by 5 minutes of closure work.[35]

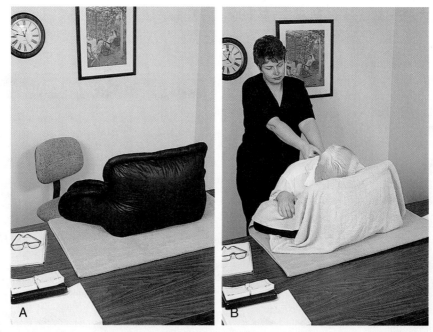

FIGURE 5-4 Seated massage may be more appropriate for the elderly client who may wish to remain clothed. **A,** A large cushion can be placed on a table or desk and draped with a cloth. **B,** The client leans on the cushion while the therapist stands behind the client to massage.

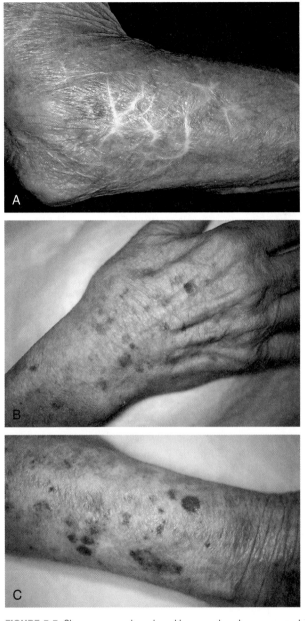

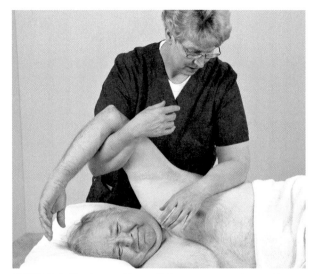

FIGURE 5-6 Gentle stretching and joint movement such as rocking are suitable for the elderly client.

FIGURE 5-5 Changes occur in aging skin, so reduced pressure and shearing force is needed to prevent skin injury. **A,** Skin thinning and atrophy on 80-year- old woman. **B,** Age spots (senile lentigines) seen on hand of 87-year-oldwoman. **C,** Bruising (senile purpura) seen on forearm of 90-year- old man.

Avoiding the Prone Position

Supine, seated, and side lying are the safest client positions for the elderly (Figure 5-7, also see Figure 5-4).[36] Many people are uncomfortable or have difficulty breathing while lying prone. Others have problems turning from supine to prone (or vice versa).

Note that medical facilities such as hospitals also avoid the prone position. To massage the back, ask the client to roll to one side if supine or to lean over slightly if seated.

Inspecting Feet

Physical limitations and visual impairments make is difficult for the elderly to inspect their feet.[14] Because foot problems are common in the elderly, the therapist can include feet inspection as part of the massage and offer valuable information to the client. If the client is wearing socks or slippers, obtain permission to remove them. Explain that you will inspect the feet before massage. Avoid any unhealthy or suspicions areas in the feet (including nails) (Figure 5-8).[12] Bring them to the attention of the client (or caregiver). Inspect, but do not use lubricant, between toes as lubricants may contribute to foot infection.[14] If any lubrication was used during the massage on healthy feet, carefully clean the feet of any traces of lubrication before moving on to the next area of the body. If socks or slippers were removed, replace them before moving to another area of the client's body.

Guard Against Chilling

Because of reduced metabolism and decreased subcutaneous fat, many elderly feel uncomfortably cold. Use heavy blankets over the client's sheet-draped or clothed body and if appropriate, an external heat source such as a portable heating unit.[14,22]

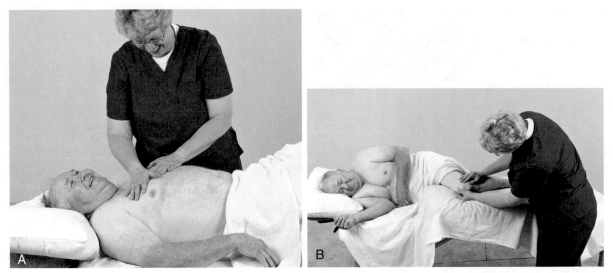

FIGURE 5-7 Supine (*image on left*), seated, and side lying (*image on right*) are the safest client positions for the elderly.

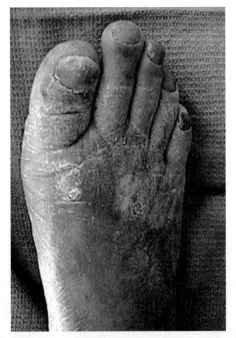

FIGURE 5-8 Avoid any unhealthy or suspicious areas in the feet (including nails). This image features the right foot of an elderly diabetic client with athlete's foot and nail fungus, which should not be massaged.

Appropriate Session Location and Time

The session location should suit the client, which means that massage might be performed at the client's residence rather than the therapist's office (Box 5-8). In

---

fact, the actual session may take place on the client's bed or sofa, especially if getting on and off the massage table is not safe for the client. Rarely is the floor a good place for massage as it may be difficult for the elderly to get up from the floor.[4]

Massage sessions should be scheduled at the safest time of the day for the client, such as during daylight hours if the client is driving to the therapist's office.[3]

Guard Against Falling

Falling is the most common safety issue for people 65 and older.[5] Several factors contribute to this. Many medications alter balance, coordination, and response time. Common examples of medications that contribute to these problems are antihistamines, sedatives, tranquilizers, hypnotics, diuretics, and antihypertensives.[4,5]

Decreased cardiac output can increase risk for dizziness (vertigo) or fainting (syncope).[17] Many elderly people experience a sudden drop in blood pressure when they move from a **recumbent** (lying down) position to an upright position, causing a loss of balance.[12] The clinical term for this is **orthostatic (postural) hypotension**. Studies have shown that over 50% of long-term nursing home residents older than 60 experience four or more episodes of orthostatic hypotension daily.[4]

To reduce the risk of falling, allow adequate time for the elderly client to change positions. If needed, assist the client in sitting or standing upright (Figure 5-9).

Since visual impairments are common in the elderly, most wear eyeglasses. These are often removed before massage. To reduce the risk of injury due to falling, replace eyeglasses immediately after treatment.

Be Patient and Reverent

The attitude in which a therapist approaches working with the elderly is often different from the approach taken with other clients. "This ain't sports massage," says Joan Lohman, a specialist in geriatric massage.[3] The therapist respects the client's slower pace rather than maximizing massage time. Schedule time in the appointment to allow for the client to undress (sometimes layers and layers of clothes have to come off); you may have to help him or her on and off the table. The client may need a time of transition after the massage or may want to share a story. If you watch and listen, you may become an honored witness to an earlier generation's wit and wisdom.

Every client will be different; every session will be different, even with a client seen every week. In Mitch Albom's best-seller *Tuesdays with Morrie,* Morrie tells Mitch that "Aging is not just decay, . . . It's growth. It's more than the negative that you're going to die, it's also the positive that you understand you're going to die and that you live a better life because of it (Figure 5-10)."[23] Each client will be in a different phase of this growth called aging. As stories are shared, some clients need to cry, some need to express anger, some need to complain, and others need to convey their fears. Provide the space for your clients to express their feelings with your attitude of compassion. Rose states that a therapist's "manner and presence are as important as the touch you give." A half hour of respectful, attentive touch helps your elderly client feel valued.[24]

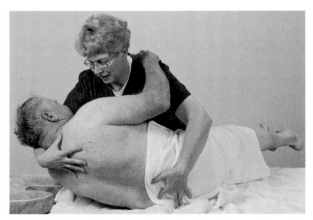

FIGURE 5-9 Be willing to assist the client in sitting up if needed. (Courtesy Anthony Iorio, DPM, MPH.)

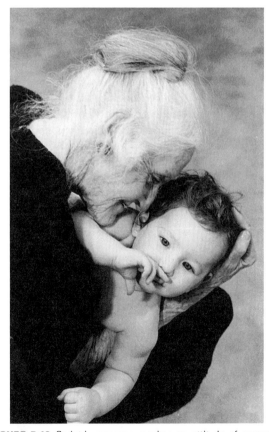

FIGURE 5-10 Geriatric massage requires an attitude of reverence for the elderly. (*From Wold GH:* Basic Geriatric Nursing, *ed 3, St. Louis, 2004, Mosby.*)

▮▮▮ IN MY EXPERIENCE

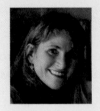

My most profound experience with geriatric massage was with a very special person, my grandmother. She began receiving massage when she was in her 80s. It was the mid-1990s and I had just completed my second training in Watsu (water shiatsu). The course addressed modifying the routine when working with the elderly. When I asked my grandmother about receiving massage in a pool of water, she seemed excited. I had located a suitable pool near my uncle's house and made arrangements to work with my grandmother there.

Since she no longer owned a swimsuit, my grandmother wore a white tee shirt and a pair of blue, jersey-knit shorts. As we approached the pool, I recall watching her walk; how her leg muscles moved under loose skin and how she glanced up to see where she was headed and then down at her feet. I reached out my hand as we stood at the top of the pool steps. She clasped it and the rail, and we slowly stepped down together into the warm water.

After a brief discussion, she closed her eyes and leaned back on my bent arm. I used my other arm behind her knees to lift her into a horizontal position. I closed my eyes and began to breathe slowly. When I felt her limp in my arms, I began to stretch and then knead her muscles.

I found myself staring at my grandmother's face, studying every detail, and burning the image of this beautiful woman in my memory. Within moments, I became overwhelmed with emotions. Tears of love began to flow gently down my face, becoming part of the water in which my grandmother lay.

Since that time, I view massaging the elderly with reverence. When the session is over, I always walk away from an elderly client with a deeper respect for humanity in all its many expressions.

TRAINING

Although several workshop programs exist in geriatric massage, the two most attended are offered through Day-Break and Comfort Touch. The Day-Break Geriatric Massage Institute currently offers level 1 and level 2 training. Level 1 focuses on the robust senior and age-appropriate massage techniques. It includes basic information about medication use, conditions that need a doctor's permission, contraindications, and ways of adapting massage around joint replacements, pacemakers, and breathing conditions. Marketing information is also provided.

The level 2 workshop offered by Day-Break moves from the age appropriate to the frail, and focuses on specific conditions commonly seen in the elderly. These include not only the basic strokes, but modifications for elderly clients with Parkinson's disease, diabetes, dementias such as Alzheimer's disease, the wheelchair bound, and bedridden client.

Comfort Touch offers a basic training in a nurturing style of acupressure focusing on the frail and the ill. The basic techniques and principles are taught and applied in a wide variety of settings and circumstances, which include hospitals, hospices, wellness centers, home-care, and long-term care facilities. Body mechanics and precautions are part of the basic training as well as client charting.

CHAPTER SUMMARY

"Old age ain't no place for sissies," said Bette Davis. And as Joan Lohman points out in her 2001 article, neither is providing massage to the elderly, "yet it is as rewarding as it is demanding.[3] It requires a genuine interest in the lives of elders, to 'get over' squeamishness about body functions and physical decline, to be willing to enter the sometimes institutionalized world of elders, and to treat our elder clients with dignity, no matter what their eccentricities or circumstances."

CASE HISTORIES

■ Case history 1: Former marathon runner

The client is an 82-year old female former marathon runner. Fitness has been her life; daily exercise, healthy diet, and a positive attitude she claims are the secret to "keeping the pep in your step." Despite her commitment, age is catching up with her. Still determined to live her life as normal, she contacts Harold, a sports massage therapist.

Failing to mention her age over the phone, Harold is surprised to meet the spunky spirit. "You still run marathons?" he asked, skeptically. "Oh, of course not, honey. Don't want to make the other kids feel bad, you know," she laughs with a twinkle in her eye. "I run daily, but thanks to my knees, it's usually only a mile." Harold grins, impressed. "I hope to be in such good shape when I'm eighty." The client, ready to get down to business, begins her instructions. "I'd like a good bit of low back work, oh, and on my hamstrings. Stretch those and give me something to help with the knees." Harold listens patiently, grinning. "I can see you're a woman who knows what she wants! I want you to understand, however, that I will have to adapt my usual methods to create a more appropriate session for you."

After reviewing all of her intake paperwork, Harold begins to write out a treatment plan, taking time to explain each step with her. "I'd like to focus on shorter sessions, 30 minutes for now. It is just a precaution, to give me time to assess your stamina. If progress goes well, we can look at extending the session time in the future. The limited time means that we'll be looking at specific work each session, rather than a full body massage. The first session we'll focus on lumbar, glutes, and hamstrings. The next week quads and reduced joint mobilization of the knee. I know it seems like slow moving, but . . ." "Oh, don't worry, "she laughs, "I know better than most that slow and steady pace wins the race." Harold nods, continuing. "The following week, we can look at lower leg issues and the feet. By that point I can reassess some problem areas and modify treatment as necessary."

Harold selects a more emollient cream to contend with the dryness of her skin. He uses primarily effleurage strokes, and opts for fulling in lieu of cross fiber friction, all with a modified pressure. He performs passive stretches, careful not to take them to end-feel. Utilizing cryotherapy and reduced joint mobilization of the knee, the client begins to notice some alleviation of her knee pain. Harold is pleased to see such progress with his one-of-a-kind client. In her fourth session she quips exuberantly, "I feel like I'm 60 again!"

■ Case history 2: The lived experience: if I had my life to live over

I would dare to make more mistakes next time. I would relax. I would limber up.

I would be sillier than I have been on this trip. I would take fewer things seriously.

I would take more chances. I would take more trips. I would climb more mountains and swim more rivers. I would eat more ice cream and fewer beans. I would perhaps have more actual troubles but I'd have fewer imaginary ones.

You see, I'm one of those people who lives sensibly and sanely hour after hour, day after day. Oh, I've had my moments and if I had it to do over again, I'd have more of them.

In fact, I'd try to have nothing else. Just moments, one after another, instead of living so many years ahead of each day. I've been one of those people who never goes anywhere without a thermometer, a hot water bottle, a raincoat, and a parachute. If I had it to do again, I would travel lighter next time.

If I had my life to live over, I would start barefoot earlier in the spring and stay that way later in the fall. I would go to more dances. I would ride more merry-go-rounds. I would pick more daisies.

Nadine Stair (from an interview at age 85)

RESOURCES

Useful Websites

Administration of Aging
http://www.aoa.dhhs.gov/

Alliance for Aging Research
http://www.agingresearch.org/

Alzheimer's Association
http://www.alz.org/

American Association of Retired Persons (AARP)
http://www.aarp.org/

American Cancer Society
http://www.cancer.org/docroot/home/index.asp

American Foundation for the Blind
http://www.afb.org/

American Geriatric Society
http://www.americangeriatrics.org/

American Heart Association
http://www.americanheart.org/presenter.jhtml?identifier=11227

American Society on Aging
http://www.asaging.org/index.cfm

Center for Compassionate Touch
http://www.compassionate-touch.org/

Chronic Illness Alliance
http://www.chronicillness.org.au/community.htm

The Colostomy Association
http://www.colostomyassociation.org.uk/

Comfort Touch Institute
http://www.comforttouch.com

Day-Break Geriatric Massage Institute
http://www.daybreak-massage.com/

Disability Foundation
http://www.reachdisability.org/

Elder Care
http://www.eldercares.net/

Elder web
http://www.elderweb.com/home/

Family Caregiver Alliance
http://www.caregiver.org/

The Fairy Godmother Foundation
http://www.fairygodmother.org/

Foundation for Health in Aging
http://www.healthinaging.org/

Gerontological Society of America
http://www.geron.org/

Gray Panthers
http://www.graypanthers.org/

The Hospice Foundation of America
http://www.hospicefoundation.org/

Institute of Gerontology
http://www.geron.uga.edu/

International Federation on Ageing
http://www.ifa-fiv.org/en/accueil.aspx

International Foundation for Research and Education on Depression
http://www.ifred.org/

Multimedia Course for Environmental Geriatrics
http://www.environmentalgeriatrics.com/multimedia_course/index.html#

National Alliance for Caregiving
http://www.caregiving.org/

National Association of Area Agencies on Aging
http://www.n4a.org/

The National Association of the Deaf
http://www.nad.org/

National Academy of Elder Law Attorneys, Inc.
http://www.naela.com/

National Council on the Aging
http://www.ncoa.org/

National Hospice & Palliative Care Organization
http://www.nhpco.org/templates/1/homepage.cfm

National Institute of Aging
http://www.nia.nih.gov/

The Rubins
www.therubins.com

Senior Health
http://www.myseniorhealthcare.com

Senior Health
http://nihseniorhealth.gov/

Universal Designers and Consultants
http://www.universaldesign.com/

Weill Cornell Center for Aging Research
http://www.cornellaging.org/

The Wheelchair Foundation
http://www.wheelchairfoundation.org/

Center for Compassionate Touch
http://www.compassionate-touch.org/

Comfort Touch Institute
http://www.comforttouch.com

Geriatric Massage Institute
http://www.daybreak-massage.com/

Touch Research Institute, Research at TRI
http://www6.miami.edu/touch-research/research.htm#MTS

US Department of Health and Human Services, Administration on Aging, A Profile of Older Americans
http://www.aoa.dhhs.gov/prof/Statistics/profile/2006/2006profile.doc.

REFERENCES

1. Dychtwald K: *Age power: how the 21st century will be ruled by the new old*, New York, 1999, Jeremy P. Tarcher/Putnam.
2. Dychtward K, Flower J: *Age wave: the challenges and opportunities of an aging america*, Los Angeles, 1989, Jeremy P. Tarcher, Inc.
3. Lohman JS: Massage for elders: an ever-growing opportunity, *MTJ* 40: No. 3, 2001.
4. Meiner SE, Lueckenotte AG: *Gerontologic nursing*, 3 ed, St Louis, 2006, Mosby.
5. Wold GH: *Basic geriatric nursing*, ed 4, St Louis, 2008, Mosby.
6. Linton AD, Lach HW: *Matteson & McConnell's gerontological nursing: concepts and practice*, ed 3, Philadelphia, 2007, Saunders.
7. Eliopoulos C: *Manual of gerontologic nursing*, ed 2, St Louis, 1999, Mosby.

8. Barstow C: *Tending body and spirit: massage and counseling with elders*, Boulder, Colo, 1985, Self-Published Manual.

9. Nelson D: Growing old with massage: in facility care, *Massage & Bodywork*, Feb/Mar 2001.

10. Heath H, Schofield I: *Healthy aging—nursing older people*, St Louis, 2000, Mosby.

11. Kahn RL, Rowe JW: *Successful aging*, New York, 1998, Pantheon Books.

12. Salvo SG. *Massage therapy: principle and practice*, ed 3, Saunders, 2007, Philadelphia.

13. Ebersole P, Hess P, Touhy T, Jett K: *Gerontological nursing and healthy aging*, ed 2, St Louis, 2005, Mosby.

14. Ebersole P, Hess P, Schmidt Luggen A: *Toward healthy aging, human needs & nursing response*, ed 7, St Louis, 2008, Mosby.

15. McCance KJ, Huether SE: *Pathophysiology: the biologic basis for disease in adults and children*, ed 5, St Louis, 2006, Mosby.

16. Damjanov I: *Pathology for the health professions*, ed 3, Philadelphia, 2006, WB Saunders.

17. Gould BE: *Pathophysiology for the health professionals*, ed 3, Philadelphia, 2006, WB Saunders.

18. Liu BA et al: Falls among older people: relationship to medication use and orthostatic hypotension, *J Am Geriatr Soc* 10:1141-5, 1995.

19. Trenter ME. From test tube to patient, Food and Drug Administration, http://www.fda.gov/oc/seniors/ Accessed 6/6/07.

20. Diego MA, Field T, Sanders C, Hernandez-Reif M: Massage therapy of moderate and light pressure and vibrator effects on EEG and heart rate, *Int J Neurosci* 114:31-44, 2004.

21. Beera MH, Berfow R: *Merck manual of geriatrics*, ed 3, Whitehouse Station, NJ, 2000, Merck Research Laboratories.

22. Worfolk JB: Keep frail elders warm! *Geriatr Nurs* 1:7-11, 1997.

23. Albom M: *Tuesdays with Morrie*, New York, 1997, Doubleday.

24. Rose MK: *Comfort touch massage for the elderly and the ill* (DVD), Boulder, Colo, 2004, Wild Rose.

25. Field T, et al: Elder retired volunteers benefit from giving massage therapy to infants, *J Appl Gerontol* 17:229-239, 1998.

26. Hernandez-Reif et al: Parkinson's disease symptoms are differentially affected by massage therapy versus progressive muscle relaxation: a pilot study, *Journal of Bodywork and Movement Therapies* 6:177-182, 2002.

27. Barnett K: A survey of the current utilization of touch by health team personnel with hospitalized patients, *Int J Nurs Stud* 9:195, 1972.

28. Montagu A: *Touching: the human significance of the skin*, ed 3, New York, 1986, Harper Collins.

29. Sloane PD, *Normal aging, primary care geriatrics: a case-based approach*, ed 3, St. Louis, 1992, Mosby.

30. Nelson D: *Compassionate touch: hands-on caregiving for the elderly, the ill and the dying*, Barrytown, NY, 1994, Station Hill Press.

31. Feldt KS: Increasing physical activity in frail, older adults: guidance for clinicians. Presentation. American Geriatrics Society 2002 Annual Scientific Meeting, May 8-12, 2002, Washington, DC.

32. Rockwood K, Song X, MacKnight C et al:. A global clinical measure of fitness and frailty in elderly people, *Canadian Medical Association Journal* 173(5):489-495, 2005.

33. Mathias M: Instructor Training for Infant Massage. Presented at workshops in Dallas, TX (1986) and Lake Charles, LA (1992).

34. Puszko S: Personal Communication, 2007.

35. Miesler DW: The ABC's of Geriatric Massage (DVD), 1999.

36. Rose MK Comfort Touch: Nurturing Acupressure Massage for the Elderly and the Ill, Massage & Bodywork magazine, December/January 2004.

37. Smith S, Gove J: Physical changes of aging, available online at http://www.edis.ifas.ufl.edu/HE019.

MULTIPLE CHOICE TEST QUESTIONS

1) Population experts estimate that what percentage of the population will be 65 or older by 2020?
   a) 5
   b) 10
   c) 17
   d) 25

2) Which of the following best describes a form of massage designed to meet specific needs of the elderly population?
   a) infant massage
   b) sports massage
   c) foot reflexology
   d) geriatric massage

3) Which of the following is a branch of medicine concerned with the diagnosis and treatment of old age?
   a) obstetrics
   b) geriatrics
   c) orthopedics
   d) pediatrics

4) Who developed the style of geriatric massage taught by the Day-Break Geriatric Institute?
   a) Dietrich Miesler
   b) David Palmer
   c) Whitney Lowe
   d) John Upledger

5) Who developed the techniques used in a style of massage called Comfort Touch?
   a) Sharon Puszko
   b) Mary Kathleen Rose
   c) Dawn Nelson
   d) Sandra Anderson

6) Who developed the style of massage called Compassionate Touch?
   a) Dietrich Miesler
   b) David Palmer
   c) Mary Kathleen Rose
   d) Dawn Nelson

7) Geriatric massage includes all of the following treatment modifications EXCEPT what?
   a) pressure and shearing is reduced
   b) reduced treatment time
   c) more time allowed for client activities
   d) vigorous stretching and mobilizations

8) Which group of the American population was born between 1946 and 1964, and constitutes approximately one third of the population today?
   a) baby boomers
   b) yuppies
   c) hippies
   d) rat pack

9) What percentage of older persons are reported to have at least one chronic condition?
   a) 20
   b) 50
   c) 75
   d) 90

10) What is the current (2008) average life expectancy?
    a) 58
    b) 65
    c) 77
    d) 89

11) Which of the following refers to the period of life from old age to death?
    a) pubescence
    b) adolescence
    c) senescence
    d) incandescence

12) According to the chapter, which age do most Americans identify as the beginning of old age?
    a) 60
    b) 65
    c) 70
    d) 75

13) Which of the following is the branch of study concerned with normal aging?
    a) archaeology
    b) genealogy
    c) etiology
    d) gerontology

14) Many elderly people experience loss of balance, resulting from a sudden drop in blood pressure, when moving from a recumbent position to an upright position. The clinical term for this is what?
   a) aphasia
   b) orthostatic hypotension
   c) hypercapnia
   d) orthopnea

15) According to the Food and Drug Administration (FDA), senior citizens purchase what percentage of all prescription drugs?
   a) 10
   b) 30
   c) 50
   d) 70

16) What percentage of the elderly is sedentary?
   a) 20
   b) 50
   c) 70
   d) 90

17) Which of the following is the LEAST safe position for an elderly person to receive massage?
   a) supine
   b) seated
   c) side lying
   d) prone

18) According to the text, which of the following is NOT one of the most commonly used medications by the elderly?
   a) cardiovascular agents
   b) selective serotonin reuptake inhibitor
   c) antihypertensives
   d) antacids

19) What is the number one chronic illness of the elderly?
   a) cancer
   b) peripheral vascular disease
   c) hypertension
   d) diabetes

20) What is the most common safety issue for people 65 and older?
   a) falling
   b) loss of driving privileges
   c) loss of hearing
   d) heart attack and stroke

Infant and Pediatric Massage

Diana Moore

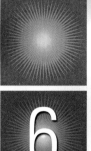

INTRODUCTION

Infant Massage

Infant massage is about love. It is more than the mere physical act of massaging a newborn, far beyond the rubbing of muscles and stretching of joints. It is among the most precious gifts you can give an infant. The very heart of infant massage involves the coming together of two beings in a divine act of loving through touching. Not only does the baby receive the tender intimacy of caresses, but the giver benefits in turn with the responses given back.

We can talk about mechanics and procedures; we can quote the results from many studies. But at the heart infant massage is a conduit for connecting parent and infant through touch at one of the most vulnerable times in development. Massaging an infant in a loving and compassionate manner can lead to frequent meaningful and responsive interactions—exactly what babies want and need. The experience begins long before birth within the mother's womb. Once birth occurs, we must continue with the touching, holding, and caressing that forms what Ashley Montagu called "the womb with a view."

"Here in the United States, which is a low-touch society, mothers and babies are apart most of the day, a fact that ranks our infants among the least held on this earth."

The above comment from Sharon Heller's book *The Vital Touch* suggests both the need and the increasing awareness in this country of infant massage.[1] Indeed, type the words "infant massage, baby massage, pediatric massage" into a search engine and you'll be rewarded with more than four million notations and page after page of websites to click on. One thing those websites tell you is that infant massage has been around for centuries.

Mothers have been practicing the art of infant massage since the beginning of time, using their innate wisdom to touch, love, and discover their **newborns** (Box 6-1). It is a traditional practice and a means of intergenerational sharing in many societies across the world—particularly in "simpler" cultures where people are accustomed to expressing their love through a form of communication that does not need words.

In India, Nigeria, and many other countries, mothers learn massage from *their* mothers and pass it along to the next generation. All over Nepal, writes Amelia Auckett, babies are massaged every day from just two to three hours old.[2] Fijian mothers carry their infants close to the body in a sling and massage them after the daily bath. A common trait among many cultures is a very close body-to-body connection maintained between mother and child, of which massage is a natural extension.

Our more "sophisticated" society can learn much from the mothers of other lands. Modern technology and busy lives provide many resources and distractions that serve to keep children and parents apart, from cribs to careers. "With our babies more often in a container than in our arms, our infants are 'at odds with their evolution', as anthropologist James McKenna put it," continues Heller.[1] "We opt for the buggy rather than the Snuglie, the crib rather than the parental bed, the swing rather than the rocking chair, because cultural values and customs discourage us from freely following our natural maternal feelings for intimacy and from responding fully to our baby's signals for closeness."

Fortunately, as all those resources on the internet seem to attest, a tide is turning toward rediscovering the importance of touch, and not just for parent-child **bonding.** Mutual dependency; in particular, has its roots in the early mother-infant symbiosis, a tension-easing relationship that begins in utero and attains its peak intensity between the first and sixth postnatal months.[3]

Infant massage in the United States today is becoming a specialty in the field of massage therapy and is further being embraced by a wide variety of professionals who work with families from those with healthy babies to those coping with such issues as low–birth-weight or high-risk newborns or those with toddlers or children who have special needs. Physical therapists, occupational therapists, nurses, infant mental health practitioners, early interventionists, and child life specialists are adding this simple, effective technique to their tools when working with young families in their homes, in hospitals, with parent support groups, and in private practice.

The Touch Language

In the most basic terms, infant or pediatric massage refers to the process of stroking the muscles of an infant using a variety of specialized massage techniques. Vocalizations, eye-to-eye contact, and other positive behavioral reinforcements are also important components of the massage.

In the United States, as around the globe, infant massage is most likely to be performed by parents (fathers as well as mothers), grandparents, and primary caregivers. Unlike elsewhere, however, the instruction on how to do it here comes not from grandmothers or societal elders but from **certified infant massage instructors** who are professionally trained by an accredited program.

The major difference between professional massage therapy and infant massage lies in the premise that infant massage is a bonding activity that is best performed by the child's primary caregiver, not by the professional. The role of the certified infant massage instructor is to gently guide the caregiver with instruction typically using a demonstration doll. This approach is very empowering and can improve the parent-infant attachment process (see Figure 6-13).

BOX 6-1 How Old is an Infant?

For consistency, this chapter uses the following, generally standard, age categories for children:

Early childhood: One year through five years. The term "child" may be used in a general way from birth on, as in discussion of the number of children in a family.

Infant: A child in the first year of life.

Neonate: A newborn up to one month of age.

Neonatal: Concerning the first 28 days after birth.

Premature infant: An infant born before the thirty-seventh week of gestation.

Toddler: A common term for a child who is learning to walk; generally between the ages of 12 and 36 months.

A growing body of experience and research also points to the therapeutic benefits of infant massage. As a result, the practice is now conducted by a wide range of medically and clinically licensed professionals who care for children outside the home. These include nurses in neonatal intensive care units who work with premature infants (see Box 6-1), physical and occupational therapists, and child life specialists who care for hospitalized children. In addition, these same professionals find it important to make the time to teach the primary caregivers the techniques.

The History of Infant Massage

It is only natural for a mother to massage her newborn as it emerges from the womb. "For more than a million years," notes Sharon Heller in *Vital Touch*,[1] "mothers have carried their infants almost continuously, slept with them at night, nursed them frequently the first to four years of life, and offered immediate comfort," including massage (Box 6-2). In the past 30 years, the United States has begun to embrace the massaging of infants in what is considered a parent-baby activity.

Much seminal work was done by Dr. Frederick Leboyer, whose highly popular 1976 book, *Loving Hands,* became the basis for most of today's infant massage training in the United States.[4] A pioneer in the study of newborn awareness and a frequent visitor to India, Leboyer captured the art from the mothers he saw in the villages there. In his poetic book, he describes the need for a baby to be fed both inside and outside. "A baby's belly is hungry, no doubt," he wrote. "But its skin is just as hungry. Its skin is craving, and so is its back, and so is its spine, craving for touch, craving for sensations. Just as its belly craves for milk."[4]

Soon after Leboyer's book came out, massage therapist's license fresh in hand, I began teaching infant

massage based on my own personal experiences and observations. As my practice began to grow, I connected with other individuals who had the same passion for this work. We joined together and formed the International Association of Infant Massage Instructors. As business director for 10 years, I helped to guide the organization, with two babies in arms, as it grew and developed worldwide. In 1992, I established the International Loving Touch Foundation, which exists today to help realize the dream of Leboyer, my grandmother, and others by furthering the art of infant massage and training new generations of infant massage instructors.

BOX 6-2 Infant Massage in 1894

One of the first recorded mentions of infant massage in the United States dates from 1894, in a book called *The Care and Feeding of Children* by Dr. Emmett Holt. Holt described some therapeutic effects of massage on young children, which was quite good advice for its time and in fact remains true today:

"What are some simple means by which constipation may be relieved? The best are diet, suppositories, and massage. . . . Massage consists in rubbing the abdomen, which may be done in two ways; Beginning at the right groin, the hand is carried up to the ribs, then across to the opposite side, then around to the left groin. The abdomen is stroked gently at first and afterward—deeper pressure used as the child becomes accustomed to it. The second method is by rubbing the deeper parts with a circular movement—the fingers not moving upon the skin—making a series of small circles, beginning at the right groin and following the same course as described above. Either method should be employed for six or eight minutes twice a day, at almost any regular time, except soon after a meal."

From Holt LE, *The care and feeding of children*, ed 6, D. Appleton, New York, 1912.

▪▪▪▪ IN MY EXPERIENCE: MY GRANDMOTHER'S HANDS

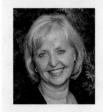

To many, including a young would-be massage therapist who had just completed her own spiritual quest to India and shared the same experiences, Leboyer's words served as a call to action. I had learned my love of the massage in early childhood from my maternal grandmother, a massage therapist since 1938 who used a loving touch regularly with her children and grandchildren. Her massage room stood at the top of the stairway in her small Portland, Oregon, home—a cheery space that clings to the memory, redolent with the fragrance of eucalyptus oil and steam-cabinet warmth.

Infant Massage Around the World

"Massage is a crucial and routine part of infant care from Africa to India and Indonesia, from Central and South America to Australia and the Soviet Union," notes The Body Shop in its 1991 book *Mamatoto: A Celebration of Birth*.[5] In tribal and nomadic cultures, it has long been customary for women to carry on their daily lives with babies supported in slings, writes Amelia Auckett in *Baby Massage: Parent-Child Bonding through Touch*.[6] "Clothing is often adapted into slings for this purpose. These babies, close to their mother's bodies, experience a rocking, rhythmical movement which can stimulate their motor and intellectual development." Here's a quick tour of some ways infant massage and touch have been used around the world, as cited in *Mamatoto*:

- In Australia, Aborigine families use touch to impart important social values to infants. "Placing her hand gently on the child's forehead, a mother or grandmother speaks softly to the infant: 'You must give, you must share everything'; on the mouth: 'Don't use bad language'; on the eyes: 'Don't concentrate your gaze on the things of others.'"
- In New Zealand, the Maori have a practice of focusing massage on knees and ankles as a means to keep the joints supple and the child graceful.
- In Bali, massage is traditionally given to relieve tummy discomfort.
- In the former Soviet Union, doctors taught mothers to massage their babies during the first day of life to help develop the central nervous system.
- In Nigeria, immediately after the birth of a Bornu baby, the mother's helpers warm their hands over a dish of hot coals and gently press the infant's body.
- In many cultures, the natural creamy coating called *vernix caseosa*, which protects the skin from uterine fluids, is rubbed into the skin when the infant is given its first massage.

MODERN PRACTICE OF INFANT MASSAGE

Infant massage is quite easy to learn: mothers around the globe have been practicing this ancient art for centuries, learning it from their elders and passing it along to their own offspring without benefit of intensive training or modern technology. It is in fact an instinctual art that can serve as an antidote to, or at least a respite from, the rush of daily life for both parent and child.

The modern practice of infant massage is adapted from these same ancient, but tried-and-true, forms of touch. As infant massage began to gain momentum in the United States, practitioners used their basic understanding of massage techniques taught in most massage schools across the country. Although everything learned in massage school applies here, there is one obvious, but critical, caveat: the recipient is an infant. This vital difference imposes specific demands, including the ability to read the behavioral cues that are a newborn's main form of communication, or "infant-speak."

The typical strokes come from the classic East Indian and Swedish massage techniques, relaxation techniques, and reflexology (zone therapy), accompanied by a strong emphasis on reinforcing parent-infant attachment and behavioral cues in the newborn. The person applying the massage—in most cases a parent or other primary caregiver—should make good eye contact and smile, sing, or hum to the infant at the same time. The massage routine should last only as long as the infant is willing to participate (Figure 6-1).

Following is an overview of techniques and other aspects of infant massage as commonly taught and practiced in the United States today.[7] Note that much of this information is structured for parents or caregivers who are not massage professionals. Much of it may seem fairly basic for massage therapists, but it's worth reviewing these issues again in the specialized context of infant massage.

Massage Techniques and Sequence

In general, infant massage should be performed in a smooth, rhythmical manner using moderate pressure and varying speeds. Slower massage strokes will produce

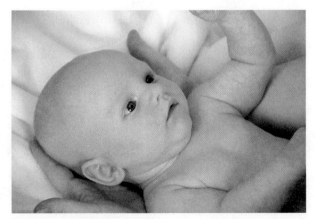

FIGURE 6-1 Making contact.

a more calming effect and faster massage strokes will be more stimulating for the newborn. Newborns prefer a simplified approach; as they grow older, they may want a more complex massage featuring a greater variety of strokes. Active toddlers often enjoy quick and vigorous movements accompanied by complementary activities such as singing and nursery rhymes to hold their attention (Figure 6-2).

The typical sequence begins with cradling the head and asking permission, making eye contact (see Figure 6-1), and getting attention. Next the feet and legs are massaged, followed by the tummy, chest, hands and arms, face, back. The sequence concludes with gentle exercises (Figures 6-3, 6-4, 6-5, 6-6, and 6-7). Keep in mind that the massage may only last a few minutes. If all is good and the interactions are positive, the massage may last longer. Once parents are comfortable with the stroking sequence, they may improvise to create a more personal experience.

Massage for babies, much the same as for adults, is the manual application of intermittent pressure to the softer tissues of the body for therapeutic purposes, which communicates the four main benefits of infant massage: (1) providing stimulation, (2) enhancing relaxation, (3) relieving pain, and (4) promoting attachment and bonding.

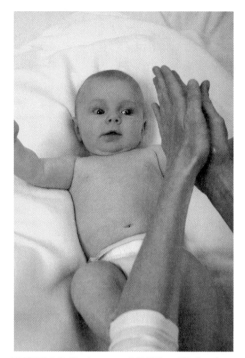

FIGURE 6-3 Getting started: Rubbing oil in hands.

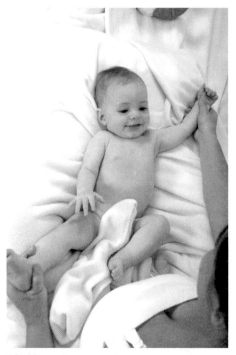

FIGURE 6-2 Playful exercise.

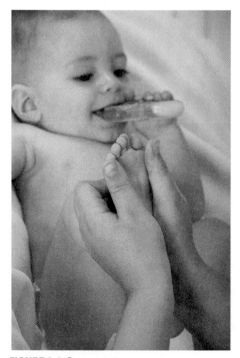

FIGURE 6-4 Foot massage.

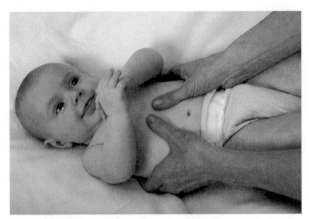

FIGURE 6-5 Tummy massage.

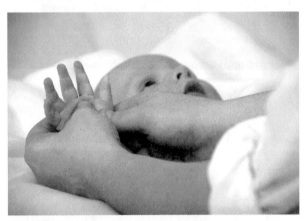

FIGURE 6-6 Hand massage.

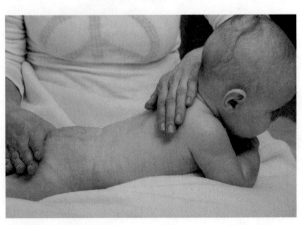

FIGURE 6-7 Back massage.

Swedish Massage

Strokes move along the extremities in the direction towards the heart. The well-baby massage routine utilizes firm but gentle pressure, "a loving touch" with strokes applied in a smooth, rhythmical, and slow manner. This is used to help increase circulation.

The typical Swedish techniques used for infants include: (1) touch in general, (2) effleurage (more commonly termed gliding strokes), (3) petrissage or kneading, (4) friction (rolling, wringing, vibration), (5) percussion movements (tapping and cupping), and (6) joint movements, which include stretching.

East Indian Massage

East Indian strokes are more calming in nature, draining tension and stress away from the body. The strokes move proximal to distal following the direction the hair grows. These outward movements are lighter in pressure than the traditional Swedish directional movements.

Reflexology

Also known as zone therapy, reflexology is applied on the feet, hands, and ears. This technique improves the responses to certain organ areas of the body and helps with such typical childhood symptoms as teething and intestinal concerns.

Conditioned Relaxation Response

The conditioned relaxation response combines a gentle shaking movement of the muscle with a verbal **cue** to relax. This technique is effective in relaxing muscle groups or an entire limb and may be termed *rhythmic mobilization*.

BEHAVIORAL STATES OF THE NEWBORN

The six **behavioral states*** of the newborn can be used to help identify the best time to communicate with an infant.[8] The quiet alert state (number 4, below) is identified in the Brazelton Neonatal Behavioral Assessment Scale as the optimal point for communication. This

---

*Credit for identifying these states belongs to Peter H. Wolff, professor of psychiatry at Harvard Medical School and senior associate in psychiatry at Children's Hospital of Boston, and a world-renowned authority on infant behavior. Among his influential writings on the subject is the 1987 book, *The Development of Behavioral States and the Expression of Emotions in Early Infancy: New Proposals for Investigation.*

state provides an optimal time for infant massage activity to begin.[9]

1. Quiet sleep
   • Smooth breathing rhythm
   • Closed eyelids with no movement
   • Muscle tone flaccid
2. Active sleep (REM rapid-eye-movement)
   • Irregular heart and respiration
   • May twitch and make facial grimaces
   • Eyes move under the eyelids
   • Associated with dreaming
   • Easily awakened
3. Drowsy or transitional State
   • State between sleep and wakefulness
   • More body movement
   • Eyes partially open and close
4. Quiet alert
   • Focused attention; eye contact is direct, mutual gaze
   • Eyes open, bright, will follow a moving object
   • Reduced body movement—inactivity
   • Cooing sounds, attentive
   • Note: If no medication is given during the birth process, the quiet alert stage lasts approximately one hour after delivery. This is an optimal time for the parents to bond with their baby. If the child has special needs, this opportunity may be delayed or postponed. Massage helps parents bond with their baby at a later time.
5. Active alert
   • Looking away, gaze aversion
   • Increased body movement
   • Signs of overarousal and overstimulation
   • Increased disengagement cues, yawning, hiccoughing
6. Fussy, crying
   • Crying noises
   • Vigorous movements
   • Skin may flush
   • Other gross motor activities

BENEFITS OF INFANT MASSAGE

Infant massage is an emerging practice in the United States that has attracted researchers to study the emotional and therapeutic benefits to infants and parents alike.

In her classic study performed on premature babies, Dr. Tiffany Field of the Touch Research Institute was able to show that massage helped facilitate weight gain, improve nervous system development, decrease levels of cortisol, increase muscle tone, and improve sleep and awake patterns.[10] These studies are still being replicated today. Global analysis of these studies revealed positive outcomes.

The Touch Research Institute has conducted a wealth of studies outlining the benefits of infant massage on such wide-ranging issues as parent-child bonding, including between fathers and infants; sleep onset problems; stress mitigation (infants and parents); physical growth and weight gain; sociability; and soothability. Infant massage has also proven helpful in the treatment of a variety of medical conditions, including premature birth, abuse (sexual and physical), asthma, autism, burns, cancer, colic, developmental delays, dermatitis, diabetes, Down syndrome, eating disorders (anorexia and bulimia), juvenile rheumatoid arthritis, posttraumatic stress disorder, psychiatric problems, and exposure to mothers with HIV, drug addiction, or depression.[11]

Here is a brief listing of recent findings by researchers working in association with the Touch Research Institute and other institutions.*

• Moderate versus light pressure massage therapy leads to greater weight gain in preterm infants.
• Mothers' depressed mood and anxiety levels are reduced after massaging their preterm infants.
• Preterm infants show reduced stress behaviors and activity after 5 days of massage therapy.
• Preterm neonates receiving massage therapy exhibit greater weight gain and increased vagal tone and gastric motility during and immediately after treatment.
• Greater increase in temperature noted for preterm infants receiving massage therapy versus a control group.
• Low birth weight infants who receive massage intervention are less likely to snore during sleep, require less feeding on waking up at night, and appear more alert during the day.
• Pilot study on the changes in mood states and salivary cortisol level show that baby massage positively affects the mood status of the mothers.
• Massage therapy facilitates mother-infant interaction in premature infants.

---

*More information, including abstracts and results, is available on-line at: http://www.sciencedirect.com and http://www6.miami.edu/touch-research/

- Massage therapy attenuates right frontal EEG asymmetry in one-month-old infants of depressed mothers.
- Massage enhances recovery from habituation in normal infants.

A wealth of anecdotal information also exists, which can be cited by any Certified Infant Massage Instructor, but it springs, especially, from the experience of parents and caregivers worldwide. My own practice, for instance, has shown the benefits of massage on behalf of children (and their parents) with Down syndrome, cleft lip and palate, colic, and sleep regulation among numerous other medical conditions.

It is well documented that some parents have difficulty in bonding with their children. Delayed or problematic bonding can be present in situations where medical intervention, difficult births, adoption, illness, or other unexpected situations may arise. A child born with a disability poses special problems for parents, perhaps in terms of acceptance, perhaps because of necessary separation for treatment, hospitalization, or other medical reasons. Postnatal depression affects about one in every five to eight women[12]; many others need help in learning how to love—how to touch their babies. Parents who have difficulty connecting with their babies, for whatever reasons, may develop a poorer set of handling techniques. Infant massage skills teach parents how to touch their infants, thus increasing their parenting confidence.

Infant massage is being used as an early intervention strategy and therapeutic tool for parents and their newborns when a derailed attachment poses a risk both for the parent and for the baby's social-emotional-cognitive development. It is well known that the first three years of life are the most crucial for health and well-being, and starting out early with infant massage can lay a solid foundation. Angela Joyce reminds us that babies "are absolutely dependent on their parents at the beginning of life. This dependency is not just for physical care, without which they would die but also for the emotional care and relating that implements and then helps sustain mental and psychic development."[13] Other physical concerns may indicate the need to refer the infant for early intervention services.

One obvious truth that needs no formal study to verify is that parents feel more relaxed with their children if they are comfortable touching them. Conversely, if they begin a natural pattern of touching, they will have a natural way of being around their children. A mother who has support and direction may not only heal in the process, but she and her infant will receive the benefits of additional loving, nurturing contact (Box 6-3).

Touch through the form of infant massage is simply a vehicle for bonding between caregiver and infant. It is a very simple tool that can be used cross-culturally, and in most situations it is the first form of communication between infant and parents. Infant massage can create great benefits for both the parents and newborn, which have been documented through many research projects. Perhaps if parents learned how to touch lovingly, they would be less likely to abuse or neglect their children later on.

BOX 6-3 Bonding Between Parent and Child

The formation of a close emotional tie between parent and infant is one of the defining purposes of infant massage. Bonding is defined as "a gradual, reciprocal process that begins with acquaintance." It is a unique and specific relationship between two people and endures across time. Bonding occurs on a different timetable for mothers than for fathers. Although mothers experience a sharp increase in bonding around the fifth month of pregnancy and have intensifying feelings throughout the pregnancy, the father's feelings usually tend to develop more slowly and become congruent after birth, when infant caretaking begins.

From Kenner et al, 2003; Krebs, 1998; Verklan MT, Walden M, editors: *Core curriculum for neonatal intensive care nursing*, ed 3, Philadelphia, 2004, Elsevier.

▮▯▯ IN MY EXPERIENCE

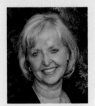

First-time parents can be overly anxious about their ability to care for their newborn(s). When parents are given clear understanding about reading their infant's cues, knowledge about development and simple ways to interact with their babies—touching, talking, massaging, holding, rocking—we will have come a long way in creating a solid foundation for bonding between parent and infant to flourish.

Potential benefits for preterm and compromised newborns, as well as children with motor problems, developmental delays, and other ailments may include the following:

- Improves weight gain
- Decreases stress hormone cortisol
- Improves sleep by increasing release of endorphins
- Leads to less crying; calms and soothes, comforts and reassures, responds to cry cues sooner
- Improves circulation: helps with immune system functioning
- Relieves colic
- Helps to relax abdominal area, which may aide in improved gastric motility and relief of constipation
- Improves parent communication, association of reading cues
- Promotes self-healing; newborns are more relaxed
- Promotes better eye contact
- Promotes body awareness
- Promotes social, emotional, neurologic, physiologic, and cognitive development
- Decreases pain response

Potential benefits for all babies may include:

- Improves general well-being
- Improves behavioral state self-regulation
- Improves circulation
- Enhances neurologic development
- Brain synapses improved IQ
- Helps child to sleep more deeply and more soundly
- Provides intimate time with parents
- Stimulates the growth hormone, which helps weight gain
- Provides all of the essential indicators of intimate parent-infant bonding and attachment: eye-to-eye, touch, voice, entrainment, smell, movement, and thermal regulation.

Potential benefits for parents may include the following:

- Provides all of the essential indicators of intimate parent-infant bonding and attachment: eye-to-eye contact, touch, vocalizations, smell, movement, and thermal regulation
- Encourages preverbal communication between caregiver and infant
- Helps parents feel more confident and competent in caring for their children
- Gives parents the tools for understanding their child's unique rhythms and patterns

- Teaches parents how to read their infant's cues and recognize their states of awareness
- Helps parents to unwind and relax, especially when made part of a daily routine

CONTRAINDICATIONS

The parent or caregiver should consult the infant's physician if there is any question about an infant's ability to receive massage. If the instructor recognizes signs of developmental delays or other medical issues, the infant should be referred to a professional therapist for treatment. Certainly, massage is not recommended in any instance in which the child is medically unstable. Likewise, precautions should be taken for those who have health issues such as skin disorders, fevers, or contagious conditions. Every precaution should be considered prior to massaging an infant born prematurely—a preterm newborn may not be neurologically prepared for interacting with the world. Premature babies born between 23 to 25 weeks have fragile skin, and although a gentle finger in the babies' palm or a touch on the leg can help make that physical connection between parent and child, the infants' skin should mature and toughen before it is touched much more than that.[14]

In cases involving infants under medical observation or treatment, a nurse practitioner or physician's order may be required so as not to conflict with diagnosis or medical procedures. If surgery has just been performed on an infant born with necrotizing enterocolitis (NEC), for instance, there should be no massaging in the stomach region.

The sensory system of a healthy, full-term newborn is turned on and ready to explore the world. If massage is applied with moderate pressure and with an awareness of the infant's cues of readiness, contraindications are few. Massage is not recommended on an infant or child who is asleep or has a full stomach, or who shows signs of stress or of being over-stimulated—which may result from the parent's gaze, voice, or touch, or by the effects of sound and light in the room (Figure 6-8). The key lies in being able to recognize and read the infant's cues. Table 6-1 includes a few examples of cues to recognize.

TREATMENT

"Treatment" seems like such a clinical term for what is in most cases a loving and highly pleasurable interaction between parent and infant—a "loving touch," in fact. In my own practice, I tend to reserve the word "treatment" for massage performed not by a parent

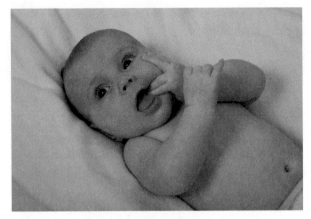

FIGURE 6-8 Over-stimulation/disengaging cues.

primarily for bonding or emotional reasons, but by a professional therapist with a higher level of skill in touch therapies for therapeutic interventions. A small issue of semantics, to be sure, but it does help point up the differences in approach and purpose between parent-infant massage and other types, whether performed on children or adults.

The following overview refers more to the "loving touch" category of well-baby massage than the "treatment" form, but many of the techniques and guidelines are appropriate for both.

THE IMPORTANCE OF BONDING

Parents—and this includes fathers and grandparents as well as mothers—should see massage as a playful and highly enjoyable experience as well as a therapeutic one, and one that supports the dynamic parent-infant relationship. The bond between parent and newborn is one of the strongest in the natural world. John Bowlby, the British psychoanalyst and father of attachment theory

(Box 6-4), spent a lifetime observing and describing the process of attachment, how it occurs and how it is disrupted. To grow up mentally healthy, he wrote in 1951, "the infant and young child should experience a warm, intimate, and continuous relationship with his mother (or permanent mother substitute) in which both find satisfaction and enjoyment."[15] Excessive separation anxiety, he found, "is usually caused by adverse family experiences, such as repeated threats of abandonment or rejections by parents . . . for which the child feels responsible."[16]

His insights are borne out in the orphanages of Romania, to cite but one example, where thousands of children suffered severe attachment disruptions during the brutal reign of Nicolae Ceausescu—problems that spiraled into a range of physical, emotional, and cognitive disabilities. Thanks to well-meaning individuals around the globe, many of these children have been rescued, but only time will tell how much they may recover of what was lost in the early, formative years of their lives since the first three years are critical for the developing child.

HOW YOUNG IS TOO YOUNG FOR MASSAGE?

The appropriate age to begin massage often depends on the disposition of the infant and the parent. Leboyer noted that in South India, the usual practice was to begin when the baby was one month old.[4] However, we have found that infant massage can be

TABLE 6-1 Cues of Engagement and Disengagement	
Cues of Engagement	**Cues of Disengagement**
Eye-to-eye contact	Gaze aversion
Smiling	Crying
Cooing	Turning away
Babbling	Arching; body
Reaching toward caregiver	Pushing away

initiated immediately after birth. Mothers have an innate biological urge to touch and caress their newborns. Certainly, the abdomen should not be massaged too close to the umbilical cord stub until it has dropped off to allow time for proper healing. Touching may begin right from the start, as long as the touches are gentle and loving, not a formal massage. Ideally, infant massage would then become a daily activity, up until the infant is developmentally active at around 6 or 7 months.

WHEN AND WHERE TO MASSAGE

Though massage can be done at any time of the day, the best time is when the infant is in the quiet alert state. Many parents like to massage before or after the bath and between feedings.

A more stimulating massage may be given during daytime hours and a more calming massage when preparing for nap or bedtime.

Preparation of the area where the massage will be given should be organized in advance to ensure the activity is enjoyable and effective for both infant and parent. Floor time is an especially suitable occasion, in that it allows the baby to safely move around—not typically a concern with adult massage. The setting should be calm, quiet, and comfortable with natural lighting, and certainly in a warm location that avoids drafts. Babies do better when the temperature is turned up, especially if the infant will be unclothed. Perhaps some lullaby or heart beat music may accompany the practice.

Choosing the right position is important as a means to facilitate close parent-child bonding. Babies are sensitive to tension transmitted by others, so the person performing the massage should be relaxed and comfortable, with back well supported. Many parents enjoy sitting on cushions or a carpeted surface with the infants placed before them face-to-face, in a position that's both comfortable and useful in providing ample room for those babies who like to squirm around. It's also helpful to use a special blanket that the infant soon associates with "massage time" and which can be used to swaddle the baby if she becomes overstimulated or gets cold. In the case of hospitalized infants, the caregiver must naturally adjust to the constraints of hospital beds and other medical equipment (Figures 6-9 and 6-10). Both infant and parent will enjoy the bonding more if not distracted by too much excessive noise. Soothing music, lullabies, or heartbeat sounds encourage relaxation.

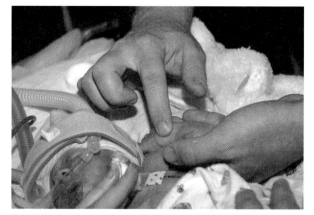

FIGURE 6-9 Massage in the NICU.

Maintaining Contact, Asking Permission

Before beginning the first stroke, it is critical to make certain the infant is ready to engage in interaction. Infant massage instructors teach parents how to read their infants' cues and recognize their states of behavior. Making eye-to-eye contact and asking permission is one way to ensure an infant is ready. Eye-to-eye contact works best at 8 to 12 inches—about the same distance a breastfeeding mother holds her infant. The International Loving Touch Foundation, Inc. (ILTF) provides these guidelines:

"[B]efore beginning, take in several deep breaths and relax your entire body. Cradle your baby's head in your hands, look into the baby's eyes, say her or his name and ask permission to begin."[7]

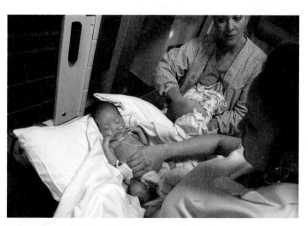

FIGURE 6-10 NICU positioning.

The exact words actually matter less than gently communicating a sense of asking permission, and then responding to the baby's behavioral cues indicating a readiness to engage in interaction—a smile, perhaps, or direct eye-to-eye contact or reaching out towards the parent.

Newborns are very good at communicating when they are not ready through signals of disengagement such as turning away or even crying (see Table 6-1 for cues). It is difficult to perform massage on an unwilling infant (see Figure 6-8).

PERFORMING THE MASSAGE

The person giving the massage should use firm but gentle pressure; light pressure should be avoided as it can be ticklish. Research studies confirm the use of deeper pressure to affect the tactile receptors. Strokes include gliding or effleurage, rolling, wringing and squeezing muscles, stretching joints, reflexology, and relaxation techniques that will provide a loving and nurturing contact.

Once the infant signals permission, the massage routine may begin. This is the time to apply a small amount of natural unscented oil to the hands and rub them together, warming the oil and letting the baby know the massage is coming (see Figure 6-3). Babies often kick out their legs towards the parent, who can then take hold and begin by gliding the hands up and down the legs and feet first, then to the stomach, chest, arms, face, and back. The strokes should be applied in a smooth and rhythmical manner. Stretches become a natural part of the massage routine as parent and infant interact. This creates a natural way for parents to communicate with their baby.

Many programs that offer infant massage apply playful names to some of the strokes so parents can easily remember them: "turn and caress" for the wringing stroke, for example, or "heart of love" on the chest for the effleurage stroke (Figures 6-11 and 6-12).

After the massage, it is nice to finish by giving the infant a warm bath—a perfect ending that will help rid the body of all tensions and, in all likelihood, send the infant off to soothing, natural sleep.

Fragile, Sick, or Premature Newborns

Professionally trained therapists should take into account current growing knowledge regarding the implication of touch therapies to fragile, sick, or premature infants. Gestational age, medical fragility, and sensitivity to touch should determine where, when, and how much to touch. It is best to

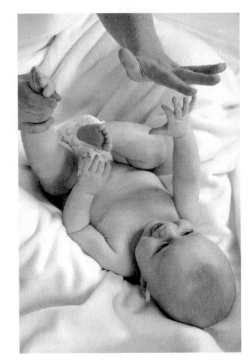

FIGURE 6-11 Airplane stroke.

begin massage when your infant is medically stable. Once your newborn is able to respond to touch, start slowly with steady, gentle but firm pressure, but not so it is a tickling type of touch. Containment or hand holds help to organize an infant. Kangaroo care or skin-to-care is an emerging practice in the neonatal intensive care unit (NICU) that encourages touch and holding of infants. Kangaroo care is a technique that places your infant against your chest with skin-to-skin contact. This is often the first

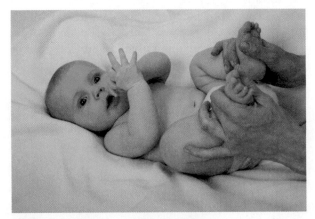

FIGURE 6-12 Stretching: pushing into abdomen.

full-body touch a parent may experience with a premature newborn.

Begin the massage by asking permission and telling the baby what is going to happen. Areas to massage may include the head, hands, legs, feet, or back. The chest and stomach areas may be oversensitive to touch, as this is where many procedures take place. Keep the massage short, one or two strokes in the beginning; a full massage would be too stimulating. Infants born preterm usually have difficulty organizing their state behaviors, but with time you will be able to recognize their cues of communicating. This will be important when beginning a regular course of massage (Figure 6-13).

LENGTH OF MASSAGE

The right length of a massage varies according to the ability of the newborn to process the sensory stimuli and the giver recognizing the states of awareness of the infant. The optimal time to massage a newborn is during the quiet alert state. Massage is done with the newborn, not to the newborn. Typical length is anywhere from 10 to 20 minutes; less for a premature infant or a newborn. Follow your infant's responses to stimulation. Toddlers will seldom lie down for a full massage. You may want to try to adapt the massage in a sitting up position. Never assume that you will be able to give a full massage to an infant. The important thing is to follow the cues the child is exhibiting. If those cues say, "Yes, engage with me," then go as long as the child is able to process the sen-

sory input. When he begins to show signs of overstimulation or disengagement—turning the head to the side, arching the back, rolling over, spitting up, crying, for example—take the cue and stop. A fussy baby has had enough massage, thank you. Cuddle and take a break.

WHICH OIL TO USE

Oil may not strictly be needed for newborns, but studies conducted at the Touch Research Institute indicate using it leads to a better response than not using it.[9] Natural cold-pressed or organic oils, such as sweet almond, apricot, sesame seed, or grape seed oil, will nourish the baby's skin and give a very smooth and pleasant feeling. Unscented oils are preferred because they enable babies to recognize their mother's scent—and because babies sometimes do put their hands in their mouths. If allergies are suspected, it's wise to perform a simple patch test: place a small amount of the oil on the infant's wrist, leave for 20 to 30 minutes. Redness may indicate a reaction. Mineral oil-based lotions, peanut oil, and baby powder should not be used.

CERTIFICATION REQUIREMENTS AND ADVANCED TRAINING

Infant massage is a global parenting practice with roots in antiquity and tradition, passed down from generation to generation. Different cultures have improvised and adapted techniques to suit the needs of their own societies and the children they massage. The growing popularity of infant massage in the United States comes largely without this background in tradition and experience. For this, and other reasons, U.S. parents, caregivers, and health professionals must have a substitute for the elders in other cultures who can teach the art in a responsible, loving, and knowledgeable manner.

There are many books, resources, and audiovisual materials available on infant massage, but the importance of learning from a properly trained and certified instructor cannot be understated. In most cases, the person who will ultimately perform the massage is a parent or caregiver, not a massage therapist, and the subject is a delicate infant or child, not an adult. Moreover, the massage will be performed, ideally on a regular basis, in the child's home. In other words, while infant massage is relatively easy to learn and delightful to share, there is a responsibility to see that these "nonprofessional" massagers get it right.

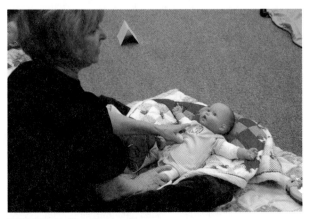

FIGURE 6-13 Floor time position.

Those who are interested in becoming certified in the field should get hands-on training through an accredited program. Infant massage pioneers in the mid-1970s created the original certification program for instructors, just as the practice was gaining acceptance in the United States.* Today, the CIMI® (Certified Infant Massage Instructor) the oldest designation for infant massage certifications is offered by two organizations, one is the International Loving Touch Foundation Inc. A number of other organizations have more recently arisen to teach and practice infant massage, though without offering the original CIMI designation.

CHAPTER SUMMARY

This chapter makes it very clear that all babies should be massaged, touched, and loved to promote their social, emotional, cognitive, and physical development. Mothers have been practicing the art of infant massage for centuries. As an early intervention strategy and therapeutic tool, infant massage is becoming a specialty therapy in the United States. It is being embraced by a wide variety of professionals who are incorporating it into their daily practices to help families cope with children with special needs. Techniques are simple and effective and are most effectively performed by parents and primary caregivers who have been taught by certified infant massage instructors. The approach is empowering and improves the parent-infant attachment process. There is a growing body of research that supports the therapeutic benefits. Infant massage is a crucial and routine part of infant care around the world and has the ability to create great benefits for both parents and the newborn.

CASE HISTORIES

■ Case history 1: Newborn with Down syndrome

The family had given birth to an infant diagnosed with Down syndrome (also called trisomy 21). The diagnosis was confirmed before birth through the chromosomal analysis known as amniocentesis. Down syndrome, a genetic condition, affects about one in 800 to 1000 babies, but is more prevalent among babies born to older

---

*In the interest of full disclosure, the pioneers who created the CIMI® designation include this writer, who is also of the International Loving Touch Foundation, Inc., and was one of the original board members who formed the International Association of Infant Massage Instructors.

women. According to Blackman, "Incidence increases with the age of the mother; one study estimates that rate for women of 40 years of age at 1 per 110 live births."[17]

This case did not involve an "older" mother, which perhaps added to the level of emotional distancing she manifested. She seemed, in fact, to be somewhat traumatized by the situation. Following delivery the infant was admitted into the NICU, where he faced specialized medical and surgical treatment for congenital heart defect.

While the mother was having difficulty dealing with her emotions over her infant's condition, the father was trying to be supportive. Upon learning that I would be available to teach and coach them about infant massage, he became very eager to learn more. We first discussed behavioral cues, watched a video, and then practiced the massage techniques on dolls. As the father gained confidence, he was able to try a little massage on his son. The mother herself became encouraged at the sight of her husband engaging in such a confident and loving manner with their son. Infant massage served as a positive strategy to help the mother and father connect with their newborn infant. As they attempted the massage together each time they touched him, they became more hopeful about the positive outcome of their son's health.

Children with Down syndrome have varying degrees of cognitive impairment, which can be coupled with low muscle tone and can lead to delays in development. Infant massage is a beneficial strategy to support the parent-infant attachment process in especially difficult situations. It is also valuable therapy for such conditions as low muscle tone and for the relief of constipation, which may itself be due to low muscle tone.

■ Case history 2: Cleft lip and palate

A lactation consultant referred the case of a mother and full-term newborn with a genetic condition called cleft lip and palate. This congenital deformity, which is caused by abnormal facial development during gestation, can result in significant feeding problems both prior to and after facial surgical procedures. "Normal development of the lip and the hard and soft palates is essential for proper eating and speech production," notes Blackman. "The front lip helps control liquids and foods during drinking and eating and helps create a suction to assist in moving liquids and food to the back of the mouth for swallowing."[17]

This anomaly is one of the most disturbing to parents as it affects the facial structure and appearance and can leave lasting facial scars. Often infants may have had as many as three surgeries before the age of one. Most mothers are not able to breast feed, which can create emotional barriers to their attachment.

Infant massage was a useful intervention for this mother to help overcome feeding issues and the emotional disruption of the mother-infant bond. I was able to teach her specific techniques that she could comfortably perform in massaging her infant's face and head. These served to fill the void and create other ways of attachment and loving interaction through body contact. Using a series of simple infant massage techniques gave her more confidence in her handling skills and assisted in her emotional alliance with her baby. By stimulating the facial muscles in a loving, sensitive, and affectionate way, she was able to overcome some of her fears in touching her infant's face, as well as help the infant reduce the sensitivity to the area after surgery.

SUGGESTED READINGS

Baby's first touch: step-by step instruction for infant massage, Portland, Oregon, 2005, International Loving Touch Foundation.

Verklan MT, Walden M, editors: *Core curriculum for neonatal intensive care nursing,* ed 3, Philadelphia, 2004, Elsevier.

Heath A, Bainbridge N: *Baby massage: the calming power of touch,* New York, 2000, DK Publishing.

Elliott L: *What's going on in there? How the brain and mind develop in the first five years of life,* New York, 1999, Bantam.

Kavanagh K: *Baby touch: massage and reflexology for babies and children,* New York, 2005, Sterling Publishing.

Meredith S, ed: *Your happy baby: massage, yoga, aromatherapy, and other gentle ways to blissful babyhood,* New York, 2006, Ryland Peters & Small.

Zeanah CH: *Handbook of infant mental health,* New York, 2000, Guilford Press.

Siegel D, Hartzell M: *Parenting from the inside out,* New York, 2003, Penquin Group.

Sinclair M: *Pediatric massage therapy,* Philadelphia, 2005, Lippincott Williams & Wilkins.

Stamm J: *Bright from the start,* New York, 2007, Gotham Books.

RESOURCES

Brain Development
www.newdirectionsinstitute.org
www.brainconnections.com

The Child Trauma Academy
http://www.childtrauma.org

Infant Cues - Nursing Satellite Child Training
University of Washington
www.ncast.org

International Loving Touch Foundation, Inc.
http://www.lovingtouch.com

Stages of Development
www.pathwaysawareness.org

World Association for Infant Mental Health
http://www.waimh.org

Zero to Three Organization
http://www.zerotothree.org

REFERENCES

1. Heller S: *The vital touch*, New York, 1997, Henry Holt.
2. Auckett AD: Baby massage in Nepal, *Whole Person* 44: 1995.
3. Campbell RJ: *Campbell's psychiatric dictionary*, ed 8, Oxford, NY, 2004, Oxford University Press.
4. Leboyer F: *Loving hands: the traditional art of baby massage*, New York, 1976, New Market Press.
5. Dunhan C, *The body shop team: Mamatoto: a celebration of birth*, London, 1991, Virago Press
6. Auckett A: *Baby massage: parent-child bonding through touch*, New York, 1992, New Market Press.
7. *Baby's first touch: step-by-step instruction for infant massage*, Portland, Ore, 2005, International Loving Touch Foundation.
8. Zeanah CH Jr, ed: *Handbook for infant mental health*, New York, 2000, Guilford Press.
9. Brazelton TB, Nugent JK: Neonatal Behavioral Assessment Scale, ed 3, *Clinics in developmental medicine 137*, London, 1995, Mac Keith Press.
10. Field T et al: Tactile/kinesthetic stimulation effects on preterm neonates, *Pediatrics* 77:654–658, 1986.
11. Available at: http://www6.miami.edu/touch-research/.
12. March of Dimes: Available at: http://www.marchofdimes.com/pnhec/188_15755.asp.
13. Baradon T et al: *The practice of psychoanalytic parent-infant psychotherapy: claiming the baby*, New York, 2005, Routledge.
14. Linden DW, Paroli ET, Doron MW: *The essential guide for parents of premature babies*, New York, 2000, Simon and Schuster.
15. Bowlby J: *Maternal Care and Mental Health, World Health Organization Monograph (serial no 2)*, 1951.
16. Montuori E, Garelli JC: A brief sketch of John Bowlby's biography (online article): http://garelli.tripod.com/bio.html.
17. Blackman G: *Medical aspects of developmental disabilities in children*, ed 3, Frederick, Md, 1997, Aspen Publication.

MULTIPLE CHOICE TEST QUESTIONS

1) Identify three countries in the world where infant massage has traditionally been used as a parenting practice:
   a) China, Nepal, and India
   b) Sweden, Norway, and Austria
   c) India, Nigeria, and Nepal
   d) United States, Canada, and Australia

2) From the book *Vital Touch,* author Sharon Heller states that anthropologist James McKenna writes about infants being "at odds" with their evolution because they:
   a) cry excessively
   b) are too independent
   c) are not kept in arms
   d) always seek attention

3) In the United States, approximately how many years has infant massage been developing as a parent baby activity?
   a) 25 years
   b) 30 years
   c) 35 years
   d) 40 years

4) The highly popular book *Loving Hands,* written by Frederick LeBoyer, was first introduced into the United States around what year?
   a) 1976
   b) 1977
   c) 1978
   d) 1980

5) One of the first recorded mentions of the use of massage in the United States occurred in a book titled *Care and Feeding of Children.* Who was that author?
   a) James McKenna
   b) Ashley Montague
   c) Angela Joyce
   d) Emmett Holt

6) In general, infant massage should be performed in what manner?
   a) smooth, fingertip touches
   b) lightly so not to hurt the baby
   c) smooth, rhythmical manner
   d) rapidly to finish quickly

7) How many behavioral states can an infant exhibit?
   a) four
   b) six
   c) average of eight
   d) too many to count

8) Tiffany Field with the Touch Research Institute did a study on the effects of massage on premature newborns. What was the strongest clinical outcome?
   a) preterm infants gained weight
   b) encouraged early discharge
   c) promoted bonding with caregiver
   d) reduced crying in babies

9) The optimal state to perform a well-baby massage is when the infant is in the:
   a) active alert state
   b) quiet sleep state
   c) drowsy state
   d) quiet alert state

10) In South India, Leboyer noted that the practice of massaging infants begins when the infant was how old?
    a) immediately after birth
    b) after the umbilical cord stub has fallen off
    c) 1 month old
    d) 2 months old

11) A cue of engagement and disengagement may include:
    a) smiling and crying
    b) cooing and babbling
    c) crying and gaze aversion
    d) arching the body, pushing away

12) An infant is considered premature if his birth occurs before how many weeks gestation?
    a) 37 weeks
    b) 38 weeks
    c) 39 weeks
    d) 40 weeks

13) What is a patch test?
    a) test for heat sensitivities
    b) test for movement restrictions
    c) test for allergic reactions
    d) test for behavioral cues

14) The most defining purpose of infant massage is:
    a) formation of a close emotional tie
    b) getting parents more connected
    c) preventing abuse or neglect
    d) treating medical conditions

15) The best type of oil or lubricant to use for giving a baby massage is?
    a) generic baby oil
    b) baby powder
    c) lavender oil
    d) natural cold-pressed oil

16) What type of music would be advantageous to accompany baby massage?
    a) any type that you like
    b) lullaby sounds or heartbeat sound
    c) no music is the best music
    d) nature sounds

17) On average, mothers feel a sharp increase in bonding with their infant around what month?
    a) first month after delivery
    b) fifth month of pregnancy
    c) about 6 months after delivery
    d) about 12 months after delivery

18) Where would be the safest place to perform baby massage?
    a) in the baby's bed
    b) on a massage table
    c) on the floor
    d) on the changing table

19) Typically how long should the massage last?
    a) varies according to states of awareness
    b) 5 minutes or less
    c) 10 to 20 minutes
    d) 20 to 30 minutes

20) Explain how you would adapt the massage routine for an active toddler:
    a) wait until they are beyond the toddler stage
    b) go slowly to avoid excitement
    c) adapt strokes in a sitting position
    d) massage only at nighttime

Lomilomi

Dane Kaohelani Silva and
R. Makana Risser Chai

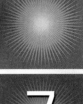

7

INTRODUCTION

Popularly known as Hawaiian massage, **lomilomi** goes beyond massage technique. Lomilomi is loving touch, aligning the body, mind, heart, and spirit to the Divine. It is ancient, but still practiced by native healers and traditionally trained practitioners in the home, at community health centers, and in the finest spas in Hawai'i and around the world. Though renowned as a means of soothing pain and relaxing tired and stiff muscles, traditionally lomilomi is a holistic health care system using massage, herbal medicine, chiropractic, osteopathy, physical therapy, colonics, sticks, stones, water, steam baths, and, most importantly, prayer, forgiveness, and reconciliation.

Lomi means to knead, to rub, or soothe, to work in and out, as the paws of a contented cat. Lomilomi has a more intensive meaning, commonly interpreted as massage. It is a system of deep work using biomechanical and energetic waves to stimulate the cells to heal and regenerate.

HISTORY

Massage arrived in Hawai'i with the Polynesian discoverers who voyaged by sailing canoes from the Marquesas Islands in the South Pacific about 1500 years ago. Their ancestors before them sailed from China, where healers practiced massage for millennia.[1] Physical therapy was essential for keeping the voyagers healthy and alive during the arduous journey and after they settled the land. Once here, lomilomi evolved into something uniquely Hawaiian and remained unaffected by outside influences until the arrival of European explorers in 1778.

Traditionally, lomilomi was practiced by every member of the family. Children performed it on adults (by walking on their backs), adults on children, and adults on each other. Everyone used it to remedy common illnesses such as headaches, colds, fevers, indigestion, sprains, back pain, rheumatic joints, and simple fractures. Medical experts *(kāhuna lā'au lapa'au)* used lomilomi as physical therapy to prevent and cure serious injury and disease, and were able to cure compound fractures in days. They also treated women during pregnancy, labor, childbirth, and postpartum.

Martial arts masters taught lomilomi to their students. It is said that lomilomi is the foundation for the training of martial arts. To learn how to incapacitate the enemy, the warrior must first know how the bones, muscles, joints, and nerves work, where the vulnerabilities are, and how to repair injuries. "You break it, you fix it."

Lomilomi was practiced by servants on the male and female chiefs, who enjoyed it as a luxury of life.

Given all these different uses, it is no wonder there are many different styles today. As an indigenous therapy, the practice has varied from island to island, from one valley to another, among 'families and individual practitioners. Traditionally, Hawaiians respected differences among practitioners. An old Hawaiian proverb says, "All wisdom is not taught in one school."[3]

In the latter part of the twentieth century, a few teachers came forward to teach their families' practices. Five received renown around the world. Each one was from a different "school." Most no longer teach, but others continue their traditions.[2]

Margaret Machado inherited family lomilomi from her grandfather and was one of the first Native Hawaiians to become a licensed massage therapist. Her strokes and draping practices have similarities to Swedish massage therapy.

Henry Auwae specialized in herbal medicine (lā'au lapa'au). He worked with clients over days or weeks using internal and external herbal remedies. He used lomilomi to hasten the effect of the medicine.

Kalua Kaiahua came from the martial arts tradition. He usually worked with the client fully clothed, lying on a table. He always started with the abdomen. He quickly squeezed and kneaded, finishing a typical treatment in 15 or 20 minutes (Figure 7-1).

Mary Fragas works with pregnant women and infants. She helps women relieve pain and prepare for childbirth, and through massage adjusts the position of the baby in the womb to prevent breech birth.

Abraham Kawai'i founded Kahuna Bodywork, known for long, flowing strokes with the forearms and fluid, rhythmic foot movements.

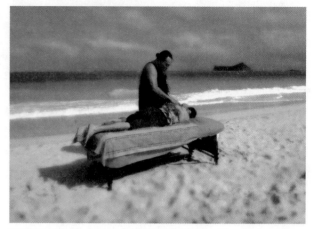

FIGURE 7-1 On deserted Waimānalo Beach, Alva Andrews uses the martial arts style of lomilomi. Alva is a teacher of lomilomi in Waimanalo who trained with Papa Kalua Kaiahua.

Differences among practitioners have traditionally been limited to the physical aspects of their practice. What makes lomilomi authentic is how it treats the mind, the heart, and the spirit.

LOMILOMI TECHNIQUE

Not unlike modern massage, lomilomi employs physical techniques of stimulating the different sensory receptors to communicate to the body-mind via the circulatory, neurologic, and myofascial systems of the body.

It uses the palms, forearms, fingers, knuckles, elbows, knees, feet, sticks, and stones, with and without lubrication. It consists of both gentle and hard techniques such as rubbing, stroking, kneading, pounding, pressing, shaking, vibrating, pushing, pulling, pinching, rolling, squeezing, slapping, digging, deep pressure point compressions, and joint manipulation.

Two techniques, though not unique to lomilomi, are an important part of the practice. Hawaiians believe the abdominal area *('ōpū)* is the center of health and vitality. Manipulation of the stomach or palpation and movement of the abdominal area frequently are used to identify and correct blockages to the healthy functioning of the abdominal organs and to enhance the elimination of body wastes. Treading—back-walking—is also popular (Figure 7-2).

However, what is unique about the physical movements is not what is done, but how it is done. Lomilomi is called sacred touch or loving touch because it is always done with prayer and intention. And it includes other forms of physical, mental, emotional, and spiritual

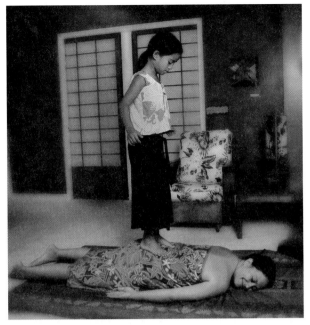

FIGURE 7-2 Kamehanaokala Ruiz carefully treads on her mom, Patricia, at Moku Ola Hawaiian Healing Center where she is learning lomilomi.

therapies as part of a holistic system of health care (Box 7-1).

From the beginning of Hawaiian history, the balanced relationship between mankind, nature, and the Creator (Akua) has been considered to be most important. This is called balance *(lōkahi)*. The healing power of ***pule*** (prayer) is used to achieve balance. Prayer had been used in massage for centuries before the arrival of the Christians and other missionaries, and it continued to be used after they arrived. Contemporary practitioners, whether Christian or of other spiritual affiliations, use prayer to establish the communication between the practitioner, the client, nature, and the Divine. Prayer is performed before, during, and after a session. Papa Henry Auwae said that 80% of healing comes from prayer. Auntie Margaret Machado taught that "lomilomi is praying work." Without prayer, it is simply a massage.

BOX 7-1 Prayer: *Pule*

"From the crown of the head to the soles of the feet, and the four corners of the body." (An expression used in prayers for healing. The four corners are the shoulders and hips; between them are the vital organs of the body.)

Breath: *Hā*

As Mary Kawena Pukui observed, "Hawaii had long observed the connection between breathing and life. Long before the missionaries arrived, Hawaiians had invested the 'breath of life' with a spiritual significance that closely paralleled Biblical references."[3]

Energetic techniques that coordinate breath or ***hā*** and spirit are integrated into the manual procedures. The patient is told to breathe at a deep, slow rate. If the patient is not able or willing to comply, a normal rate and rhythm are acceptable. Clients are told they may experience temporary exacerbation of their pain when the tender points and areas are treated. But they are not advised to "breathe into the point of pain" because doing so may facilitate a holographic image of pain that may make it more difficult to eradicate. Clients should, however, be encouraged to accept their condition. A practitioner may, for example, direct a client to "look into the point of pain and observe it flow out of your body like the smoke from a snuffed candle. With each breath, see the smoke flow out of the point of pain."

This movement of pain occurs with systematic treatment over time. Each layer of pain, discomfort, stiffness, or weakness is peeled away at each subsequent session.

The practitioner uses the breath to facilitate the movement of blocked and stagnant energy (pain) during the treatment session. Clients exhale while the practitioner applies pressure to an area or tender point and/or projects energy into the site. They are asked to visualize the breath flowing into the area, causing the stagnant energy to billow outward from the tender points and into the environment, like smoke.

Forgiveness: *Hoʻoponopono*

Hoʻoponopono is a traditional system for restoring balance or harmony within the client and the client's family. Many practitioners are trained in the basic aspects of this art. Hoʻoponopono means "setting to right," "forgiveness," "reconciliation," or "family counseling."

Early Hawaiians knew what modern medicine has now proved—holding grudges makes you sick. They identified sickness that came from "within"—not within the body, but within the family. When a person has done something that creates a loss of balance in their relationship within themselves or with significant others, a process of forgiveness and reconciliation is necessary for optimal healing.

Ho'oponopono is a meeting of the entire family with a precise structure of multiple phases involving questioning, reflection, confession, discussion, requesting forgiveness, making amends, and reconciliation. The process may take hours or days. Each session starts and ends with prayer, and prayer is resorted to whenever tempers flare. Prayer sets the tone, generating trust and good feelings (Box 7-2).

Hot Stones: *Pōhaku Wela*

Smooth, round *pōhaku wela,* or hot stones, may be heated in a fire or in a container of water, wrapped in leaves, and placed on the patient to relieve back pain and spasms. The leaves used include kava *('awa),* ti *(kī),* Indian mulberry *(noni),* and castor oil plant *(koli).* One unique method is to place a leaf of the ti plant on the body and rub the heated stone across the leaf.

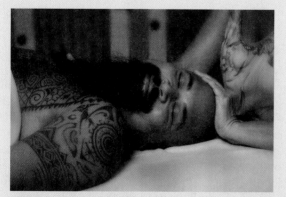

FIGURE 7-3 In the hands of lomilomi teacher Noelani Bennett, Maluhia La Pierre of the band, Ooklah the Moc, finds complete acceptance.

A bare, hot stone may be massaged on scar tissue to soften and smooth it. The attachment of the levator scapulae muscle to the scapula is a good location for this type of hot stone therapy. Therapists should use caution, taking care not to burn the skin: the importance of safety cannot be overemphasized.

Small stones may be placed in a cloth bag and used to gently pound areas on the surface of the patient's body such as the hamstrings. When heated, this bag also may be placed on the abdomen for relief of abdominal cramps.

Lomi Sticks — *Lā'au Lomi*

Lomi sticks or *lā'au lomi* are used in a variety of ways. A thick stick about 12 inches long with a tapered end can be used by the practitioner to compress pressure points. A pole 6 feet in length is used for balance while back-walking and may also be used to move the extremities of a patient lying on the floor. A 3-foot long stick with a foot-long branch angled at 45° can be used by the patient to compress places on the back (Figure 7-4).

Traditional practitioners search for the wood themselves, carve the stick into shape, and polish it for use. Over time, being used with prayer and intention, the stick accumulates spiritual energy *(mana).*

Steam: *Pūholoholo*

The steam bath, or *pūholoholo,* is a favored form of therapy that is used to stimulate circulation and to assist in the cleansing process. The first Hawaiians discovered natural steam baths at the volcanoes. A little hut made with hau tree branches arched over at the top would be constructed over steam vents or areas of heated stones. They also created steam by heating water in a bowl or gourd and placing it with the patient under a bark cloth blanket. Herbs may be placed in the container for the patient to inhale the vapor. Modern steam bathers use a sauna or sweat lodge.

Water and Sunlight: *Waiola*

Waiola refers to the healing properties of water and sunlight (Figure 7-5). Along the Eastern coast of the island of Hawai'i, practitioners use pools of geothermally heated water for their healing powers. The warm, buoyant water soothes the muscles and arthritic joints and reduces the full effects of gravity. While patients are immersed, practitioners may administer physiotherapy including exercises and massage.

A gentle waterfall relaxes stiffness and relieves pain. Cold water that seeps through the lava tubes from the mountains to pour into ponds at the shore is used to stimulate deep circulation. Immersion in fresh water is often the final part of a course of treatment.[3]

Both physical and spiritual rituals of restoration and purification may be performed using either sea water or fresh water with salt dissolved in it, mixed with turmeric *('ōlena),* and sprinkled onto the patient.

Sunbathing is another part of the restorative treatment and is usually accompanied or preceded by the application of herbal potions or liniments to the body. The juice of the black nightshade *(pōpolo)* leaves may be used on swollen tendons, for example, followed by sunbathing.

Closing Feast: *Pani*

At the conclusion of a successful program, a ***pani*** or special meal may be held with patients and their families, usually featuring food from the sea. It not only celebrates the closing of the treatment, but also physically reminds them that the illness is in the past.

TREATMENT OVERVIEW

A session can be as simple as a 10-minute chair massage or as long as a treatment plan requiring continuing care over a period of days, weeks, or months. A typical protocol for extended treatment could include:

- Preparation of sacred space
- Prayer
- Assessment
- Lā'au lapa'au (medicinal herbs)
- Drink tea
- Apply herbs externally
- Lay down/meditate/drink medicine
- Exercise may be prescribed (walk to mountains or sea)
- Diet may be prescribed (e.g., eat lū'au greens and limu seaweed)
- Cleanse
- Steam bath
- Bowel movement
- Ho'oponopono (forgiveness, make things right)
- Lomilomi
- Complete the circle
- Clearing ceremony ***(kala)***
- Cut away the bad, leave the good ('oki)
- Closing meal (pani)
- Prayer

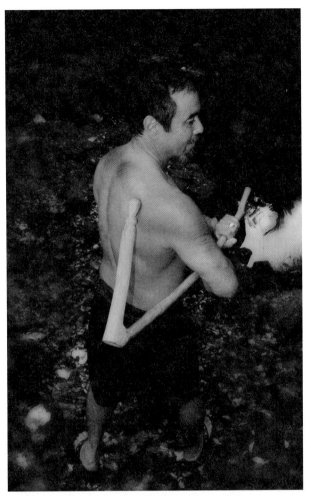

FIGURE 7-4 Koni demonstrates one way to use a lomi stick. He crafts them from guava wood found on the island of Hawai'i.

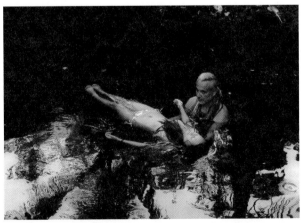

FIGURE 7-5 Author Dane Silva treats his daughter, Shelle, in the hot pond on the island of Hawai'i.

PREPARATION OF SACRED SPACE: *HALE OLA*

Hawaiians know the land itself is healing. Certain areas possess special healing powers. Practitioners historically and today often give treatments outdoors so patients can see the mountains, feel the warm caress of the breeze, smell the flowers, hear the waves, and taste the salt air. If this is not possible, treatment is given in the *hale ola* or place of healing.

The environment may be warm, filled with a calming scent and relaxing music. The natural light may be dimmed. The surface that supports the one who is receiving the treatment may be firm but yielding. Air circulates freely. It is conducive to the flow of healing energy (Figure 7-6).

Sheets are spread on the mat or table, and a sarong, sheet, or blanket covers the patient. It offers warmth and modesty and can be adjusted to cover the parts of the body not being treated at that moment.

Plants may be used within the hale ola. Ti plants are renowned for their protective and healing properties. The maile plant or lei may be used to add the subtle scent for which it is beloved. This plant is also known for its use in sacred rituals.

Water is a necessary element to have available in the house of healing. A container may be filled with fresh water. Sea salt and turmeric may be added to the water, or sea water may be used when available. This is used to bathe the hands after energy passes from the patient

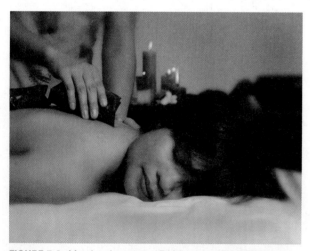

FIGURE 7-6 After heating stones, Eri Mahealani Sakai Virden wraps them in healing ti leaves and places them along the spine. Notice the use of candles in this hale ola, Lomilomi Hana Lima in Kailua on Oʻahu.

into the hands of the practitioner. The water drains this energy and allows it to flow out of the hands and into the bowl of water. This water is poured over the ground outside or around one of the plants within the space.

Sometimes it is necessary to use a flame from a source, such as a large candle, in order to release and transmute the potent energy that may be drawn off a patient and into the hands. It is important to release this energy into the fire, where it may be converted into light and heat and recycled into the environment.

PRAYER: *PULE*

The pule, or prayer, is a ritual act of preparation that is an integral part of the healing process. It opens the way for the exchange of healing energy. A clear channel of energy is more effective than one that is blocked.

First we pray for harmony and healing within ourselves, asking for a blessing and divine guidance. This initial moment of calm meditation and receptivity is a ritual act of humility and acceptance of our role as the one who brings forth and shares the gift of the healing touch of aloha or love.

As we release our own energy blocks and focus our life force, we prepare ourselves for the act of helping to preserve the health of the people. We concentrate on the one who is to receive. We ask for guidance and assistance in recognizing the blocks that do not belong in the body-mind and need to be released. We ask for assistance in releasing the life force to flow within and to bring in love and light. We focus on the restoration of harmony within the environment of their body, mind, and spirit.

We ask for spiritual protection for ourselves, the patient, and for the place of healing. A prayer may also include a visualization of a powerful field of energy surrounding the space and all of the participants (Figure 7-7).

PRINCIPLES OF ASSESSMENT: ʻALAWA

Five principles are taught in the Hawaiian culture as part of the process of mastery of any art. These principles are modified by each school or teacher in order to specifically address the needs of the art. For example, when applied to hula they are defined within the specific context of the dance. In the art of lomilomi, we apply these principles as part of the assessment process.

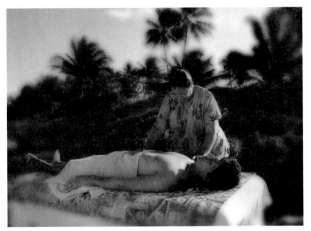

FIGURE 7-7 Lomilomi teacher Haunani Hopkins of Mapuna Waiola on the Big Island begins with prayer. She says, "Ke Akua God guides our hands through our hearts."

Nānā: To Look, Observe

The art of observation is applied by the practitioner with regard to several aspects of the patient. Some of the physical aspects noted are posture or shape of the body. The observer also notes the relative size, symmetry, and coloration of different parts of the body such as the face, shoulders, arms, elbows, forearms, hands, chest, abdomen, back, pelvis, legs, knees, lower legs, ankles, and feet. The presence of observable lumps, lesions, colored spots, spasm, loss of muscle tone, tremors, or paralysis, as well as abnormalities in hair color, teeth, or gait, etc., are noted. Blackened skin around the feet of an adult, for example, may indicate the presence of diabetes. Or uneven shoulders may indicate that a patient has a curvature in the spinal column, with shortened muscles and fascia, affecting the function of the spinal nerves, which communicate with all of the body parts, including the internal organs.

Two perspectives of observation may be employed. The observer can look at the entire person using a wide-angled view known as the "big picture," or look at the details of asymmetries or anomalies using a telescopic or microscopic view known as the "little picture." Our focus may be wide at one moment, and it may change as we zoom in on something of interest. It is also possible to look at the "aura" of the patient. The presence or absence of the *'aumakua* may be noted. The *'aumakua* are the personal or family gods, including deified ancestors who may have become transmogrified into animal forms.

Ho'olohe: To Listen, Obey

In the hula school, the teacher may say *"lohe lohe,"* listen and obey. In the lomi school, we apply the phrase "ho'olohe." In the context of assessment, this means to listen to the patient. Listen to their speech. Is it strong or weak? Slow and calm or fast and frenetic? These findings may indicate the presence of stress, concussion, or mental disease. Listen to the body. Is the breath short and ragged or deep and clear? Can you hear the heart beat? Is it regular and rhythmic or irregular? Do the bowels make noises? Do the joints pop or grind when the patient moves? Can you hear clicking sounds coming from the teeth or jaws? These findings may indicate the presence of arthritis, asthma, heart problems, or other conditions.

In a spiritual context, ho'olohe means to close the two ears and listen with the "middle ear." Communication may be obtained in a telepathic sense, either in the form of words or images. Words or sounds may come from the patient's body or from their spiritual form. They may correspond to images perceived with eyes open or closed.

Nīnau: Question, Interrogate

We ask a patient where it hurts and to point out the location. We ask how and when they acquired the problem, if they have had this problem more than once, and if there have been previous treatments, whether successful or not.

In the Hawaiian culture, genealogy is very important. Patients are questioned about their personal lives and the lives of the members of their family. They are questioned about diet, exercise, work, and play habits. We interrogate them and sometimes other members of the family until we have as clear and complete a picture of their personal and family history as is feasible.

The health history or cause of illness or death of each member of the immediate family is an important part of the assessment process. It may indicate a genetic disorder or occupational hazard that has affected members of the patient's family over several generations. The time allotted for intake is more than the typical 10 minutes allowed within a health maintenance organization. A key element of lomilomi is not to be restricted to a brief intake. It is allowable to spend an hour or more, perhaps over the course of several visits.

Pa'a ka waha: Close the Mouth

Pa'a ka waha means that practitioners should be aware of their own tendency to talk too much. It means the patient is the focus. When we talk too much we lose the focus necessary for our work. It also means to maintain confidentiality of those things that we have learned in the process of assessment.

Hana lima: Work with the Hands

Hana lima is a perfect description of the art of palpation. We use our hands to assess the patient. The hands may press the skin to detect places of heat, density (hard, soft, mushy), or texture (rough, scaly, dry, moist). We may press around the abdomen to gather information about the internal organs. For example, constipation in the large intestine may be noted. Inflammation in the large intestine may also be noted at the angles near the liver or the spleen or the sigmoid colon. An enlarged liver may be noted. When pressing with the hands, ask the patient to let you know when a painful area is located. Body parts such as the joints of the spine and extremities may be moved while stiffness or pain may be noted. Abnormal structures such as soft tissue masses or hard, bony masses may be noted in the body.

Herbal Medicine: *Lā'au Lapa'au*

Bruises, strains, sprains, spasms, and pain are often treated with lā'au lapa'au combined with massage. Turmeric root is an antiinflammatory agent that may be finely ground and ingested in a capsule or tea. If externally applied absorption is limited, although effect may be noted in the relief of edema, reduction of redness, or some pain relief. However, this plant, also known as yellow ginger, is a natural dye and will permanently stain sheets and clothing.

The leaves of the kava plant may be applied as a poultice to block pain. It may be brewed as a tea to reduce stress or treat insomnia. The powdered root of the plant may be ingested in a capsule or tea. Inhaling the smoke of this plant or steam from a hot poultice can cause drowsiness and a feeling of intoxication. It is not unusual to feel numbness wherever the plant touches, internally or externally.

A pack made of the fresh leaves of the castor oil bush may be applied to the joints of a patient with back pain. The leaves are heated before application. Arthritic joints, bruised muscles, or areas of sprain or strain may be wrapped in Indian mulberry (noni) or candlenut tree *(kukui)* leaves. Headaches may be treated with ti or 'awa leaves wrapped around the forehead or temple. Fevers are also treated by wrapping the head and/or body with ti leaves. Fresh leaves replace the old ones when they change texture and become dry or clammy. A hot pack may be made by heating salt wrapped in cloth. Salt draws out the pain.

Colon Cleansing and Diet: *Ho'oma'ema'e* and *'Ai*

The ancient Hawaiian system of healthcare included the use of diluted seawater and herbal juice to cleanse and purge the body, called ***ho'oma'ema'e***. Modern practitioners using purified seawater continue to treat patients with 10-day intensive programs for internal cleansing in combination with herbs and abdominal manipulation. Extended programs for seasonal or year-long cleansing may be recommended for patients with chronic conditions.

A patient who is under the care of a native healer is given strict guidelines in the consumption of *'ai* food and drink. This is done in the belief that certain foods can enhance the healing process and that other foods slow or block the process. Liquids that hydrate the body or contribute to the amount of blood that is created are part of the diet.

Lubricant: *'Aila Hamo*

Before beginning the lomilomi a lubricant may be prepared, although some practitioners do not use lubrication. A variety of ***'aila hamo*** lubricants may be used, including water-based potions, oils, or creams. Different lubricants amplify the sensory stimuli of texture. They may be warmed or subtly scented with the essence of flowers or herbs. Aromatherapy may serve to stimulate the breathing process.

Lomilomi has a long history of using the oils from the kukui nut, the coconut, and the fat of the turtle. Sandalwood powder, ground turmeric root, noni juice, or 'awa may be added to the oils to enhance the health of the skin, relieve pain and inflammation, and reduce myofascial spasms. Salves or creams may also be prepared that contain some of the herbs in combination with beeswax.

The oils reduce friction, stimulate the senses (especially smell and touch), and nourish the skin. Kukui nut oil, for example, contains significant amounts of soothing vitamin E.

Lomilomi has been used successfully for centuries with aromatic oils, *'alaea* (a red colloidal ocherous earth), or herbs to enhance the facial features. In this regard, it shares some of the effects of other popular forms of beauty and wellness care.

While preparing the oil, the practitioner prays to add the spiritual component and amplify its healing power.

LOMILOMI PROTOCOL

In a 1934 booklet on Hawaiian physiotherapy, native researcher Mary Kawena Pukui discussed the range of lomilomi protocols:

"Various modes of procedure have been described to me—starting at centers of pain or congestion and working outward along veins, tendons, muscles (all called *a'a*), or bones *(iwi)*, starting at the top of the head and working down the front and then up the back, starting at the feet and working up to the chest, and so on. The procedure is naturally determined by the case under treatment."[2]

Auntie Mona Kahele learned a protocol from her great-grandfather, who was the grandfather and teacher of Auntie Margaret Machado:

"He said, 'You never start where the pain is. You start from the head, even if the pain is down below, you never start there, but you start working from the tip of their head and end at the tip of their toe. That's how it should be.' Because they believe that when you get to the tip of their toe, sickness goes out."[2]

Kalua Kaiahua always began treatment with *'ōpū huli,* literally "turning stomach" (Figure 7-8).

A lomilomi practitioner sometimes starts with a power stroke. Gentle and flowing strokes are applied to the upper body, generating a wave starting at the shoulders and rippling down alongside the spine onto the hips. From there, the therapist's hands create a wave in the trunk, as he brings them back up toward the shoulder blades. An outward stroke toward the arms is immediately followed by a gliding movement toward the neck, where a final wave is created in the cervical spine. This power stroke is repeated at least three times. The first sequence is performed at a shallow level of pressure. The second sequence is performed at a middle level of pressure. The third sequence is performed at a deep level of pressure. This initial technique sends a soothing vibration throughout the body, in preparation for subsequent stimulation of the soft and boney tissues.

Complete the Circle

Hawaiians traditionally mark the ending of a treatment. This is to close the way to the past and move into the present. This simple protocol is one of the ways to complete a session.

Visualize the Flow

Stand at the feet, holding one foot in each hand. Visualize the smooth flow of energy from the patient's head to the toes, into your hands, through your body, into your feet, and into the earth. As your intent is to assist in the restoration of a balance of energy in the body, you exert a pulling force, a force of atraction, that creates a current through your own body. This can assist in the movement of stagnant or sluggish energy flow through the client.

OPTIONAL PATIENT VISUALIZATION

Ask the client to imagine a flow of energy coming from above and into the top of the head. As the pulsating, vibrating, flowing light pours into the body, the client should visualize the energy filling every cell, tissue, organ, and space. As the energy completely fills the body, it overflows. The excess energy flows into the client's feet, from the feet, and into your hands.

Release

Perform the meditation for a few minutes, then disengage your hands. Your intent is to cut the energy connection between yourself and the client.

Rebalance

Place your hands in a bowl of water or under flowing water. Pray that any unbalanced energy that may be in your body, or which may have passed into your body, be passed into the water to be recirculated into the environment.

Clearing Ceremony: *Kala*

A ritual of clearing is used after a treatment has been performed. In energetic terms, **kala** is "cutting the cord"

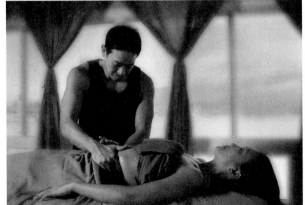

FIGURE 7-8 Kaliko Chang gives 'ōpū huli at Moku Ola Hawaiian Healing Center on O'ahu.

that connects the practitioner to the patient. This is a protective technique that allows the healer and patient to continue their lives independent of the spiritual influence of each other.

Many therapists have acknowledged that they have a gift for healing. This gift allows for the transfer of energy between the patient and the healer. This follows the principle of "energy flows from a place of higher concentration to a place of lower concentration." The healer's energy may be clear and powerful and useful for healing. Unfortunately, the disorganized and turbid energy of the patient may also flow from a place of higher concentration (the patient) to a place of lower concentration (the healer).

Some healers complain of "getting the same disease" as the patient following a therapy session. The kala ritual is helpful for those healers who have that problem on occasion. The ritual clearing is used to prevent the continual drain of energy from the therapist to the patient. It is also used to prevent the continual transfer of energetic disharmony from the patient to the therapist.

Traditionally, one way this was done was for the practitioner to go to the shore and make a lei of a seaweed called "kala" (a type of *Sargassum*). The practitioner would immerse in the sea and the lei would float off into the water, symbolizing the release of emotional stress or pain, as well as spiritual entanglements. The practitioner also would vocalize or "primal scream" while under water.

One version of the kala ceremony done today has three phases. Each phase is activated by a prayer. The first phase consists of a symbolic cutting of the cords that connect the healer to the patient. This is called *'oki* and is done by moving the hand in a cutting fashion over the three *piko* or navels of the patient (the top of the head, the navel, and the genital area). The second phase is a cleansing protocol where a bundle of ti leaves dampened in salt water with turmeric is brushed across the body of the patient. The third phase is for empowerment, where energy is amplified for use by the healer. This is called *ho'omana*. These three phases of cleansing, forgiveness, and empowerment are spiritual components of the healing process.

IN MY EXPERIENCE

People come with a specific complaint or request for help. When this complaint is resolved, another condition or layer of disease is revealed. After that complaint is resolved, still another condition or layer is exposed. This pattern of layers of complaints by the same patient is a common situation.

When a patient suffers from a syndrome of overlaid pain, swelling, stiffness, or loss of functions, it may reveal a state of chronic inflammation that affects multiple sites in the body. It follows that the patient will complain of each site until the inflammation has decreased throughout the entire body.

INDICATIONS FOR LOMILOMI

The immediate effect of the rituals and techniques of lomilomi is to induce a state of profound relaxation and sublime soothing of the mind, body, and spirit. At the mental level, lomilomi can help ease the effects of depression or sadness.

At the physiologic level, lomilomi has profound antiinflammatory benefits. The immune system is supported and stabilized. Typical complaints of head, hand, knee, or backaches due to injuries or arthritis are relieved. Muscle spasms, which affect the flexibility and alignment of the joints, are relieved, increasing circulation (lymphatic, arterial, venous) throughout the body, enhancing respiratory, digestive, and eliminative functions, and stimulating the sensory and motor compo-

nents of the nervous system. Abdominal manipulation directly affects the internal organs.

In the Hawaiian culture, lomilomi has been used for centuries to soothe the pregnant mother as well as the newborn child. This practice continues to nurture the new generations of residents in Hawai'i (Figure 7-9).

At the spiritual level, lomilomi aids in achieving an intuitive state of awareness and aloha or love.

CONTRAINDICATIONS FOR LOMILOMI

Although it is correct to simply say that specific conditions such as hemorrhage, tumor, infection, and fracture warrant a policy of avoidance due to contraindications, that would be overly simplistic and not

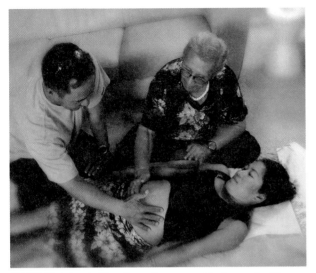

FIGURE 7-9 Auntie Mary Fragas is renowned for her work with pregnant women. Here she shows a husband how to give lomilomi to his wife and child.

offer due justice to the levels of wisdom and skill of an advanced lomilomi practitioner. Each client is treated on a case-by-case basis, with due diligence being given for local and national standards of care. Whenever appropriate, a referral is provided for the client to consult another health care professional.

There are multiple levels of contraindications. These levels apply to the degree of knowledge and experience of the practitioner. A beginner would be advised to avoid a specific condition, whereas an advanced practitioner would be able to manage the client in the treatment of the same condition. For example, the presence of a lump (benign tumor) might be reason for avoidance by a beginner but an opportunity for further exploration and understanding by an expert. Skin infections are avoided by the beginner but may be addressed by the expert who also uses herbal medicine. A fracture is a cause of referral to a physician but may also be healed with prayer and laying on of hands or *lā'au kahea*.

CERTIFICATION REQUIREMENTS

Historically, knowledge of lomilomi was a closely held secret within the family. Traditionally, a child would be picked at the age of 5 or so to learn it. A child is chosen based on several signs: upon birth, the signs in the heavens and the earth are observed for any potential correspondence to the future of the infant. For example, the presence of a comet, a storm, or a large earthquake may be signs to consider. An elder or seer of the family examines the infant for markings on the body, or skin

coloration, especially around the fontanel and sutures of the head. These observations are continued during the growth and development of young children. Their behavior with other children is noted. It is said that if they show compassion when their playmates are injured, perhaps they have the soul of a kahuna lapa'au. Their relationships with the parents, grandparents, siblings, and other family members are noted, for only those who are good and kind could be given the knowledge.

Children studied for 10 or 15 years, and then spent the rest of their lives perfecting the art. Those who practiced lomilomi along with herbal medicine might be trained in a healing temple, or *heiau* (Figure 7-10).

Experienced practitioners of ancient times often received knowledge revealed in dreams by the 'aumākua or ancestral gods. These detailed visions could be instantaneous, transmitting a body of information to the practitioner in a flash. Modern teachers continue this tradition of extensive practical training and inspirational visions.

Lomilomi can be learned only from a teacher, not a book. Although today there is no established curriculum or length of time for training, traditional teachers are saddened that unscrupulous "teachers" purport to teach it in a weekend (or less) after they themselves have taken a weekend workshop.

The Hawaiian Lomilomi Association (HLA) was founded to certify teachers and practitioners and has been endorsed by Margaret Machado, Henry Auwae, Kalua Kaiahua, Mary Fragas, and many more Native Hawaiian practitioners. A list of members from around the world is on its website.

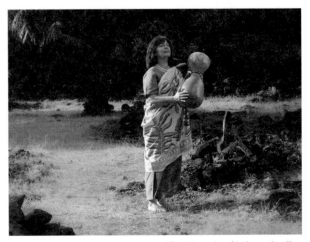

FIGURE 7-10 At the ruins of Keaīwa (The Mysterious) heiau, a healing temple on O'ahu, lomilomi teacher Brenda Mohalapua Ignacio prays. Medicinal trees and herbs surround the temple.

There are many wonderful instructors who are not members of HLA. In choosing an instructor for yourself, there is a saying in Hawaiian, *"Nānā i ke kumu."* Look to the source. Go to the teacher who was closest to the original teacher. If someone claims to be a favored student of one of the renowned kumu, you can easily check with the family of the kumu to be sure. Sadly, some "teachers" have been known to misrepresent their education and experience.

CHAPTER SUMMARY

Lomilomi is part of a comprehensive health care system that includes prayer, assessment, and herbal medicine. Long before medical studies proved the value of forgiveness, the Hawaiians had perfected the art in their ho'oponopono process. They knew what science has now proved, inflammation is a major source of disease and correct physical manipulation reduces inflammation. For people without access to modern medical care, lomilomi can be a useful alternative. At the same time lomilomi can be simply a wonderful restorative massage.

CASE HISTORY

A public health nurse referred a 19-year-old 440-pound diabetic male patient for treatment of a gangrenous lesion on his lower leg. The primary care physician had recommended amputation to prevent the infection from spreading to the upper leg. The referral for lomilomi from the concerned nurse was a last-case scenario for the young man.

After first praying for his health, my assistant and I gave him a sponge bath on the entire body, using salt water with powdered turmeric. We then performed lomilomi. We combined our strength and skills to decompress his joints, which had been stiffened due to his heavy bodyweight. Working primarily on the ankle, knee, and hip joints we applied traction, flexion, extension, and circumduction until the edematous fluids could flow back toward the heart.

I applied an herbal remedy onto the gangrenous lesion. One week later he returned for a second treatment, and the same protocol was followed. After the second treatment, his physician proclaimed he was healed and able to return to work.

SUGGESTED READINGS

Chai RMR, Zak JCK: *Hawaiian massage lomilomi: sacred touch of aloha*, Kailua, Hawaii, 2007, Hawaiian Insights.

Chai RMR: *Nā mo'olelo lomilomi: the traditions of Hawaiian massage and healing*, Honolulu, 2005, Bishop Museum Press.

Chun MN: *Ho'oponopono: traditional ways of healing to make things right again*. Honolulu, 2006, Curriculum Research & Development Group, University of Hawai'i.

Chun MN, trans and ed: *Must we wait in despair: the 1867 report of the 'ahahui lā'au lapa'au of Wailuku, Maui on native Hawaiian health*, Honolulu, 1994, First People's Productions.

Gutmanis J: *Kahuna lā'au lapa'au*, Aiea, Hawaii, 1999, Island Heritage.

Kahalewai NS: *Hawaiian lomilomi: big island massage*, Mountain View, Hawaii, 2005, Island Massage Publishing.

Zak JCK: *Hawaiian healing* (DVD), Kailua, Hawaii, 2004, Zak West Productions.

Zak JCK: *Pule wailele* (waterfall prayer) (DVD), Kailua, Hawaii, 2006, Zak West Productions.

RESOURCES

Hawaiian Lomilomi Association
www.hawaiilomilomi.com

R. Makana Risser Chai
www.lomilomibook.com

REFERENCES

1. Calvert RN: *The history of massage: an illustrated survey from around the world*, Rochester, Vt, 2002, Healing Arts Press.
2. Chai RMR, Zak JCK: *Hawaiian massage lomilomi: sacred touch of aloha*, Kailua, Hawaii, 2007, Hawaiian Insights.
3. Chai RMR: *Nāmo'olelo lomilomi: the traditions of Hawaiian massage and healing*, Honolulu, 2005, Bishop Museum Press.

Photographs by John C. Kalani Zak from the book *Hawaiian Massage Lomilomi: Sacred Touch of Aloha*.

MULTIPLE CHOICE TEST QUESTIONS

1) The roots of lomilomi are found:
   a) in Hawai'i, where it was invented
   b) with the voyagers who came to Hawai'i from the Marquesas
   c) in China
   d) in Tahiti

2) Who did not practice lomilomi in old Hawai'i?
   a) children
   b) servants of the chiefs
   c) martial arts masters
   d) all of the above practiced lomilomi

3) What two techniques are particularly important in lomilomi?
   a) stomach and foot massages
   b) foot and back massages
   c) back walking and stomach massage
   d) salt scrubs and steam baths

4) Which one of these aspects is the least important in determining if a particular style of lomilomi is authentic?
   a) mental
   b) physical
   c) emotional
   d) spiritual

5) How are herbs used in Hawaiian healing?
   a) as poultices
   b) to create oil
   c) for aromatherapy
   d) all of the above

6) Ti leaves are used in all of these ways except:
   a) for their aroma
   b) for spiritual protection
   c) for medicinal properties
   d) as poultices

7) How are sticks used in lomilomi?
   a) for balance when back walking
   b) for compression
   c) for self-massage
   d) all of the above

8) What safety concerns are there for the use of hot rocks?
   a) excessive weight
   b) burning the skin
   c) scratching the skin
   d) all of the above

9) Every session of lomilomi begins with:
   a) a chant
   b) rubbing with herbs
   c) prayer
   d) drinking water

10) Why is ho'oponopono part of lomilomi?
   a) Hawaiians believe holding grudges causes illness.
   b) The answer is kept secret.
   c) It is part of the tradition.
   d) To cleanse the body of evil spirits

11) What does a practitioner tell the client about breathing?
   a) "Exhale with each stroke"
   b) "Observe the pain flow out on each breath like smoke"
   c) "Breathe into the pain"
   d) "Breathe with me"

12) How did Hawaiians historically create steam baths?
   a) They erected huts over volcano vents.
   b) They built huts over hot rocks.
   c) They covered themselves and a gourd of hot water with a blanket.
   d) All of the above.

13) When creating a sacred space, which of the following are required?
   a) plants
   b) candles
   c) bowl of water
   d) none of the above

14) Which of the following is not important in making an assessment?
   a) visual observations of the patient's body
   b) telling the patient about similar cases you've seen
   c) asking questions of patients and their families
   d) palpating with the hands

15) Where is the best place to start the physical strokes?
   a) at the head
   b) at the abdomen
   c) away from the place of pain
   d) It depends on the case.

16) Why might clients complain of different problems at each session?
   a) They are drained of energy.
   b) As major chronic problems are resolved they become aware of underlying issues.
   c) An emotional or spiritual problem needs resolution.
   d) all of the above

17) What is the most important factor in determining contraindications for lomilomi?
   a) the experience of the practitioner
   b) the nature of the condition
   c) the patient's preference
   d) a medical doctor's opinion

18) Why is the "cutting the cord" ritual performed?
   a) to protect the practitioner
   b) to protect the patient
   c) to cleanse the environment of the patient's energy
   d) to symbolically end the treatment

19) How long does it take for lomilomi teachers to be trained?
   a) a few hours
   b) a weekend
   c) a month
   d) years

20) What is the best way to find a qualified lomilomi teacher?
   a) Google "lomilomi."
   b) Ask anyone who practices lomilomi.
   c) Check the Hawaiian Lomilomi Association website.
   d) Move to Hawai'i.

Manual Lymphatic Drainage (MLD)

Robert Harris

STUDENT OBJECTIVES

Upon completion of this chapter, students will be able to do the following:

- Describe the history of the Dr. Vodder method of MLD.
- Understand the major and minor components of lymph.
- Define and describe individual structural components of the lymph vessel system.
- Understand the role the lymph vessel system plays in maintaining normal physiologic conditions.
- Describe the various techniques of the Dr. Vodder method of MLD.
- Describe the major effects of MLD.
- Understand which main conditions are indicated and contraindicated for MLD.
- Comprehend an overview of treatment using MLD.

KEY TERMS

Collector lymph vessel
Combined decongestive therapy (CDT)
Initial lymph vessel
Lymph
Lymph-obligatory load (LOL)
Lymphedema (swelling)
Manual lymph drainage (MLD)
Precollector lymph vessel
Sympathicolytic effect

INTRODUCTION

There are several different manual techniques in current use in the massage and manual therapy fields that affect the lymph system. The most well known of these is the Dr. Vodder method of **manual lymph drainage (MLD).** It is a gentle, light, rhythmic manual technique that can have dramatic effects in the body if performed correctly. The Dr. Vodder method of MLD is a well-researched technique and is taught worldwide. It was developed and documented in France in the 1930s by a Danish couple, Emil and Estrid Vodder. This was the first time that a systematic method of manually affecting the lymphatic system had been described although others had mentioned the use of massage in treating swelling.[1]

Since the 1930s, MLD has been developed for use in many different conditions ranging from **lymphedema (swelling),** orthopedic applications, sports injuries, dermatologic indications, and stress. A thorough understanding of the lymph vessel system enables an understanding of how MLD can affect various systems in the body. Beginning with the history of the development of MLD, this chapter will describe the lymph vessel system and how MLD can affect it. The various strokes and techniques will be described in detail and then the effects of MLD discussed. With this basic knowledge, the reader will be able to understand the effects and indications for MLD.

HISTORY

Manual techniques to affect the lymph system have been described in the literature since the late 1800s. Von Winiwater[1] described massage for swollen limbs as follows:

"It is best to start with the manual treatment of those parts of the body which are in the immediate vicinity of the root of the swollen extremity. In order to influence lymphatics and veins, the extremity itself is treated only later on. Dependent upon what the aim of the treatment is: to crush or to divide hardened infiltrates, or to help reabsorption, or to move a stagnant tissue fluid centrally, various forms of massage can be used. Those masseurs who boast about all their force and proudly inflict bruises on their patients are of lesser help than a clever layman! After every massage treatment, passive movements of the swollen extremity should be performed methodically."

More specifics about the treatment of swelling will be described later in the chapter, but it is of interest to note that massage techniques were already recognized as being effective in the 1800s for reducing swelling.

Emil Vodder was born in 1896 in Copenhagen, Denmark. Dr. Vodder initially studied biology and then medicine in Brussels, Belgium. In1928 he was able to complete his studies and was awarded a PhD in philosophy by the University of Brussels.

He worked with his wife, Estrid Vodder, a trained naturopath, treating patients in Cannes, France, in a physical therapy institute from 1929 to 1933. During this time they studied what little was known about the lymph system using anatomical charts and medical texts that had little information about this important system. They were firm believers in treating the whole person. Partly through their studies and partly through intuition, they developed the techniques that are still used today to affect lymph flow in the body. The Vodders accumulated experience with patients, especially those suffering from upper respiratory tract problems such as rhinitis and sinusitis. In 1933 they moved to Paris and continued their studies into the lymph system. They presented their techniques at a health conference in Paris in 1936, which was the first time the Dr. Vodder method of MLD was exposed to the world. Newspapers reported on lymph drainage as a revolutionary skin treatment. Dr. Vodder wrote an article on MLD for the Parisian journal *Santé pour Tous* in 1936.[2,3]

The Vodder's MLD treatment techniques were gentle, rhythmic, circular motions that focused on the lymph nodes. The Vodders found that they were able to reduce swelling and congestion of areas drained by these nodes. They later established the Dr. Vodder Center in their native Denmark, where they utilized these treatments.

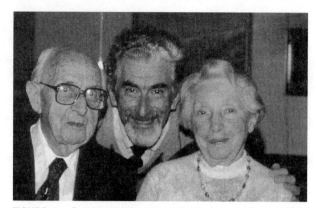

FIGURE 8-1 Emil Vodder, Guenther Wittlinger, Estrid Vodder, 1984. (Courtesy, Professor Hildegard Wittlinger.)

In 1965, the Vodders met Hildegard and Guenther Wittlinger, massage therapists, as well as a German physician, Dr. Asdonk. Together, they developed specialized Vodder techniques for use in medicine (Figure 8-1). Clinics were established in Austria and Germany.

The technique was so successful in Germany in the treatment of edema, especially lymphedema, that it was recognized by the national German medical insurance and then prescribed by physicians. It has since become the most prescribed physical therapy technique in Germany.

Dr. and Mrs. Vodder legally designated Hildegard and Güenther Wittlinger to be their successors and authorized them to teach and to train teachers in the original Dr. Vodder Method of MLD. In 1971 the Wittlingers established the Dr. Vodder School and Clinic in Walchsee, Austria. It is an internationally recognized study center for this method. The Wittlingers have taught extensively in North America and established the Dr. Vodder method as the premier lymphatic drainage technique. The Dr. Vodder method of MLD was first taught in the USA by the Wittlingers in 1972 at a conference in New York and then in Canada in 1982 in Toronto.

▚▚▚ IN MY EXPERIENCE

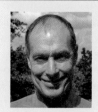

In my 25 years (2008) as an MLD therapist, I have experienced the joys and challenges of treating patients with lymphatic problems as well as training therapists in an exacting yet very rewarding field of therapy. When I started working as a massage therapist in 1980, I had no particular plan in mind and happened to notice the MLD training offered in Toronto in our professional journal (Ontario Massage Therapist Association). After enquiring among the few therapists who had taken the training the previous year, I decided to take the first level of the training ("Basic" course with Hildegard and Guenther Wittlinger). The science behind the practice made sense to me, coming from a science background, and I decided to follow through with the next level of the training (Therapy I) in Toronto the following year. Slowly the results with my patients convinced me that this light gentle touch could have a dramatic effect on the body. I was inspired to complete the training (Therapy II and III) in Austria in 1984, and at that time these courses were not offered in English.

After completion of the second level of the training, I had a young patient who had broken his nose in a cycling accident. It was the day after the injury, and he suffered from painful swelling and bruising, blood-shot eyes, and general unease and tension in his body. I performed MLD on his neck and face daily with special attention to the nose and eyes. Within a week his swelling and bruising had disappeared, as had the blood-shot eyes. The main effect that he noticed was the decrease in pain. A month later he had to have corrective surgery for the nose, and I did MLD for a few days before surgery and a week after surgery. Again the results were dramatic, especially the pain reduction.

However, the main insight after years of training therapists is regarding the importance of quality in treatment. No matter how many therapists are trained, in the end it is not about numbers, but about the quality of our hands. From my experience training gifted and bright therapists, I have seen that the best hands are those belonging to therapists who have dedicated themselves to proper training and then worked on maintaining and improving their skill level. It is a big commitment to devote ourselves to a particular field of therapy.

I remember a presentation by a young Dr. Vodder–trained massage therapist at one of our updating courses (Review). She had graduated 4 years prior to the updating course and quietly described how she and another Vodder-trained therapist had treated a patient with severe lymphedema in a hospital setting. The patient weighed over 500 lb and they successfully reduced the patient's limb edema so that he could walk again. The treatment had taken place over a 3-year period, but they had dedicated themselves to help this man and in so doing had altered the course of his life.

Due to the growing demand for properly trained MLD therapists in the USA and Canada, the Dr. Vodder School International was established by Robert Harris in 1994 with the guidance and approval of the Dr. Vodder School in Walchsee, Austria, and the Dr. Vodder Center in Denmark. This is now an international school—and therapists and teachers are trained in many different countries around the world including the USA, Canada, Australia, New Zealand, Singapore, Japan, and Ireland.

LYMPH VESSEL SYSTEM ANATOMY

In order to understand the effects of MLD, it is very important to have a thorough understanding of the lymph vessel system. MLD targets the flow of lymph through the lymph vessels. Importance of the lymph vessel system has often been underestimated, but it plays a primary role in enabling our bodies to function well. We need an active, healthy lymph vessel system to carry off wastes, toxins, proteins, viruses, bacteria, excess water, and dead cells, etc., from the interstitium. Any fluid and substances that cannot be removed by the bloodstream from the interstitial spaces should be removed by the lymph vessel system. Collectively, these substances are described as **lymph-obligatory load (LOL).**[4] The lymph system is required to remove these substances as they generally cannot be carried away by the venous capillaries. The LOL can be divided into major and minor components.

- Major components: water, proteins, cells, and fats from the intestines
- Minor components: pathogens, inorganic matter (e.g., dyes and dusts removed from the interstitium)

Once these major and minor components are taken up by the lymph vessels they are collectively referred to as **lymph.**

Collection of the LOL from the interstitium is a vital function, just as the blood circulation and nervous system are vital to our health. The most important function of the lymph vessel system, according to Prof. A. Guyton, is the removal of proteins from the interstitium by the lymphatics.[5] Blockage or damage to the lymph vessels or nodes can result in swelling (lymphedema), congestion, and eventually pathology. The congestion may not be obvious or palpable. Professor S. Curri describes disturbances in the microcirculation in the interstitium resulting in small edemas and congestion that eventually lead to pathology.[6]

STRUCTURE OF THE LYMPH VESSELS

Originating in the loose connective tissue and terminating in the venous system close to the heart, the lymph vessel system is a one-way system transporting fluid and substances from the tissues back to the venous system. Imagine for a moment a tree with fine branches leading to thicker, larger branches and eventually into a large trunk. The smallest branches represent the first

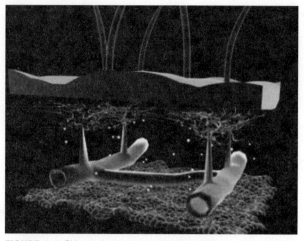

FIGURE 8-2 Skin and subcutaneous tissues showing arrangement of initial, precollector, and collector lymph vessels. *Piller NB:* The vital Essence: Understanding the lymphatic system in health and disease (professional version), (*Adelaide, 2003, Flinders Medical Centre.*)

lymph vessels, known as **initial lymph vessels,** or capillaries. The thicker branches represent the **precollector lymph vessels** and then the **collector lymph vessels** (Figure 8-2). The trunk of the tree represents the largest lymph vessels—i.e., ducts or trunks.

INITIAL LYMPH VESSEL

The LOL is collected by thin-walled, initial lymph vessels. These vessels are found primarily in the skin and are arranged in groups of finger-like projections. Fluid is channeled toward these initial lymph vessels via prelymphatic pathways in the interstitium. The initial lymph vessels drain into precollector and then collector lymph vessels.

The walls of the initial lymph vessels are made of a single layer of overlapping endothelial cells with gaps between the cells that allow fluids, cells, and dissolved substances to enter the vessel (Figure 8-3). Similar to blood vessels, there is a basement membrane surrounding the endothelial cell layer.

The outer covering of the initial lymph vessels is comprised of elastin and collagen fibers that are interwoven and connected to the endothelial cells and intimately connected to fibers throughout the connective tissue. Consequently, any movement or force on these fibers translates all the way back to the initial lymph vessels, causing movements of the endothelial cells, separating them and allowing fluids to enter. Fluids can leak back out into the interstitium again, depending on pressures inside and outside the vessels. The initial lymph vessels are approximately 0.5 mm in length with a diameter of 15 to17 μm.

PRECOLLECTOR LYMPH VESSEL

The role of the precollector lymph vessels is to drain lymph from the initial lymph vessels and funnel it into the collector vessels. The walls of the precollectors are similar to those of the initial lymph vessels, with an inner layer of endothelial cells surrounded by basement membrane and then connective tissue fibers. Progressing down the precollectors, rudimentary, bicuspid valves begin to appear as well as a type of smooth muscle cell in the wall. Precollectors can also be permeable allowing fluids to move in and out of the walls. They then drain their lymph into the collector lymph vessels.

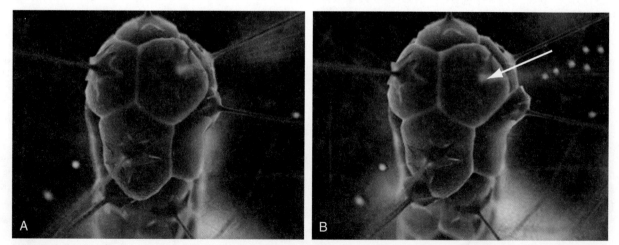

FIGURE 8-3 A, Initial lymph vessel, valves closed. **B,** Initial lymph vessel, valves opened. *Piller NB:* The vital Essence: Understanding the lymphatic system in health and disease (professional version), (*Adelaide, 2003, Flinders Medical Centre.*)

COLLECTOR LYMPH VESSEL

The collector vessels (Figure 8-4) are fine, silklike structures that are made of consecutive units called angions. An angion is the unit of a lymph vessel from one bicuspid valve to the next. The collector vessel walls have three layers. The internal layer (intima) is comprised of endothelial cells surrounded by a basement membrane. The middle layer (media) is a type of smooth muscle, innervated by sympathetic nerve fibers. The outer layer (adventitia) is connective tissue with collagen and elastin fibers.

There are intrinsic mechanisms such as stretch receptors that help the smooth muscle to contract. When the walls are stretched, for example, by internal filling of the vessels, the stretch receptors are stimulated and they elicit a firing along a nerve that connects with other nerves to cause contraction of the smooth muscles. When the muscle fibers contract, they help to propel the lymph forward in the direction of the valves. Collector lymph vessels have a baseline contraction rate of approximately 6 to 8 times per minute though this may increase up to about 20 times per minute if the lymphatic load increases.[7] In addition there are extrinsic factors such as skeletal muscle movements, arterial pulsations, breathing, and peristalsis that all help to promote lymph flow, essentially by providing a massaging action on the lymph vessels. These angion units can function independently although they tend to work in unison and shift lymph from one unit to the next through one-way, bicuspid valves. Each angion unit is approximately 0.1 to 1 mm in length, with a diameter of 50 to 120 μm.

Some collector vessels are designated "afferent collectors," which means that they bring lymph to the lymph node. Others are designated "efferent collectors," which means they transport lymph away from the lymph node.

LYMPH NODE

Eventually the lymph is funneled through afferent collectors into one of more than 600 lymph nodes throughout the body, where it is cleansed and concentrated (Figure 8-5). Up to 50% of the water and some dissolved substances can be reabsorbed into the venous system in the lymph nodes. Efferent collector lymph vessels then take lymph from the nodes and transport it to further lymph nodes or large collecting vessels and trunks. Eventually lymph flows to either the thoracic duct, the largest lymph vessel in the body, or the right lymphatic duct. These two vessels join the large veins entering the heart and empty approximately 2 to 4 liters of lymph every 24 hours back into the venous system at the venous arch.

Lymph Vessel System Physiology

As mentioned previously, removal of tissue proteins is considered to be one of the most important functions of the lymph vessels system. Tissue proteins generally cannot return to the bloodstream once they have left the capillaries. By removing proteins from the interstitium, the lymph vessels system helps to maintain an osmotic balance in the tissues and thus prevents the excess accumulation of fluids. If the proteins are not removed, they become stagnant and attract water toward them causing more congestion and edema. These stagnant proteins also gradually start to break down and an inflammatory process is initiated. The body reacts to this by stimulating fibroblast activity, and hardening or fibrosis of the tissues may eventually occur.

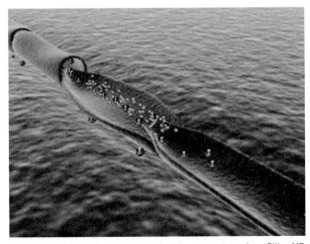

FIGURE 8-4 Collector lymph vessel with cut-away section. *Piller NB: The vital Essence: Understanding the lymphatic system in health and disease (professional version), (Adelaide, 2003, Flinders Medical Centre.)*

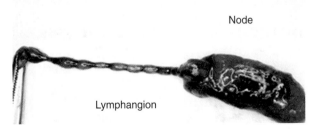

Node

Lymphangion

FIGURE 8-5 Lymph node with attached collector lymph vessel showing angions. *Piller NB: The vital Essence: Understanding the lymphatic system in health and disease (professional version), (Adelaide, 2003, Flinders Medical Centre.)*

The lymph vessel system also removes water from the tissues through the pumping action in the lymph angions. Normally this pump draws fluids along the collector vessels, which, in turn, drains precollectors and thus initial lymph vessels. This allows initial lymph vessels to accept more fluid from the surrounding tissues. By continually draining fluid from the tissues and keeping them in a so-called "dry state," the distances between blood capillaries and cells are kept at a minimum. Short distances mean that nutrients and wastes can be transported relatively quickly, and thus the health of the cells is maintained at an optimal level. If the distances increase, then the time taken for diffusion greatly increases and cell health deteriorates. A functioning lymph vessel system can increase its activity by up to 20 times normal capacity, enabling a much greater fluid removal, as occurs for example during intense skeletal muscle activity during peripheral exercise.

Many immune reactions occur within the lymph vessel system. Both B and T lymphocytes constantly circulate through the lymph vessels and nodes. When an antigen (e.g., bacteria or virus) is recognized by a lymphocyte, B cells are activated and move to germinal centers in the nodes. Antibody-producing plasma cells are formed that migrate to the medullary cords in the nodes, and swelling may occur. T lymphocytes help to control cell-mediated immunity and the development of B lymphocytes. They have many different subsets, such as killer T cells, cytotoxic T cells, and memory T cells. They circulate through the skin, lymph vessel system, and back into the bloodstream. A healthy, functioning lymph vessel system is key to this circulation.

The lymph vessel system also plays a role in the removal of fats from the small intestines. Lymph vessels known as lacteals in the villi (folds) absorb fats that are too large to be taken up by the blood vessels. The gap between the endothelial cells in these lymph vessels is sufficiently large to allow large fat molecules to pass through.

DESCRIPTION OF DR. VODDER'S MLD

The best way to understand Dr. Vodder's MLD is to receive a treatment from a certified therapist. This section of the chapter will describe the technique in words, but this is only a one-dimensional view of the technique.

Imagine a gentle wave lapping at your feet and legs while you are lying at the edge of the ocean. As a wave comes in, there is a gentle increase in pressure on the skin starting at the feet and progressing in a proximal direction. Repetitive waves washing over the skin create alternating pressure. This is similar to how a correctly applied MLD feels.

Basic Techniques

There are four basic techniques taught in the Vodder method, and there are many adaptations to specific tissue conditions. In a patient with a normal, functioning lymph vessel system, the techniques stretch the skin in the direction of lymph flow. See below for an explanation of why this is important. The maximal pressure used is extremely light, yet very precise. There is an alternating pressure and release phase in every stroke, and typically the pressure applied is equivalent to the weight of a quarter on the skin (approx. 30 mm Hg). The minimum pressure is 0 mm Hg.

Movements are generally repeated in sets of five when performed with one hand or both hands moving together. If the hands alternate from one to the other, the sets are repeated six times (three movements with each hand). No oil is necessary when performing MLD, unless the skin is very hairy, in which case a few drops of oil can be used. Sometimes corn starch or talcum powder is used if the therapist's hands or patient's skin are moist.

The descriptions and explanations are intended to help the reader understand the concepts of lymph drainage and do not replace supervised classroom instruction by a certified and qualified instructor. Taking appropriate training in MLD is strongly recommended before utilizing it as a therapeutic modality.

Stationary Circles

The skin is twisted and torqued in a specific manner.

Using the Thumbs. Thumb circles can be achieved using the pad of the thumb to engage the skin and using the wrist to move the skin. The pad of the thumb is laid flat on the skin and pushed in one direction then twisted in another direction, using the wrist. Generally the thumb is moved in a 45° twist, and then the skin is released while continuing the movement through to 90° (Figure 8-6).

Using Flat Fingers. The concept is the same as the thumb circle, but this time all the fingers engage the skin, up to the metacarpal phalangeal (MCP) joint (Figure 8-7). The skin is moved by the fingers, which just engage the skin but do not compress it. The fingers are moved by the arm, and there is no finger or wrist

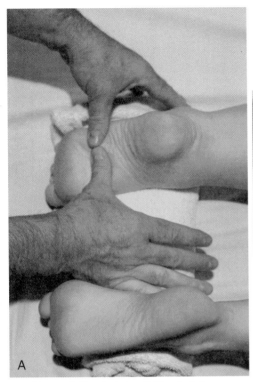

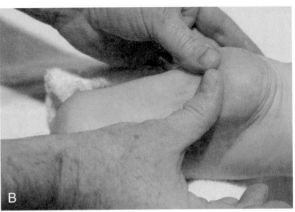

FIGURE 8-6 A, Thumb circles. **B,** Thumb circles.

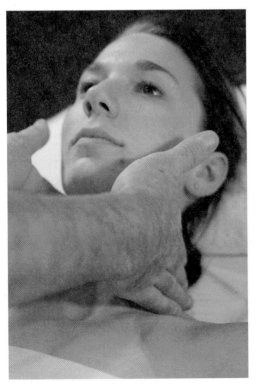

FIGURE 8-7 Stationary circles using fingers.

movement. The skin is stretched in a circular fashion without sliding over it. Each circle has an increasing stretch phase and a decreasing stretch phase (visualize a crescent moon, with the thickest part of the curve at the maximum stretch of the skin). There is also a zero phase in the circle where no pressure is applied but the fingers remain in contact.

Pump Technique

The wrist drives this movement, and the hand and fingers are passively moved. If your hand is placed on an arm or leg, the palm of your hand contacts the skin and the fingers hang loosely on one side of the arm or leg and the thumb on the other side. This is the start position for the pump technique (Figure 8-8). The wrist is then raised, lifting the palm off the skin but keeping the fingers and thumb in contact with no gripping pressure. The fingers and thumb are perpendicular to the arm or leg at this stage. Now the wrist is lowered and the skin is gently stretched, first slightly perpendicular and then forward in the direction of lymph flow, using the palm of the hand to engage and move the skin. Once the skin has been stretched to its maximum, yet still very lightly, the palm is slightly

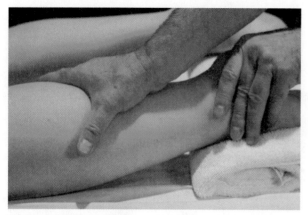

FIGURE 8-8 Pump technique.

disengaged, allowing the skin to return under the palm to its original position.

Scoop Technique

This involves the use of the palm of the hand to engage the skin rather than the fingers. Contact can begin at the MCPs but should involve the whole palmar surface to fully engage the skin to be moved. The palm is placed flat on either the lower arm or back of the calf for example. The first direction of movement is perpendicular to the arm or leg (Figure 8-9). Once the maximum stretch is achieved, the wrist moves the palm with a slight twist proximal. At the maximum stretch, the palm disengages the skin, which then slips back to its original position under the palm. It is important that the palm not recoil with the skin as this will prevent a forward progression of lymph up the limb. With the skin disengaged, the wrist is then ulnar deviated, pivoting around the thumb until the start position is reached again.

Rotary Technique

The hand is placed flat on the skin, with the palm and fingers engaging the skin fully. The thumb is fully approximated against the radial side of the flat hand. Now the wrist is flexed, lifting the palm off the skin while keeping the finger pads in contact. Using the arm, the hand is moved forward in the direction of lymph flow, sliding the fingers gently over the skin while keeping the thumb pad in the same position. The thumb is now at 90° in relation to the hand (Figure 8-10). The wrist is extended, lowering the palm gently back onto the skin. Using the arm and wrist, the palm stretches the skin in the direction of the fingers, but also a slight ulnar deviation is added. The skin is stretched to its

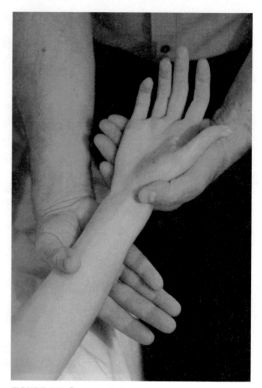

FIGURE 8-9 Scoop technique.

maximum, and then, keeping the wrist extended and the hand flat, the skin is disengaged from the palm by very slightly lifting the palm. Now the skin returns to its original position, but the hand is already in a new position. The last part of the stroke involves releasing the thumb and allowing it to go from 90° back to an approximated position against the radial side of the hand.

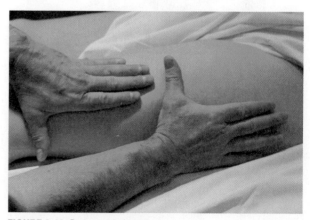

FIGURE 8-10 Rotary technique.

SUMMARY OF QUALITIES OF DR. VODDER'S MLD TECHNIQUES

- Light pressure
- Alternate pressure and release phase in each stroke
- Slow, rhythmic strokes
- Engage and move the skin rather than sliding over it
- Work in direction of lymph flow
- Begin proximal and progress distal
- Should not cause pain or reddening of skin (erythema may be possible with sensitive skin)
- Elicit a sense of deep relaxation in patient

Dr. Vodder's MLD is performed according to anatomic and physiologic principles and follows the normal lymphatic flow unless there is damage to the lymph vessel system. In cases where the lymph system is damaged, fluid movement is directed around the damaged or blocked areas. The techniques are selected for each body part, according to anatomic suitability. For example, the pump technique is most often used on the arm and leg as the hand conforms best to these body parts. The rotary technique is used on the back because it can cover large surface areas most efficiently.

The neck is always treated first to enhance drainage of the major lymph ducts into the venous arch. After the neck, localized affected areas are treated and, in general, treatment patterns progress from proximal to more distal parts of the body. However, each section undergoing treatment is worked in a distal to proximal direction. Treatment times are usually a minimum of 30 minutes and may last up to 90 minutes. The frequency of treatment depends upon the condition being treated. For example, patients with lymphedema may require daily treatment for a 2- to 4-week period. To achieve success with treatment, it is optimal to have a warm, comfortable, soothing environment when receiving MLD. The less distraction during treatment, the more a patient is likely to be able to relax and encourage the parasympathetic system to predominate (see section on Effects of MLD).

OTHER LYMPHATIC DRAINAGE METHODS

Although the Vodder method is well known and is taught extensively by the Dr. Vodder School, other methods of lymphatic drainage have also developed. The purpose of this chapter is not to comment on these versions but to educate the reader on manual lymph drainage. However, the reader should be aware that all methods have different effects and outcomes that can be dependent on the method and also on the individual practitioner. Box 8-1 includes details on the other methods of lymphatic drainage.

EFFECTS OF MLD

It is important to have a thorough understanding of the science behind MLD in order to understand how it can affect different systems in the body, and more importantly how it can affect pathologies. We often associate MLD with the treatment of swelling (edema) through its drainage effect, yet it can be used for a wide variety of conditions such as burns, dermatologic indications (e.g., acne, eczema), venous ulceration, orthopedic applications (such as frozen shoulder, hip replacements, arthritic joints), and more. Apart from these more clinical applications, the original method is also very well suited to preventive and wellness programs and can be used in the spa setting for detoxification and rejuvenation.

How Manual Lymph Drainage Works

One of the reasons that the original Vodder method is so versatile and thus applicable to massage therapy is that it impacts different systems in the body.

1. **Effect on the nervous system**

The technique is a very light, gentle manual technique, and patients often feel a sense of deep relaxation during treatment. This has been described by Wittlinger[3] and is beneficial for patients suffering severe stress such as those undergoing cancer therapy.

BOX 8-1 Other Lymphatic Drainage Methods

In Australia there is a method developed by Drs. John and Judith Casley-Smith that involves effleurage-like techniques. Dr. Bruno Chickly from France has developed a Lymph Drainage Therapy that involves "mapping" the lymph system in order to manually attune the specific rhythm, pressure, quality, and direction of the lymph flow. There are also variations and versions of the Vodder method taught by instructors and training programs throughout the world. In Germany, for example, there are the Foeldi, Asdonk, Feldberg, Damp, and other training programs, each teaching versions of the Vodder method. In the USA there are the Klose, Norton, Academy of Lymphatic Studies, and other training programs.

The technique also helps to elicit a **"sympathicolytic" effect.** This term was coined by Professor Dr. P. Hutzschenreuter at the University of Ulm in Germany, who has researched this effect of Dr. Vodder's MLD.[9] The term refers to a lowering of sympathetic nerve firing in the body. In a sympathetic state, skin is moister and thus more conductive to electricity. When the sympathetic nerve firing is lowered and the patient goes into a more parasympathetic state, the skin is drier and thus less conductive to electricity. The sympathicolytic effect of MLD can be proven by measuring the resistance of the skin to electric current.

In experiments testing patients' resistance to a small electric current passed through the skin, Hutzschenreuter demonstrated that the Dr. Vodder method of MLD increases the resistance, which is an indicator of a lowered sympathetic state. This has important consequences on other systems in the body, especially those innervated by the autonomic nervous system.

Another effect on the nervous system is the interruption of pain pathways. When it is applied correctly (i.e., with gentle, rhythmic strokes in the direction of lymph flow), MLD can be used for its analgesic effect. It is especially used in the treatment of recent trauma such as sports injuries, whiplash, migraines, and headaches but also in the treatment of pain-related conditions such as reflex sympathetic dystrophy and fibromyalgia.[10]

2. **Effect on smooth muscles of the blood and lymph vessels**

Prof. P. Hutzschenreuter has demonstrated that MLD increases the speed of blood flow.[11] This is thought to occur through an increase in vasomotion caused by a contraction of arteriole smooth muscle. A relaxation of the precapillary smooth muscle sphincter in the arterioles is mediated by the sympathicolytic effect described above, which also results in an increased blood flow.

Unlike deep tissue massage, MLD is very light and does not create an increased local blood pressure, but rather an increased speed of blood flow. Because the pressure used in deep tissue massage is much greater than MLD, it tends to increase blood pressure in the local area proximal to the direction of pressure. MLD will not increase congestion in a tissue and may cause a temporary decrease. Therefore it is beneficial to patients with congested tissues such as those with lymphedema who have an increased amount of interstitial fluid. An increased blood flow without increased congestion is also beneficial to patients with circulatory disturbances such as those with Raynaud's syndrome marked by abnormally cold hands and/or feet.

MLD also has an effect on the smooth muscles of the collector lymph vessels. These are the main channels in the body that conduct lymph from the superficial initial lymph vessel (lymph capillary) network to the lymph nodes and then on to the larger ducts. As described in the section on lymph vessel anatomy, the walls of these vessels contain a type of smooth muscle arranged in a circular or longitudinal manner. One way that this muscle contracts is through a stretch-receptor reflex. When the walls are stretched, for example by internal filling of the vessels, the stretch receptors are stimulated and they elicit a firing along a nerve that eventually results in contraction of the smooth muscles. The specific and precise movements of Dr. Vodder's MLD enable a specific stretching of the lymph vessels that increases the frequency and amplitude of contraction. By mechanically pushing the lymph forward, MLD may also increase the filling of the lymph vessels ahead of the therapist's hand.

The smooth muscle of the lymph collectors is innervated by the autonomic (involuntary) nervous system, specifically sympathetic nerves. A lowering of sympathetic nerve firing will also cause dilation or filling of the vessel. MLD has been shown to have such an effect on the sympathetic system and the smooth muscles by Hutzschenreuter.

A similar mechanism is found in the gastrointestinal tract and when the walls of the intestines are stretched, a peristaltic wave of contraction is initiated. Mislin has described how specific stretching forces stimulate the lymphatic motor system.[12]

3. **Effect on drainage**

By increasing both the filling capacity of the lymph vessels and the contraction rate in the walls of the collectors, MLD has a positive effect on draining tissues of excess fluids (i.e., edema fluid in the interstitial spaces). Protein removal into the lymphatic system is enhanced, and consequently the colloid osmotic pressure in the tissues is lowered. Colloid osmotic pressure is the water-attracting force of proteins. Water tends to move toward a higher concentration of proteins. If there are fewer proteins in the tissues, then less water is attracted toward the tissues and the edema is reduced. The main use for this drainage effect is in the reduction of edema caused by intervention in cancer therapy—e.g., post-mastectomy lymphedema, or in the treatment of patients with primary congenital lymphedema (Figure 8-11). However, the original Vodder method of MLD is used with other types of edema too, such as venous edema or after trauma such as sports-related injuries.[13]

Professors H. Mislin in Switzerland and P. Hutzschenreuter in Germany have both demonstrated an

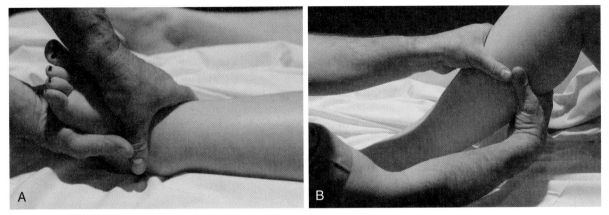

FIGURE 8-11 A and **B,** Treatment of a patient with primary leg lymphedema.

increased speed of blood flow after MLD treatment. This effect is beneficial to patients with lymphedema as an increased blood flow without an increased blood pressure will not increase congestion in a tissue.

INDICATIONS FOR THERAPY

MLD is used in the treatment of many different pathologies. In the Dr. Vodder School training program, a physician trained in lymphology teaches the theory behind various pathologic indications and applications that enable the therapist to fully understand the pathologies and implications of treatment. For example, lymphedema can be caused by surgery after cancer, irradiation of lymph nodes and vessels, congenital defects in the lymph system, parasites, infections, or injuries. It is a recognized complication of many skin disorders including acne, rosacea, cellulitis (erysipelas), leg ulcers, and chronic dermatologic disorders.[8] A thorough understanding of the patient's pathology in relationship to treatment enables the therapist to provide appropriate care. Treatment may often be carried out in association with or under the guidance of the patient's physician. In the training program, typical treatment scenarios are discussed and practiced to enable the therapist to competently apply manual lymph drainage to a wide variety of disorders.

For further reading on the indications of MLD, refer to Ingrid Kurz, MD, the former medical director of the Dr. Vodder School in Austria, who has written an excellent text on applications for MLD.[14] This text covers many indications that have pushed the boundaries of treatment and encouraged applications of MLD. Another text by Renato Kasseroller, MD, who was also

a medical director of the Vodder School in Austria, describes the applications for MLD.[15]

The main applications for MLD include:

- Orthopedic: posttrauma, fractures, strains, inflammation in joints (e.g., osteoarthritis), ligament and tendon injuries.
- Neurologic: neuropathic pain, complex regional pain syndrome (CRPS), facial nerve paralysis, fibromyalgia, paralysis, stroke.
- Edema: lymphedema (primary and secondary), venous insufficiency edema (an excess fluid accumulation in the interstitial spaces caused by increased venous blood pressure), and lipedema (an abnormal, symmetrical fat deposition with accompanying edema).
- Dermatologic: acne, rosacea, dermatitis.
- Connective tissue disorders: lupus erythematosus, scleroderma.
- Digestive disorders: constipation.
- Wellness: spa, as an adjunct therapy during cleansing, rejuvenation, and fasting.

Therapeutic success can be defined in many ways. For example, one patient with lymphedema may be happy with a reduction in pain, increased mobility, and ability to function whereas another may be dissatisfied unless a significant volume reduction in edema is attained. Defining goals and working toward realistic outcomes can help patients achieve realistic results. Recognizing our own involvement as therapists in the healing process of our patients, apart from the hands-on therapy we provide, is also an important component to consider in patient treatment. As a therapist I am very grateful to my mentors who inspired the confidence in me to try MLD with many different patients. In particular, Professor Hildegard Wittlinger who inspired me to "just do it."

MANUAL LYMPH DRAINAGE IN THE TREATMENT OF LYMPHEDEMA

One of the most common uses of the Dr. Vodder method of MLD is in the treatment of patients with a swelling-related condition known as lymphedema. This is a common condition that may arise spontaneously in patients with congenital malformations of the lymph vessel system (primary lymphedema), or subsequent to damage or obstruction of the lymph vessels (secondary lymphedema). For example, in breast cancer patients who have undergone lymph node dissection and/or radiation therapy, the prevalence of lymphedema can range from 6% to 44%.[17] The average onset of this lymphedema is 3.5 years from the date of cancer treatment, dependent on the type and degree of intervention.

MLD is incorporated into a management strategy for lymphedema, known as **combined decongestive therapy (CDT).** This is also referred to as complex decongestive physiotherapy. CDT can be divided into two stages, the first being an intensive treatment phase and the second phase a maintenance phase. The patient is initially assessed and the appropriate treatment plan devised (Figure 8-12, *A*).

Treatment Phase

Treatment is performed daily during the intensive phase (5 days per week) with at least one or two 60-minute sessions per day lasting over a 2- to 4-week period. This is very important in order to achieve good results in volume reduction, which appear to be accumulative. Assessment methods including volumetric measurement are made several times during the phase to monitor the progress, and changes to the treatment plan may be made accordingly.

MLD is the cornerstone of this phase. It is adapted specifically to the patient's needs, and edema-reducing strokes are used (see Figure 8-12, *B*). If hardened areas of fibrosis are encountered then the pressure of strokes is usually increased (see Figure 8-12, *C*). Adjacent and proximal areas are treated first and then affected areas, directing fluids away from blocked or congested areas toward open pathways. There are numerous reports in the literature about the use of MLD in lymphedema treatment.[7,18] During this phase of treatment, the patient is bandaged using a low-stretch compression bandage system in order to maintain the reductions obtained by MLD and to prevent worsening or refilling of the limb. The skin is kept clean and free of infections, and any wound care

issues need to be addressed. The patient is taught specific remedial exercises in order to activate remaining lymphatics and assist removal of fluid. Depending on factors such as age, duration of the lymphedema, skill of the therapist, patient compliance, and risk factors, lymphedemas may reduce by 40% to 50% during this intensive phase.

Maintenance Phase

Once a suitable reduction or outcome has been achieved, according to the goals of treatment, the patient enters the maintenance phase. In order to maintain the reduction attained during the intensive treatment and prevent refilling of the limb, it is important for patients with lymphedema to wear a compression garment. Toward the end of the intensive phase, a patient is fitted for a compression garment. Sleeves or stockings are usually custom made from a low-stretch, flat-knit material that conforms to the shape of the reduced limb. In some cases of mild edema, an off-the-shelf garment may be used.

The patient may continue receiving less-frequent MLD and may be taught self–lymph drainage techniques. Remedial exercises are continued and the skin is closely monitored for changes. Lymphedema is a lifelong condition with no cure, so patients do need to maintain self treatment and occasionally go back to their therapist for follow-up intensive treatment. Patients are usually checked every 6 months for a follow-up treatment as their garments need to be replaced at least every 6 months.

Many patients are informed that there is little that can be done for them once they have lymphedema. However with correctly applied combined decongestive therapy from a well-trained therapist, a good reduction in lymphedema volume can be achieved and the quality of life improved for these patients.

CONTRAINDICATIONS TO MANUAL LYMPH DRAINAGE TREATMENT

Manual lymph drainage is a "safe" modality if applied correctly by properly trained therapists. However, as with all therapeutic modalities, the potential for harm is possible if attempts are made to treat patients without the proper understanding, assessment skills, and appropriate procedures and precautions being utilized. A patient's safety is the prime consideration.

There are generally considered to be four major contraindications to Dr. Vodder's MLD, although each patient must be evaluated as an individual with specific

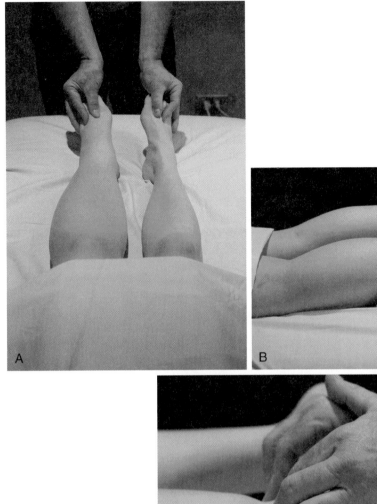

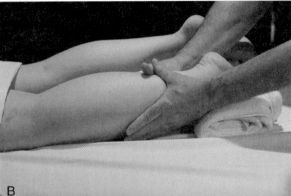

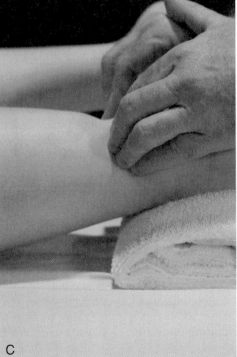

FIGURE 8-12 **A,** Initial assessment of lymphedema patient. **B,** Treatment of edema in a patient with lymphedema, and **C,** Treatment of fibrosis in a patient with lymphedema.

health care requirements and precautions. Patients with the following conditions need to be carefully evaluated before treatment:

- Untreated metastatic cancer. This is a contentious issue, and there appears to be no evidence linking MLD to the spread of cancer.[16] However, as a precaution, MLD is generally not used with patients who have untreated cancers, especially close to the tumor site. There may be exceptions in palliative cases.
- Untreated thrombosis. There is a potential risk of dislodging a thrombus and causing an embolus if tissues are moved close to the site of a thrombus.
- Acute inflammation with infection. The danger here is of spreading an infection and worsening the condition. In acute inflammatory episodes, the body has a natural reaction to close the proximal lymph collectors and prevent the spread of infection. MLD could force pathogens through these closed areas.
- Cardiac insufficiency (congestive heart failure). By moving fluids back to the heart via the lymph vessels and back to the venous system, MLD can increase the load on an already congested heart. The heart is unable to manage these extra fluids because it is already compromised and consequently, fluid leaks into the lungs, creating pulmonary edema.

OVERVIEW OF TREATMENT

MLD can be a very relaxing and calming treatment for the therapist to give. It does not require muscle strength to provide the very gentle pressures involved. It does, however, require a lot of focus and attention. For a typical MLD treatment session, the patient begins in a supine position and the lymph pathways of the neck and shoulders are addressed first. This is where the lymph system terminates (joins the venous system), and by clearing these pathways first, fluid can be accepted from more distal regions. The therapist then progresses gradually to more distal regions of the body, depending on the condition presented by the patient. If the lymph pathways and nodes are intact, then the therapist follows the normal flow and fluid is directed towards the regional collector lymph nodes. If there is a disruption of these pathways, then fluid has to be redirected toward adjacent, open pathways. Each body part is treated in a precise and logical manner, according to the lymph pathways.

For example, the normal leg treatment is started at the proximal end of the thigh first by draining toward the inguinal lymph nodes. The therapist then gradually progresses to the knee, then the lower leg, directing fluid toward the popliteal and medial pathways around the knee. Lastly the ankle and foot are addressed. Each section of the leg is treated in a distal to proximal fashion. The logic behind this is that by moving fluid forward along the collector pathways, the proximal lymphangions are activated.

Typical treatment time is 60 minutes although it may be shorter or longer, depending upon the condition being treated. After the treatment session is concluded, the patient is encouraged to rest and enjoy the benefits of deep relaxation for several minutes. Care should be taken with patients getting off the table as they may find their blood pressure has lowered slightly and they may be prone to fainting or dizziness. Patients are encouraged to drink extra fluid to help "flush" their systems, and patients will often find that they need to urinate immediately after treatment.

CERTIFICATION

Although many massage therapists may have received an introduction to lymph drainage techniques in their undergraduate studies, the treatment of patients with pathologies requires specialized and expert knowledge to be able to assess and treat patients appropriately. A fully trained MLD therapist will have undertaken additional, postgraduate training in this specialized field. For example, in order to successfully treat lymphedema patients, it is important to learn specialized MLD techniques that are appropriate for this condition including compression bandaging, adapted exercises, skin care, and compression garment use. Courses should include instruction from a physician trained in lymphologic problems who has experience in and knowledge of treating lymphatic conditions. The Dr. Vodder School offers an international program and trains massage, physical, and occupational therapists and nurses as well as other health care professionals in these procedures. The training is divided into 5-day segments and has 160 contact hours, including 15 hours of pathology taught by a physician. An updating class is offered (Review or Recertification) where therapists present case studies, new information is shared, and therapists update all their skills learned in the 160-hour training. A full description of the training program and courses can be found on the Dr. Vodder School website. The website lists certified therapists for referral who have attended updating courses every 2 years since their original certification as MLD therapists. In the USA, Canada, and other countries there are also various associations that can refer patients to therapists. Please refer to the list of resources at the end of this chapter.

Conclusion

The popularity of a technique is a measurement of its success. Judging by the rapid growth in awareness and demand for the Dr. Vodder method of manual lymph drainage, it has proven to be a successful technique. In North America, there were a handful of therapists in the early 1980s and now there are many thousands. These are dedicated and committed therapists who have invested a great deal of time and energy in their education to attain a high level of quality in order to treat their patients in an appropriate manner. Good techniques will produce good results but excellent techniques will produce excellent results, and this underlines the philosophy in training quality hands and therapists with the Dr. Vodder School.

CHAPTER SUMMARY

This chapter describes the Dr. Vodder method of manual lymph drainage (MLD). An overview of the history of MLD is given from the founding of this technique by Emil and Estrid Vodder in 1932 to the present day. To help the reader understand the impact of MLD, the anatomy of the lymph vessel system is described in detail from the initial lymph vessels in the interstitium of the skin to the major lymph ducts returning lymph into the main veins entering the heart. The importance of the lymph vessel system is described in terms of its physiologic function: maintaining homeostasis in the tissues.

The various techniques of the Dr. Vodder method of MLD are then described. The effects of MLD on the nervous system, on tissue drainage, and on the smooth muscles of blood and lymph vessels are described. Applications of MLD to therapy are outlined including the treatment of lymphedema, the most widely known application for MLD. The major contraindications to MLD are included. The chapter finishes with an overview of the certification process required to become a Vodder-certified MLD therapist.

CASE HISTORY

AC was a 74-year-old retired male who had suffered from chronic venous stasis in both legs for several years and resultant pitting edema. In addition he had osteoarthritis in his left knee and wore a brace to support the joint. His left leg also had prominent varicosities. His mobility was limited, and he was doing some swimming pool exercises. Ten months prior to visiting me he was diagnosed with prostate cancer and underwent radiation for 6½ weeks followed by hormone therapy. Radiation was in the inguinal and pelvic areas. His physician had referred him to me for massage therapy.

He experienced pain and swelling in both legs. On a score of 1 to 10, his pain level was experienced as 8 to 9. He also experienced decreased mobility, tingling, bursting, and heaviness in both legs.

Significant and palpable swelling, which was pitting upon pressure, was present in both legs. Leg volume was estimated using a calculation from circumferential tape measurement at 4 cm intervals up the leg from malleolus to upper thigh. Areas of hardness were noted in his lower right leg. Suprapubic edema was also present. There was limited range of movement in the left knee.

Diuretics had been prescribed to control the edema in his legs. These were discontinued under his physician's guidance, during treatment with CDT. Extra-strength Tylenol® was taken when pain prevented walking.

This patient was experiencing a lot of pain in his legs, and as a result his mobility was very limited. His goal in therapy was to reduce the edema as much as possible and hopefully reduce the pain. Complicating factors were the left knee brace, which may have impeded lymph outflow from the lower leg; the radiation for prostate cancer, which would have caused damage to the inguinal and pelvic lymph nodes, restricting outflow from the legs; and the lack of mobility, which also slows down lymph fluid transport. It was not possible to direct fluid from the legs into the groin area, which normally I would do if they are intact, because of the damage to the inguinal and pelvic lymph nodes. Instead, I needed to redirect fluids to the axillary lymph nodes.

After assessing this patient carefully and taking a thorough case history as well as measuring the limbs, I decided that the best course of action was an intensive course of combined decongestive therapy, including MLD, bandaging, skin care, and exercises. It was anticipated that this treatment plan would take 3 to 4 weeks of daily treatment. Once the limbs had stabilized, he would be fitted for compression stockings to maintain the reduction.

Twelve MLD treatments were performed over a 3-week period. Areas treated included the neck, axilla, thorax wall, abdominal skin, and anterior legs in supine position. The thorax wall, hip area, and posterior legs were treated in prone position. All treatments attempted to redirect fluid from the legs to the axillary nodes in the armpit, in order not to congest the inguinal/pelvic areas. Treatment sessions lasted from 60 to 90 minutes. At the end of each treatment the patient's legs were treated with a hydrating moisturizer and then bandaged, using short-stretch bandages. The patient was asked to remove the bandages should the legs become painful, especially at night time when he was not mobile. Home exercises were given and the patient encouraged to do these within his tiring tolerance.

The patient noted a decrease in swelling. At the end of treatment, the decrease in the right leg volume was 700 ml and 437 ml in the left leg. The suprapubic edema had also decreased. His mobility improved enabling him to walk greater distances. Pain levels also decreased and he was thus able to take less Tylenol®. At the end of the treatment series, AC was fitted for a Juzo® Varin compression garment to maintain the reductions attained.

Pain was certainly a big factor for this patient, and reducing this enabled a better quality of life as well as greater mobility. The light, gentle pressure of MLD is known to have a strong pain-reducing effect and this patient would not have tolerated deep tissue massage pressure. A lower reduction in volume of the left leg was to be expected due to the constriction of the leg brace and this was the case here. A significant reduction in limb volume was measured in the right leg, and most of this occurred in the thigh (600 ml). This may have indicated that while the whole limb had reduced, more time could now be spent in the lower leg. Suprapubic edema is a consistent finding for patients who have undergone radiation therapy to the pelvic lymph nodes, and as this is the most proximal edema, we always try to resolve this before moving more fluids into the pelvic/abdominal areas. The compression garment fitted for this patient is suitable for venous stasis edema patients. However, because of the probable lymphedema component, due to pelvic/inguinal node radiation, a more suitable garment may have been a flat-knit, low-stretch garment that does not cause any strangulation in the skin.

This case is an example of how MLD can be employed successfully with a complex patient and may be more appropriate to address the symptoms than using deep tissue massage.

SUGGESTED READINGS

American Cancer Society: *Lymphedema*, Atlanta, 2006, ACS.

Foeldi M: *Textbook of lymphology*, ed 2, London, 2007, Elsevier.

Weissleder H, Schuchhardt C: *Lymphedema diagnosis and therapy*, ed 3, Koeln, Germany, 2007, Viavital.

Zuther JE: *Lymphedema management: the comprehensive guide for practitioners*, New York, 2005, Thieme.

RESOURCES

Dr. Vodder School International
PO Box 5121
Victoria, BC
V8R 6N4 Canada
Tel: (250) 598-9862
Fax: (250) 598-9841
info@vodderschool.com
www.vodderschool.com

Dr. Vodder School and Clinic, Austria
Alleestr. 30,
A6344 Walchsee, Austria
Tel: (43) 5374 5245
Fax: (43) 5374 5245 4
office@vodderschule.com
www.vodderschule.com

Lymphology Association of North America (LANA)
P.O. Box 466,
Wilmette, IL
60091
Tel: 773-756-8971
lana@clt-lana.org
www.clt-lana.org

Lymphovenous Association of Ontario
PM Postal Box 55241
1800 Sheppard Avenue East
Toronto, ON
M2J 5A0 Canada
Tel: 416 410-2250
lymphontario@yahoo.com
www.lymphontario.org

Lymphatic Research Foundation
100 Forest Drive
East Hills, NY 11548
Tel:(516)625-9675
Fax:(516) 625-9410
lrf@lymphaticresearch.org
www.lymphaticresearch.org

National Lymphedema Network
1611 Telegraph Avenue, Suite 1111
Oakland, CA 94612-2138
Tel: (510) 208-3200
Fax: (510) 208-3110
nln@lymphnet.org
www.lymphnet.org

North American Vodder Association for Lymphatic Therapy (NAVALT)
P.O. Box 920658,
Houston
TX 77292-0658,
TN/Fax 281-971-5990 or 1-888-462-8258
blang2626@sbcglobal.net
www.NAVALT.org

REFERENCES

1. Von Winiwater A: Die elephantiasis. In *Deutsche chirurgie*, Stuttgart, 1892.
2. Vodder, E: Le drainage lymphatique, une nouvelle methode therapeutique, *Santé et beauté pour tous*, Paris, 1936.
3. Wittlinger G, Wittlinger H: *Textbook of Dr. Vodder's manual lymph drainage*, ed 7, Stuttgart, 2004, Thieme.
4. Kurz I: *Textbook of Dr. Vodder's manual lymph drainage*, ed 4, Heidelberg, 1997, Haug.
5. Guyton AC: *Textbook of medical physiology*, ed 11, Philadelphia, 2007, Saunders.
6. Curri SB: *Oedem, lymphoedem und perivaskulaere grundsubstanz*, Heidelberg, 1988, Haug.
7. Weissleder H, Schuchhardty C: *Lymphedema diagnosis and therapy*, ed 2, Koeln, Germany, 2001. Viavital.
8. Aloi F et al: The clinicopathologic spectrum of rhinophyma, *Journal of the American Academy of Dermatology* 42:468–472, 2000.
9. Hutzschenreuter P, Ehlers R: Effect of manual lymph drainage on the autonomic nervous system, *Z Lymphol* 10:58–60, 1986.
10. Asplund R: Manual lymph drainage therapy using light massage for fibromyalgia sufferers: a pilot study, *Journal of Orthopaedic Nursing* 7:192–196, 2003.
11. Hutzschenreuter P, Brummer H, Eberfeld K: Experimental and clinical studies of the mechanism of effect of manual lymph drainage therapy, *Z Lymphol* 13:62–64, 1989.
12. Mislin H: Die Lymphdrainage als biotechnisches problem, *Erfahrungsheilkunde* 9:573–577, 1984.
13. Wittlinger D: Einfluss der manuellen lymphdrainage und der klassischen massage auf das laktatverhalten unter belastung bei einem leistungssportler (The influence of M.L.D and classical massage on the lactate reaction to exertion in a competitive athlete), *Physikalische Therapie*, Dec 1988.
14. Kurz I: *Textbook of Dr. Vodder's manual lymph drainage, vol 3, Treatment manual*, ed 3, Heidelberg, 1996, Haug.
15. Kasseroller R: *Compendium of Dr. Vodder's manual lymph drainage*, Heidelberg, 1998, Haug.
16. Godette K et al: Can manual treatment of lymphedema promote metastasis? *J Soc Integ Oncol* 4:1, 2006.
17. Shuneman H, Willich N: Lymphoedema nach mammakarzinom (Lymphedema after breast cancer), *Deutsche med Wschr* 122:536–541, 1997.
18. Harris RH, Piller NB: Three case studies indication the effectiveness of manual lymph drainage on patients with primary and secondary lymphedema using objective measuring tools, *Journal of Bodywork and Movement Therapies* 7:213–223, 2003.

MULTIPLE CHOICE TEST QUESTIONS

1) Lymph angions are the units of vessels found in which type of lymphatic structure?
   a) initial lymph vessels
   b) precollectors
   c) collectors
   d) nodes

2) Manual lymph drainage techniques described by Dr. Vodder are best defined as which type of stroke?
   a) effleurage
   b) heavy kneading
   c) petrissage
   d) light circular motions

3) A major component of lymph is:
   a) protein
   b) pathogens
   c) red blood cells
   d) carbohydrates

4) MLD causes a sympatholytic effect which is understood as a lowered:
   a) blood flow
   b) lymph flow
   c) parasympathetic nerve firing
   d) sympathetic nerve firing

5) Colloid osmotic pressure is the water-attracting force of:
   a) fats
   b) hormones
   c) vitamins
   d) proteins

6) The main use for the drainage effect of MLD is in the treatment of which type of edema?
   a) lipedema
   b) venous edema
   c) lymphedema
   d) cardiac edema

7) The intima of all lymph vessels is made of which type of cell?
   a) epithelial
   b) endothelial
   c) B lymphocyte
   d) T lymphocyte

8) Which is a contraindication to MLD?
   a) acute infections
   b) swelling
   c) postsurgical pain
   d) constipation

9) MLD increases contraction rate in lymph vessels by using:
   a) heavy force
   b) specific stretching
   c) constant pressure
   d) fast movements

10) The most important function of the lymph vessel system in the interstitium is:
   a) circulation of fats
   b) distribution of vitamins
   c) removal of proteins
   d) supply of nutrients and oxygen

11) Which Dr. Vodder MLD technique is best for treating large surface areas?
   a) rotary
   b) thumb circles
   c) pumps
   d) scoops

12) Which is not a quality of the Dr. Vodder method of MLD?
   a) slow and rhythmic
   b) begin distal and progress proximal
   c) light pressure
   d) work in direction of lymph flow

13) Lymphedema is which type of edema?
   a) low protein
   b) high protein
   c) pulmonary
   d) dynamic

14) Lymphedema management using combined decongestive therapy involves the use of:
   a) deep tissue massage
   b) heat
   c) contrast bathing
   d) compression

15) The volume of lymph returning to the heart via the right lymphatic duct and thoracic duct every 24 hours is normally about:
    a) 24 liters
    b) 10 liters
    c) 2 to 4 liters
    d) 100 ml

16) Approximately how many lymph nodes are found in the body? More than:
    a) 60
    b) 100
    c) 600
    d) 1000

17) Which year was the Dr. Vodder School established in North America?
    a) 1936
    b) 1972
    c) 1982
    d) 1994

18) Lymph is taken from the lymph nodes by which lymph vessels?
    a) initial
    b) precollectors
    c) afferent collectors
    d) efferent collectors

19) Lymphedema is a recognized complication of:
    a) rosacea
    b) arthritis
    c) nephritis
    d) chondromalacia

20) Which is not a cause of lymphedema?
    a) congenital defects
    b) venous disease
    c) parasites
    d) irradiation

Myofascial Release

Keith Eric Grant and Art Riggs

9

INTRODUCTION

Myofascial release (MFR) is a collection of approaches and techniques that focuses on freeing restrictions of movement that originate in the soft tissues of the body. The benefits of this work are diverse. Direct bodily effects range from alleviation of pain, improvement of athletic performance, and greater flexibility and ease of movement to more subjective concerns such as better posture. More indirect goals include emotional release, deep relaxation, or general feelings of connection and well-being. Rather than being a specific technique, MFR is better understood as a goal-oriented approach to working with tissue-based restrictions and their two-way interactions with movement and posture.

The umbrella of MFR methods focuses heavily on how postural habits, specific activities or lack of activity, and compensations for prior injuries result in chronic stress and avoidance of full range of movements. These in turn result in both shortening of muscular units and **adhesions** between layers of **fascia.** Fascia forms the passive structural definition of our bodies. Adhesions are places in which separate fascial layers or fibers have bonded together dysfunctionally. The application of controlled and focused force, applied in a purposeful direction, acts to stretch or elongate the muscular and fascial (myofascial) structures toward the goals of restoring the fluid/lubricative quality of

DVD To better understand concepts in this chapter, watch *Myofascial Release video on the* **DVD** found at the back of this book.

149

BOX 9-1 Learning MFR

Learning best occurs when one reflects on personal experience with awareness but without self-criticism. The former guides our path; the latter impedes our progress. On shifting to a more myofascial approach, the work and techniques may seem strange or uncoordinated, especially if you are used to using a lot of lubrication, following a fixed massage sequence, or keeping to a fixed tempo of strokes. This feeling of strangeness is simply a necessary stage of learning and integrating new kinesthetic skills. As with all who practice and master such skills, you will someday look down to find your body and hands performing skills of myofascial release without conscious thought or effort. Although a single chapter cannot truly provide "How To" instruction, it is hoped that with a clearer understanding of fascia and some of the approaches to working with it, the reader will automatically expand his/her touch and intention to include myofascial work into whatever form of bodywork they perform.

---

the fascial tissue, the mobility of tissue, and normal joint function.*

Erik Dalton, an advanced Rolfer and bodywork author and instructor, has described our society as a culture of "flexion addicts." He notes, "The last century has witnessed a dramatic acceleration in our culture's flexion addiction. This pervasive and insidious condition is primarily due to the population's generational transition from an active group of movers to a sedentary bunch of sitters."[1]

Apart from acute injury, the genesis of pain and restriction is commonly the long-term effect of chronically flexed (i.e., shortened) positions. As noted by Cantu and Grodin,[2] **Wolff's Law** (the adaptation of bone to repeated patterns of applied force) applied to soft tissue (i.e., **Davis's Law**) implies that "all connective tissue seeks metabolic homeostasis commensurate to the stresses being applied to that particular tissue." Tissues habitually held short become physically shortened, both in the contractile elements of the muscle cells and in the more static collagenous elements of fascia that support the muscles. Lack of movement and lines of stress from tension and opposition to gravity facilitate formation of adhesions and fibrosis. Antagonists of chronically activated muscles can be overworked or neurologically inhibited and become fibrotic or weak. Ultimately,

pain and dysfunction occur—conditions that myofascial release aims to address by a combination of directly applied pressure, recruitment of neurologic reflexes, and relearning of movement potential. Because our (human) bodies are collections of interacting systems—connective tissue, neurologic, chemical-immune, and emotional—we have multiple paths that we can combine to effect positive changes. We follow suit with Cantu and Grodin's classification of myofascial approaches as being reflexive, mechanical, or movement-oriented,[2] having used combinations of these in our own work. We distinguish this combined approach from one confining itself to consideration of the purely physical application of force to fascia. An additional subtle but important component of the work is facilitation of the body's own tendency toward healing and a positive homeostasis when tissues are normalized and dysfunctional habits are retrained.

HISTORY

In the multiple professions in which manipulation of soft tissue arose in the twentieth century, myofascial release (MFR) became a term of convenience for a wide range of subtly differing but highly valued "goods" of healing and commerce.

Much confusion is saved by remembering that myofascial release is a generic term. MFR is an umbrella term used to describe various approaches, with considerable variation in philosophies and techniques, sharing a common focus of freeing fascial restrictions. Depending upon the personality, training, and skills of the practitioner; the type and degree of restriction or dysfunction; and to a very large extent, the makeup of the client, different techniques may have varying degrees of success. Any technique that works to free fascia is a form of myofascial release, and what works well for one client may not be as effective on another.

The recorded history of the term "myofascial release" is as much a linguistic history as it is a comprehensive gathering of the history of practice. For as long as massage has been practiced in its many forms, and long before dissection demonstrated a separate tissue defined as fascia that surrounds and permeates all muscles and organs, any accomplished practitioner would have felt the distinct properties of fascia as being very different from those of muscle tissue. Simply from tactile distinction, practitioners, consciously or intuitively, would quickly have developed techniques for releasing fascial restrictions that were different from those used to ameliorate purely muscular dysfunctions.

---

*The restoration of joint function occurs where such function has been adversely affected by the dysfunction of the surrounding myofascial tissue. The authors differentiate this from dysfunctions intrinsic to the joint itself, which are beyond the scope of our consideration.

Robert Ward, an osteopath, is attributed with coining the term *myofascial release* in the 1960s.[3] Since then, John Barnes, a physical therapist, has become a well-known writer and teacher of MFR as a separately identified study.[4-6] MFR, however, has been considered by Ward and other authors to be a "bridging technique" that ties together a number of different approaches toward relieving pain and restrictions of movement.[7] Another way of looking at this is that MFR is not so much a technique in itself, as a goal orientation that successfully weaves a number of techniques together. We thus find the underlying "framework" for the development of MFR coming from a number of different treatment traditions involving direct pressure, neurologic facilitation of muscles, and reeducation of learned neuromuscular patterns of posture and movement.

Philip Greenman mentions that "fascia has received attention from such individuals as the osteopathic physician William Neidner, who used twisting forces on the extremities to restore fascial balance and symmetry."[7] Ward also suggested that the direct method, called fascial twist, came from the osteopathy school in the 1920s by Neidner.[8] Also according to Ward, myofascial release originated from concepts used by Andrew Taylor Still, the founder of osteopathic medicine in the late nineteenth century.[8,9] Ward further comments that he was using "combinations of isometric, isotonic, functional indirect, and MFR concepts since the early 1950's, since they were taught by Wilbur Cole and Esther Smoot."[8] Long before this osteopathic thread of the early twentieth century, we can surmise that the human tendencies toward touch[10] had led to noticing the effects of organized pressure on tissue as well as its abilities to sooth anxiety and reduce pain. The techniques used would have been kinesthetic, observational, and palpation skills passed on as a direct tradition from master to apprentice with little written down (Box 9-2). Techniques would likely have been refined and propagated by traveling practitioners.

BOX 9-2 Pattern Recognition

One of the threads weaving through much of the writings on myofascial release is the concept of following the palpated "sense" of the tissue. This is a sense that springs forth of its own volition from our past practice and guided experience, not from a process of conscious analysis and rational thought. Its use relies not on what we "know" but on what we have previously done and sensed. The skill of the therapist is often in recognizing causative factors or sensing tissue restrictions intuitively rather than depending upon rigidly prescribed protocols. Two quotes, the first from a scientific text on computer-based pattern recognition and the second from a book on neurologic research and the workings of the human brain, illustrate how deeply human are these unconscious skills. They also illustrate the growing scientific basis for our trained but unconscious skills of reaction to subtle patterns.

"The ease with which we recognize a face, understand spoken words, read handwritten characters, identify our car keys in our pocket by feel, and decide whether an apple is ripe by its smell belies the astoundingly complex processes that underlie these acts of pattern recognition. Pattern recognition—the act of taking in raw data and making an action based on the 'category' of the pattern—has been crucial for our survival, and over the past tens of millions of years we have evolved highly sophisticated neural and cognitive systems for such tasks."[17]

"Your neocortex is a complex biological auto-associative memory. During each waking moment, each functional region is essentially waiting vigilantly for familiar patterns or pattern fragments to come in.... Your brain constantly makes predictions about the very fabric of the world we live in, and it does so in a parallel fashion. It will just as readily detect an odd texture, a misshapen nose, or an unusual motion. It isn't immediately apparent how pervasive these mostly unconscious predictions are, which is perhaps why we missed their importance for so long. They happen so automatically, so easily, we fail to fathom what is happening inside our skulls. I hope to impress on you the power of this idea. Prediction is so pervasive that what we 'perceive'—that is, how the world appears to us—does not come solely from our senses. What we perceive is a combination of what we sense and of our brain's memory-derived predictions."*

Even beyond such human capabilities of pattern recognition and prediction, modern neurologic research is opening new windows through which we can view learning and perception and by which we start to have a concept of how we create our innate sense of having a body.[†‡§] It is interesting to speculate, for example, if such research will eventually show that the clinical observations leading to Chinese meridian theory stem not from a direct physiologic property of our bodies, but from within the innate processing of the brain that creates our sense of body from the myriad of sensory information we produce internally. Particularly on the neurologic side, we are only now beginning to understand our full range of functioning as embodied human beings.

---

*Duda RO, Hast PE, Stork DG: *Pattern classification,* ed 2, New York, 2001, Wiley Interscience, ISBN 0-471-05669-3, p. 1.

†Blakeslee S, Blakeslee M: *The body has a mind of its own*, New York, 2007, Random House, ISBN 1-400-06469-4.

‡Hawkins J, with Blakeslee S: *On intelligence*, New York, 2004, Times Books.

§Melzack R: Pain and the neuromatrix in the brain, *Journal of Dental Education* 65 (12): 1378-1382, 2001.

Another contribution to myofascial thought, also in the 1920s, came from Mabel Ellsworth Todd. In her book, *The Thinking Body,* Todd examines the postural support of the human body and the physical and neurologic pattern basis for our body's amazing abilities to learn and use movement.[11] The book was first published in 1937 but has its roots in Todd's earlier 1929 teaching syllabus titled "The Balancing of Forces in the Human Being." Todd was well aware of the habitual and learned nature of postural patterns of unconscious muscle activation and of the supporting and adaptive role of fascia. She comments, "Fascia constitutes a general interstitial connective-tissue network, traversing all parts of the body, and thickened in various regions to form more or less definitive supporting and protective structures for other parts, whether visceral, bony or muscular. The fascial sheets vary greatly in their density, sometimes being quite tenuous or loosely webbed, containing fat, and sometimes forming dense, glittering sheets resembling the expansions of certain tendons, and like them termed aponeuroses.... Fascial structures, like tendons and ligaments, thicken in areas where extra strength is needed for muscular action, or for support. Fascia, tendons, and ligaments, which are all types of tough connective tissue, function together intimately." Todd's work captured the state of awareness of postural issues at the cutting edge in the 1920s and 1930s and became the basis of a school of work based on retraining of movement and postural patterns. The work, which has extensively influenced dance training, has been carried forward into the twenty-first century by Lulu Sweigard,[12] Irene Dowd,[13] and Eric Franklin.[14] A conceptual line from Todd to Franklin, which became known as **ideokinesis,** tells us that what we visualize—how we conceive our social position and how that affects our body self-image—has profound effects on our posture and movement patterns. Conversely, our posture and movements play back on our internal images and self-image. Change the way a person inhabits his or her body, and you change the person.

From the 1930s up to her death in 1979, Ida P. Rolf developed and taught her work directed at freeing of fascial planes. Rolf began her work in structural integration in the 1940s using yoga postures.[15] She later studied and further developed osteopathic methods. Tom Myers comments, "Rolf studied and worked with a number of osteopaths (reportedly including William Garner Sutherland, the originator of cranial osteopathy). One could consider the Structural Integration system she developed to be a soft-tissue subset of the general osteopathic inquiry, with the exception that SI

looks for general systemic improvement, rather than specific correction of **lesions.**[†] In this, she was more in step with the original ideas of Still and Sutherland, but a bit off from the thrust of osteopathy at that time, which was seeking more legitimacy through demonstrating its ability to deal with specific pathologies as well as structural issues."[15]

In contrast to the early osteopathic twisting methods, such as those of Neidner, Rolf's work was unique in being along straight lines of fascia, to increase congruence with gravity. Rolf's work also fed back into the line of osteopathic work. Erik Dalton recalled a conversation with Robert Ward in which Ward commented on drawing extensively from Rolf.[§] Tom Myers notes that, in the 1960s and 1970s, Rolf turned from teaching her techniques to medical professionals to those coming from a diversity of holistic and alternative treatment backgrounds.[15] Myers himself is notable both as a structural integration instructor and for bringing concepts of fascial force connection to a wider, massage-oriented audience in works such as his book *Anatomy Trains.*[16]

To convey her approaches to those with a more holistic orientation, Rolf came to teach at Esalen Institute, where she would create the nucleus of later structural integration practitioners and provide a juxtaposition of concepts and techniques that created other offshoots. Rolf's residence at Esalen also provided her work with a juxtaposition and conversation with the human potential movement and the Gestalt work of Fritz Perls.

One merging of somatic techniques at Esalen resulted in what came to be known as *deep tissue.* Brita Ostrom describes this evolution.[17] "As practitioners began receiving Rolfing® structural integration (Ida Rolf's Structural Realignment 10-session series of deep, intense bodywork, which she taught at the institute), they became curious about fascia alignment and deeper work. Vicki Topp and others studied anatomy and Al Drucker's offshoot, Esalen Deep Tissue Work, uniting intuitive massage with more physiological know-how. A massage class kept the meditative atmosphere but began to include muscle description and discussion on the physiology of breath." While there is, as with myofascial release, variance in matching technique with vocabulary within the profession, it is this lineage from Rolf's work and its fascial emphasis that sets

---

[†] Throughout this chapter, the term "lesion" is used in the orthopedic sense of a "myofascial lesion" or "soft tissue lesion"—a focal area of tissue abnormality or dysfunction resulting in pain or movement restriction.

[§] Erik Dalton, private communication, September 2007.

the framework for both "direct myofascial work" and "deep tissue massage" within this chapter. In short, the authors of this chapter take these two terms as being synonyms. We also adamantly differentiate this work from simply doing a "standard massage" with greater pressure, ignoring the changes in intent and anatomical specificity.

ANATOMY AND PHYSIOLOGY FOR MYOFASCIAL WORK

In order to understand the practice of myofascial release as it has evolved and as it is taught in its many forms as a therapeutic tool, we first need to have a clear perception of what fascia is and how it differs from muscle tissue. The largest practical difference between fascia and muscle is that fascia is not capable of voluntary contraction. Although there is some exciting new research reported by Schleip et al. that demonstrates some contradictions to the following,[18] for practical purposes fascia lacks the circulatory and neurologic capacity to actively shorten and lengthen.

Fascia surrounds each muscle fiber (endomysium), surrounds bundles (fascicles) of muscle fibers (perimysium), individual muscles to differentiate them from adjacent muscles (epimysium), and, as shown in Figure 9-1, is also present in broad sheets to add support to the body. Fascia defines surfaces between structures and acts as adaptable but passive structural support, creating connections between fibers as shown in Figure 9-2. Without fascia and the support it creates in such areas as the plantar region of the foot, the iliotibial band along the knee, along the lateral thigh, and in the lumbar back, the muscles would need to be in a constant (and exhausting) state

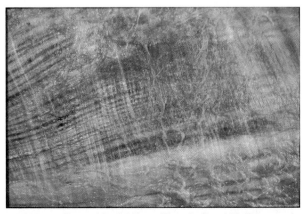

FIGURE 9-1 Sheet of fascial fibers. (Photo by Ronald A. Thompson.)

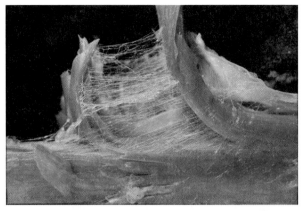

FIGURE 9-2 Gossamer strands of fascia between structures. (Photo by Ronald A. Thompson.)

of contraction just to hold the body upright. Instead, the fibers of fascia act to create and support the basic shape of our tissues.

The adaptability of fascia is both its blessing and its curse. Our bodies, although seemingly static in structure, are highly adaptable to what we do and—equally—don't do. We adapt to the stresses on our tissues from how we move and to the habitual postural positions we adopt in the field of our planet's gravity. This ability to adapt over time allows us to structurally strengthen both in bone and soft tissue to sustain, for example, long-distance running. Increasing activities too quickly (>10% per week), thus not allowing time for such adaptation, can lead to tendinosis (soft tissue breakdown) and to stress fractures. Equally, however, inactivity and chronic dysfunctional stress applied to our tissues can cause them to adapt in dysfunctional ways, resulting in atrophy, fibrosis, shortened tissues, and adhesions between tissues.

When our tissues, both soft and hard (bone), resist gravity or another force they undergo **physical stress.** We often tend to think of **emotional stress** when we hear the word stress. This might be loosely defined as our sense of burden in coping with activities occurring in our lives. Physical stress, on the other hand, is technically defined as force exerted on a material per unit area of the cross-sectional area perpendicular to the force. Thus, for something like a tendon, the physical stress is the force pulling on the tendon divided, at each increment of length along the tendon, by its area at that point. A further nuance is that stress can have two components: **tensile stress** along the length of something like a tendon as just described, and **shear stress.** Shear stress occurs when side-to-side force is applied in different directions to adjacent areas of tissue. In response to stress, a material lengthens. The fraction of lengthening (change in length divided by initial length) is the definition of **strain.** When fascia has stress applied to it, it first lengthens elastically. If the force is removed at this point, the connective tissue returns to its original length. It's thought that this elastic region occurs as the **crimp,** or natural physiological zigzagging in the tissue, is removed. This is analogous to pulling on a piece of the rickrack trim used in sewing. If greater force is applied to fascia, it begins to plastically deform, lengthening but creating microtears within the tissue. If the force is further increased to the **tensile strength** or **shear strength** of the tissue, a tear occurs, resulting in discernable injury. In combination, a conception model capturing both the initial elastic phase and the latter plastic or viscous phase is known as a **viscoelastic model.**[2]

If the amount of stress we incur increases gradually, to a great extent we adapt. Davis's Law for soft tissue and Wolff's Law for bone state that tissue is laid down along lines of stress.[19] This is the key to both functional and dysfunctional adaptations. Tom Myers presents the theory that the mechanism for adaptation is not an increase in the rate at which tissue is actually deposited by fibroblasts and osteoblasts, but a reduction in the rate of resorption or removal. The reduction in removal is thought to be induced by a piezoelectric field resulting from the applied stress.[16] Since both deposition and removal occur continually, a piezoelectric suppression of removal changes the local balance toward more accumulation of tissue. Similarly, lack of regular applied stress changes the balance toward loss of tissue. This concept motivates the use of weight-bearing exercises, for example, to help prevent osteoporosis.

As mentioned in the brief description above, Dalton has described our society as a culture of "flexion addicts," being sedentary compared with our ancestors and often staying in sitting positions that shorten our anterior torsos, lumbar spines, and hamstrings. While it is often our posture and lack of movement and use that drive us into dysfunction, the specific changes also are based on deeper physiologic properties of muscular fibers.

Professor Vladimir Janda, a Czechoslovakian physician and rehabilitation specialist, provided insight into common patterns of dysfunction with his classification of muscles as being postural or phasic. Postural muscles tend toward "slow-twitch" fibers that contract more slowly but also fatigue more slowly. Phasic muscles, containing more "fast-twitch" fibers, are designed to power more explosive movements. To simplify, it's the distinction between sprinters and marathoners. The important difference for myofascial work, the key noted by Janda, is that postural muscles tend to shorten into dysfunction while phasic muscles tend to weaken. Postural muscles can become short and hypertonic (which does not necessarily imply stronger), while their phasic antagonists become inhibited and weak.[20] In order for the weakened phasic muscles to be effectively strengthened and reeducated, in order for a client to be able to move toward a better posture, chronically shortened and hypertonic postural muscles must first be normalized, a process that requires addressing both the muscle activity and the fascial restrictions (Box 9-3).

In particular, Janda pointed out two common patterns of myofascial dysfunction, the upper-crossed syndrome and lower-crossed syndrome.[20,21] In upper-crossed syndrome, the pectoralis major and minor, upper trapezius, levator scapulae, and sternocleidomastoid all tighten and shorten. Simultaneously, as described above, the lower and middle trapezius, serratus anterior, and rhomboids all weaken. The result is a posture with shoulders and head forward and a compensatory shortened posterior neck, as shown in the left half of Figure 9-3. In lower-crossed syndrome, the iliopsoas, rectus femoris, tensor fasciae latae, short adductors of the hip, and the erector spinae group of the trunk all tighten and shorten. At the same time, the abdominal and gluteal muscles weaken. The typical result is the posture with an anterior pelvic tilt and an accentuated **lordosis** (i.e., anterior curve) of the lumbar spine as shown in the right half of Figure 9-3 (see Case History 1).

Generally, little can be done to strengthen and improve the usage patterns of the weakened muscles before the shortened muscles and associated fascia are normalized. **Sherrington's law of reciprocal innervation/inhibition** states that the antagonist to an activated muscle will be inhibited.[7,20] According to this, the normal tonus of the weakened phasic muscles is due not only to lack of use but also to this neurologic inhibition from the tightened side. In addition, fascia that surrounds muscle compartments or is in broad superficial sheets has a tendency to shorten in areas of stress, causing problems in mobility and joint function. It is incredibly strong and relatively resistant to lengthening, so when postural patterns, injury, or other issues shorten fascia, techniques to release this shortening are required. These techniques are more anatomically specific and more directional dependent than those needed for general massage work.

BOX 9-3 Postural and Phasic Muscles

As practitioners move from more relaxation-oriented work into more clinical work, the techniques used are the simpler part of the learning. More difficulty lies in gaining mastery of organizing a plan of exploration and treatment to meet a particular client's needs. The choice of techniques should flow from the needs of the work rather than the work being framed to practice the last learned set of techniques. But there's the catch, How do we understand what needs to be done for the client who stands before us?

Vladimir Janda's concept of postural and phasic muscles is one of several biomechanical models discussed by Chaitow and DeLany* that provide insights for working with three-dimensional dysfunctions. Postural muscles are composed of "slow-twitch" fibers. These fibers contain more mitochondria for ongoing energy production, fatigue slowly, and are mainly involved in lower-force actions needed for stabilization and maintaining posture. Postural muscles tend to shorten into dysfunction and include the gastrocnemius, soleus, hamstrings, short adductors of the thigh, psoas, piriformis, tensor fascia lata, quadratus lumborum, erector spinae, latissimus dorsi, upper trapezius, sternocleido mastoid, levator scapulae, pectoralis major, and the flexors of the arm.† To a large extent, these distinctions should be taken to be comparative relationships between muscles rather than absolute properties, many muscles having dual functions for maintaining posture and the also an ability to power rapid motion.

In contrast, phasic muscles contain more "fast twitch" fibers, needed for bursts of activity. Such fibers depend largely on the more immediate energy sources of creatine and glycolysis and fatigue relatively quickly. Phasic muscles tend to weaken in dysfunction. Phasic muscles also tend to be neurologically inhibited by hypertonic postural antagonists.

While it would be expected that shortened, hypertonic muscles would become fibrous, it might appear that weakened, stretched muscles would not be. For example, we would expect a shortened hamstring to be fibrous, but what about long and weak rhomboids? Muscles that tend to weaken, such as the rhomboids, can still be under stress. Davis's Law tells us that tissue is laid down along lines of stress without requiring the tissue to be the source of the stress. Thus, after we normalize the shortened, hypertonic muscles, it is often the case that both shortened and weakened muscles will need to be treated for fibrosity and adhesions. Rhomboids can be stretched tight (rather than contracted tight), fibrous, painful, and long, because they are losing the battle with the more important flexors in the anterior body.

We can add to this consideration by looking at additional models of dysfunction discussed by Chaitow and DeLany.* These include Robert Ward's biomechanical model of "tightness" and "looseness" and Karel Lewit's "loose-tight" thinking. Quoting from Ward, "Tightness suggests tethering, while looseness suggests joint and/or soft tissue laxity, with or without neural 'inhibition'. These barriers (tight and loose) can also be seen to refer to the obstacles which are sought in preparation for direct (toward bind, tightness) and indirect (towards ease, looseness) techniques." Lewit notes that pain is often experienced on the "loose" side.‡ Chaitow and DeLany* then bring the concepts together with a comment on "pain and the tight-loose concept." "Pain is more commonly associated with tight and bound/tethered structures, which may be due to local overuse/misuse/abuse factors, scar tissue, reflexively induced influences or centrally mediated neural control. When a tight tissue is then asked to either fully contract or fully lengthen, pain is often experienced." Paradoxically, as pointed out by Lewit above, pain is also often noted in the "loose" rather than the "tight" areas of the body, which may involve **hypermobility** and **ligamentous laxity** at the "loose" joint or site. In cases with hypermobility, muscle hypertonicity and tissue restrictions may be a protective response to increase stability. When this is the situation, freeing dysfunctional restrictions will need to be done within a context of strengthening exercises to replace the needed stability. A cohesive treatment plan clearly requires looking at interrelations between muscles.

* Chaitow L, DeLany JW: *Clinical application of neuromuscular techniques: the upper body*, Edinburgh, 2000, Churchill Livingstone.
† Chaitow L: *Muscle energy techniques*, New York, 1996, Churchill Livingstone.
‡ Lewit K: *Manipulative therapy in rehabilitation of the locomotor system*, ed 2, London, 1991, Butterworth-Heinemann.

DEFINING MYOFASCIAL RELEASE

Because the term myofascial release, literally "release of muscles and fascia," is so encompassing and because the roots and application of MFR are so diverse, we encounter a problem of definition and differentiation of the work. Cantu and Grodin take a useful approach in differentiating joint mobilization from myofascial work.[2] They note that joint work strictly follows arthrokinetic rules based on joint structure.

In contrast, myofascial work is less predictable and can occur along different lines and planes that have little to do with the direction of actual joint motion. While myofascial work needs to retain a basis of analysis of the symptoms and their potential sources, its more unpredictable nature requires an ability to sense and respond to the tissue itself. This ability comes not from analysis but from experience and awareness—in short, putting the miles of touch into your hands.

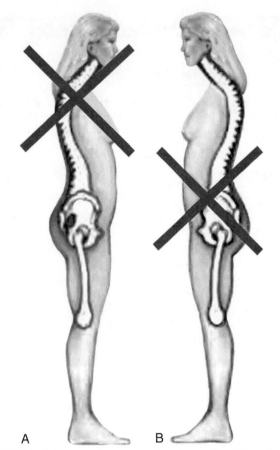

FIGURE 9-3 Upper and lower crossed syndromes. Lines **(A)** are lines of shortening. Lines **(B)** are lines of weakening. (Used with the permission of Erik Dalton.)

This aptitude, while often considered to be "intuitive," more scientifically draws on the amazing pattern-matching abilities of the human brain (see Box 9-2). Greenman[7] and Chaitow[22] both provide exercises for improving and refining palpation skills.

For our purposes, myofascial release will also be restricted within the bounds of hands-on manual therapy. Thus we eliminate from our concern surgical procedures such as a lateral release of the knee. This procedure is frequently recommended by orthopedists to free fascial restrictions around the iliotibial band and knee retinaculum that cause knee pain due to the patella tracking too laterally. While technically a "myofascial release," it lies beyond our domain of practice.

There are several forms of myofascial release that are entirely applicable for our purposes. The following section of the chapter will explain some of the major techniques according to the actual manual skills that are applied; a later section will speak to the effectiveness of some of these techniques in paradigms of larger

goals such as treatment of injuries, "structural integration" or body alignment, improvement of performance in athletics or dance, or other areas such as the psychologic realm. Although there can be great overlap, myofascial release can be practiced anywhere along a continuum from very gentle indirect release to considerably more pressure applied in direct procedures.

INDIRECT RELEASE TECHNIQUE

This philosophy proposes an inherent ability of the body to "self-correct" and applies unwinding techniques that tend to follow in the direction that fascia seems to move when gentle pressure is applied. This natural tendency toward tissue homeostasis is referred to as the **inherent force.** The tissue is stretched and the therapist applies slow, steady pressure in the direction that the fascia can be felt to allow greatest ease of movement. The therapist may hold the tissue at the end range of stretch for up to several minutes until the tissue appears to reconfigure itself, allowing greater range of movement or movement in a new direction. Although he certainly teaches more direct methods, Barnes orients much of his teaching around such indirect methods.

DIRECT RELEASE TECHNIQUE

Proponents of this approach, also often referred to as deep tissue work, practice a more aggressive manipulation of fascia, often applied in opposition to the direction that the fascia may freely allow movement. They establish where the fascia is short and lengthen it in opposition to this shortness. Folklore often describes the more direct approach as painful, but such painfulness results more from a too immediately deep or too impatient use of pressure than from a necessity of the direct technique itself. Although some discomfort may be experienced, the amount of pressure can be relatively gentle and its application slow and at an oblique angle. The primary distinction between the direct and indirect techniques is that direct release uses less unwinding and "following" of release tendencies and more directly encourages the fascia to release in a direction the practitioner feels will improve function or posture.

COMBINED DIRECT AND INDIRECT TECHNIQUES

There unfortunately has been some history of a polarization between respective practitioners of the direct and indirect methods. At times, this has led to strident criticism of the opposing view, with each side convinced that it possessed "the answer." From the authors' mutual perspective, the reality is that different people respond better to different approaches. Clients with very sensitive central nervous systems or particularly low pain thresholds may feel disoriented or overwhelmed by too much direct input. In contrast, more muscular and physically active clients often prefer the aggressiveness of more direct methods, said techniques being in fact substantially less invasive than their own training regimens.

Often direct-release techniques will offer immediate change at a faster pace, so clients experience more noticeable benefits in a shorter period of time. In contrast, some people release more quickly if allowed to follow their own patterns. If too much pressure is applied and the work is overly intense or painful, the tissue will resist and less will be accomplished. Additionally, for some already near their adaptive limits of fatigued or stress, too aggressive sensory input or too much microtissue damage might provoke an immune response resulting in subsequent malaise, aches, or cognitive fog. Many therapists thus find advantage in alternating between methods depending upon the individual needs of their clients or the amount of restriction in a specific area. For efficient use of time, it is sometimes advisable to first attempt direct methods to see if they will work easily and quickly, but to move to slower, more indirect methods if these initial attempts are not satisfactory or if client is uncomfortable.

COMPRESSION WITH MOVEMENT

The basic concept of compression with movement is well-captured by the generic name "pin and stretch." The distinctions among what is used and taught by various practitioners involve whether the movement is active or passive, and the direction and speed in which the compression is applied. Oblique pressure with active movement has been a fundamental technique of structural integration from its inception with Rolf. Over 50 years ago, Rolf instructed her students to "put the tissue where it belongs and ask for movement." Sports massage practitioner and instructor Benny Vaughn has taught active movement with compression as "compression with active engagement"[‡‡] Whitney Lowe uses "compression with active movement." British sports massage practitioners, such as Mel Cash and Stuart Taws, call it "soft tissue release," or STR. Michael Leahy has developed and marketed, particularly to the

medical and physical therapy communities, codified application protocols for the technique as "Active Release Technique®" or ART.[§§] Leahy's training is extensive and offers many excellent protocols for treatment of specific injuries or areas of the body. Before discussing application, however, let's backtrack for a moment to look at the anatomical basis for the technique.

When movement occurs, muscles, tendons, fascia, and nerves also have to move. Some of this movement will occur relative to other fiber bundles in the same muscle, some across other tissue structures. If layers of tissue that need movement across each other are adhered to each other, movement will be restricted, as symbolized in the "fascial sweater" of Figure 9-4. If tissues within a muscles structure can't freely elongate, movement will be restricted. If, as a muscle shortens, fibers can

---

[§§] See Greenman's use of the acronym ART for "Asymmetry, Range of motion, and tissue Texture."[7] Craig Liebenson has used "Active Muscular Relaxation Techniques" or AMRT to describe techniques based on postisometric relaxation and reciprocal inhibition.

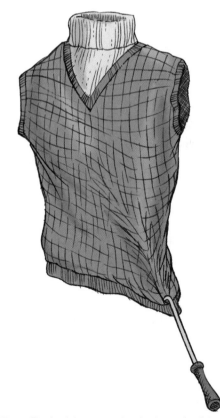

FIGURE 9-4 The fascial sweater, showing how a fascial restriction in one area will strain areas away from the restriction. (Reprinted from Rolf I: *Rolfing: the integration of human structures* with permission of the Rolf Institute of Structural Integration © 1977.)

[‡‡] From notes from a class Benny Vaughn taught at Heartwood Institute, Garberville CA in October 1998.

broaden and separate laterally from each other (i.e., they are cross-linked together), movement will be restricted. If nerve tissue elongation is adhered to or impeded by other tissue, the nerve tissue will either suffer **impingement** (compression against an underlying structure) or **adverse neural tension** (dysfunctional stretching). So how does compression with movement help?

As a muscle lengthens, it has movement along its length (longitudinal) between its own fibers and also relative to other tissue structures. Compression along the muscle as it is lengthened (actively or passively) localizes the stretch. Pressure applied longitudinally against the lengthening locally increases the stretch within the muscle tissue. Pressure applied longitudinally with the elongation increases the **shear stress** on any adhesion, binding the lengthening muscle to adjacent structures. Conversely, when a muscle shortens, it is also forced to broaden. A direct or cross-fiber compression applied to a broadening muscle will flatten it, forcing fibers to spread transversely apart (think of pressing on a bundle of uncooked spaghetti), breaking adhesions between fibers. The compression, properly directed, thus assists the tissue movement required, allowing the tissue to free itself from adhesions. It is this latter property of self-tendency that also tends to make compression with active movements more effective than passive movements.

With these techniques, the therapist anchors restricted fascial or muscular areas, with the knuckles, fist, forearm, elbow, or braced fingers, while having the client move an adjacent joint so that the muscle, tendon, or fascia is slowly stretched from the anchor point. This focuses the stretch at a precise point rather than having the stretch dissipated over the entire length of the muscle. Muscle tightness is rarely equally distributed over the entire length of a muscle, so focused anchoring eliminates the tendency of the more flexible areas of the muscle adapting to stretch while allowing tight and fibrous areas to remain short. The practitioner uses palpation and visual observation to evaluate adhesions restricting movement and anomalous tissue texture. Abnormal tissues are treated by combining precisely directed tension with very specific active or passive movements.

Finally, the addition of active client movements adds the elements of neuromuscular reeducation, neurologic reinforcement of techniques, and making the practitioner-client teamwork stronger and more explicit. For example, Lewit noted that using eye movements in the direction of release would produce additional gains from postisometric relaxation.[21] This concept of subtle neurologic enhancement also finds support in the visualization approaches developed in ideokinesis.[11-14] Asking for active client movement may reveal aberrant movement patterns and fascial strain patterns not seen in static or neutral positioning, enabling the practitioner to "track" muscles and fascia into proper position and length. Active movement against gentle practitioner resistance can enable clients to relearn joint proprioception lost from disuse or injury. Techniques can be synchronized with respiration to gain added release from this core human cycle. Finally, having the client perform active movements is both a very explicit reinforcement of working together and a form of gaining client commitment.***

ADJUNCT METHODS

The effectiveness of myofascial release can often be increased by folding in other, synergistic methods. Techniques commonly used as adjunct methods include trigger point/neuromuscular therapy, positional release/strain-counterstrain, and various forms of postisometric relaxation. Chaitow's integrated neuromuscular inhibition technique (INIT) is a case in point.[23] In INIT, Chaitow uses direct pressure, positional release, and muscle energy technique (MET) to effectively target dysfunctional soft tissues. From a trigger point perspective, the additional techniques ensure a more complete release of the involved tissues. From the perspective of myofascial release, reflex techniques such as positional release (i.e., positioning to take all stress off of the targeted muscle) and MET can be used to reduce muscle hypertonicity before addressing fascial adhesions. This avoids working against the client's muscular tension. In chronic cases, it may be advantageous to alternate between reflex and direct methods. Where an involved muscle is too painful for the direct isometric contraction of MET, isometric contraction of the antagonist will gain release via reciprocal inhibition (RI). Positional release can also be used in such cases.

***In his book *Influence: Science and Practice* Robert B. Cialdini devotes substantial discussion to the powerful behavioral aspects of commitment and consistency. While this material is beyond the scope of this chapter, it nevertheless provides a sociological basis for understanding how client involvement can increase treatment effectiveness.

APPLICATION OF MYOFASCIAL RELEASE
General Technique

In spite of the differences in definition of myofascial release, there are threads of intent, skill, and technique that remain consistent throughout the fabric of interpretation. The authors strongly feel that the subjective elements of a powerful yet nurturing touch is the key element in carrying out the goals of any deep fascial work. No matter how effective a particular modality may be, if the practitioner has a harsh or ineffective touch, the effectiveness of the work will be greatly compromised. For the core of myofascial technique, Michael Stanborough provides an excellent and concise description of application[24]:

- Land on the surface of the body with the appropriate "tool" (e.g., knuckles, or forearm).
- Sink into the soft tissue.
- Contact the first barrier/restricted layer.
- Put in a "line of tension."
- Engage the fascia by taking up the slack in the tissue.
- Finally, move or drag the fascia across the surface while staying in touch with the underlying layers.
- Exit gracefully.

Figure 9-5 provides a visual representation of the goal of engaging a layer of fascia. Notice the white color of the tissue, demonstrating the lack of vascularization, and the wrinkled appearance of the fascia. The intention of the stroke would be to "iron" out the wrinkles and lengthen the sheet. It also is obvious that simply kneading the fascia would have little effect on such smoothing and lengthening. The key to successful work is in engaging the fascia and "ironing" it with longitudinal intention.

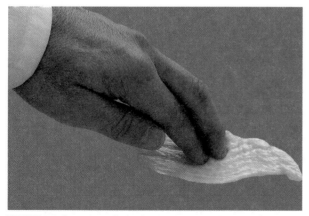

FIGURE 9-5 Pressure applied to fascia with braced fingertips. (Used with the permission of Robert Schleip.)

Probably the most obvious difference that clients first notice between conventional massage and myofascial release techniques is that the therapist uses less or even no lubrication. Because the emphasis is upon lengthening fascia rather than kneading muscle tissue, it is necessary to "grab" the tissue rather than sliding over it. Just as it is difficult to open a tight jar lid or turn a doorknob with slippery wet hands, it is also difficult to grab and lengthen short fascia if using too much lubrication. As with the jar lid, much more effort is necessary to provide the necessary friction. Exerting such effort by pressing too hard on tissue can easily translate to discomfort or pain for the client and fatigue or risk of injury for the practitioner.

From the experience of our classes, the authors feel that one of the most important skills to teach students is that of sinking through tissue to reach the level of fascial restriction, rather than beginning work at layers that don't need work. Many new therapists spend unnecessary time warming up outer layers with superfluous or ineffective work. Others create pain by beginning intense work as soon as they contact the body. A good rule is *"sink ... and then work,"* with the sinking occurring as the body responds to applied pressure and intent rather than being forced or hurried by the practitioner.

After sinking to the first fascial barrier, the therapist chooses the proper tool (fingers, knuckles, fist, forearm, elbow) depending upon the precision and power needed to address the fascia and the space of the location on the client's body. The novice practitioner will benefit from realizing that skill in such palpatory exploration comes as a result of practice with awareness. In time, it becomes an unconscious process (see Box 9-2), but in the beginning the practitioner must consciously feel for differences in tissue direction, texture, tension, and temperature. Similarly, while choice of the body surface used to apply pressure is later automatic, in the beginning the novice must consider which area needs application, the size of their own body "instruments," pressure required, and the relative wear and tear on their own body. Using direct or indirect techniques, it is now necessary to clarify the goals of working with the fascia. Do you want to lengthen fascial sheets in the direct line of muscle pull, apply force diagonally to correct torsion forces, or separate fascial compartments? On a deeper level, it may be necessary to sink through superficial tissue with direct downward pressure before encountering the layer needing work. After sinking, force is then applied in a more oblique stretching direction, using either direct or indirect intention.

Often, myofascial work goes beyond addressing individual layers of shortened fascia. Different muscle compartments or fascial layers or envelopes may have adhered to each other. Precise work with fingers or knuckles may be appropriate to separate these layers or envelopes for the muscles to properly slide by each other and allow free movement.

Although they are very different tissues, muscle and fascia are inextricably linked. The therapist is always working with both of these tissues with varying emphasis. By the same token, a massage practitioner can be working with fascia while doing relaxation massage and a myofascial specialist can be relaxing the contractile elements of muscles pursuant to releasing facial restrictions.

Next to the minimal use of lubricants, the speed of strokes is one of the most noticeable differences between massage and myofascial release work. Fascia releases in two stages, each stage completing much more slowly than it takes for contractile muscle tissue to release. The first release or "melt" is from the elastin and the collagen crimp, which allow the fascia to lengthen along with normal muscle lengthening. After this initial release, the therapist waits for the more stubborn collagen and ground substances to reconfigure to gain the more permanent viscous lengthening and smoothing of texture. Clients often describe a slight burning feeling during this release but also comment on the lasting effect of the work. They describe the sensations as "feeling like their muscles are clay that is being molded." Clients immediately notice that the work is performed much more slowly. Some therapists, after taking up the slack by stretching the fascia to its end range, wait for 4 or 5 minutes while holding tension for the second release or for a feeling of heat to indicate that the fascia is stabilizing into a lengthened position.

A brief description with photographs may prove helpful in understanding some of the different approaches to performing myofascial release work. We turn now to a series of applied variations of the core technique just described.

Skin Rolling

Starting our specific applications with the most superficial, we turn first to skin rolling. It is motivated by the observation of adhesions between the skin and the layers of fascia immediately beneath the skin or between superficial and deeper layers of fascia. At times, the pull of such adhesions will be observed as a "puckering" of the skin. The first work at releasing these adhesions often produces a strong burning sensation. Once the adhesions are cleared, further work at this superficial level is generally free of adverse sensations.

To implement skin-rolling, the practitioner grabs a "roll" of skin and subcutaneous fascia between his/her fingers and thumb and rolls this skin or scar tissue while lifting it away from the body. Over the years of the authors' clinical experience numerous clients have extolled the virtues of skin rolling after having previously tried virtually every other form of bodywork to help with pain in such areas as the elbows, knees, shoulders, and, especially, the sacrum and low back. While skin-rolling is generally a very limited part of myofascial methods, it can provide substantial relief where indicated. Lewit describes skin stretching to take up the slack and engage a hyperalgesic zone (HAZ), which may be a cause of pain and is notable for lacking a springy resistance at the end-position of the stretch.[21] The stretch is gently held until resistance weakens and normal springing is restored. This variant extends the concept of skin-rolling into small areas in which it is difficult to "roll" the skin.

To release the fascial restrictions causing strain around a joint, the practitioner needs to go deep enough to grab the subcutaneous fascia along with the epidermis. If one imagines the torsional (i.e., twisting) strain upon a joint, especially around the sacral area, it seems quite logical that freeing "stuck" fascia in the area would allow for better movement and improvement of imbalance. Skin rolling is usually limited to specific painful areas rather than applied as a broad integration technique. It can be very intense or even painful on the initial session and certainly does not lend itself to a long bodywork session. Its effectiveness is also limited to working with superficial fascial restrictions rather than with deep fascial restraints between muscle compartments or in the viscera.

MFR Direct Technique

In these examples the therapist may use forearms, palms of the hands, or any broad surface. Remember that it is important to expedite the stretch to the fascia by either using body positioning to elongate the myofascial component (place the tissue in enough stretch to elongate the muscles without so much tension that it is difficult to penetrate to the proper level) or by anchoring with the other hand to localize the stretch to the specific area needing lengthening. This is demonstrated in Figure 9-6 by the stretch placed on the iliotibial band with the left hand while the fascia is stretched away from the anchor with the right forearm.

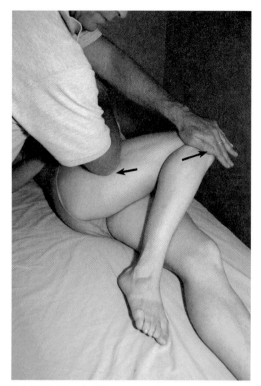

FIGURE 9-6 Working the ITB on a stretch.

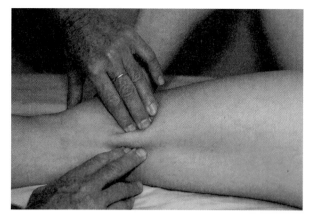

FIGURE 9-7 Differentiating the iliotibial band.

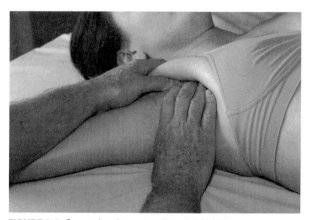

FIGURE 9-8 Separating the pectoralis and deltoid.

Separation of Compartments

These techniques are very useful in working with many areas including the pectoralis major, the small muscles in the forearm, the trapezius, and anywhere different muscles overlap. The lateral leg easily demonstrates this principle, working along the lateral border of the iliotibial band and the vastus lateralis, as shown in Figure 9-7, or separating the hamstring compartment from more anterior or lateral muscles. Pressure should be applied with relatively sharp or precise tools such as fingers or knuckles, slowly moving up the border of the muscle or fascial compartment visualizing gently prying the compartments apart. Asking for active movement on the part of the client will expedite the process. As a second example, Figure 9-8 shows separating the pectoralis and deltoids by lifting the pectoralis with the fingers.

Lifting or Rolling Muscle Compartments

These strokes depend upon bringing the muscle to the end range of easy movement and waiting to feel the release when the muscle rolls away from restrictions either adjacent to or deep to the muscle being worked. Although it is handy for use with large muscles, such as the pectoralis major or gluteus maximus, this technique is most often used for long muscles such as the quadriceps, biceps, triceps, and calf muscles. Slowly lift the muscle away from the bone and roll it until resistance is felt, as shown for the gastrocnemius in Figure 9-9. Then wait for the muscle to slowly release in the direction of force. This technique is very useful to improve "tracking" of joints that are disrupted by torsion—forces that occur when muscles are not exerting their force in the proper line in relation to the joint. The sternocleidomastoid muscle needs to be free from adhesions to adjacent muscles in order to properly shorten and have a clear line of pull to turn the head. Lifting the muscle with fingers (or knuckles) and rolling or mobilizing with shearing force is demonstrated in Figure 9-10.

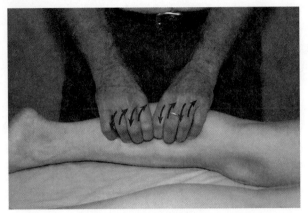

FIGURE 9-9 Lifting and rolling the gastrocnemius with the fingers.

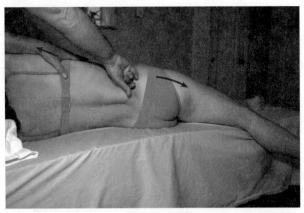

FIGURE 9-11 Working the quadratus lumborum on a stretch, leg off the table and slightly posterior.

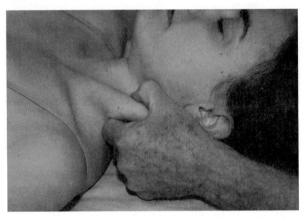

FIGURE 9-10 Lifting and rolling the sternocleidomastoid to free adhesions.

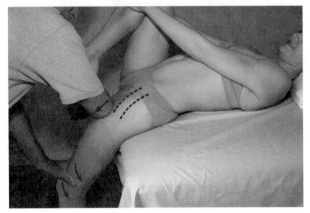

FIGURE 9-12 Working the quadriceps on a stretch in the position of a Modified Thomas Test.

Placing Muscles into Stretched Position

As long as the muscles are not placed in so much stretch that they are hard to penetrate or the stretch receptors are innervated causing the muscle to contract, the therapist will have the advantage of beginning work at the end range of fascial stretch instead of exerting effort to take up the slack. Additionally, the release that occurs at the end range of the relaxed stretch provides valuable neurologic input to the stretch receptors, helping to reprogram a "learned" dysfunction of shortness. In Figure 9-11 the quadratus lumborum is released by extending the leg down and posterior while securing the lower rib cage.

The position creates a stretch, while an open fist is used to directly work the tissue. A similar gravity-assisted position is also used to release the quadriceps in Figure 9-12. The client positioning is identical

to that for a Modified Thomas Test, with the client securing the contralateral (i.e., opposite) leg in hip flexion to stabilize the pelvis and low back (i.e., to prevent the pelvis from tilting anteriorly). The practitioner's free hand secures the worked leg above the knee to augment the stretch from gravity. The hip extension stretches both the rectus femoris and the iliopsoas. Having the knee flexed on the leg being worked increases the stretch on the rectus femoris relative to that on the iliopsoas, the rectus femoris crossing both the hip and knee joints (i.e., being a two-joint muscle).

Anchor and Stretch Strokes

This is the first of two examples of applications of compression with movement. With the anchor (or pin) and stretch strategy, the force of the movement or stretch is localized at specific areas of thickening or adhesions. Rather than attempting to place the entire muscle in a stretch, the therapist relaxes (shortens) the muscle by flexing the joint, anchors on the area that is fibrotic, and then extends the joint so that the stretch is focused at a precise point where the force is applied. It is crucial that the therapist anchor the point rather than sliding over in a conventional massage manner. Figure 9-13 demonstrates use of the anchor and stretch technique on the anterior compartment of the leg to anchor at a localized source of fascial restriction while stretching the tibialis anterior in the opposite direction.

Expedited Lengthening Strokes

Another variant of the application of compression with movement is expedited lengthening. This variant is particularly helpful in teaching clients to work with tracking issues and movement patterns. As with anchor and stretch strokes, the muscle is placed in a relaxed or shortened position. Instead of stretching the muscle against resistance, however, the therapist works in the direction of muscle lengthening and guides the myofascial compartment to efficiently lengthen in the most expedient direction for the joint. In Figure 9-14 the therapist's pressure and direction create a proximal-to-distal stretch of the quadriceps. This positioning can be further enhanced by dropping the leg off the side of the table, allowing the knee to flex to create an additional stretch on the quadriceps. The client can be instructed to lower the leg slowly, timing the movement to synchronize with the work being done. Compare with the Modified Thomas Test position in Figure 9-12. Note that the stretch is directed distally in the example. Many therapists have been

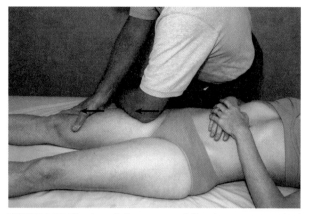

FIGURE 9-14 The therapist's pressure and direction create a proximal to distal stretch of the quadriceps.

instructed that *all* strokes should be directed in the direction of venous blood flow back to the heart. The authors feel that this edict is greatly overemphasized in early massage training, precluding many benefits of directing strokes in different directions as tissue indicates. In Figure 9-14 the distal direction of the stroke has the advantage of decompressing the hip joint and lengthening the quadriceps against the usual direction of shortening. The pressure is oblique: thus the amount of pressure applied depends on the angle of application, the pressure required to reach the desired layer of tissue, and the rate at which the client's tissue allows forward movement without inducing self-protective resistance.

BENEFITS OF APPLICATION

The major benefits of myofascial release are increased freedom and ease of movement and freedom or reduction of pain associated with tissue restrictions. For many people, freeing postural or holding patterns in the body will bring feelings of physical well-being. Changing restricted postural patterns may also free emotional holding patterns, allowing clients to better experience their feelings. For those involved in coordinated movement activities, such as athletics and dance, myofascial release will improve functional use of the body. Facilitating athletic endeavors underscores that therapeutic bodywork need not always be performed to help solve clinical problems or conditions. Much benefit can be achieved in working to improve and maintain bodies that are already functioning well. Particularly with such athletes, who are used to pushing their physical

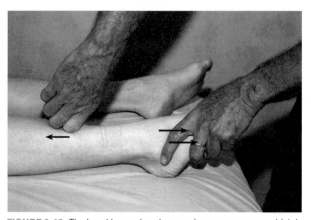

FIGURE 9-13 The knuckles anchor the anterior compartment, which is then stretched by plantar flexing the ankle.

boundaries and limitations, the practitioner may find the MFR direct technique/deep tissue massage to be straightforward. Because of their psychological conditioning, athletes will, more often than the general public, be able to relax into relatively intense deep tissue work.

Conditions and injuries responding well to myofascial release include:

- Adhesions and scar tissue from sprains, strains, surgical procedures, minor injuries, overuse, and chronic postural strain.
- Fibromyalgia and myofascial pain syndrome[†††]
- Myofasciitis—particularly plantar fasciitis
- Tendinosis or tenosynovitis—either by working on the inflamed area or tight muscles that cause strain on the tendon
- Low back pain
- Neck pain
- Osteoarthritis

In 2004 *Consumer Reports* conducted a survey involving 34,000 of its readers to determine the benefits that different alternative care modalities (chiropractic, physical therapy, deep tissue massage, prescribed exercises, prescription medication, acupuncture, acupressure, and diet) provided for various conditions or complaints.[25] For relieving back pain and neck pain, deep tissue massage was virtually tied with chiropractic for those respondents who felt "much better," and deep tissue work led with those that reported that they felt "somewhat" better. For fibromyalgia and osteoarthritis, deep tissue massage provided the greatest extent of relief for both "significant" and "somewhat better" improvements. Physical therapy and exercise were also rated highly. In general, for the conditions mentioned above, both the "significant" and "somewhat better" categories for massage ranged from 35 percent to 45 percent of respondents with combined levels averaging around 80 percent.[26] The Cochrane Review of massage for low back pain also reported evidence for effectiveness.[27] While the review concluded that acupressure massage was more effective than Swedish massage, this is as likely due to

the specificity of the work and the tissue addressed as to particular style.

CONTRAINDICATIONS

The adage "One man's medicine is another man's poison" certainly applies to the contraindications of myofascial release. Any technique that is powerful enough to create significant benefits has the potential to create problems. However, because MFR can be performed with varying levels of pressure and with varying amounts of directness, it is highly adaptable to many client limitations. Some conditions, such as rheumatoid arthritis, are often listed as contraindications because clients may have a significant increase of symptoms if work is performed too vigorously. At the same time, such clients may report benefits from gentle or indirect myofascial work from the improvements in joint alignment and relaxation of myofascial components around the joints. Such changes may help or work with other lifestyle and nutritional changes. It is important to remember that, as therapists, we are working on more than just tissue and that any individual may have other contributing factors to dysfunction such as lifestyle, emotions, diet, and genetic/congenital factors.

The best course of action is to openly discuss the procedures with your clients and receive medical clearance before working on any of the following conditions. Remember that there is a difference between a contraindication and a precaution. Always err on the side of caution, but remember that many people find that myofascial release offers them relief when other treatments have failed.

The following list contains situations listed as either contraindications or requiring great care and experience in treatment. Some are contraindication only for a limited local area of the body rather than general contraindications precluding any treatment.

- Acute inflammation.
- Client use of anticoagulant medications (medical consent, medication increases susceptibility to bruising). Pressure and depth should start conservatively and the client should be monitored/queried for bruising. The practitioner is reminded that MFR is about intent toward specific tissue not about blatant pressure. MFR can be adapted as needed to facilitate the client.

[†††]The practitioner should start conservatively with shorter sessions and less intense pressure, planning progressions based upon client response, over multiple sessions. The response of clients with fibromyalgia can be highly individual. There is wide variation in response to these conditions, with some individuals reporting considerable improvement, while others experience increased symptoms.

- Cellulitis (immediate medical referral). Cellulitis is a potentially serious bacterial infection of the skin. Cellulitis appears as a swollen, red area of skin that feels hot and tender, and it may spread rapidly. Left untreated, the spreading bacterial infection may rapidly turn into a life-threatening condition, particularly in consideration of recent strains of antibiotic resistant bacteria (e.g., methicillin-resistant *Staphylococcus aureus* [MRSA]). This would be a general contraindication until the condition is medically controlled and cleared.
- Deep vein thrombosis. Obtain medical consent. Refer immediately with unexplained pain or edema of unknown cause in legs.
- Fractures of bones (local).
- Heart attack symptoms. **Immediately assist client in accessing emergency medical care.**
- Hematoma (local).
- History of an aneurism (medical consent).
- History of arterial dissection (medical consent).
- Hypermobility of joints (local).
- Malignancy (local, medical consent).
- Osteomyelitis (infection).
- Osteoporosis, especially in ribs and vertebrae (cautionary).

- Rheumatoid arthritis (cautionary, medical consent).
- Severe edema (cautionary, medical consent). Treating lymphedema in general requires substantial training in lymphatic drainage technique and knowledge of pressure bandaging. MFR would only be appropriate in unaffected areas and when the cause of the edema is known and diagnosed (e.g., as a side effect of surgery or radiation treatment).
- Skin sensitivity (cautionary).
- Acute strain or sprain (local).
- Stroke indications (dizziness, unexplained sharp headache, visual distortions). **Immediately assist client in accessing emergency medical care.**
- Varicose veins (local). Varicose veins are veins that have become enlarged and twisted. The term commonly refers to the veins on the leg, although varicosities occur elsewhere. To avoid damage, avoid direct work through varicose veins. However, many people with varicose veins need not miss out on badly needed work to the muscles deep to the veins. Tissue below such veins can usually be accessed by coming in from the side.

▢▢▢▢ IN MY EXPERIENCE: KEITH ERIC GRANT

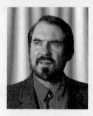

It is rather astounding to me to look back and realize that I first signed up for a massage class over 27 years ago. At the time, I was a graduate student in physics, struggling to complete a thesis, and simply seeking to rebalance my life a bit. Little did I know when signing up for that first class how large a role massage was going to play in my life. While I did complete that thesis and have continued with a physics career, I also continued to expand my knowledge and skills in massage, for, once invoked, massage would not let me go so easily. Eventually that led me to teaching massage, and that in turn has led me on to writing about massage.

As a runner, folk-dancer, and backpacker, I naturally gravitated to the forms of massage that would help me and those around me. At Scottish and Scandinavian dance camps, I have worked with minor injuries of overuse on both dancers and fiddlers, sometimes on an actual massage table on a "free" afternoon and sometimes at midnight on whatever surface we could cobble together. Sometimes those I worked with were local talent, and sometimes they had been hand imported from Sweden or Norway as teachers or musicians. There is something both gratifying and deeply humbling about being able to help people function or keep functioning simply with one's hands and a bit of knowledge of how our bodies work and move.

I have tried to appreciate those who taught me well by passing on what knowledge and skills I can to others. One learns in many ways by teaching, particularly in an area as interactive as massage. That also continues to be both a gratifying and humbling experience. This chapter is a continuation of that process of giving and receiving. Part of that has been the pleasure of working with my coauthor, Art Riggs, with the back-and-forth of thoughts and ideas. Ultimately, however, the true test of this chapter will be up to you, the reader. If it aids you in your search for usable knowledge and skills, then we have written well. While we are not there to teach you in person, we are there with you in spirit. May our words convey that hope.

■□□ IN MY EXPERIENCE: ART RIGGS

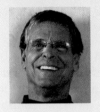

I could wax on about how experiencing bodywork that addressed fascial restrictions changed my life, first by providing the most beneficial therapeutic results I had ever experienced, and next, led to a career change to a profession that provides rewards, both financial and emotional, that I never would have thought possible. I can honestly say that I cannot imagine any profession that would make me happier for its combination of excellent income, satisfaction for the appreciation that my interesting clients express, and the always interesting puzzles that the miraculous human body presents.

However, after teaching deep tissue massage and myofascial release for 20 years, I must say that the most appropriate subject for this chapter would be the gratification I receive from seeing some students make the paradigm shift to working with myofascial restrictions as either an adjunct to their present massage practice or as a specialty.

The phenomenal increase in popularity of massage is both a blessing and a curse for the aspiring bodyworker. As public awareness of the power of massage expands, the mushrooming field becomes increasingly competitive. Statistics indicate that 80% of all massage school graduates are out of the profession within two years—victims of burnout from working at massage mills, the inability to sustain a full private practice, and often, the lack of genuine enthusiasm for their work because of a stroke-oriented and cookie-cutter approach to bodywork instead of a fresh, problem-solving approach to each client.

In the field of massage, it is very difficult to distinguish one's self from the masses of competition as being "better." Yet, a large percentage of the students I encounter are shackled by a restrictive definition of massage that they received in their first massage trainings. They attempt to distinguish themselves from competitors who are all working with tissue in essentially the same way. Instead of competing with the same "product," the successful therapist is well advised to distinguish himself or herself from the masses by being "different," offering more, and leaving a lasting impression on clients.

The reality is that even if a client comes for relaxation massage, most everyone has some complaint or desire for improvement. Many of these issues are a direct result of myofascial strain patterns, and practitioners who are able address these restrictions are often able to counter the common complaint by clients: "I felt good during the massage and possibly for a short time afterwards, but the results didn't last."

Since fascia permeates all levels of muscle, we all are influencing fascia when we work; it behooves all of us to work with this component with intelligence and intention. Working with myofascial restrictions in no way necessitates a large shift in your present practice and, since the skills are incrementally learned, acquisition of myofascial skills does not require a quantum leap in learning or in expensive training. Learning to work with fascia as part of any bodywork specialty, from general relaxation massage to specialized therapeutic work, can be the key to distinguishing yourself as a professional with exceptional skills.

As beneficial as myofascial release work has been for me in dealing with my personal issues and as much as I enjoy performing the work, both as a Rolfer and in general bodywork, I must say that the frequent feedback from students is one of my biggest gratifications.

One of the largest rewards of teaching this work is the frequent feedback from students who report a dramatic transformation of their entire practice when they altered their intention to stretching and releasing fascial restrictions. Long-time regular clients immediately comment on the lasting benefits and feelings of change in their bodies. Word of mouth referrals increase dramatically, and as practices evolve into solving problems, the work becomes more interesting and rewarding.

TRAINING REQUIREMENTS

There is no single path to competence in this area of work. It is relatively obvious, however, that the student wishing to pursue such work needs to look toward gaining a functional knowledge of how the human body moves, skills of palpation, skills of assessment based on the former two skills, and the kinesthetic skills of applied pressure and neurologic facilitation to evoke change. The authors also are strongly in agreement that this is not a matter of all or nothing. The ability to work effectively is a repeating interactive process of learning, practicing, and gaining clinical experience. Whatever the gain from training, it comes not from passive learning, but from the opportunity to actively observe how those with substantial experience organize information from multiple senses and translate that into effective benefit for clients.

In the authors' experience, many massage practitioners have expressed hesitancy or trepidation about moving their relaxation-based massage into a more therapeutic deep tissue practice working with fascia. Some fear that the nurturing aspects that their clients love will be lost and that regular clients will not be happy to have their relationship altered away from the massage they are accustomed to. In reality, moving to a more fascial approach is almost always appreciated by clients who experience more-lasting benefits and love the connection of working together that deeper work brings. There is no need to drastically alter your massage by adding more specific skills. Virtually every client will have some areas that would benefit from myofascial work. Rather than spending an entire massage on deep work (which often is too much for the client to integrate), simply choose a couple of areas in each massage that can benefit from a more myofascial intention.

Other therapists express a lack of confidence in their fascial abilities and are somewhat intimidated by the expensive and extensive educational requirements. Many assume that the absence of specific protocols for work and a structural paradigm means that myofascial work is not the domain for untrained massage therapists.

By all means, the best way to learn a myofascial approach is to take continuing education seminars, since there is no substitute for seeing and experiencing the work in real time. There is much to be gained, however, from any means of watching experienced practitioners at work. Technology continues to offer up new opportunities for learning from the work of both current practitioners and those once filmed but now retired or deceased. Mastery in myofascial techniques and philosophies, and especially the intangible skills of a soft and powerful touch, are not, however, gained overnight. There are excellent programs offered in structural and therapeutic protocols that may speed the process, but rather than suddenly transforming a massage practice, it is recommended that one adds skills incrementally.

Students must first gain the specific manual skills required to release fascial restrictions. These include both skills of palpation and the use of different tools such as fists, elbows, knuckles, and the use of fingers to grab and stretch tissue rather than just to compress or knead. If the importance of learning proper touch is not emphasized, any specific protocols for integrating a myofascial approach into therapeutic or medical massage will be less effective or possibly even dangerous. The subtleties of touch are best learned in a hands-on teaching environment with enough personal attention for the teacher or assistants that all students can experience how myofascial release feels in their own bodies and have proper guidance when working.

CHAPTER SUMMARY

This chapter provides an historical background of the varied threads of work contributing to modern techniques of myofascial release. It also provides the essential anatomy and physiology for understanding and motivating this work. No single chapter can be definitive: we have left out far more than we could have possibly included. Nonetheless, both authors feel that this chapter provides an introduction to MFR that enables a massage practitioner to begin to incorporate myofascial techniques into their existing set of skills.

As the public becomes more informed on the benefits of massage that specifically addresses fascial dysfunctions, whether named by the practitioner as myofascial release or deep tissue massage, it seems worthy of some additional attention as a modality that the authors feel depends, in large part, upon the practitioner's ability to develop MFR kinesthetic skills. Although there are many myofascial release variants that were covered in this chapter, the vast majority of practitioners who will use myofascial skills will perform them in a more generic massage setting. Most spas and private massage therapists performing therapeutic work now charge higher rates for deep tissue massage, but there is little continuity in what is expected by the public or is practiced by therapists. Although some clients may just expect a more intense massage and assume that the extra charge is for the therapist working harder, this is far from what should be the case.

Properly performed, deep tissue massage is not simply doing a "regular" massage while pressing harder or using tools such as elbows or knuckles. In addition to more precise focus on the depth (not how hard one presses) at which restrictions are held, MFR involves a substantial change in intent. The client and practitioner are mutually positioned to allow a focus on specific myofascial elements and stretching tissue. This contrasts with simply sliding over the skin surface and broadly compressing the tissue beneath it, differentiating direct technique/deep tissue work from more relaxation-based massage. The specificity and slower tempo of the work also imply that MFR would not be the sole modality of a whole body massage. If covering the body is a goal, the practitioner would work deeply where indicated and in other area use broader brush techniques from other modalities, such as Swedish or sports massage.

Barnes writes that "The separation of a fascia from its muscular component and their influence on each other is imaginary. In other words, we have been evaluating and treating an illusion. Reality demands that we consider both [muscle and fascia] by understanding their characteristics and using this information in our evaluation and treatment regimens."[5] Virtually every teacher of any form of body therapy (and most things in life) will emphasize the importance of "intention"—having a purpose and focus behind the physical pressure of strokes.

This subtle quality of intention is what separates manual massage from machines that can knead, vibrate, or press tissue. Since we all work with fascia whether we intend to or not, it behooves any therapist to include myofascial release as an intention behind the work whatever form of bodywork is being performed. Rather than leaving the results of intervention to serendipity or, in the worst case, possibly causing a counterproductive effect, the results are thus guided by the practitioner's conscious fascial intention toward the desired end of a substantial benefit to the client's body and life.

ACKNOWLEDGEMENTS

The authors wish to acknowledge the thoughts and comments of Eric Dalton and Jan Sultan that have increased or confirmed our historical perspective.

CASE HISTORIES

■ Case history 1

Virtually any manual therapist can cite numerous examples of clients who have been greatly helped by their work. Especially when our clients have been unsuccessful in finding relief through more conventional medical channels, these experiences are extremely rewarding and a large reason why so many therapists come to the work and continue to work well past the time that many people retire. In our discussion of anatomic and physiologic issues, we considered patterns of postural dysfunction—in particular, upper-crossed and lower-crossed syndromes. We draw this case from the work of one author (AR) with a Rolfing® client rather than from a case purely focused on myofascial technique.

John (pseudonym) was a 50-year-old ex–college football player who complained of constant neck and shoulder pain. Pictures to illustrate his posture were taken before his first session and after his tenth treatment, as shown in Figure 9-15. The postural issues and fascial adaptations are quite complex. The explanation we present illustrates the benefits of a well–thought out evaluation of fascial tension as a preliminary to creating balance in the body and mitigating the causes of pain. We differentiate this approach from simply relaxing painful areas and obviously hypertonic muscles to give temporary relief.

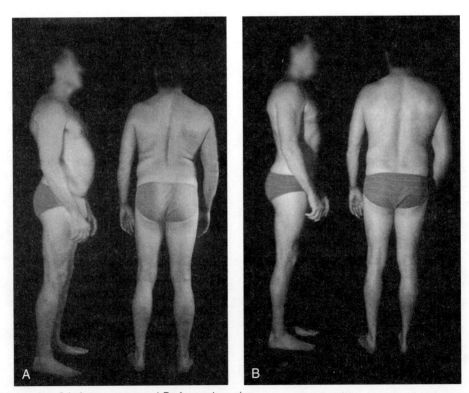

FIGURE 9-15 Pictures taken *A,* before treatment, and *B,* after tenth session.

John's severe lordosis is both a cause and result of many imbalances in his body. The anterior lumbar vertebrae give the appearance of a large abdomen. The anterior tilt of the pelvis and lumbar lordosis pull his weight forward so that he needs to pull his shoulders back for vertical balance; however, his neck and head are then pulled forward to counterbalance the shoulders. His gluteal muscles are hypertonic in response to the pelvic tilt. He exhibits a functional right side bending of his upper lumbar spine as a compensation for some of his rotational patterns. (A functional pattern results from posture and habitual muscular activation rather than stemming from a defect or imbalance in the bony structure of the body.)

In a case with multiple postural compensations, the skill in determining a plan for treatment comes in deciding which shortness patterns are driving the imbalance and strain on the body. Is a specific short and tight fascial area the primary cause or is it a compensatory pattern for a dominant pattern elsewhere? There are, of course, situations in which an initial dysfunction results in compensations that modify the original dysfunction, creating a "chicken/egg" relationship. In this example, however, one needs to determine if the anterior tilt of the pelvis is causing the shoulder tightness or visa versa.

Deciding that pelvis issues were crucial and causative prompted a strategy aimed at lengthening areas that contribute to an anterior tilted pelvis. The rectus femoris was pulling the pelvis anterior at the anterior inferior iliac spine (AIIS), so that was a primary target area for lengthening. The next focus was the shortened lumbar fascia that was pulling the lumbar spine and the pelvis like a bow string. Finally, work was directed at relaxing the psoas, which was pulling the lumbar spine forward—a typical lower-crossed mode. As John's pelvis began to level, his shoulders no longer needed to be pulled so far back and his rib cage leveled. This, aided by myofascial work to his rhomboid area and anterior neck muscles, enabled his head to drop back. All of this work was solidified and supported by work to balance weight on his legs and feet, so they could adapt to the changes upstairs.

After the sequence of treatment, John's legs became more comfortable beneath his pelvis. His gluteals, aided by ample myofascial work along with work to the deep rotators, no longer needed to grab to stand upright. John's pelvis had leveled, and his lumbar spine displayed less lordosis. As a result, John's abdomen appeared much smaller because it wasn't pushed forward by his spine. His spine had decompressed and elongated so that the horizontal lines formerly visible in mid back were less apparent. There was better left-to-right balance in spinal rotation so his side-bending pattern had lessened. His neck and shoulders were no longer "at war" with each other due to better front to back balance so his neck had lengthened and no longer jutted forward, and his head was level.

Prior to these treatments, John had tried numerous massage sessions. While they provided temporary relief from pain, they had not addressed the myofascial causes of his strain patterns.

Following the work described, John was very happy with the absence of tightness and pain in his shoulders and neck. Moreover, he remained pain free thereafter. The permanence of benefits always depends on many factors, including body awareness, flexibility exercises, lifestyle and exercise, and, to a large extent, motivation. Pain is a great motivator and even temporarily removing a client from pain can provide the hope to become proactive, rather than simply assuming that pain is natural.

■ Case history 2

These two comparative cases are drawn from relatively direct treatments that were accomplished during classroom technique demonstrations by one of the authors (KEG). They are used here to point out the influence that time of an injury's existence can have on treatment. Both cases involve restrictions or pain in movements at the shoulder that were external to the glenohumeral joint capsule. The injuries thus evidenced simple restrictions rather than the capsular patterns of restriction determined by Cyriax.[28]

Patricia had driven from southern California to the Bay Area the day before. The drive had been uneventful except for her having to compensate for a strong crosswind during much of the trip. Arriving in class, Patricia was unable to abduct her left arm above 90°. A passive range of motion test confirmed the restriction. Since there was no history of prior injury, the author concluded that the adductor muscles had been trained into a restricted length by constant stabilization during the previous day's drive. The condition responded within minutes to several repeated applications of muscle energy technique (i.e., postisometric relaxation). Because the reflex dysfunction was fresh and didn't involve a macroscopic acute injury, no dysfunctional changes in the actual tissue had occurred. Accordingly no direct tissue work was required. This was one of those rare occurrences when a relatively simple intervention achieved seemingly magical results.

In contrast, Kate had incurred a "shoulder injury" several years prior. The injury resulted in ongoing pain and restriction during movements of reaching upward or horizontal extension. Passive range of motion tests coupled with palpation revealed fibrotic tissue in the anterior deltoid and around the attachments of the biceps brachii (short head), the coracobrachialis, and the pectoralis minor at the coracoid process. Direct oblique pressure was coupled with active movements by the client in the direction of the restricted movements. The work was based on the hypothesis that adhesions had formed between fiber bundles and between layers of tissue. A substantial increase in available range of motion and corresponding decrease in pain was achieved within several minutes. Kate experienced some discomfort during the work but remained relaxed and emotionally comfortable with the process throughout and was happy with the result. Even as a practitioner herself, she was surprised at the effectiveness of a few minutes of very directed treatment.

SUGGESTED READINGS

Barnes J: *Healing ancient wounds: the renegade's wisdom*, 2000, MFR Treatment Centers & Seminars.

Calais-Germain B: *Anatomy of movement*, Vista, Calif, 1993, Eastland Press.

Chaitow L: *Muscle energy techniques*, New York, 1996, Churchill Livingstone.

Clay J: *Basic clinical massage therapy*, ed 2, Hagerstown, Md, 2006, Lippincott Williams & Wilkins.

Dalton E: *Advanced myoskeletal techniques*, Huntington Beach, Calif, 2005, Freedom From Pain Institute.

Hedley G: *Integral anatomy series, vols 1 and 2 (DVD)*, Westwood, NJ, 2006, Integral Anatomy Productions.

Hedley G: *Reconceiving my body*, Philadelphis, 2000, Xlibris.

Lowe W: *Orthopedic assessment in massage therapy*, Sisters, Ore, 2006, Orthopedic Massage Education and Resources Institute.

Lowe W: *Orthopedic massage*, St. Louis, 2003, Mosby.

McAtee R: *Facilitated stretching*, ed 3, Champaign, Ill, 2007, Human Kinetics.

Myers T: *Anatomy trains*, New York, 2001, Churchill Livingstone.

Riggs A, Myers T: *Deep tissue massage, revised: a visual guide to techniques*. ed 2, Berkeley, Calif, 2007, North Atlantic.

Stanborough M: *Direct release myofascial technique: an illustrated guide for practitioners*, London, 2004, Churchill Livingstone.

RESOURCES

Guild for Structural Integration
www.rolfguild.org
PO Box 1559
Boulder, CO 80306
303-447-0122
800-447-0150

Hellerwork International
www.hellerwork.com
PO Box 17373
Anaheim, CA 92817
714-873-6131

International Association of Structural Integrators (IASI)
www.theiasi.org
PO Box 8664
Missoula, MT 59807
406-543-4856
877-843-4274

International School of Structural Integration (ISSI)
www.theissi.org
8000 Madison Blvd
Madison, AL 35758
256-772-0669

Kinesis Myofascial Integration (KMI)
www.anatomytrains.com
318 Charles Love Rd.
Walpole, ME 04573
888-546-3797
207-563-7121

REFERENCES

1. Dalton E: Simplifying the pain puzzle (article online): http://erikdalton.com/articlepainpuzzle.htm. Accessed August 5, 2007.
2. Cantu RI, Grodin AJ: *Myofascial manipulation—theory and clinical application*, Gaithersburg, Md, 1992, Aspen Publishers.
3. Knaster M: *Discovering the body's wisdom*, New York, 1996, Bantam.
4. Barnes J: Myofascial release in treatment of thoracic outlet syndrome, *Journal of Bodywork and Movement Therapies* 1: 53–57, 1996.
5. Barnes JF: Myofascial release—the missing link in traditional treatment. In Davis, CM, editor: *Complementary therapies in rehabilitation*, Thorofare, NJ, 1997, Slack.
6. Barnes JF: Myofascial release. In Hammer WI, editor: *Functional soft tissue examination and treatment by manual methods—new perspectives*, ed 2, Gaithersburg, Md, 1999, Aspen Publications.
7. Greenman PE: *Principles of manual medicine*, Baltimore, 1989, Williams & Wilkins.
8. Ward RC: Integrated neuromusculoskeletal release and myofascial release. In Ward RC: *Foundations for osteopathic medicine*, ed 2, Philadelphia, 2003, Lippincott, Williams and Wilkins.
9. Ward RC: Myofascial release concepts. In Basmajian V, Nyberg R, editors: *Rational manual therapies*, Baltimore, 1993, Williams & Wilkins.
10. Montagu A: *Touching—the human significance of the skin*, ed 2, New York, 1978, Harper & Row.
11. Todd ME: *The thinking body*, Hightstown, NJ, 1980, Princeton Book.
12. Sweigard LE: *Human movement potential—its ideokinetic facilitation*, Lanham, Md, 1974, Harper & Row.
13. Dowd I: *Taking root to fly—articles on functional anatomy*, New York, 1995, Irene Dowd.
14. Franklin E: *Dynamic alignment through imagery*, Champaign, Ill, 1996, Human Kinetics.
15. Myers TW: Structural integration—developments in Ida Rolf's recipe—I, *Journal of Bodywork and Movement Therapies* 8:131–142, 2004.
16. Myers TW: *Anatomy trains—myofascial meridians for manual and movement therapists*, Edinburgh, 2001, Churchill Livingstone.
17. Ostrom B: Esalen massage: bodywork with a place in history, *Massage Magazine* 66:29, 1997.

18. Schleip R, Klingler W, Lehmann-Horn F: Active fascial contractility: fascia may be able to contract in a smooth muscle-like manner and thereby influence musculoskeletal dynamics, *Medical Hypotheses* 65:273–277, 2005.

19. Tippett SR, Voight ML: *Functional progressions for sport rehabilitation*, Champaign, Ill, 1995, Human Kinetics.

20. Chaitow L, DeLany JW: *Clinical application of neuromuscular techniques: the upper body*, Edinburgh, 2000, Churchill Livingstone.

21. Lewit K: *Manipulative therapy in rehabilitation of the locomotor system*, ed 2, London, 1991, Butterworth-Heinemann.

22. Chaitow L: *Palpation skills—assessment and diagnosis through touch*, New York, 1997, Churchill Livingstone.

23. Chaitow L: *Muscle energy techniques*, New York, 1996, Churchill Livingstone.

24. Stanborough M: *Direct release myofascial technique: an illustrated guide for practitioners*, London, 2004, Churchill Livingstone.

25. What alternative treatments work, *Consumer Reports*, August 2005.

26. The healing touch, *Consumer Reports*, August 2005.

27. Furlan AD, Brosseau L, Imamura M, Irvin E. Massage for low-back pain, *Cochrane database of systematic reviews* 2002, issue 2, art no: CD001929. DOI: 10.1002/14651858. CD001929.

28. Cyriax JH, Cyriax PJ: *Cyriax's illustrated manual of orthopaedic medicine*, ed 2, Oxford, 1993, Butterworth-Heinemann.

MULTIPLE CHOICE TEST QUESTIONS

1) In general, modern humans spend too much time:
   a) overextending themselves
   b) moving around
   c) sitting in flexed positions
   d) unnecessarily lifting heavy objects

2) Myofascial release specifically helps with problems of:
   a) movement restrictions from tissue adhesions
   b) obsessive-compulsive behavior
   c) pain from a hyperlordotic lumber spine
   d) tendinosis at the attachments of tendons to the periosteum

3) A major advantage of coordinating postisometric relaxation with MFR is that:
   a) it helps to reactivate a weakened antagonist muscle
   b) it provides an alternative to working directly against hypertonic muscles
   c) it is easier on both client and practitioner than painful trigger point work
   d) it is easier to do with very athletic clients

4) What is NOT an explicit goal of MFR?
   a) alleviation of pain
   b) greater flexibility and ease of movement
   c) improvement of posture
   d) all of the above are usually goals of MFR

5) Erik Dalton describes our society as a culture of:
   a) flexion addicts
   b) extension addicts
   c) overexercise and overactivity addicts
   d) contracted and short muscled couch potatoes

6) The authors of this chapter feel that MFR:
   a) should be for the most part confined to the skilled application of force to fascial adhesions
   b) may be a combination of approaches including mechanical, neurologic, and movement-oriented approaches
   c) should only be practiced after taking specific courses to teach the skills so that it may be practiced safely
   d) has the advantage over generic massage of having consistent protocols that work for virtually all people

7) Although MFR has been practiced for as long as therapeutic hands-on work has existed and has many contributors to its genesis, the term *myofascial release* is most often credited to:
   a) Robert Ward
   b) John Barnes
   c) Ida Rolf
   d) Andrew Still, the founder of osteopathic medicine

8) The concept that what we visualize as our social position affects our body self-image, which in turn profoundly affects our posture and movement patterns, is given the name:
   a) postural/emotional synthesis
   b) mind/body integration
   c) ideokinesis
   d) emotional Darwinism

9) Although her work had many effects upon bodywork, Ida Rolf's major legacy with her myofascial work was:
   a) the broadening of Rolfing® into deep tissue massage work
   b) clarifying the intention of her bodywork to work on fascia rather than muscle
   c) emphasizing the holistic concepts of treating the entire body for balance rather than just the areas of pain or dysfunction
   d) working along lines of fascial shortening to increase congruence with gravity

10) What is an accurate physiologic description of fascia?
    a) it surrounds each individual muscle fiber
    b) it surrounds bundles of individual muscle fibers and individual muscles to differentiate them from other muscles
    c) it exists in broad sheets to add support to the body so individual muscles do not need to be in a state of contraction to stabilize the body
    d) all of the above

11) What is NOT a correct statement about postural and phasic muscles?
    a) postural muscles contain more "fast twitch" fibers
    b) phasic muscles contain more "fast twitch" fibers
    c) postural muscles tend to shorten into dysfunction
    d) phasic muscles tend to weaken into dysfunction

12) Indirect MFR tends to work with "unwinding" of fascia in the direction that it tends to release because of a belief in the natural tendency of the body to self-correct. What best describes the philosophy of Direct MFR?
    a) Manipulation of fascia is always applied in the direction of least initial restriction.
    b) Direct MFR is always more intense and sometimes painful but generally works more quickly.
    c) Practitioners of Direct Release MFR usually try to determine where fascia is short and then lengthen in opposition to the shortness and restriction.
    d) Direct MFR strokes are performed more quickly than indirect methods.

13) What is the major *physical* advantage of "compression with movement" techniques?
    a) Asking for active movement from your client enables a closer relationship based on working together rather than the client passively accepting the work.
    b) Movement throughout the session keeps the client from getting stiff from being in one position for too long.
    c) Compression of the muscle localizes the stretch to specific areas of restriction.
    d) All of the above are true and equally important.

14) What is a difference in application between myofascial release and conventional massage?
    a) MFR uses broader, vigorous cross-fiber strokes.
    b) With MFR much less lubrication is used.
    c) Clients seeking MFR are more serious.
    d) MFR usually requires a series of sessions to be effective.

15) A common postural dysfunction of the upper body is:
    a) lower-crossed syndrome
    b) anterior line shortening syndrome
    c) rotator cuff injury
    d) upper-crossed syndrome

16) Within the MFR paradigm, in what direction should strokes be made?
    a) In the direction of venous return to the heart (distal to proximal).
    b) The direction of strokes should be dictated by the tissue specific goals, such as lengthening a muscle against its pattern of shortness.
    c) In the direction of arterial blood flow away from the heart (proximal to distal).
    d) Cross fiber strokes are most effective in releasing fascial restrictions.

17) According to Wolff's Law for bone and Davis's Law for soft tissue, tissue is laid down:
    a) along lines of stress
    b) in cross-linked patterns to best support us
    c) while we are actively moving
    d) all of the above

18) Cellulitis is:
    a) a type of fatty cell often found on people's thighs
    b) a condition of dry, peeling skin
    c) a serious and potentially life-threatening bacterial infection
    d) a sensitivity that bodyworkers can develop to chemicals in oils and lotions

19) In learning and performing MFR skills, the authors recommend that students:
    a) take several years of training before attempting to practice MFR because of the high risk of injury
    b) always work in shorter sessions where you can perform MFR during the allotted time frame without exhausting your clients
    c) convince your clients that MFR would be the most beneficial technique for them
    d) learn the skills gradually and incorporate them into your existing practice as you gain expertise

20) If a client comes in with dizziness, slurred speech, and/or a sharp headache, you should:
    a) work the suboccipital muscles because they likely have a migraine
    b) help them to lie down on the table to avoid the potential liability of their falling
    c) recognize that these are symptoms of a stroke and access immediate medical care
    d) not work on the lateral neck because that might trigger a vasovagus response and make them even dizzier

Neuromuscular Therapy

Judith DeLany

10

INTRODUCTION

Neuromuscular therapy (NMT) offers a series of regional treatment protocols that are built upon a foundational platform based in science and clinical evidence. It uses time-tested, hands-on protocols that integrate well into any practice setting. With the increased emergence of complementary and alternative medicine,[1] NMT is now often included in mainstream medicine and multidisciplinary clinics worldwide.

Simply defined, NMT is a precise, thorough examination and treatment of the body's soft tissues using step-by-step regionally oriented protocols. Clients generally present with chronic pain, a condition for which NMT is highly effective. Although some of the techniques can also be applied to acute injuries, all of them can be applied for preventive purposes. NMT is sometimes inaccurately labeled as "deep tissue massage." It is important to clarify that, although NMT is sometimes used on deeper tissues of the body, the superficial and intermediate tissues must also be assessed in an attempt to ascertain precisely where the problem lies. For instance, lower back pain often

DVD To better understand concepts in this chapter, watch *Neuromuscular Therapy* video on the **DVD** found at the back of this book.

stems from the psoas muscle, which lies on the anterior surface of the spinal column, undoubtedly "deeply placed." However, trigger points in rectus abdominis, the most superficial muscle of the anterior abdomen, has a target zone of referral into the lower back. Active trigger points in rectus abdominis can result in lower back pain that may be confused with that produced by psoas.

NMT assessments and examinations usually consider **ischemia** (tight tissue with reduced blood flow), **myofascial trigger points** (hypersensitive points within muscles that give rise to referred phenomena, including pain),[2] **neural entrapment** (pressure on nerves by muscles and other soft tissues), and **nerve compression** (pressure on nerves by osseous and other bonelike tissues, such as disks). Also of primary consideration are the elements uncovered in a **postural assessment** (assessment of the position of the body as a whole) and the implications of dysfunctional **gait** patterns (manner of movement when walking) as well as other perpetuating factors, such as nutrition, breathing patterns, and psychologic stress.[3-5]

HISTORY

NMT emerged on two continents almost simultaneously well over a half century ago.[5,6] The European term "neuromuscular technique" evolved from techniques developed in the early twentieth century, stemming primarily from the work of Stanley Lief and Boris Chaitow (see history later in this chapter). North American "neuromuscular therapy" also derived from a variety of sources, including massage, chiropractic, and myofascial trigger point therapy. The two NMT methods are philosophically similar and differ primarily in hands-on application, which is discussed later in this chapter. European NMT uses a slow-paced, thumb-drag method whereas NMT American version™ uses a medium-paced thumb- or finger-glide. There is also a slightly different emphasis on the manner of application of **ischemic compression** (pressure applied to force blood from tissues) for deactivation of **trigger points,** a common source of referred pain. Additionally, American NMT offers a more systematic method of examination and treatment. European methods utilize less detail in palpation of deeper structures and more focus on superficial tissue textures.[2-4]

Both European and American methods of NMT emphasize the value of self-care applied at home and the client's participation in the recovery process, which might include lifestyle changes that help to eliminate precipitating factors that may be contributing to the condition. Both versions support the use of hydrotherapies, movement, and self-applied therapies. Education may also be offered to train clients to make healthy nutritional choices and to increase awareness of habits of use in work/recreational settings.

Over the last 70 to 80 years, neuromuscular therapy techniques have emerged throughout the world with unifying theoretic foundations and subtle differences in palpation methods.[7] NMT has bridged multiple professions to be integrated into a variety of settings, including massage therapy, chiropractic, osteopathic, sports medicine, occupational therapy, physical therapy, nursing, health spas, professional sports, and conventional medicine. NMT has served as a powerful tool in the treatment of injury, surgery, or repetitive trauma, as well as a preventive procedure for assessing and removing the potential sources of myofascial dysfunction. It has gained in popularity in the last two decades as complementary medicine has emerged within mainstream health care.

Between the mid-1930s and early 1940s, European-style NMT first appeared through the work of Stanley Lief and Boris Chaitow. These cousins, trained in chiropractic and naturopathy, practiced in Lief's world-famous health resort, Champneys, at Tring in Hertfordshire, England.[7] They developed and refined "neuromuscular technique," which was their means of assessing and treating soft tissue dysfunction found in the patrons of the healing center. Many osteopaths and naturopaths have since contributed to the evolution of the European NMT techniques, including Peter Lief, Brian Youngs, Terry Moule, Leon Chaitow, and others.[6]

Following the development of European NMT, a step-by-step system began to emerge in America, not only from European roots, but also from modalities within chiropractic, traditional massage, and classic medicine. In the *Receptor Tonus Techniques* newsletter, Raymond Nimmo and James Vannerson wrote of their experiences with what they termed "noxious nodules."[8,9] They called their modality "Receptor-Tonus Technique," though it is commonly referred to today as the "Nimmo method." While Nimmo continued to research, write about, and train practitioners to treat the noxious points that had come to be known as trigger points, his students began teaching their own treatment protocols, which were closely similar to his. Today, Nimmo's original method is commonly incorporated in chiropractic settings and remains the basis for a number of other protocols in American NMT methods.

Nimmo's and Vannerson's struggle to support their theoretic platform was eased by the writings and research of Janet Travell and David Simons, two pioneers in the field of myofascial trigger point therapy. Travell and Simons' work with myofascial TrPs[2,10] was rich in documentation, research, and references, and provided a new field of medical study, the basis of which is presented in Chapter 20 of this text. Trigger points soon became a central focus of both European and American neuromuscular techniques as clinicians gained access to Travell and Simons' documentation and published work.

Paul St. John, a massage therapist who was one of Nimmo's students, developed his own NMT method in the late 1970s.[7] St. John added detailed palpation to Nimmo's basic routine and developed new techniques for the treatment of a number of muscles not included in Nimmo's training. In the mid-1980's, Judith DeLany (then Judith Walker) became St. John's first approved additional instructor of his method of neuromuscular therapy. She assisted St. John in the development of NMT techniques and protocols for massage therapy from 1984 to 1989, when they blended Nimmo's protocols with Travell and Simons' insights. They also added the emphasis on applied manual pressure as Prudden discussed.[11] (See also Chapter 20 of this text.) In 1989, the two separated the work into two styles—NMT St. John Method and NMT American version.[7] These two prominent NMT methods still today retain a strong focus on Nimmo's original protocols. While both systems feature significant focus on trigger points, both developers have significantly influenced his/her own particular style with unique insights and new techniques. A number of other teachers throughout the world have also developed their own systems of NMT based primarily on the work of Chaitow, DeLany, and/or St. John.

The differences between European and American styles of NMT were first compared within a text in *Modern Neuromuscular Techniques*.[12] In 2000, Chaitow and DeLany published the first volume of a set of comprehensive, anatomy-based, strongly referenced textbooks that blend the European regional exams with the American step-by-step NMT protocols. *Clinical Application of Neuromuscular Techniques, Volume 1—The Upper Body*[3,5] and its companion Volume 2 for the lower body[4] also incorporate osteopathic and massage principles and integrate examination and assessment routines with treatment protocols. They also include positional release, muscle energy techniques, regional anatomy, and substantial discussions regarding the physiology of the development of dysfunction in soft tissues. A practitioner may prefer one method over another; however, such preferences are likely purely personal. When practiced, either method will work equally well to locate and release somatic dysfunctions, and each can be seamlessly integrated with the other to the benefit of both client and practitioner.

FOUNDATIONAL PRINCIPLES OF NMT

Most factors in illness as well as in healthcare applications can be easily grouped under general headings of biomechanical, biochemical, and psychosocial factors, with the interface between these being profoundly related.[13] Although an impact can be made by applying an intervention from only one of these categories, a synergistic, often very significant change is seen when several are incorporated. The following contains examples for each of these categories and is not intended to be fully encompassing.

Biomechanical factors include a number of conditions that influence movement and structural stability. These may be solely present or may be present in combination and/or relationship to each other.

- Ischemia is found in tight myofascial tissues that have a reduced flow of blood. It produces a **local energy crisis,** which is a lack of sufficient ATP within the associated muscle(s). Ischemic tissues alter joint relationships, apply pressure to neurovascular structures, and give rise to the development of trigger points.
- It is hypothesized that trigger points (TrP) may occur in muscles, skin, fascia, ligaments, periostium, joint surfaces, and, perhaps, in visceral organs. Only those that occur in myofascial tissue are considered myofascial trigger points, the formation of which is believed to relate to actin and myosin filaments, and is the focus of considerable research. They give rise to three levels of referred sensations—sensory (often moderate levels of pain), motor disturbances (including taut bands), and sympathetic (hydrosis, goose bumps, etc.). Each produces responses in other body tissues, the "**target zones,**" which are moderately predictable regions to which a trigger point refers.[2] An **active TrP** refers to a pattern of common complaint while a **latent TrP** refers to one that the person does not recognize (see Chapter 20).

- Mechanical pressure on neural structures may be imposed by osseous or disk (compression) structure, or by muscle, tendon, ligament, fascia, and skin (entrapment). These "mechanical interfaces" interfere with normal neural transmission and produce a variety of symptoms.[14] The skilled practitioner will consider the entire neural pathway and perform an assessment (or refer for assessment) when any neural impingement condition is suspected. Manual methods may often be used to modify or correct for neural impingements and should be considered prior to surgical intervention.
- Postural positioning and habits of use greatly influence skeletal and muscular components.[4] Of particular interest is **fascia,** a fibrous tissue that envelops the body as a whole as well as encases individual muscles and muscle groups. While many practitioners examine standing or upright **posture** (static alignment in a fixed position), assessment should also be made while the person moves and consideration made as to the positions taken when working, sitting, during sleep, or during recreation. As to "perfect posture" and "correct" alignment, experts, including Feldenkrais[15] and Hanna,[16] point out that a degree of asymmetry is normal; the information uncovered in examination must be cast against the person's ability to handle the imposed stresses. Unless it is excessive, within "imbalances" there should occur **adaptation,** the innate ability of the body to adjust to change.[13] Adaptation provides for "normal" functional accommodation, the extent of which is based to some degree upon factors of age, genetics, and preexisting conditions.[3-5]
- Trauma (major, minor, and repetitious) can result in tissue damage, edema, and necessary tissue repair that can produce adhesions and scar formation.
- Congenital conditions and "wear and tear" are not easily recognized without a specific test, such as an x-ray or MRI.
- Joint dysfunction may stem from misalignment, osteoarthritis, or joint deterioration. These may not be obvious and may affect the body locally and globally.
- "Use" syndromes, including overuse, misuse, disuse, and abuse, are often insidious sources of destruction.
- Of particular importance to overall structural health is the foundation of the body, the feet.[4] Examination of each foot should be conducted to search for calluses, bunions, patterns of pronation and supination of the foot, and, particularly, for the health of the **plantar vault,** a dome-shaped cavern (commonly referred to as the arch of the foot) that maintains structural integrity of the foot when it bears weight.[4]
- Gait assessment can be included by those who understand walking, running, jumping, and other advanced concepts of dynamic posture. Visually based gait analysis is moderately subjective. Computerized methods can measure points of weight-bearing, pelvic tilt, and rotation more accurately as well as other elements that are not usually clearly determined by visual assessment. The use of computerized methods and measuring devices enters (or at least fringes upon) the diagnostic realm and is likely out of the scope of practice of massage therapists in most settings. However, experienced practitioners of NMT who understand compensatory structural patterns, the various aspects of the gait cycle, and patterns of muscle substitution may gain insights from gait observation. It should always be borne in mind that postural assessment and gait analysis are complex concepts. To misrepresent either as a simple process is to clearly misunderstand the complexities of adaptation and compensation.

Biochemical factors include those that influence local and/or body wide chemistry. They include localized ischemia, dehydration, nutrition, endocrine function, chemical exposure, use of medication, inflammatory processes, and many others. Referral for assessment and treatment may be needed in order to remove perpetuating factors of pain production.

- Sound nutrition is especially important for chronic pain clients. It includes ingestion, digestion, absorption, and assimilation of nutrients necessary for cellular metabolism, repair, and normal reproduction of cells in the body. Avoidance of toxic agents, such as chemical exposure, caffeine, smoke, etc., which are stimulating or irritating to the nervous system or which create body toxicity in general, is strongly suggested.
- Hydration is critical for brain function, healthy myofascial structures, and for many of the body's other systems.

- Obvious or hidden allergies, food intolerances, or environmental pollutants may increase nociception (perception of pain) and lymphatic congestion. This can produce "allergic myalgia," a form of muscle pain stemming from environmental factors, including intolerances to food, inhalants, and other irritants.[17]
- Vitamin and mineral deficiencies may perpetuate the existence of ischemia, trigger points, and neuroexcitation[2,5] and may serve as a critical factor in pain management.
- Endocrine dysfunction (most particularly thyroid in the case of myofascial pain)[18-20] can contribute to local and general inflammatory processes. Leptin hormone resistance, as produced by adipose tissue, has been definitively linked to systemic inflammation and the development of a number of diseases, including cardiovascular disease, diabetes, and cancer.[21]
- Additionally, the balance between oxygen and carbon dioxide in the body is of critical importance. It is intimately connected to breathing patterns and has huge psychosocial overlays. For instance, upper respiratory breathing mechanics (overbreathing or hyperventilation) results in excessive exhalation of CO_2. As CO_2 decreases, this can produce a Bohr effect, which includes a rise in alkalinity. As the bloodstream and tissues increase in alkalinity, the hemoglobin molecule binds more firmly to the oxygen it is carrying, releasing it less efficiently, which leads to hypoxia and a reduction of serum calcium and red cell phosphate levels. Additionally, as part of the renal compensation mechanism for correcting alkalosis, there is a loss of intracellular Mg^{2+}. The function of motor and sensory axons will be significantly affected by lower levels of calcium ions, and these sensitive neural structures will tend toward hyperirritability, negatively affecting motor control. With increased sensory and motor discharges, muscular tension, spasm, and spinal reflex activity result. There will likely be heightened perception of pain, photophobia, and hyperacusis (exceptionally acute hearing), as well as muscles becoming more prone to fatigue, altered function, cramping, and trigger point evolution.[5,22]
- On a local level, ischemia reduces blood flow, oxygen, and nutrients, resulting in an accumulation of metabolic waste products. As these neuroirritants accumulate within the tissue, they increase neuroexcitability,[23] which can become self-perpetuating.

Psychosocial factors, including emotional elements and stress management, all influence the musculoskeletal system, beyond doubt.[3,24] "Stress" includes overload of physical, emotional, financial, and other less-recognized sources of burden to the central nervous system and the peripheral tissues.

Anxiety, guilt, fear, depression, unresolved emotions, work-related pressures, and other burdens may result in somatization. This can result in expression of a psychologic burden or disorder as recurring physical symptoms.

While alleviating the stress burden is ideal, the role of the practitioner may often be seen to involve teaching and encouraging the individual to handle their psychological load more efficiently or to refer elsewhere when scope of practice and (lack of) training indicates. The degree to which anyone can be helped in regard to somatoemotional stress may relate to how efficiently adaptation is occurring. Whether the stress is self-generated or externally derived may determine how much of the load can actually be removed.

Biomechanical, biochemical, and psychosocial factors synergistically interface and, rather than producing single modifications, potentially provoke a multitude of changes. In fact, their interaction with each other is quite astounding. The following are examples of their profound interface.

- Hyperventilation creates feelings of anxiety and apprehension, modifies blood acidity, influences neural reporting (initially hyper and then hypo), and directly impacts on both muscles and joints of the thoracic and cervical region.[25]
- Hypoglycemia, acidosis, and other factors that alter chemistry affect mood directly while altered mood (depression, anxiety) changes blood chemistry, muscle tone, and (by implication) trigger point evolution.[26]
- Altered structure modifies function (for example, posture alters breathing) and, therefore, impacts on chemistry (e.g. O_2: CO_2 balance; circulatory efficiency, and delivery of nutrients, etc.), all of which impact mood.[25]

Neuromuscular therapy assesses the person's condition for as many of these factors as the practitioner is capable of handling. Referral to appropriate healthcare professionals can be used when needed measures lie outside the practitioner's scope of practice.

The practitioner and client together may address as many of these (or additional) influences on musculoskeletal pain as can be identified, so long as they avoid excessive demands on the individual's adaptive capacity. In other words, for each intervention applied, the body must adapt—to a new posture, new muscle length, increased fiber in the diet—sometimes in a number of ways. For the most comprehensive recovery to be achieved it may be necessary to remove or modify many etiologic and perpetuating influences.[2] However, since local and general adaptation will likely be involved for each, a delicate balance of application of techniques and principles must be maintained to produce beneficial change without overwhelming the body's adaptation mechanisms. Otherwise, results may be unsatisfactory,[27] confusing, or frustrating for both client and practitioner.

Additionally, a home care program will be individually designed to help promote awareness of poor habits of use and posture, as well as to improve use through appropriate stretching, retraining, and frequent breaks from long-term strain. Positions of sitting, standing, and sleeping are considered as well as the items that contact and influence the body, such as shoes, clothing, and items that are carried.

European and American Versions: Similarities and Differences

Similarities as well as differences between the European and American methods of NMT are definable. While the differences lie mainly in palpation methods, the similarities (as discussed previously) are foundational and philosophically encompassing. The two methods share ultimate goals to normalize the tissues, uncover the precipitating and perpetuating factors, and teach skills to the person to prevent recurrence. The incorporation of other modalities, such as hydrotherapies, stretching methods, and rehabilitation of the tissues, also commonly occurs in both versions.

One of the common goals in both versions of NMT is to cause a thixotropic response in the matrix of the fascia. **Thixotropy** is a property of **colloids** (the ground substance that makes up fascia is an example) that allows it to become more fluid when heated, shaken, or stirred or when mechanical tension is applied to it, such as during **effleurage** (applied gliding strokes), compression (applied pressure), and stretching (elongation of fibers). The colloidal matrix also has the ability to reset to a gel state when allowed to stand.

In general, both European and American styles of NMT aim to[3,5]:

- Relax and normalize tense fibrotic muscular tissue
- Simultaneously offer the practitioner diagnostic information
- Deactivate myofascial trigger points
- Follow deactivation of TrPs with elongation of associated taut band and muscle tissues (manual, passive, or active)
- Enhance lymphatic drainage and general circulation
- Offer reflex benefits
- Prepare for other therapeutic methods, such as stretching, exercise, or manipulation
- Prepare the person to recognize behaviors and patterns of use that stress the tissues
- Offer the person alternative functional patterns and choices with the aim of reducing perpetuating factors

NMT American version techniques place a strong emphasis on differentiating between **central TrP** (one that develops at the midfiber region) and an **attachment TrP** (one that develops at the musculotendinous juncture or periosteal attachment). Central TrPs (CTrPs) are treated by applying static or increasing pressure (commonly called **trigger point pressure release**) for at least 8 to 12 (or up to 20) seconds, during which time the referred sensation associated with the trigger point begins to fade away. After tissue has rested, the applied pressure techniques are repeated. Applications of heat or cold (as appropriate) may be alternated with the pressure techniques on a central TrP. An attachment TrP (ATrP) usually resolves when its associated CTrP is deactivated. Applications of ice are appropriate for ATrPs. If appropriate, the tissues should be stretched, either manually or with range of motion, following the release of a trigger point.

European NMT offers a variation that applies the appropriate pressure to the trigger point that is sufficient to produce the referral pattern for approximately 5 seconds, followed by an easing of pressure for 2 to 3 seconds. This alternation is repeated for up to 2 minutes, or until the referred sensation diminishes (or is discontinued if it increases, which is rare). Pulsed ultrasound, application of hot towels to the area (followed by effleurage), or positional release for 20 to 30 seconds can further ease the hyperreactive patterns of a trigger point, after which a lengthening procedure is applied.

European NMT offers Integrated Neuromuscular Inhibition Technique (INIT), which combines several techniques, such as muscle energy techniques, positional release, and stretching of tissues in combination. Similarly, American NMT also seamlessly moves from one inhibitory method to another until release is achieved or until it becomes obvious that no further improvement will be achieved within the session.

TREATMENT TOOLS

Hot and cold packs can be used effectively within the session and at home between sessions. American version NMT uses both hot and cold, sometimes alternating between them. European version primarily uses cryotherapy, by applying cold packs to local tissues and by incorporating cold in systemic applications, such as cold-water bathing.

It is important that the practitioner and patient be aware of appropriate use of hot and cold. Unless contraindicated by excessive tenderness, redness, heat, swelling, or other signs of inflammation, application of heat can be used. This can increase blood flow to an area and enhance the thixotropic response, thereby softening the fascia, and allowing fluids to move more freely into the tissues. When heat is intolerable or when inflammation is suspect, applications of ice (cryotherapy) may be used. This is especially appropriate on attachment TrPs due to the inflammatory response caused by constant stress of tension from a taut band at the attachment site.[2,28] When in doubt, ice is the appropriate choice rather than heat.

While the hands remain the primary treatment tools in NMT, a number of other tools can be incorporated to help preserve the practitioner's thumbs and in order to more easily access attachments that lie under or between bony protrusions. Each tool should be assessed for its unique qualities and degree of effectiveness, and a practitioner should avoid using tools that might be harmful to the practitioner's hands or the client. All tools that touch the skin should be scrubbed with bacterial soap after each use or cleaned with cold sterilization or other procedures recommended by their manufacturers.

Pressure bars are hand-held tools, apparently first introduced by Dr. Nimmo in his Receptor Tonus Techniques, which have remained popular in NMT for several decades (Figure 10-1). The flat tipped bar is used to apply pressure into tissues while the bevel tip bar is designed to scrape tendons or to work under bony ledges or between bones. In order to safely use pressure bars, tableside training with a knowledgeable instructor (and subsequent practice) is strongly suggested.

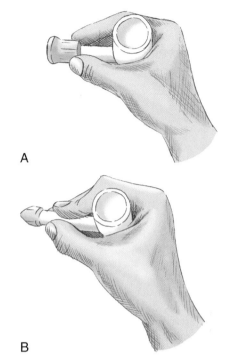

A

B

FIGURE 10-1 Stress on the practitioner's thumbs may be reduced with properly held treatment tools, such as the pressure bars shown here. (From Chaitow L, DeLany J: *Clinical application of neuromuscular techniques, vol 1, The upper body,* ed 2, Edinburgh, 2008, Churchill Livingstone.)

A variety of self-help tools has been created for purposes of releasing tissue more easily, reaching hard to reach spots, or enhancing attempts at client home care. They are also useful to increase client awareness of various areas of tight and tender tissues. Tools that create oscillation or vibration, such as the Thumper™, assist in providing a thixotropic effect, while the Backnobber® replaces a commonly used doorframe for clients to access those "favorite spots" on the posterior torso. Although a bit pricey, massage chairs that have a variety of "techniques" built into their motorized components can offer daily relief and benefits, at least to certain regions of the body. These and other tools can be incorporated during treatment and are useful in "homework" applications.

CHARACTERISTICS OF NMT AMERICAN VERSION

The use of a lubricant and repetitious gliding techniques (effleurage) is one of the distinguishing features of NMT American version (Box 10-1). These

BOX 10-1 Summary of NMT American Version Assessment Protocols

Glide where appropriate.
- Assess for taut bands using pincer compression techniques.
- Assess attachment sites for tenderness, especially where taut bands attach.
- Return to taut band and find central nodules or spot tenderness.
- Elongate the tissue slightly if attachment sites indicate this is appropriate or tissue may be placed in neutral or approximated position.
- Compress CTrP for 8 to 12 seconds (using pincer compression techniques or flat palpation).
- The client is instructed to exhale as the pressure is applied, which often augments the release of the contracture.
- Appropriate pressure should illicit a discomfort scale response of 5, 6, or 7.
- If a response in the tissue begins within 8 to 12 seconds, it can be held for up to 20 seconds.
- Allow the tissue to rest for a brief time.
- Adjust pressure and repeat.
- Passively elongate the fibers.
- Actively stretch the fibers.
- Appropriate hydrotherapies may accompany the procedure.
- Advise the client as to specific procedures which can be used at home to maintain the effects of therapy.

From Chaitow L, DeLany J: *Clinical application of neuromuscular techniques,* Edinburgh, 2000, Churchill Livingstone.

- To most effectively glide on the tissues, the practitioner's fingers are spread slightly and "steady" the thumbs.
- The fingers support the weight of the hands and arms, which relieves the thumbs of that responsibility. As a result, the pressure exerted by the thumb is more easily controlled and can be changed as varying tensions are matched in the tissues.
- The fingers stabilize (steady) the hands while the thumbs are the actual treatment tool in most cases.
- The wrist needs to remain stable so that the hands move as a unit, with little or no motion in the wrist or the thumb joints. Excessive movement in the wrist or thumb may result in practitioner's joint inflammation, irritation, and dysfunction.
- When two-handed glides are employed, the lateral aspects of the thumbs are placed side by side or one slightly ahead of the other with both pointing in the same direction, that being the direction of the glide (Figure 10-2).
- Pressure is applied through the wrist and longitudinally through the thumb joints, not against the medial aspects of the thumbs, as would occur if the gliding stroke were performed with the thumb tips touching end to end (Figure 10-3).

Clinical experience indicates that the best result usually comes from gliding on the tissues repetitively (6 to 8 times) before working elsewhere. The author's experience indicates that gliding repeatedly on areas of hypertonicity:

lubricated, gliding strokes serve to warm the tissues, flush lymphatic waste, and increase circulation. They simultaneously serve as assessment strokes to examine the underlying tissues for ischemia, taut bands suspect of housing trigger points, and areas of congestion or fibrosis. They allow the practitioner to rapidly become familiar with the individual quality, internal (muscle) tension, and degree of tenderness in the tissues being assessed.

In the American version, the thumbs lead and the entire hand moves with the stroke. The thumb usually applies the pressure, however, sometimes the fingers (or the palm or forearm) apply the pressurized stroke instead. The fingers (usually spread) serve to stabilize the glide. This differs significantly from the European version (discussed later). The following description[3,5] applies to the use of the thumb as the treatment tool.

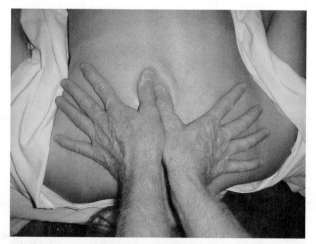

FIGURE 10-2 The fingers offer support and enhance control as the thumbs apply pressure or glide. (From Chaitow L, DeLany J: *Clinical application of neuromuscular techniques, vol 1, The upper body,* ed 2, Edinburgh, 2008, Churchill Livingstone.)

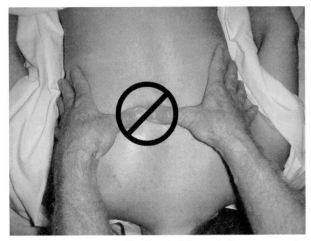

FIGURE 10-3 Incorrect application of gliding techniques stresses the thumb joints. (From Chaitow L, DeLany J: *Clinical application of neuromuscular techniques, vol 1, The upper body,* ed 2, Edinburgh, 2008, Churchill Livingstone.)

- Often changes the degree and intensity of the dysfunctional patterns
- Reduces the time and effort needed to modify them in subsequent treatments
- Tends to encourage the tissue to become more defined, which particularly assists in evaluation of deeper structures
- Allows for a softening of the surrounding tissues that will eventually provide a more precise localization of taut bands and trigger point nodules
- Encourages hypertonic bands commonly found to become softer, smaller, and less tender than before

A moderate speed is used during the gliding stroke, covering 3 to 4 inches per second, which allows the hands to more easily feel what is present in the tissues. When a rapid pace is used, the hands may pass over congestion and other changes in the tissues, fail to identify individual muscles, and, in some cases, cause unnecessary discomfort. When the tissue is excessively tender or sensitive, a slower pace and reduced pressure are suggested. The gliding strokes are performed repetitiously in an attempt to increase blood flow and to soften fascia for further manipulation.

The tissues that have been treated in this manner are then left alone for a brief period, say 5 minutes, while the practitioner works elsewhere. When they are reassessed, they are usually found to be softer, less tender, and tolerant of more pressure. The region of ischemia is usually reduced. If, instead, the taut bands have become more tender, this might indicate an underlying inflammatory process. Such conditions may be aggravated by heat, friction, effleurage, or the application of aggressive stretching or other techniques that may irritate the tissues and spread the inflammation. In such cases, the application of ice and other cryotherapy techniques, gentle myofascial release, positional release, lymphatic drainage, and other antiinflammatory measures would be appropriate. Should the region continue to exhibit signs of inflammation at future sessions, referral for assessment is suggested.

CHARACTERISTICS OF EUROPEAN NMT

While American NMT gliding techniques move the hand as a whole with the thumb being the assessment tool, the use of the thumb in European NMT differs greatly. The following points regarding European applications distinguish it from its counterpart.

- With the palm arched and the hand spread for balance and control, the tips of the fingers provide a fulcrum, or "bridge." The thumb contacts the tissues to be assessed and is stroked in a direction that takes it away from the practitioner's body and toward the finger tips, causing it to pass under this bridge (Figure 10-4). The thumb always remains behind the stable fingers, the tips of which rest just beyond the end of the stroke.
- A light, nonoily lubricant is often used to facilitate easy, nondragging, passage of the palpating digit.
- The hand and arm remain still, while a single stroke of the thumb, applying variable pressure, covers between 2 and 3 inches (5 to 8 cm) and lasts approximately 4 to 5 seconds.
- The arm should not be flexed at the elbow or the wrist by more than a few degrees in order that pressure/force be transmitted (via the long axis of the extended arm) directly to its target. The transferred force (practitioner's body weight) travels in as straight a line as possible to the thumb tip.
- The thumb and hand seldom impart their own muscular force unless dealing with fibrotic "nodules" or small, localized **contractures** (taut bands found within muscles that commonly house TrPs).

The versatility of this thumb position enables it to modify the direction of imposed force and, depending upon the indications of the tissue being tested/treated, deliver varying degrees of pressure. For less localized and less specific contact, the broad surface of the distal phalange of the thumb is often used whereas contact by the very tip may be employed for more focus.

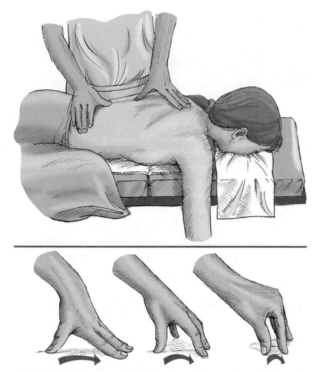

FIGURE 10-4 European NMT thumb technique. (From Chaitow L, DeLany J: *Clinical application of neuromuscular techniques, vol 1, The upper body,* ed 2, Edinburgh, 2008, Churchill Livingstone.)

The medial or lateral aspect of the tip can make contact with angled surfaces, or provide access to spaces between bones, such as intercostal structures.

European NMT'S Finger Technique

When the thumb's width prevents successful positioning, the middle or index finger can usually be substituted. The finger technique is also a useful approach to curved areas, such as the area above and below the pelvic crest, or on the lateral thigh, and is usually applied from a contralateral position of the practitioner (Figure 10-5).

European NMT protocols[3,5] suggest:
- The middle or index finger should be slightly flexed and, depending upon the direction of the stroke and density of the tissues, should be supported by one of the adjacent digits.
- The angle of pressure to the skin surface should be between 40° and 50°.
- As the treating finger strokes, with a firm contact and a minimum of lubricant, a tensile strain is created between its tip and the tissue underlying it. The tissues are stretched and lifted by the passage of the finger, which, like the thumb,

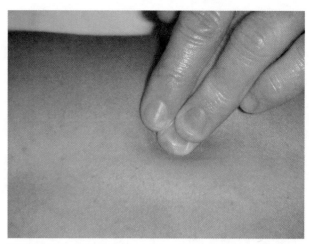

FIGURE 10-5 NMT finger technique. (From Chaitow L, DeLany J: *Clinical application of neuromuscular techniques, vol 1, the upper body,* ed 2, Edinburgh, 2008, Churchill Livingstone.)

should continue moving unless, or until, dense indurated tissue prevents its easy passage.
- These strokes can be repeated once or twice as tissue changes dictate.
- The fingertip should never lead the stroke but should always follow the wrist, the palmar surface of which should lead as the hand is drawn toward the practitioner.
- It is possible to impart a great degree of traction on underlying tissues, and the client's reactions must be taken into account in deciding on the degree of force being used.
- Unlike the thumb technique, in which force is largely directed away from the practitioner's body, in finger treatment the stroke is usually toward the practitioner. The arm position therefore alters, since elbow flexion is necessary to ensure that the stroke of the finger across the lightly lubricated tissues is balanced.
- Unlike the thumb, which makes a sweep toward the fingertips while the rest of the hand remains relatively stationary, the whole hand will move when a finger stroke is applied.
- Some variation in the degree of angle between fingertip and skin is in order during a stroke, and some slight variation in the degree of "hooking" of the finger may be necessary.
- The treating finger should always be supported by one of its neighbors.

With pain being an indicator of abnormal physiology, most sensitive areas are interpreted as indicating some degree of associated dysfunction (local or reflex). Although the presence of transient pain and/or mild discomfort is to be expected, it is important to record their presence so that reexamination at a future session becomes part of the treatment plan.

APPLICATIONS OF PRESSURE

While NMT is notably effective at reducing chronic pain, during NMT examination and treatment the recipient can also experience mild to moderate discomfort. This is because one common objective in NMT is to locate localized tender areas and then to introduce an appropriate degree of pressure. Feedback from the client during this process is needed in order to use appropriate pressure. The amount of pressure to use during applied strokes as well as during sustained pressure will vary from person to person and even from tissue to tissue within the same person. The degree of pressure used will be influenced by the nature of the tissue being treated, the degree of tissue damage, overall health of the individual, and many other factors (Box 10-2).

The pressure can be moderated by feedback from the client regarding the discomfort level. By using a "discomfort scale" from the client, coupled with the practitioner's experience with tissue response, the practitioner can determine the appropriate pressure on a moment-to-moment basis. The client should not feel pain, however, and should report immediately to the practitioner when the discomfort scale rises too high.

The amount of pressure to use is not measured in ounces, grams, kilograms, or pounds of pressure. Instead, an attempt is made to precisely meet and match the tissue resistance. This requires the pressure to be constantly varied in response to what is found during palpation. To encourage the tissue to release, a slightly increased pressure can then be applied, the degree of which is always determined by client feedback.

Using a Discomfort Scale

Important information, such as the condition of the tissues, location of taut bands, and the degree of tissue involvement, is discovered by the practitioner while assessing the tissues. From this, the practitioner determines the appropriate next step in treatment. One choice is trigger point pressure release, which is formally known as ischemic compression. This applied compression of specific tissues, when maintained for several seconds, is thought to cause the following effects:

BOX 10-2 Effects of Applied Compression

When digital pressure is applied to tissues it is believed to simultaneously cause a variety of effects.

1. A degree of localized ischemia results due to interference with circulatory efficiency, a reverse of which can be expected when pressure is released.[2]
2. A sustained barrage of efferent information resulting from the constant pressure creates neurologic inhibition.[33]
3. As the elastic barrier is reached and the process of "creep" commences, mechanical stretching of tissues occurs.[34]
4. A thixotropic effect occurs when shearing forces are applied, altering relatively gel-like fascial tissues toward a more "sol" state.[35]
5. Mechanoreceptors are stimulated, which is thought to cause an interference with pain messages (gate theory) reaching the brain.[30]
6. A reduction in pain perception occurs as local endorphin release is triggered along with enkephalin release in the brain and CNS.[36]
7. Direct pressure often produces a rapid release of the taut band associated with trigger points.[2]
8. Acupuncture and acupressure concepts associate digital pressure with alteration of energy flow along hypothesized meridians.[3]

After Chaitow L, DeLany J: *Clinical application of neuromuscular techniques,* Edinburgh, 2000, 2008, Churchill Livingstone.

- Reduce inappropriate degrees of hypertonicity in taut band, apparently by releasing the contracted sarcomeres in the TrP nodule[2]
- Induce a mechanical stress on the colloidal matrix, thereby producing a thixotropic effect[29]
- Reduce spasms by overriding neural reflex mechanisms, possibly through gating mechanisms[2,30]
- Blanch the tissues, which is followed by enhanced blood flow that brings with it oxygen and nutrients[12]
- Release of endorphins and enkephalins,[30] the body's own natural pain modulators

A "discomfort scale" can usefully be established to help encourage the application of appropriate pressure. This method will also involve the patient in the treatment and allow the patient a degree of control over the process, both of which may produce a positive psychologic effect. Melzack and Wall suggest a scale in which[30]:

- 0 represents no pain
- 10 represents unbearable pain

- In regard to pressure techniques, it is best to avoid pressures that induce a report of a pain level of 8 to 10.
- The person is requested to report, when questioned or when desired, if the level of perceived discomfort varies from what is judged as 5 to 7.
- Below 5 usually represents inadequate pressure to facilitate an adequate therapeutic response from the tissues. Prolonged pressure or pressure that elicits a report of pain above a score of 7 may provoke a defensive response from the tissues, such as reflexive shortening or exacerbation of inflammation.

TRIGGER POINT RELEASE TECHNIQUES

A trigger point (TrP) is a tender, hyperirritable spot within a muscle that, when provoked, refers pain and other sensations to a (fairly predictable) target zone.[2] TrPs are prevalent in the body as a common source of acute and chronic pain. TrPs are often overlooked as a primary or secondary source of pain. A neuromuscular therapist has a heightened awareness of trigger points, their locations within muscles, and how to treat them. Examination for and treatment of TrPs remains a key factor in NMT (see Chapter 20).

In the palpation methods previously discussed and in those that follow, a main goal is to uncover taut bands within ischemic tissue. These are palpable during a transverse movement across the taut fibers. Once defined the practitioner searches for nodules within the taut band at midfiber region. An appropriate degree of sustained pressure is then applied on any centrally located nodules, which are usually associated with central trigger points.

A number of TrP treatment options exist that can be used to deactivate the fibers housing a TrP.[2-5] Among the most well known are:

- Trigger point pressure release, which uses precisely applied sustained pressure
- Chilling techniques, such as spray and stretch technique that applies a vapocoolant spray and elongation of fibers
- Dry needling, which can be applied with acupuncture needles, or wet needling, which included injection methods using procaine, botox, or other chemicals (performed by those who are duly licensed and precisely trained)
- Positional release methods

- Muscle energy techniques
- Myofascial release, broadly placed or precisely applied

It is also important to address additional factors that might be associated with trigger point formation and to assist in home care. This might include:

- Correction of associated osseous (skeletal) malalignment, possibly involving a variety of osteopathic or chiropractic mobilization methods
- Education to correct perpetuating factors, such as posture, hormonal discordance, nutritional factors, stress, and habits of use
- Teaching self-applied treatment for trigger point release as discussed by Davies (see Suggested Readings list)
- Offering other self-help strategies that can be applied at home, such as stretching, hydrotherapies, changes in habits of use, etc.

Therapeutically, NMT aims to encourage a restoration of normal function by modifying dysfunctional tissue. A particular focus is placed on myofascial trigger points, and much of the treatment time is spent locating and deactivating them. NMT also aims to uncover perpetuating factors that cause TrPs to form, whether based on structural misalignments, habits of use, or habits of health, such as diet and stress.

INDICATIONS AND CONTRAINDICATIONS

While the primary application of NMT regards chronic pain syndromes, it is also valuable in the management of postsurgical and posttrauma recovery and in rehabilitation. NMT can also be applied to the apparently healthy body to assist in injury prevention by removing musculoskeletal stresses before they become painful, long-lasting dysfunctions. It has been successfully applied to people of all ages, from newborns to the elderly.

NMT is contraindicated in initial stages of acute injury. During the acute phase following injury, the body often will produce swelling and splint the injured area.[23] This natural response helps reduce hemorrhaging in torn tissues and prevent movement that might further traumatize the fibers. During the initial 72 hours following injury, application of principles of *Rest*, *Ice*, *Compression*, and *Elevation* (RICE) is appropriate.[31] Since NMT increases blood flow and helps to increase mobility, it should not be used on the recently injured tissues while they initiate the first phase of repair. NMT may be applied, however, to other parts of the body, which are often compensating for the injured area. Application of other techniques, such as lymphatic drainage and certain movement therapies that are appropriate for acute injuries, may be used when a medical evaluation has determined it is safe to proceed.

NMT helps to reduce spasm and ischemia, encourage drainage, cautiously elongate the tissues, and tone and strengthen the muscles. It can usually be safely introduced after the acute phase has passed. This may sometimes occur at the first treatment session; however, moderate pain should always be respected as a signal that whatever is being done is inappropriate. The "discomfort scale" presented earlier in this chapter is the primary indicator regarding application of techniques, especially regarding recent injuries.

Consultation with the attending physician is suggested when the practitioner has any doubt of the safety of treatment. When symptoms of neurologic involvement are present, when unidentified objects are palpated (such as cysts, tumors), or when the person presents with unusual symptoms that seem inconsistent with the case history, it is best to refer to a physician for an evaluation. Ignoring symptoms that the practitioner does not understand is a risky practice, at best.

When active or passive movements initiate a painful response, especially when that pain is elicited with little provocation, dysfunction of joints associated with that movement needs to be considered. Pain that returns for no apparent reason, despite adequate therapy and home care, may be the sign of joint dysfunction or even visceral pathology. Appropriate assessment should not be delayed.

BOX 10-3 Summary of Rehabilitation Sequencing

- Decrease spasm and ischemia, enhance drainage, deactivate trigger points.
- Restore flexibility (lengthen).
- Restore tone (strengthen).
- Improve overall endurance and cardiovascular efficiency.
- Restore proprioceptive function and coordination.
- Improve postural positioning, body usage (active and stationary), and breathing.

From Chaitow L, DeLany J: *Clinical application of neuromuscular techniques,* Edinburgh, 2000, 2008, Churchill Livingstone.

Palpation of open sores, postsurgical healing sites, segmental neuropathies (shingles), skin lesions, swelling, bruising, or other abnormal tissues should be postponed until those conditions have been examined by a physician and approved for treatment. Special attention should be paid to enlarged (swollen) lymphatic nodes or lymphedema[32] and, unless the practitioner has been suitably trained, treatment of associated tissues should be avoided until the lymphatic condition has been fully assessed and medically addressed.

SEQUENCING OF NMT PROTOCOLS

The stages of healing are defined by more than just the length of time since the injury. The degree of current pain and inflammation within the injured tissues should always be borne in mind when applying manual techniques. Once acute inflammation subsides, the following order of rehabilitation is suggested (Box 10-3).[31]

NMT protocols[3,5] suggest:

1. Appropriate softtissue techniques should be applied with the aim of decreasing spasm and ischemia, enhancing drainage of the soft tissues, and deactivating trigger points.
2. Appropriate active, passive, and self-applied stretching methods should be introduced to restore normal flexibility.
3. Appropriately selected forms of exercise should be encouraged to restore normal tone and strength.
4. Conditioning exercises and weight-training approaches should be introduced, when appropriate, to restore overall endurance and cardiovascular efficiency.
5. Normal proprioceptive function and coordination should be assisted by use of standard rehabilitation approaches.
6. Methods for achieving improved posture and body use should be taught and/or encouraged as well as exercises for restoring normal breathing patterns. Posture, body usage, and breathwork may be addressed at any stage along with the other approaches listed above.

The last two of these steps may be started at any time; however, the first four should be sequenced in the listed order. When the suggested order is not followed, clinical experience suggests that symptoms may be prolonged and recovery compromised. For example, if exercise or weight training is initiated before contractures are eliminated and trigger points deactivated, the existing referral patterns may become intensified or new pain patterns initiated. In cases of recently traumatized tissue, deep tissue work and stretching applied too early in the process could further damage the recovering tissues.

NMT protocols are taught as a step-by-step procedure, the consistent order of which is encouraged. Assessment, examination, and treatment of each muscle that may be associated with a particular pain pattern, restricted movement, or chronic syndrome are incorporated within the "routine." These associated tissues include synergists, antagonists, and trigger points related to painful target zones. While the protocols offer a generalized framework, they also offer flexibility for alternative or additional treatment approaches, the use of which will depend upon the practitioner's training and skill. In many situations, several manual techniques may be equally effective in easing pain, improving range of motion, or in releasing excessive tone. Some may be more effective with certain conditions whereas combinations of techniques may significantly and synergistically build upon each other. On the other hand, excessive therapeutic intervention might induce a negative effect and create inflammation or reflexive spasms. Finding the right combination for each situation to "unlock" the patterns of dysfunction is sometimes the greatest challenge for the practitioner.

Based on clinical experience, the following is suggested by the author to be used as a general guideline when addressing most myofascial tissue problems[3,5]:

- The most superficial tissue is usually treated before the deeper layers.
- The proximal portions of an extremity are treated ("softened") before the distal portions are addressed so that proximal restrictions of lymph flow are removed before distal lymph movement is increased.
- In a two-jointed muscle, both joints are assessed; in multijointed muscles, all involved joints are assessed. For instance, if triceps is examined, both glenohumeral and elbow joints are assessed; if extensor digitorum, then wrist and all phalangeal joints being served by that muscle would be checked.
- Most myofascial trigger points either lie in the endplate zone (midfiber) of a muscle or at the attachment sites.[2]
- Other trigger points may occur in the skin, fascia, periosteum, and joint surfaces.
- Knowledge of the anatomy of each muscle, including its innervations, fiber arrangement, nearby neurovascular structures, and overlying and underlying muscles will greatly assist the

practitioner in quickly locating the appropriate muscles and their trigger points.

Where multiple areas of pain are present, a general "rule-of-thumb," based on clinical experience, is suggested:

- Treat the most proximal,
- Most medial, and
- Most painful trigger points first.
- Avoid overtreating the whole structure as well as the individual tissues.
- Treatment of more than five active trigger points at any one session might place an adaptive load on the individual, which could prove extremely stressful. If the person is frail or demonstrating symptoms of fatigue and general susceptibility, common sense suggests that fewer than five active trigger points should be treated at any one session.

USING NMT PALPATION TECHNIQUES

NMT palpation techniques refer to the application of lubricated or nonlubricated gliding strokes, friction, and specifically applied pressure. Occasionally, special tools (pressure bars) or other body parts (elbows, palms, forearms, knuckles) may be used. However, most of the techniques are performed by the thumb, fingers, or combination of thumb and fingers (as in pincer-type grasp).

NMT can be applied with the client in a variety of positions (seated, supine, prone, or side-lying). The techniques may be focused generally (as when associated with posture) or specifically (regarding specific pain patterns or joint dysfunctions). Usually the sequence in which body areas are addressed is not regarded as critical so long as the proximal portion of an extremity is treated before distal and superficial layers are addressed before deeper tissues.

Skin palpation has tremendous value in NMT application. Assessment can include palpation of the skin's freedom of movement from underlying tissues and palpation of the quality of the skin itself. When the skin is slid over the underlying fascia of a dysfunctional tissue or when the skin over a suspicious area is lifted and rolled between the fingers and thumb (as in connective tissue massage or bindegewebsmassage (German)), it is often found to be adherent or "stuck" to the underlying tissue. This lack of skin flexibility helps to confirm a suspicious zone, which may be housing a trigger point or may be a trigger point target zone. When the skin itself is assessed, it is often found to have increased hidrosis (sweatiness), a "sandpaper" texture, or a cutaneous temperature that is hotter or cooler than the surrounding skin. Skin rolling techniques and myofascial release, when appropriately used, often dramatically soften and loosen the skin from the underlying fascia and may cause a profound softening of the involved muscles deep to the "stuck" skin.

In *flat palpation* (Figure 10-6) the whole hand, finger pads, or fingertips are slid through the skin over the underlying fascia to assess for restriction. When pressure is increased, the tissue is compressed against underlying bony surfaces or muscles that lie deep to those being assessed. At that point, congestion, fibrotic qualities, indurations, and tone of the tissue become apparent. While taking the slack out of the tissues, the palpating digit or hand will meet tension within the tissue. Attempt to closely match that tension. The discomfort scale, as previously discussed, assists in avoiding excessive discomfort. The examining fingers, thumb, or hand search for evidence of healthy, normal tissues and quickly uncover trigger point nodules (usually exquisitely tender points), congestion, fibrosis, or otherwise-altered conditions.

Flat palpation is used primarily to assess muscles that are difficult to lift and closely adherent to the body (such as the rhomboids). It also may add information to that received from pincer compression techniques, such as to the width of the discovered band. As pressure is applied to the tissues, particularly if the taut bands are deeply situated, the tissues may tend to shift or roll away from the applied pressure. A more carefully applied pressure may be needed to precisely palpate the tissue. Pressure applied at an angle of around 45° to the surface, while offering slight "support" to prevent the tissue from escaping the hands, may offer an advantage.

Pincer compression requires that the practitioner grasp and compress the tissue between the thumb and fingers with either one hand or two, in either a broad or a specific manner. A broad general compression is provided by the finger and thumb pads as they are flattened (like a clothespin) (Figure 10-7) while a more precise pincer compression of specific tissue is provided by the fingertips when the fingers are curved like a C-clamp (Figure 10-8). In either of these techniques, static pressure can be applied. The tissues can also be manipulated by sliding the thumb across the fingers with the tissue held between them or rolling the tissue back and forth between the thumb and fingers.

Snapping palpation (Figure 10-9) is used to elicit a **local twitch response** (LTR), a momentary spasmodic contraction of fibers when they are properly provoked. Snapping palpation is extremely difficult to apply correctly and to adequately assess. A local twitch response confirms the suspicion of a trigger point when that tissue meets the minimal criteria for a trigger point diagnosis (a nodule located in a taut band which, when properly provoked, produces a referral pattern). While the lack of an LTR does not rule out a trigger point, especially because of the extreme skill needed to correctly apply it, its presence confirms the existence of a trigger point when other diagnostic criteria are present.

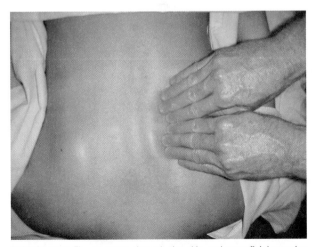

FIGURE 10-6 Fingers press through the skin and superficial muscles to evaluate deeper layers against underlying structures using deep flat palpation. (From Chaitow L, DeLany J: *Clinical application of neuromuscular techniques, vol 1, the upper body,* ed 2, Edinburgh, 2008, Churchill livingstone.)

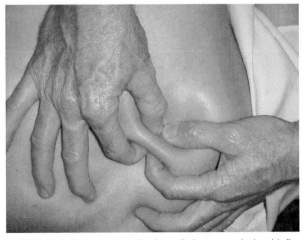

FIGURE 10-7 Pincer compression is applied more precisely with fingertips. (From Chaitow L, DeLany J: *Clinical application of neuromuscular techniques, vol 1, The upper body,* ed 2, Edinburgh, 2008, Churchill Livingstone.)

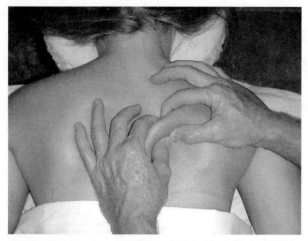

FIGURE 10-8 Pincer compression is applied with the finger pads in a c-clamp for a more general release. (From Chaitow L, DeLany J: *Clinical application of neuromuscular techniques, vol 1, the upper body,* ed 2, Edinburgh, 2008, Churchill Livingstone.)

To perform snapping palpation, the fingers are placed at midfiber level and quickly snapped transversely across the taut fibers, in a manner similar to plucking a guitar string. Snapping palpation can serve as a useful skill in clinical research where precise diagnosis of a trigger point location is crucial. Surface electromyography can be used to record the twitch response. Snapping palpation can also be used repetitively as a treatment technique, which can be effective in reducing fibrotic adhesions.

USING LUBRICANTS

Lubrication sometimes provides the distinct advantage of reducing friction on the skin when the practitioner needs to glide smoothly over the skin surface. However, it is not always advantageous and, in fact, at times inhibits the practitioner's ability to lift and manipulate tissues. Both the European and American versions of NMT call for use of lubrication during some of the technique applications, though the American version uses it far more often than its European counterpart.

When lubrication is used, a suitable amount of oil/lotion allows smooth passage of the palpating digit. When too much oil is applied, the essential aspect of slight traction by the thumb/finger will be reduced and a great deal of palpatory information might be lost. Procedures, such as myofascial release, skin rolling, or other techniques used to lift, stretch, or manipulate the tissues, should be performed prior to lubrication. If the area has already been lubricated, a tissue, paper towel, or thin cloth may be placed between the palpating digit and the skin to prevent slippage or the oil can be removed with an appropriate alcohol-based medium.

With or without lubrication, the practitioner may best locate taut bands by sliding the palpating digit transversely across the fibers. Once located, the fibers may be assessed longitudinally to locate the approximate center of the fiber where central trigger points form. The attachment sites should also be assessed to

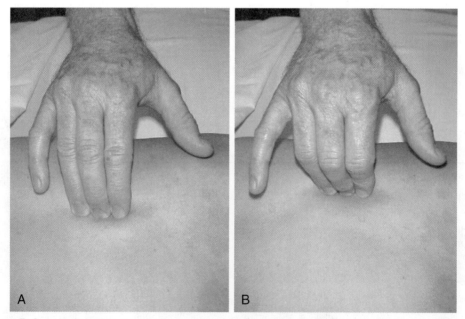

FIGURE 10-9 **A** and **B**, Snapping palpation may sometimes elicit a local twitch response (confirmatory of a trigger point location) and may be useful on more fibrotic tissue as a treatment technique when (if appropriate) it is applied repeatedly to the same fiber. (From Chaitow L, DeLany J: *Clinical application of neuromuscular techniques, vol 1, the upper body,* ed 2, Edinburgh, 2008, Churchill Livingstone.)

determine the degree of tenderness and the possibility of inflammation. Any number of procedures may be incorporated as the practitioner moves from one tissue site to the next. These may include:

- A light, superficial stroke in the direction of lymphatic flow
- Direct pressure along or across taut fibers
- Direct pressure or traction on fascial tissue
- Sustained or intermittent "inhibitory" pressure

The practitioner can efficiently move from assessment to treatment and back to assessment without interruption. Trigger points will be more easily located when taut bands are assessed, reduced in size and density, and then examined. The trigger points may then be treated by means of compression (trigger point pressure release), fiber elongation (stretching, with or without vapocoolants), heat and/or ice (when appropriate), vibration, or movement, all of which usually encourage the release of the taut fibers that house the trigger point.

COMMUNICATION DURING THERAPY

During a treatment session, clear communication is important for both the practitioner and the person being treated. It enables the person to better assist and become involved in understanding his/her body. When the practitioner understands what has brought on the condition and what helps to relieve it, this can be communicated to the person so that he/she can assist in changes in habits that will alter the condition. The practitioner can benefit from a case history with full medical background of the condition. From this appropriate protocols can evolve for treatment and avoidance of steps that are contraindicated. The following questions are frequently used to help guide the session.[31]

- *What is tender upon palpation?* Healthy, flexible tissues are not tender with appropriate pressure. Ischemic tissues and TrPs are usually tender when provoked. It is important to chart tender tissues and return to them for further inspection.
- *Are there referred sensations of pain, heat, tingling, cold, numbness, itching, or any other sensations to other body parts when the tissues are pressed?* TrPs will refer sensations to other parts of the body. The location and target zones of referral as well as the type of referred sensations are important to know and to chart. These should be compared to the client's chronic pain patterns and should be reassessed at subsequent treatment sessions.
- *Is there a reduction of discomfort produced by applied trigger point pressure release?* This will help determine

if the desired results are being achieved. TrPs and ischemia may be reduced and, ultimately, normal tonus and tissue health restored to the area.

An astute practitioner records clinical findings, including areas of dysfunction, referral patterns, postural assessments, client symptoms, and all other relevant material onto a case card or into a case file. The client's medical history and reports of findings of other healthcare professionals should also be reviewed. Out of this substantial information base, a picture will emerge from the viewpoint of the client's and from this a therapeutic plan can be formed.

TRAINING AND CERTIFICATION

A solid foundation of palpable anatomy instruction, understanding of myofascial physiology, and development of skills in locating trigger points form the foundation of neuromuscular therapy. Additionally, an emphasis on contraindications and precautions is crucial in any course that teaches NMT techniques. Although many of the protocols may be practiced without supervision, when practicing certain techniques (such as anterior cervical work), tableside assistance with qualified instructors is imperative.

Both NMT American version™ and NMT St. John method offer certification training that has successfully been conducted in short course seminar events. Completion of a number of weekend courses (4 to 6) is usually required with suggested time allowed between each course for the trainee to practice the techniques offered in the curriculum. Once all the required courses are completed, the trainee may take a certification examination that includes a written and a practical test. There are no required continuing courses to maintain the basic certification, although advanced courses and seminars offering new developments within the field are often available.

NMT American version™ has also been successfully taught in massage schools in the United States. The NMT courses are taught within the school's curriculum by qualified NMT instructors. These courses use the same NMT course manuals and protocols that are offered in the graduate level short courses but are taught more slowly than in the short course version. Additionally, the student has almost daily access to the instructors and assistants, who can recheck the techniques learned previously. The graduating student receives his/her NMT certification along with the massage school diploma and is ready to enter the job market as a certified neuromuscular therapist.

▪▪□□ IN MY EXPERIENCE

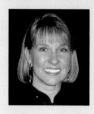

As a clinician as well as an educator, I have found neuromuscular therapy to be a highly effective modality that can be incorporated into any manual techniques setting. The steps used in European NMT are easy to learn and can be quickly performed. The regionally oriented NMT American version™ offers detailed and thorough assessment protocols that are simple to learn due to their "routine" format. Trigger points are often overlooked as a source of chronic pain or other softtissue dysfunction. Skills that assist the practitioner in locating and treating TrPs are very valuable and worth the time and effort that it takes to master them.

When NMT protocols are appropriately performed and the condition does not quickly improve, it is advisable to look for other causes for the problem. This might include joint dysfunction, or might be associated with systemic or visceral pathologies. In such cases, to delay appropriate treatment by continuing palliative care might be dangerous.

It is important to recognize conditions where NMT and other softtissue techniques might be beneficial to a person's presenting condition. It is equally important to recognize conditions where referral to another health care practitioner is warranted.

The European version of NMT is taught as a standalone module on undergraduate schemes, in the School of Integrative Health, University of Westminster. The NMT course involves 12 4-hour lecture and practical classes, spread over a semester. It is an elective module, available on the 3-year BS degree course in *Therapeutic Bodywork* offered by the university. It is available as a stand-alone course to suitably qualified manual therapists who receive a certificate of proficiency on successfully completing the course and its knowledge and skills evaluation examinations.

Clinical Application of Neuromuscular Techniques [3-5] offers step-by-step protocols of neuromuscular techniques as well as foundational anatomy, supporting modalities, and information pertinent to the practice of NMT. The texts do not replace the need for hands-on, supervised training. Instead, it moves the training of NMT into a new realm, supported by study guides and computer interactive programs. By incorporating reading from the textbooks, the trainees can study the material prior to taking an NMT class and enter the course with a stronger foundation of understanding. Reviewing the texts after the class can help solidify comprehension of the materials taught within the course.

At the time of writing, there are no national requirements for certification or licensure to practice NMT. It is important to remember that each state in the U.S. has its own requirements for a license to practice touch therapies. Within each license, there may also be restrictions as to the practitioner's right to treat certain areas of the body. For instance, some states allow intraoral protocols to be performed by a massage therapist while other states restrict this treatment to the dental profession and its employees. Conversely, the practicing

dentist is usually confined to the area cephalad to the clavicles, even though the primary cause of TM joint dysfunction clearly may lie within a pelvic distortion. It is important that each practitioner understand his/her scope of practice and the legal boundaries that limit that practice. Building a referral network with other qualified practitioners is advantageous when proposed treatment lies outside the practitioner's scope.

Practitioners seeking training in neuromuscular therapy are encouraged to contact the groups listed at the end of this chapter for the current standards of training and requirements for certification by each group. There are organizations that specifically train palpation and treatment of trigger points without endorsing particular protocols, and information offered in these additional courses may be of substantial value, especially when built upon the basic foundational knowledge offered in the NMT curriculum. Treatment of trigger points alone is usually not sufficient to produce long-term results. It is only one of many components addressed in an NMT practice.

CASE HISTORIES

▪ Case history 1

A 42-year-old female presented with pain in the cervical spine region and considerable loss of range of motion (ROM), both of which she reported had been present for a number of years. She also complained of chronic headaches, neural sensations in the arms and hands, and a midthoracic pain near her left scapula that felt like "a knife in the back." A previous medical examination had revealed (through MRI) that two cervical disks were bulging into her spinal canal with slight encroachment onto the thecal sac. Her doctor was planning to remove the two disks and had referred her for softtissue work in preparation for the surgery and in hopes of reducing some of her pain prior to surgery.

After a review of her case history and assessment of ROM, the cervical routine of NMT American version™ was performed. ROM was assessed after each step of the routine in order to ascertain precisely which step gained movement if any was achieved. After the third step of a nine-step routine, cervical rotation was at full range; however, carefully performed minor neck flexion still produced sensations in the upper extremity. After the completion of the routine, full range of motion was restored with no pain during movement. The midthoracic pain remained.

It was suggested that the person immediately consult her physician to discuss the changes in her mobility. The practitioner was concerned about the profound changes in ROM for a number of reasons, including the following:

- The muscles that had been released were likely to be weak and in need of rehabilitation therapy.
- Although range of motion had been increased, the previously damaged posterior elements of the disk and posterior longitudinal ligament remained weak and unable to adequately support the structure.
- Increased ability to move the head and neck could place the structures under greater stress that might result in increased protrusion of the disk into the cord space.
- The physician might want to reassess the region and reconsider the need for surgery.

At subsequent sessions, the client reported that her headaches had ceased and that she had retained the ROM. The sensations in her upper extremity were gone, prompting her physician to cancel her surgery and suggest specific exercises to strengthen the cervical muscles without risking excessive movement of the region. He also suggested that a cervical collar be worn temporarily in order to avoid excessive movement (particularly cervical flexion) until the muscles became stronger. The client was advised against activities that might result in further injuries to the area, such as roller-skating, water or snow skiing, or riding on jet skis.

It is not unusual to see a rapid improvement when neuromuscular therapy is appropriately applied. However, in this case, it was also important to recognize the risks involved when the range of motion was dramatically improved. Consultation with the physician was absolutely warranted to protect the client from the potential results of increased ROM.

■ Case history 2

A 55-year-old female who has had been previously treated with NMT for back pain presented with considerable pain and significantly decreased ROM 8 weeks following bilateral mastectomy stemming from breast cancer. She also complained of upper and lower back pain. After updating her medical history and reviewing the procedures used for her cancer treatment, a very gently applied assessment of the soft tissues of both shoulders revealed bilateral involvement of every muscle that crossed each shoulder joint. Since she was unable to lie prone, supine, or side-lying due to pain at her surgical sites, modifications were made in the NMT routines so that they were performed while she was seated. Some steps were performed with her upright, while others were performed with her leaning forward onto a pile of extremely soft pillows to allow access to posterior torso muscles.

Several immediate precautionary flags were noted. Unique features of her reconstruction plan were discussed that would influence her NMT sessions.

- Because pain medication was masking the person's perception of pain, the pressure used in palpation was adjusted to avoid excessive pressure.
- One of her upper extremities (the side where lymph nodes were removed) was notably larger than the other side at midhumeral region. Since this situation likely stemmed from lymphatic congestion and possibly from damage to lymph vessels, the practitioner determined that it was best not to increase blood flow distal to the shoulder joint (which most certainly would occur if NMT was applied to the arm, forearm, or hand) until further investigation could determine the status of lymph flow.
- During the mastectomy surgery, scar tissue formation was provoked below the breast region in order to build a "shelf" to help support an implant that would be inserted during the rehabilitation process. In this case, it was important to let inflammation run its course rather than providing antiinflammatory measures, such as ice packs, to this pink, swollen region.
- Prior to the placement of the implant that would help to normalize the appearance of the breasts, expanders would be used to gradually stretch the tissues to allow room for the implant. In this case, the expander would be inserted deep to the pectoralis major. Fluid would be injected through a special valve on a weekly basis to stretch the overlying tissues. NMT sessions were scheduled to coincide with the injections to relieve the predictable spasms that usually result from this tissue stress.
- A number of other issues were discussed concerning plans for radiation, chemotherapy, and other aspects of her treatment and rehabilitation. Questions were prepared for her physicians and a treatment plan designed that would interface as a support during this process.

When any person is receiving medical care in conjunction with NMT, it is important that the practitioner be informed as to what has been done and what the rest of the treatment plan will encompass. Whenever the practitioner is not familiar with a procedure, drug, diagnosis, or other factor of the client's care, it is important that he/she seek advice from the physician or other sources to determine the best course of action for that case.

What is best for one person is not necessarily best (or even safe) for another, even when they have a similar diagnosis. Being fully informed is the practitioner's responsibility, regardless of the modality used.

SUGGESTED READINGS

Chaitow L: *Modern neuromuscular techniques*, ed 2, Edinburgh, 2003, Churchill Livingstone.

Chaitow L, DeLany J: *Clinical application of neuromuscular techniques, vol 1, the upper body*, ed 2, Edinburgh, 2008, Churchill Livingstone.

Chaitow L, DeLany J: *Clinical application of neuromuscular techniques, vol 2, the lower body*, Edinburgh, 2002, Churchill Livingstone,

Chaitow L, DeLany J: *Clinical application of neuromuscular techniques, case study exercises*, Edinburgh, 2005, Churchill Livingstone.

Davies C: *The trigger point therapy workbook: your self-treatment guide for pain relief*, Oakland, Calif, 1999, New Harbinger.

Fernandez F: *Deep tissue massage treatment—a handbook of neuromuscular therapy*, St. Louis, 2006, Mosby.

Sharkey J: *The concise book of neuromuscular therapy*, Berkeley, 2008, North Atlantic Books.

Simons D, Travell J, Simons L: *Myofascial pain and dysfunction: the trigger point manual, vol 1: Upper half of body*, ed 2, Baltimore, 1999, Williams & Wilkins.

Travell J, Simons D: *Myofascial pain and dysfunction: the trigger point manual, vol 2, The lower extremities*, Baltimore, 1992, Williams & Wilkins.

RESOURCES

NMT American version™

NMT Center, Judith DeLany, Director
900 14th Avenue North, St. Petersburg FL 33705
(727) 821-7167
E-mail: nmtcenter@aol.com
www.nmtcenter.com

St. John Method of NMT

St. John Seminars
6565 Park Blvd., Pinellas Park FL 33781
1-888-NMT-HEAL
E-mail: info@stjohnnmtseminars.com
www.stjohnseminars.com

For an updated a list of schools offering NMT American version, European NMT, and other NMT training in their curricula, visit the NMT Center at www.nmtcenter.com

REFERENCES

1. Punzo A: Foreword, *Techniques in Orthopedics* 18:1-2, 2003
2. Simons D, Travell J, Simons L: *Myofascial pain and dysfunction: the trigger point manual, vol 1, Upper half of body*, ed 2, Baltimore, 1999, Williams & Wilkins.
3. Chaitow L, DeLany J: *Clinical application of neuromuscular techniques, vol 1, The upper body*, Edinburgh, 2000, Churchill Livingstone.
4. Chaitow L, DeLany J: *Clinical application of neuromuscular techniques, vol 2, The lower body*, Edinburgh, 2002, Churchill Livingstone.
5. Chaitow L, DeLany J: *Clinical application of neuromuscular techniques, vol 1, The upper body*, ed 2, Edinburgh, 2008, Churchill Livingstone.
6. Chaitow L, DeLany J: *Modern neuromuscular techniques*. In Coughlin P, editor: *Principles and practice of manual therapeutics*, New York, 2002, Churchill Livingstone.
7. Chaitow L: *Modern neuromuscular techniques*, ed 2, Edinburgh, 2003, Churchill Livingstone.
8. Nimmo R: Receptors, affectors and tonus, *Journal of the American Chiropractic Association* 27:21, 1957.
9. Nimmo RL, Vannerson JF: *The collected writings of Nimmo & Vannerson, pioneers of chiropractic trigger point therapy*, Pittsburgh, PA, 2001, self-published.
10. Travell J, Simons D: *Myofascial pain and dysfunction: the trigger point manual, vol 2, the lower extremities*, Baltimore, 1992, Williams & Wilkins.
11. Prudden B: *Pain erasure: the Bonnie Prudden way*, New York, 1980, Ballantine.
12. Chaitow L: *Modern neuromuscular techniques*, Edinburgh, 1996, Churchill Livingstone.
13. Chaitow L, DeLany J: Neuromuscular techniques in orthopedics, *Techniques in Orthopedics* 18:74-86, 2003.
14. Butler D: *Mobilization of the nervous system*, Melbourne, 1991, Churchill Livingstone.
15. Feldenkrais M: *Awareness through movement*, New York, 1972, Harper & Row.
16. Hanna T: *Somatics*, New York, 1988, Addison-Wesley.
17. Randolph T: *Stimulatory and withdrawal and the alternations of allergic manifestations*. In Dickey L, editor: *Clinical ecology*, Springfield, Ill, 1976, Charles C Thomas.
18. Ferraccioli G: Neuroendocrinologic findings in fibromyalgia and in other chronic rheumatic conditions, *Journal of Rheumatology* 17:869-873, 1990.
19. Lowe J, Honeyman-Lowe G: Facilitating the decrease in fibromyalgic pain during metabolic rehabilitation, *Journal of Bodywork and Movement Therapies* 2:208–217, 1998.
20. Lowe J: *The metabolic treatment of fibromyalgia*, Boulder, Colo, 2000, McDowell Publishing.

21. DeLany J: Leptin hormone and other biochemical influences in systemic inflammation, *Journal of Bodywork and Movement Therapies* 12:121-132, 2008.
22. Lum L: Hyperventilation syndromes. In Timmons B, Ley R, editors: *Behavioral and psychological approaches to breathing disorders*, Plenum Press, 1994, New York.
23. Cailliet R: *Soft tissue pain and disability*, ed 3, Philadelphia, 1996, FA Davis.
24. Latey P: Feelings, muscles and movement, *Journal of Bodywork and Movement Therapies* 1:44-52, 1996.
25. Gilbert C: Hyperventilation and the body, *Journal of Bodywork and Movement Therapies* 2:184-191, 1998.
26. Brostoff J: *Complete guide to food allergy*, London, 1992, Bloomsbury.
27. DeLany J: Clinical perspectives: breast cancer reconstructive rehabilitation: NMT, *Journal of Bodywork and Movement Therapies* 3:5-10, 1999.
28. *Stedman's electronic medical dictionary*, version 4.0, Baltimore, 1998, Williams & Wilkins.
29. Juhan D: *Job's body: a handbook for bodywork*, ed 2, Barrytown, NY, 1998, Station Hill.
30. Melzack R, Wall P: *The challenge of pain*, ed 2, Harmondsworth, England, 1988, Penguin.
31. DeLany J: *NMT course manuals: applications pack*, Saint Petersburg, Fla, 1994, NMT Center.
32. Chikly B: *Silent waves: theory and practice of lymph drainage therapy with applications for lymphedema, chronic pain and inflammation*, Scottsdale, Ariz, International 2001 Health and Healing.
33. Ward R: *Foundations of osteopathic medicine*, Baltimore, 1997, Williams & Wilkins.
34. Cantu R, Grodin A: *Myofascial manipulatio.*, Gaithersburg, 1992, Aspen Publications.
35. Barnes J: Myofascial release in treatment of thoracic outlet syndrome. *Journal of Bodywork Movement Ther* 1(1):53-57, 1996.
36. Baldry P: *Acupuncture, trigger points and musculoskeletal pain*, Edinburg, 1993, Churchill Livingstone.

MULTIPLE CHOICE TEST QUESTIONS

1) Neuromuscular therapy:
   a) is only for use in medical offices
   b) can be integrated into a variety of practice settings
   c) should only be performed by physical therapists
   d) is only for use in home care

2) NMT examinations usually include all of the following except:
   a) ischemia
   b) myofascial trigger points
   c) postural assessment
   d) bone density tests

3) Contributors of techniques from which NMT evolved include:
   a) Stanley Lief
   b) Boris Chaitow
   c) Raymond Nimmo
   d) all of the above

4) Biomechanical factors in health include all of the following except:
   a) postural positioning
   b) joint dysfunction
   c) emotional stress
   d) "use" syndromes

5) Biochemical factors in health:
   a) include endocrine function, hydration, and mineral levels
   b) have no influence on chronic pain
   c) are of no consideration in NMT
   d) none of the above

6) Biomechanical, biochemical, and psychosocial factors:
   a) are of little concern to manual practitioners
   b) synergistically interface to provoke a multitude of changes in the body
   c) have virtually no influence on softtissue health
   d) should all be referred for diagnosis

7) Colloids become more fluid when:
   a) heated
   b) shaken or stirred
   c) allowed to stand still
   d) a and b only

8) A central trigger point:
   a) cannot be treated without injections
   b) develops at the midfiber region
   c) rarely causes pain
   d) is best treated with cross-fiber friction

9) Trigger point pressure release:
   a) is rarely useful in the treatment of trigger points
   b) is only used at the attachment site
   c) is only applied once to each trigger point
   d) is an effective technique used to deactivate central trigger points

10) European and American versions of NMT:
    a) have unique differences, primarily in positions and use of hands
    b) share common foundational platforms
    c) neither a nor b
    d) both a and b

11) Which of the following tools are commonly used in NMT?
    a) pressure bars
    b) hot packs
    c) cold packs
    d) all of the above

12) When applying gliding strokes in NMT American version™:
    a) the thumbs are usually the treatment tool
    b) the fingers are always the treatment tool
    c) the thumbs are placed tip to tip
    d) none of the above

13) "Deep tissue massage" is:
    a) another name for NMT
    b) never used in NMT sessions
    c) always the best NMT technique
    d) sometimes mistakenly used as another name for NMT

14) Gait assessment is:
   a) a simple technique that corrects walking patterns
   b) easily performed by any practitioner with very little training
   c) seldom of any clinical value
   d) moderately subjective when conducted without computerized equipment and other diagnostic tools

15) When the person being examined with NMT states that a sensation of pain, heat, tingling, cold, or numbness, or when itching is being felt in another body part when the practitioner presses in the center of a muscle's belly, the primary suspicion is that:
   a) attachment trigger points are present
   b) a central trigger point has been located and provoked
   c) a nerve is being pressed on by a disk
   d) the client should be referred to another practitioner

16) As the practitioner applies an appropriate degree of steady pressure to a central trigger point:
   a) the person should only report a sensation of pain
   b) the person might report that a referred sensation is fading away
   c) the referred sensation usually will grow in intensity
   d) pain in the local region will be the only indication that a trigger point has been located

17) NMT protocols:
   a) always incorporate lubricated gliding strokes
   b) rarely incorporate lubricated gliding strokes
   c) provide a step-by-step process for examining the tissues within a region
   d) are only used in hospital settings

18) Pincer palpation and snapping palpation are:
   a) very similar and usefully interchangeable
   b) very different and used for different purposes
   c) the only two techniques needed by manual practitioners
   d) techniques that should be avoided when trigger points are present

19) Skin palpation:
   a) assesses the skin's freedom of movement from underlying tissues
   b) has tremendous value in NMT application
   c) can include palpation of the quality of the skin itself
   d) all of the above

20) Which of the following is *not* part of the general guidelines for practice of NMT?
   a) the most superficial tissue is usually treated before the deeper layers
   b) the proximal portion of an extremity is addressed before the distal portions
   c) most myofascial trigger points lie in the end-plate zone (midfiber) of a muscle or else at attachment sites
   d) in two-jointed muscles only the proximal joint needs to be assessed

Orthopedic Massage

Whitney Lowe

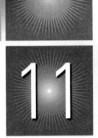

11

STUDENT OBJECTIVES

Upon completion of this chapter, students will be able to do the following:

- Describe the four primary components of orthopedic massage.
- Describe the difference between assessment and diagnosis.
- Explain the importance of assessment in treatment of softtissue disorders.
- Explain treatment adaptability.
- Identify several types of softtissue pathologies and describe massage techniques that might be appropriate to address them.

KEY TERMS

Assessment

Compression broadening technique

Deep longitudinal stripping

Diagnosis

Kinesiology

Musculoskeletal disorder

Orthopedic conditions

Orthopedics

Rehabilitation protocol

Static compression with active shortening/lengthening

Static compression with passive shortening/passive lengthening

Treatment adaptability

INTRODUCTION

Orthopedic massage is a relatively new modality practiced by massage therapists. It is a systematic approach to treating pain and injury conditions and incorporates other specific forms of clinical massage. As a broader category, orthopedic massage applies to treatment of conditions resulting from any number of activities, such as work, sports, or accidents. Using massage to treat pain and injury conditions has not been a major part of Western medical practice in the last 50 to 60 years. However, this is changing. Studies by Drs. David Eisenberg and Daniel Cherkin demonstrate increased use and acceptance of massage by the public.[1,2]

One of the primary reasons for massage's popularity is the success massage has had in therapeutic applications. In the last 50 years massage has gone from being primarily for relaxation and stress release to a therapeutic modality applied to complicated **musculoskeletal disorders.** Orthopedic massage offers practitioners working in medical/clinical settings an organized and effective approach to handling the greater needs of today's clients. Orthopedic massage practitioners work with professional sports and dance teams, in occupational therapy settings, and with physical therapists, chiropractors, and osteopaths. In many cases, massage is proving to be more effective than other modalities for treating certain conditions. In fact, millions of people have sought complementary care for musculoskeletal problems.

To date, two texts, both published in 2003, have defined systems of orthopedic massage: Tom Hendrickson's *Massage for Orthopedic Conditions* and my own *Orthopedic Massage: Theory and Technique.* Orthopedic massage courses are taught in massage schools and as continuing education courses. While there are distinct differences among these systems, there are also fundamental similarities, particularly in the emphasis on **assessment,** treatment variability, and knowledge of common pain and injuries. The discussion that follows describes the basic components integral to a general understanding of orthopedic massage. These components are increasingly emerging as a generally accepted model of orthopedic massage as evidenced in trade journal publications and courses taught in schools. Orthopedic massage offers practitioners a systematic and effective approach to treating pain and injuries and allows them to integrate skills they already possess.

HISTORY

Massage has been used for treating various ailments for centuries. Yet, it fell from frequent use in the U.S. and most Western medical systems with the rise of pharmaceutical medicine and physical therapy modalities. In the U.S. the application of massage in the field of sports set the stage for a resurgence of interest in massage's use as a treatment modality. By the late 1980s, there was increasing use of massage in the clinical and sports medicine environments for the treatment of pain and injury conditions. Most of the practitioners involved in this movement were calling their work sports massage, although that term also referred to the use of massage at athletic events to enhance performance and improve recovery. Those working more extensively in the clinical application of massage for general injury management gradually started to use other terms to refer to their work, such as clinical or rehabilitative massage.

The term *orthopedic massage* has been increasingly used since the mid-1990s to describe treatment of pain and injury conditions with massage therapy. Many practitioners who have worked in sports massage have started to refer to their practice as orthopedic massage, as the term is more encompassing. The first published educator to apply the term orthopedic massage to their softtissue treatment approach was Tom Hendrickson, who began using it in the early 1980s. After training with physical therapist Lauren Berry, Hendrickson used the term to describe the system he developed that was influenced by Berry and his own chiropractic and softtissue training. I began referring to the treatment system I developed as orthopedic massage in the early 1990s. Training and then working with Benny Vaughn in the sports massage environment from the mid-1980s to the mid-1990s greatly informed my work. In addition, working and studying in the orthopedic setting during this time moved my work toward broader orthopedic applications.

There was a recognized need to establish a broader reference for pain and injury treatment that went outside of the sports setting. Because **orthopedics** refers to the locomotor tissues (those associated with creating or limiting movement), orthopedic massage seemed a natural reference for the use of massage in treating softtissue pain and injury conditions. Subsequently, other educators and practitioners also working with pain and injury conditions began using orthopedic massage to refer to their work. However, there are no fully agreed upon standards for orthopedic massage, due to several factors. In particular, similar to sports massage, orthopedic massage refers primarily to a generalized system of massage in a certain setting, in this case massage for pain and injuries. Also, each educator's version of orthopedic massage is characterized by that person's history, knowledge, and expertise. These educators may or may not incorporate the entire systems of other earlier promoters of orthopedic massage.

At the same time, students emerging from schools who use textbooks from the key promoters of the modality will understand orthopedic massage as a particular system. Those who have published textbooks used in schools or trade journal publications, as well as those who taught the system early in the modality's development, tend to have the key elements of their systems adopted by students and educators using their works. As a result, some of these systems' components are starting to be found in other educators' teachings and writings.

The discussion below highlights the key elements in Whitney Lowe's system. They are used increasingly by orthopedic massage educators and provide a starting point for a generalized description of orthopedic massage.

DESCRIPTION

Orthopedics is the "branch of medical science that deals with prevention or correction of disorders involving locomotor structures of the body especially the skeleton, joints, muscles, fascia, and other supporting structures such as ligaments and cartilage."[3] Thus, orthopedic massage is a modality that seeks to address **orthopedic conditions**—those pains and injuries affecting the locomotor soft tissues. Any orthopedic massage approach has at minimum three main components: orthopedic assessment, treatment technique variety, and adequate knowledge of pain and injury conditions. The degree to which these components are emphasized in any orthopedic massage practice depends on the expertise and training of the practitioner.

A study on the practice patterns of U.S. massage therapists in 2005 found that about 60% of visits to massage therapists were for musculoskeletal symptoms.[4] A conservative estimate would suggest over 100 million office visits to massage therapists each year address musculoskeletal disorders (MSDs).[5] This number is likely to increase significantly with the aging of the baby boomer population.

MSDs are one of the most pervasive health care issues in the United States. These conditions include a wide array of softtissue problems such as strains, tendinosis, sprains, myofascial trigger points, nerve entrapment, and the ever-present host of biomechanical problems resulting from chronic muscle tightness. MSDs are the second-most common reason for seeing a family practice physician, infectious conditions being the first.[6] Ineffective treatment for MSDs in the traditional medical system has driven millions of Americans to seek better care through complementary and alternative medicine (CAM) approaches, such as massage therapy. Orthopedic massage is ideally suited to address many of these conditions and has the potential to offer clients a more affordable, accessible, and effective treatment option.

COMPONENTS OF ORTHOPEDIC MASSAGE

Orthopedic massage is often referred to as a "comprehensive system." This means that an orthopedic massage approach moves beyond a focus on a particular technique to include a more comprehensive approach to rehabilitation. As discussed previously, the general understanding of orthopedic massage includes several important components in order to be an orthopedic massage approach; these include assessment, treatment technique variety, and knowledge of conditions and physiology. Effective treatment of orthopedic conditions requires sufficient understanding of **kinesiology,** the study of human movement, anatomy, and physiology of healthy and injured tissues.

This section provides a discussion of the components of orthopedic massage set out in *Orthopedic Massage: Theory and Technique.*[7] The four primary components of the following system are: 1) orthopedic assessment, 2) matching the physiology of the tissue injury with the physiologic effects of treatment, 3) treatment technique variety, and 4) appropriate use of the **rehabilitation protocol** (see Box 11-1).

Assessment

A critical component to any orthopedic massage system is assessment and evaluation. By assessment I am not referring to the abbreviated interviews that many massage therapists learn in their initial training. Massage practitioners who treat clients with either mild or more severe pain or injuries must develop the skills necessary to assess the nature of the client's condition and continue to evaluate it through the progression of treatment. Over the years, clients have increasingly sought massage for treatment of aches and pain. As massage practice has become able to accommodate these needs, the expectations placed on practitioners

have also increased. A practitioner cannot immediately assume that a client's pain is the result of simple tension or mild stress. Instead, practitioners today must be able to make initial assessments to evaluate the appropriateness of massage. Subsequently, they need to perform more thorough assessment if they choose to treat a client with more than simple pain presentations. Assessment is a critical component of any application of orthopedic massage, and of massage in general.

Without assessment, treatment will be based on guesswork and assumptions rather than critical thinking and analysis—not a good approach to treating pain and injury conditions. Sufficient and valid knowledge and understanding of the locomotor system, its tissues, and common pain and injury conditions are a prerequisite for orthopedic massage. Without adequate understanding of how the soft tissues function and their key roles, treatment may be at minimum futile and at worst complicate the condition.

Assessment, put simply, is the systematic process of gathering information to make informed decisions about treatment. To address pain and injury conditions the practitioner must be able to assess the nature of the condition(s) and understand its physiologic characteristics. Assessment skills help answer fundamental questions about the condition and allow the practitioner to make educated treatment decisions. Basically, assessment reveals the tissues most likely involved in the condition, how they are involved, and what their status is. In the simplest terms, the practitioner should know what tissues are involved (e.g., muscle, fascia, tendon, ligament, joint capsule). In addition, the practitioner will evaluate the type of dysfunction in the tissue (e.g., tear, hypertonicity, myofascial trigger point, nerve conduction impairment).

Treatment should be based on the nature of the tissue pathology. Assessment enables the practitioner to aim treatment at reducing symptoms and improving function in the tissues involved. Assessment also allows the practitioner to determine if massage is in fact appropriate for the condition or to refer the client to another healthcare provider if massage is contraindicated. Even when a client is referred with a physician's **diagnosis,** treatment approaches cannot be filtered down to simplistic recipes. The individual characteristics of the client's condition must be explored with assessment.

There is a distinct difference between assessment and diagnosis. A physician uses information gathered during assessment to make a diagnosis, but the process of assessment in and of itself is not diagnosis. A medical diagnosis is a licensed medical professional's identification and labeling of a disease, illness, or condition. With this information a basic idea of the client's condition can be formed that allows the practitioner to create a clinically sound treatment plan.[8]

There are several basic functions of assessment. First, assessment helps to determine the tissues involved. There are numerous types of soft tissues. In massage the tissues of most concern are muscle, tendon, ligament, joint capsule, nerve, cartilage, bursa, and fascia. A second function of assessment is to identify the type of injury these tissues have suffered. The most common include strain, sprain, tears, hypertonicity, tendinosis, nerve compression, and arthritis. Assessment helps evaluate the biomechanical forces that produce these tissue effects.

Gauging the client's pain levels and symptoms is another function of assessment. Initial evaluation provides a baseline against which progress is measured. It allows the practitioner to keep track of their client's progress and make educated decisions about continued therapy approaches. In addition, both the initial and ongoing evaluations can supply information to other healthcare professionals working with the client. Skilled assessment can build the client/practitioner relationship, further enhancing treatment.

It is important to note that though assessment answers many important questions, it is not an exact science. There are no specific evaluation techniques that can provide 100% positive or negative results in establishing the tissues and dysfunction involved. In some cases the nature of the client's pain is fairly straightforward. In other cases, it may be far more complex. For example, with neck and arm pain it might be fairly easy to establish that the client has hypertonicity in the upper back and neck from doing a job requiring a repetitive task, such as data entry. But the client's irregular arm symptoms of paresthesia and numbness may require more thought and evaluation.

While skill development will improve the accuracy of the practitioner's assessment, there are always exceptions and caveats. This is why ongoing assessment is important. It is extremely important that immediate assumptions are not made. Numerous conditions have symptoms that mimic each other. And in some cases, a reason for the client's complaint simply cannot be established, regardless of the practitioner's experience or knowledge. In this case, continued exploration and monitoring—and possibly referral to another professional—are the best approaches.

> ### BOX 11-1 HOPRS Method
>
> The basic assessment tools:
> - History
> - Observation
> - Palpation
> - Range-of-motion and resistance testing
> - Special tests

Treatment Adaptability

In addition to understanding the nature of the client's condition, the practitioner should be skilled in the treatment techniques most frequently used for pain and injury massage. The second common component included in most systems of orthopedic massage is **treatment adaptability.** Clearly, with the diversity of problems that clients may present, the practitioner should not rigidly adhere to any one particular technique. Relying on prescribed treatment routines ignores the uniqueness of the particular presentation and blinds the practitioner to what could be essential information for addressing the client's complaint. Although there are suggested applications and therapeutic approaches that work in many cases, it does not mean these methods will work in all cases. There are simply no recipes for treating pain and injury conditions.

Practitioners must use their assessment and critical thinking skills to choose and adapt treatment methods or techniques to address the unique situation of each individual client. Orthopedic massage practitioners tend to keep a diversity of methods in their massage tool kit in order to have the most options for treatment. The practitioner can then choose from a wide variety of treatment approaches to find the approach that is most appropriate for each client's unique rehabilitation needs. The best treatment plan for a condition is often based not on special techniques but on the best technique for that particular tissue injury and client.

Matching Treatment to Injury

This third component essential to effective treatment of pain and injuries with massage is to match the physiology of the injury with the physiologic effects of the treatment technique. The massage practitioner has at his or her disposal any number of therapeutic techniques. However, practitioners must understand how their techniques interact with tissues involved in pain or an injury condition. Understanding the physiologic effects of a technique means knowing physiologically how and in what ways a technique is helpful for a particular tissue dysfunction.

Additionally, practitioners will find that there are no set rules when applying a technique to a tissue dysfunction. In one instance with a certain client a particular technique might work well, while with slight variation in injury and with a different client the technique is not appropriate. In certain cases, techniques may be ill advised or contraindicated given their effects on particular pain or injury conditions. Informed treatment decisions come not from the simple amassing of techniques, but more from being able to apply knowledge and critical thinking skills to the unique presentations of their clients.

For the most effective treatment, technique effects are matched to the physiologic nature of the pain or injury condition and the client. For example, deep transverse friction massage applied to myofascial trigger points in the posterior cervical muscles could aggravate the tissues, making the condition worse. A massage technique that would more effectively match the physiology of the condition might be static compression or longitudinal stripping to the affected muscles, thus leading to a decrease in dysfunctional activity of the myofascial trigger points.

PROPER USE OF THE REHABILITATION PROTOCOL

The last component in this system of orthopedic massage is called the rehabilitation protocol.[8] The rehabilitation protocol is the course of injury management used to support recovery. Rehabilitation follows a general pattern regardless of tissue type (muscle, tendon, ligament, or other tissue). A proper rehabilitation approach is important for recovery; in some cases it can mean the difference between recovery and permanent impairment. Massage can play an integral role at various stages of this process, particularly in normalizing tissues and regaining flexibility. The degree to which softtissue practitioners are involved with managing a client's protocol will depend on their skills and qualifications. However, the orthopedic massage practitioner can play an important part in the rehabilitative process with a wide range of pain and injury conditions. Understanding and working appropriately within the rehabilitation protocol are necessary for successful recovery.

The rehabilitation protocol is a four-step process, though the steps often overlap. For tissue injury recovery each step will be necessary. Working through each of the steps is particularly important for clients working in occupations or activities that will resubject them to the conditions that caused the dysfunction initially. For example, athletes who must return to their respective activities after injury will benefit from following through with all the rehabilitation steps. This is true for those working in particular occupations as well, such as construction or data entry. Motivation, time pressures, and psychologic factors must be inserted into the equation to determine the most effective way to utilize the protocol with each individual.

The four steps of the rehabilitation protocol are:
- **N**ormalizing soft tissue dysfunction
- **I**mproving flexibility
- **R**estoring proper movement patterns
- **S**trengthening and conditioning

The first step is to normalize the softtissue dysfunction. This step requires that the practitioner understand the function and nature of the injured tissues when the tissues are in a healthy state. The goal is to return the tissues to a condition resembling their function when healthy. While normalizing softtissue dysfunction seems like a common first step, it is often overlooked in an effort to get someone back to activity or out of rehabilitation as soon as possible. A variety of modalities might be used to achieve this step's goal, including massage.

Improving flexibility is the second stage of the rehabilitation protocol. The timing of this rehabilitation step depends on the client's condition and other factors. Flexibility, like exercise, may or may not be beneficial in the early stages of recovery. In some cases, stretching is not recommended. For example, if a client has severe carpal tunnel syndrome, any attempts to stretch the flexor muscles of the wrist may cause severe pain and aggravate the condition by stretching the median nerve. In this instance flexibility training is not appropriate until a later stage in the treatment. Knowledge of the condition, client history, and the stage of rehabilitation is critical (see Assessment above).

Dysfunctional compensating neuromuscular patterns develop as a result of most injuries. Along with regaining normal function and flexibility, rehabilitation should include reintegrating proper movement patterns. Dysfunctional patterns involve protective muscle spasm or biomechanical imbalance that result from compensation. The law of facilitation reminds us that neuromuscular patterns are more likely to be adopted when they are frequently repeated.[9] Rehabilitation protocols generally incorporate methods to encourage the client to return to proper movement patterns. Biomechanical corrections such as postural change are an example. Massage can play a role in this aspect of rehabilitation as well. In an ideal situation, the tissue dysfunction is normalized and flexibility is restored prior to this step; however, this is not always possible and this step becomes interspersed with steps 1 and 2.

Strength training and conditioning for specific activities are the last stage of the rehabilitation protocol. Rehabilitative exercises and stretching should only be performed when the tissues are able to accomplish these activities without being further injured or impaired. The average client is not always inclined to follow through with this aspect of recovery on their own, but this step remains important. Those in professional sports understand the critical role of conditioning. The physical demands from many occupations and weekend activities are enough to warrant the client's following through on a conditioning regimen. Massage therapy, to make an applicable example, is a physically demanding occupation. These practitioners would benefit from a strength training and flexibility program—in addition to using good postural form—to achieve career longevity.

Though the steps above often follow a sequential pattern to some degree, the steps are not necessarily distinct and frequently overlap. One step need not be fully complete before moving on to the next. An example would be chronic muscle tightness from myofascial trigger points. The first goal would be to neutralize the trigger points and normalize muscle tone, ultimately leading to reduction of pain and restoration of normal activity. Often at the same time, stretching is encouraged to promote flexibility. In this case, step one is likely to overlap with steps two and three until the client is prepared to begin conditioning. In contrast, in a more acute injury, tissue healing would likely need to occur prior to steps two through four.

Therapists who understand the rehabilitation protocol and can follow the different stages of their client's progress are much more likely to know how best to participate in the client's recovery process. When the practitioner's skills are most helpful is determined through assessment, consultation with the client, and/or communication with other healthcare providers involved in the client's rehabilitation. The degree to which the practitioner engages with the client's rehabilitation will also depend on the practitioner's training. Understanding the rehabilitation protocol is an important, but sometimes overlooked, aspect of pain and injury treatment with massage.

SPECIFIC TECHNIQUES USED

Any number of massage techniques and systems can be integrated into a practitioner's orthopedic massage practice. In fact, it is this variability and flexibility that make the orthopedic massage system so appropriate for treating the myriad individual presentations of soft-tissue dysfunction. However, there are basic massage techniques that massage practitioners should have in their tool bag when working with clients having pain and injury conditions. The following techniques are particularly useful for disorders involving muscle or fascia. The first two, compression broadening and deep longitudinal stripping, are especially effective when combined with passive or active movements. These techniques are discussed below.

Compression Broadening

The **compression broadening technique** comes out of sports massage and is a basic component of the orthopedic massage practitioner's tool bag. It has numerous applications and is often adapted into other, more specialized techniques. A healthy, fully functioning muscle is able to completely contract and elongate. When a muscle contracts, it also broadens due to the overlapping of sarcomeres within the fiber.[10] This technique is designed to help spread and broaden muscle fibers so the muscle can regain flexibility and tonus. Enhancing muscle broadening also reduces the likelihood of adhesions within the muscle tissue and helps reduce overall muscle tension. This stroke is particularly effective when used as part of the active engagement methods described later.

In this technique the practitioner applies pressure to the muscle being treated and simultaneously performs a broad cross fiber stroke (Figure 11-1). The compression can be applied with a broad contact surface such as the palm of the hand in areas of large muscle mass like the quadriceps. In other regions, such as the wrist flexors and extensors, the region to be treated is much smaller and the thenar aspect of the hand and thumb may be more appropriate (Figure 11-2).

Deep Longitudinal Stripping

Deep longitudinal stripping is also sometimes called deep tissue massage and is a basic stroke used in neuromuscular therapy and other modalities. It is a slow gliding stroke along the direction of the muscle fibers applied with the primary purpose of encouraging elongation in the muscle tissue. Deep longitudinal stripping is another basic massage stroke for pain and

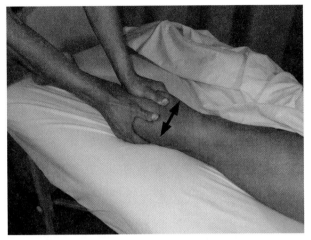

FIGURE 11-1 Compression broadening stroke applied to the gastrocnemius and soleus muscles. In this region pressure is applied with the thumbs and base of the hand and then the thumbs are spread apart.

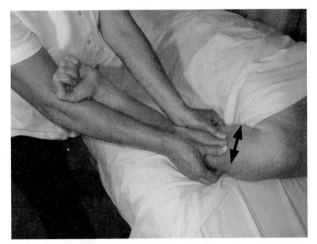

FIGURE 11-2 Compression broadening stroke performed with the thumbs in a smaller muscle group area.

injury treatment because it is an excellent method for reducing hypertonicity and increasing pliability in muscles. It is also considered the most effective way to inactivate myofascial trigger points when using a direct manual approach.[11]

Deep longitudinal stripping is not as easy to perform as it looks. Pressure is moderate to deep when this technique is applied, and the clinician must be skilled in reading the response of the client's muscle tissue to gauge what the appropriate pressure level should be for the client. A detailed knowledge of anatomy and muscle fiber direction is also required to perform this technique correctly. The technique is performed in the direction of the muscle fibers being treated, usually from one

tendinous attachment of the muscle all the way to the other. Longitudinal stripping can be performed with a broad application of pressure such as the palm, fist, or forearm, which may be helpful prior to more specific muscle treatments so that tension in the superficial tissues can be reduced. The most effective pressure level is at the threshold between pleasure and pain. Clients often report that this treatment "hurts in a good way."

Following the broad application of pressure, the practitioner may want to treat individual muscles more specifically. More specific treatment is performed with small contact surfaces of pressure. Examples include the thumbs, fingertips, knuckles, elbow, or pressure tools (Figure 11-3). The general guidelines of following circulatory flow and working toward the heart should be considered when performing these techniques on the extremities.

The deep pressure and stripping motion of this technique have an effect on resetting the tension levels registered by the muscle spindle cells and helping to elongate shortened sarcomeres.[12] The pressure level should be adjusted to a level the client can tolerate. The result is a reduction in tightness of the muscle fibers. The added benefit of stripping vs. applying pressure without movement (static compression) is the movement along the direction of the softtissue fibers. When this technique is applied to muscle fibers, it helps to encourage lengthening and elasticity leading to a reduction in hypertonicity (muscle tightness) and increased flexibility.[12] The practitioner should be aware that in the course of a stripping technique that exceedingly tight or tender spots may be present in the

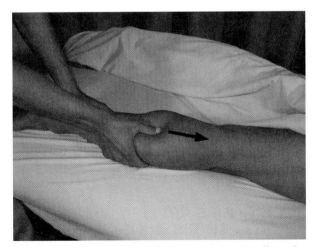

FIGURE 11-3 Deep longitudinal stripping applied to the calf muscles with the thumb.

muscle, so immediate adjustment of pressure levels is sometimes necessary to accommodate the different levels of muscular tenderness.

MASSAGE WITH ACTIVE AND PASSIVE MOVEMENT

The methods used above can be used in combination with active and passive movements to achieve greater results. Massage techniques applied during active and passive movements can produce more profound effects than when the techniques are used alone. These techniques magnify the neurologic and mechanical responses in the muscle. The following techniques incorporate static compression, compression broadening, and deep longitudinal stripping in combination with active or passive movements of a muscle. These techniques are applied while a muscle is either being shortened or lengthened. Compression can be performed with the palm, knuckles, thumb, fingers, elbow, or a pressure tool.

Proper application of these techniques requires a sound knowledge of kinesiology. Different variations and positions can be used for a wide variety of treatment options. These techniques are not universally applicable to every condition or with every client. As discussed previously, the practitioner, through assessment, must make the determination if and when these techniques would be useful for a particular case and client. For example, the techniques involving massage with active engagement can be more uncomfortable for the client if there is a softtissue injury because more muscle fibers are engaged during the technique. In those cases it is best to keep this technique for the later stages of the rehabilitation process.

Massage with Passive Movement

The massage practitioner can use a variety of massage techniques in conjunction with passive movement of the area being treated. Incorporating movement along with massage helps mobilize soft tissues thereby enhancing freedom of movement and improving myofascial function. The techniques below incorporate static compression or deep longitudinal stripping while the muscle is passively moved into either a shortened or lengthened position.

TECHNIQUES APPLIED WITH MUSCLE SHORTENING

There are several techniques that can be applied to a muscle while it is in a shortened position. This technique is very similar to procedures that go by the name of positional release or strain/counterstrain.[13] Moving a muscle to a shortened position, instead of trying to lengthen it, may help decrease tension, trigger point activity, and neuromuscular dysfunction in that muscle. Static compression is particularly helpful in situations of severe muscle spasm, such as those which occur following an acute injury. The primary effect of **static compression with passive shortening** is a reduction in neurologic activity in the muscle. The intensity of pressure from the static compression technique is decreased when the muscle is shortened, and thus there is less tension on the muscle fibers. As a result, pain is reduced and the neurologic system responds by reducing muscle tightness. The final shortened position of the muscle may be held for longer periods to achieve a better neurologic release. There are different theories about how long the position should be held for the most benefit, ranging from about 20 to 90 seconds.[14]

The practitioner applies static compression to an area of the muscle that has a heightened neurologic response, such as a myofascial trigger point, an area of restricted fascial movement, or muscle tightness. Once static pressure is applied over the area, the tissues underneath the pressure are shortened by the practitioner moving the affected joint passively so that the muscle is in a shortened position (Figure 11-4). Most clients will feel a decrease in painful sensations as the tissue is brought into a shortened position.

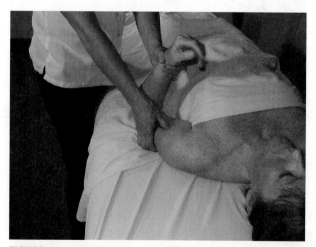

FIGURE 11-4 Massage with passive movement (shortening stroke) is applied to the biceps brachii. Pressure is placed on the muscle while the elbow is extended, and then the elbow is passively flexed while pressure is maintained on the muscle.

TECHNIQUES APPLIED WITH MUSCLE LENGTHENING

Static compression and deep longitudinal stripping techniques used along with **passive lengthening** are effective for mobilizing connective tissue, improving flexibility, and increasing elongation in the myofascial tissue. In addition, they help reduce adhesions within the muscle. The pressure applied to the tissue while it is being elongated helps to stretch connective tissue and contractile elements within the muscle.

Static Compression with Passive Lengthening

The target muscle is placed in a shortened position. The practitioner applies static compression to a particular area of the muscle tissue while it is in the shortened position. While applying continuous pressure, the practitioner elongates the tissues underneath the pressure by passively moving the limb so the muscle is then lengthened. This technique is also called pin and stretch (Figure 11-5).

Deep Longitudinal Stripping with Passive Lengthening

The target muscle is placed in a shortened position. The practitioner performs a deep longitudinal stripping technique on the target muscle while moving the joint passively to lengthen the muscle (Figure 11-6). This method can be repeated several times working in parallel strips on the muscle until the entire area is treated.

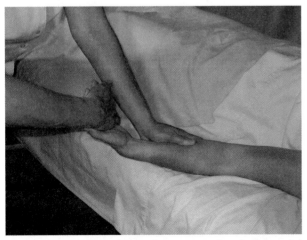

FIGURE 11-5 Massage with passive movement (lengthening stroke) applied to the wrist flexor muscles. The wrist is flexed to begin, and then pressure is applied to the wrist flexor muscles. With pressure maintained on the wrist flexor muscles, the practitioner passively extends the client's wrist, stretching the wrist flexor muscles.

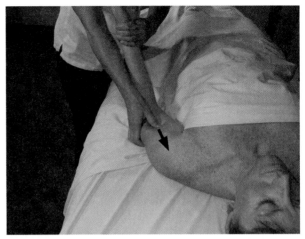

FIGURE 11-6 Massage with passive movement (lengthening stroke) applied to the elbow flexors with deep stripping performed simultaneously. The practitioner places the client's elbow in a flexed position to begin. Then as the practitioner passively extends the client's elbow, a deep longitudinal stripping technique is applied to the elbow flexors moving toward their superior attachment.

MASSAGE WITH ACTIVE ENGAGEMENT

Any number of massage techniques can be used in conjunction with active movement. Incorporating movement along with massage helps mobilize soft tissues thereby enhancing freedom of movement and improving myofascial function. The techniques below incorporate static compression, compression broadening, or deep longitudinal stripping while the muscle is actively moved into either a shortened or lengthened position.

The primary effects of active engagement techniques are both neurologic and mechanical. Applying pressure while a muscle is under contraction helps to reduce excessive muscle spindle activity and decrease overall muscle tension. Pressure during active contraction also helps mobilize some of the deep fascia surrounding muscles. In addition, using active engagement allows more access to otherwise hard-to-reach tissues, as well as making treatment more effective. For example, with muscles that are tight and also deep, it is hard to apply effective pressure when doing a longitudinal stripping technique without using a great deal of force, which is extra effort for the practitioner. By having the client actively engage the area, the pressure is magnified because the density of the tissue is increased when the muscle is engaged in active contraction.

The amount of muscle contraction can be varied by adding additional resistance. Additional resistance

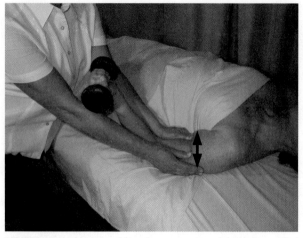

FIGURE 11-7 Massage with active engagement (shortening stroke) with additional resistance. The practitioner is performing a compression-broadening stroke on the client's elbow flexors as the client actively flexes the elbow while holding a weight.

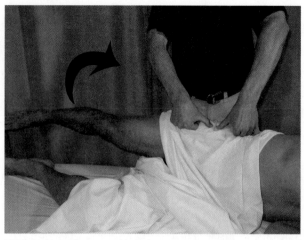

FIGURE 11-8 Massage with active engagement (shortening stroke) is applied to the hip abductor muscles. The client begins with the hip in an adducted position. The practitioner applies pressure to the hip abductor muscles, and then the client actively abducts the thigh while the practitioner maintains pressure on the abductors.

recruits a greater number of muscle fibers and makes the pressure level more effective. Practitioners can increase muscular effort by providing resistance with their hands, resistance bands, weights, or manual resistance (Figure 11-7). If resistance bands or weights are used, both hands are freed to perform the technique.

TECHNIQUES APPLIED WITH MUSCLE SHORTENING

In the techniques that follow, static compression and broadening techniques are used during active shortening of the muscle. These techniques enhance the broadening of the muscle during concentric contractions, thus reducing adhesions and tension and helping the muscle return to normal function.

Static Compression with Active Shortening (Concentric Contraction)

Static compression is applied to an area in the muscle that is hypertonic, contains myofascial trigger points, or appears restricted or tender due to excess tension. Once static compression is applied (only a moderate amount of force is needed), the client is instructed to concentrically contract the affected muscle. Pressure is maintained during the shortening phase of the contraction. Pressure can be maintained or released as the client returns the affected area to the original position. The static compression technique can be applied with a broad base of pressure like the palm or a small area of pressure like a thumb, knuckle, or pressure tool (Figure 11-8).

Compression Broadening with Active Shortening

A more effective method to broaden a muscle during concentric contraction is to use compression broadening strokes through the contraction or **active shortening.** With this broadening technique the cross fiber movement performed with pressure helps to spread and broaden muscle fibers thereby decreasing any intramuscular adhesions and enhancing pliability. The technique is started with the target muscle in a lengthened position. The client is instructed to actively contract (shorten) the affected muscle. During the client's concentric contraction the practitioner performs a compression broadening technique on the muscle (Figure 11-7 and 11-9). The practitioner releases pressure as the client returns to the starting position. This process is repeated moving along the length of the muscle until the entire muscle has been treated. Timing and coordination are important. The practitioner should start the compression broadening technique at the same time of the client's movement and time the stroke so that it finishes as the client reaches the fully shortened position of the muscle.

TECHNIQUES APPLIED WITH MUSCLE LENGTHENING

Static compression and deep longitudinal stripping techniques used along with **active lengthening** are effective for enhancing elongation of the muscle, stretching the myofascial tissues and decreasing tightness

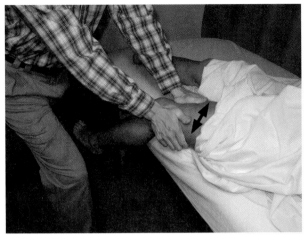

FIGURE 11-9 Massage with active engagement (shortening stroke) applied to the quadriceps muscle group. A compression broadening technique is applied to the quadriceps while the client actively extends the knee.

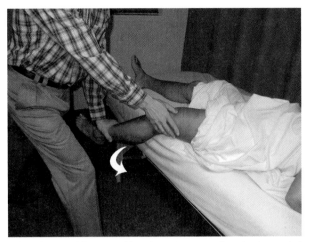

FIGURE 11-10 Massage with active engagement (lengthening stroke) with static compression applied to the quadriceps group. The client engages an isometric contraction of the knee extensors against the practitioner's resistance. The practitioner applies static compression to the quadriceps muscles and then instructs the client to slowly let go of the contraction. The practitioner pushes the client's leg into flexion while maintaining the static compression on the quadriceps.

in the muscular fibers. These techniques are more commonly utilized in the later stages of the rehabilitative process or with individuals whose muscles are in moderately good tone to begin with. The techniques are begun with the muscle in its shortest position. Some muscles, such as the hamstrings, will have a tendency to cramp if contracted in their shortest position. For these muscles use a more neutral position to engage the initial isometric contraction.

Static Compression with Active Lengthening

This procedure is similar to the lengthening technique performed with passive movement (pin and stretch) with the only difference being the eccentric contraction in the muscle as opposed to passive elongation. The technique begins with the client establishing a moderate level of tension in the muscle with an isometric contraction. This isometric contraction should be engaged close to the shortest position of the muscle as long as that muscle is not prone to cramping in this short position. Muscles prone to cramping in a fully shortened position are usually multijoint muscles such the hamstrings. The practitioner applies static compression to the muscle during the isometric contraction and holds the pressure throughout the procedure. The client is instructed to slowly let go of the contraction while the practitioner offers resistance, creating an eccentric contraction in the target muscle. The practitioner continues to hold static compression on the target area of the muscle (Figure 11-10).

Deep Longitudinal Stripping with Active Lengthening

Deep longitudinal stripping with eccentric contraction is even more effective than static compression (above) at reducing muscle tension and enhancing myofascial elongation. The practitioner has the client engage an isometric contraction of the affected muscle from a shortened position just as in the procedure above. Be careful about performing this contraction in muscles that are prone to cramping. The client is then instructed to slowly let go of the contraction while the practitioner offers resistance, creating an eccentric contraction in the target muscle. During the eccentric contraction the practitioner performs a deep longitudinal stripping technique on the target muscle (Figure 11-11). In most cases, especially on the extremities, the stripping is performed toward the heart. This technique magnifies the effects of deep stripping techniques.

BENEFITS OF ORTHOPEDIC MASSAGE

Orthopedic massage is an organized and comprehensive approach that provides the practitioner with the flexibility to work with a wide variety of conditions. Orthopedic massage is showing enormous possibilities and successes in treating a wide range

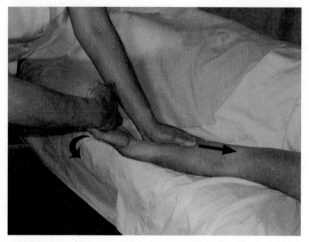

FIGURE 11-11 Massage with active engagement (lengthening stroke) with deep longitudinal stripping to the wrist flexor group. The client engages an isometric contraction of the wrist flexors against the practitioner's resistance. The practitioner instructs the client to slowly let go of the contraction and applies a deep longitudinal stripping technique to the flexors as the client's wrist is slowly extended.

of common musculoskeletal disorders. These conditions include an array of softtissue problems such as strains, tendinosis, sprains, myofascial trigger points, nerve entrapment, and biomechanical problems resulting from chronic muscle tightness. Orthopedic massage provides a viable and effective intermediary or adjunct therapy that can allow the client to avoid more invasive solutions. In cases of conflicting or confusing symptoms, orthopedic massage can provide a noninvasive treatment approach through which conditions can be further clarified and alternative treatments found. In addition, when other modalities fail massage is often able to successfully intervene.

There is also increasing evidence that massage can reduce or even eliminate the need for surgery. For example, many clients with herniated disks, low back pain, carpal tunnel and thoracic outlet syndromes, and rotator cuff disorders have shown improvement and been saved from the painful and lingering disability that comes from surgery or other invasive procedures (such as steroid injections) for these conditions. A prime example of the use of massage as a noninvasive but successful treatment approach is with carpal tunnel syndrome. Carpal tunnel syndrome is widely diagnosed today, with many of those patients having surgery. Yet research indicates that myofascial techniques can effectively treat carpal tunnel syndrome, alleviating the need for surgery in many cases.[15]

Orthopedic massage is particularly beneficial for demystifying symptoms and clarifying the client's condition. In situations where symptoms mimic those of other conditions, the palpatory and assessment skills of the orthopedic massage practitioner can provide valuable information to guide appropriate treatment. For example, pronator teres syndrome can mimic carpal tunnel syndrome. In many cases the pronator teres involvement is not identified and the nerve compression symptoms persist because the condition is not properly treated. Through its emphasis on effective assessment, orthopedic massage can help clarify these conditions and is an excellent intervention for a diversity of dysfunctions.

CONTRAINDICATIONS

Orthopedic massage is a modality used for working with a wide variety of pain and injury conditions. Consequently knowledge of appropriate contraindications that would prohibit treatment or warrant referral to another health professional is important. Contraindications can be divided into two categories: absolute and relative. Absolute contraindications are those where it is very clear that massage should not be used under any circumstances. Examples would include any type of direct contact massage on open wounds or extensive range-of-motion stretching methods on an acute and severe ligament sprain. A basic understanding of pathology is usually sufficient to understand absolute contraindications to massage. However, there are occasions where a client's symptoms are suppressed yet the injury is severe enough that assessment is required to determine that massage is absolutely ill advised.

A relative contraindication includes situations in which massage might be inadvisable under certain circumstances, but its use is not ruled out completely. In cases where massage is not obviously contraindicated, assessment is critical for accurately evaluating the nature of the condition and the role massage might play. The use of massage can be either or both condition- or client-specific in terms of contraindications. For example, in general, treating fibromyalgia with deep massage is contraindicated because it can exacerbate pain and disturb sleep. Yet some clients with the condition are able to eventually tolerate this level of therapy, particularly after receiving treatment for some time. In other situations, the client is never able to move beyond more superficial strokes. Consequently what might be a contraindication for one client and his or her condition may not be for another: this is why the contraindication can be relative.

When determining if massage is contraindicated practitioners must also evaluate their own limitations. For example, a practitioner might not be comfortable treating a client with a painful shoulder condition if he or she is unable to accurately determine the tissues involved or is not sure what is causing the client's problem. A more experienced practitioner with more advanced skills might be able to accurately identify the problem and might recognize specific types of massage approaches that would be helpful for this stage of the client's rehabilitation. Thus, skill and experience of the practitioner alone can make massage contraindicated or appropriate. In cases where practitioners are unsure of the dysfunction or their ability to help, it is best to follow the axiom *"when in doubt, refer it out."*

A Sample Application of Orthopedic Massage

Orthopedic massage is a system of skills, rather than a specific technique, and can be integrated into any massage practice. The student can conduct an orthopedic massage session in a variety of ways, depending on initial client evaluation and need. What orthopedic massage training students have had will also influence how they practice the approach. Like other massage modalities, orthopedic massage skills are developed over time and require practice. Recent massage therapy graduates or those with less experience will need to learn these new skills just as they did their entry-level training. With practice, practitioners will become more at ease in applying these procedures. Practitioners with more healthcare or massage experience will find the learning process and integrating these techniques into their practice easier.

Below is an example of applying orthopedic massage concepts in practice applied to a client diagnosed with tennis elbow. This example is a fairly straightforward case; evaluation and treatment complexity depend on the client and his or her condition. Assessment, treatment analysis and development, the rehabilitation protocol, and knowledge of condition specifics are all employed. Identifying the nature of the client's condition is necessary so that an appropriate treatment plan can be developed. Depending on the stated needs of the client, this step can range from a brief evaluation to a full-on assessment with special orthopedic tests. Blindly following a routine is ill advised in massage where symptoms indicate pain or injury. Knowing *why* the practitioner's choice of treatment could help is a goal for learning proper treatment of pain or injuries and orthopedic massage. Beginning to approach the client's pain and injury complaints in this manner will help build student's conceptual and clinical skills.

While the following is a simple example, one can extrapolate how well the orthopedic massage approach works as a comprehensive system for pain and injury treatment. See Box 11-3 for a sample exercise on orthopedic massage.

Example A: Choosing an appropriate treatment strategy.

Case description: A client presents with lateral elbow and forearm pain. The client states that her physician diagnosed her pain as a case of mild tendinosis (commonly called tennis elbow or lateral epicondylitis) seeming to be from chronic overuse at work. The physician recommended massage.

Assessment: The first thing the orthopedic massage practitioner should do is to ensure he or she understands the nature of the client's complaint. In this case, the client has come with a diagnosis. However, assessment skills are still employed to clarify the pathology and the particulars of the tissues involved. In some cases, a practitioner may find that her evaluation produces results that differ from those originally diagnosed by the physician. It is not within the massage practitioner's scope of practice to diagnose any condition. However, the practitioner can and should relay

---

BOX 11-2 Building the Healthcare Team

Orthopedic massage practitioners work specifically with soft-tissue pain and injury conditions. As their practices and skills develop they will begin to have a greater number of client referrals from other healthcare professionals. In addition these practitioners will likely be sending some of their clients to other health professionals when the client's condition is outside their scope of expertise. These other healthcare professionals become part of a network of colleagues, and it is important to build strong relationships with them. There are many different health professionals the orthopedic massage practitioner might work with. It will be particularly valuable to establish a consulting and referral network with orthopedists, osteopaths, physical therapists, occupational therapists, chiropractors, acupuncturists, and other physical medicine specialists. Sometimes this is done through the client, such as when the client is referred. Referring clients to other health professionals is also a valuable way to help them learn about the benefits of orthopedic massage approaches, thereby increasing future contact and referrals.

BOX 11-3 Softtissue Disorders and Treatments

Below is a list of common softtissue disorders. For each disorder listed describe in detail the following:
- The physiology of the condition (what is actually occurring).
- Several signs or symptoms that would most likely be apparent when you evaluate the condition with a detailed client history, palpation, or any range-of-motion evaluations.
- Important physiologic aspects of the condition. Possible relevant physiologic aspects of the injury, how it might have occurred (biomechanics).
- Whether massage would be appropriate for the condition in most cases. What techniques or methods could address the condition.
- What the client can learn or do at home or work to enhance the rehabilitation process.
- What type of relative or absolute contraindications to watch out for with these conditions.
  Answer the above questions for these conditions:
- Myofascial trigger points in the posterior neck muscles
- Patellar tendinosis (commonly called tendinitis)
- A mild hamstring muscle strain
- Carpal tunnel syndrome

---

any relevant clinical findings back to the diagnosing physician that suggest a cause for reevaluation.

In this case the client was told she has tennis elbow and the physician recommended massage. The practitioner performs an initial evaluation to ensure that she has the skill and knowledge to address the complaint.

The practitioner's evaluation begins with a comprehensive medical history that includes the onset of symptoms and as much pertinent information about the client's condition as the practitioner can draw out. Following the history the practitioner palpates the area and performs a number of evaluation procedures including active motion, passive motion, and manual resistive tests for the affected region. If lateral epicondylitis is present, the practitioner assumes she will see a characteristic pattern of responses to these evaluation procedures. For example, it would be common for the client to express pain when the affected tendons are stretched in either active or passive wrist flexion. It would also be common for pain to occur in resisted wrist extension when the muscles of the affected tendons are contracted. After the range-of-motion and resistance tests, the practitioner uses special orthopedic tests, such as the tennis elbow test, to further investigate the condition. A skilled

practitioner can accomplish the above fairly quickly, and be more selective with tests to save time.

Treatment: If the practitioner chooses to treat the client she or he will consider the physiology of tennis elbow to determine treatment. This condition is a common tendinosis (tendon dysfunction) complaint that is rarely inflammatory. It results from chronic overuse of the wrist extensor muscles, which might occur with a repetitive task such as typing. This stage in treating this condition is to normalize the primary tissue dysfunction (remember the first stage of the rehabilitation protocol). Tendinosis is a breakdown of the collagen matrix in the tendon. Normalizing the tissue dysfunction means addressing the dysfunctional tendon tissue as much as possible by encouraging the healing process. Deep friction massage is particularly effective at stimulating fibroblast production to help heal the damaged collagen in the tendon.[16-18] In addition to treating the collagen breakdown in the tendon, the practitioner will address the stress on the tendon that led to the problem in the first place. Deep longitudinal stripping as well as active and passive engagement techniques to the wrist extensor muscles are helpful in decreasing muscular tension.

Rehabilitation: In conjunction with massage on the forearm region, it will be helpful to encourage the client to engage in regular stretching and look at ways to cut down on the chronic overload of these muscles at work (see rehabilitation protocol). This could mean the client evaluates the ergonomics of her work station or begins to vary tasks during her day to give her forearms a break from repetitive motions. A skilled practitioner might be able to recommend specific exercise and stretching techniques or refer out for these aspects of the rehabilitation.

TRAINING REQUIREMENTS

Orthopedic massage classes are beginning to appear in some entry-level massage school programs, but most orthopedic massage training is advanced course work that is acquired in continuing education programs. A number of organizations offer a certification in orthopedic massage, but there is no consistency or standard as to what is involved in certification. One organization's certification requirements and standards may be very different from another. Most orthopedic massage training incorporates the general components laid out here that comprise orthopedic massage. Resources for additional training in orthopedic massage are listed at the end of the chapter.

■■□□ IN MY EXPERIENCE

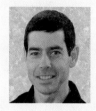

A client once came to me for treatment of a carpal tunnel syndrome that had been diagnosed by her physician. At that time, I was also treating another client with the same condition. However, this second client's carpal tunnel syndrome was so far advanced that she could not open doorknobs, hold silverware, or do many functions of daily living. The first client was having hand pain, but it was nowhere near as severe as the second client. As a result, the type of treatment I used with each client was very different, even though their diagnosed conditions were identical. The second client could only tolerate a very light touch the first several times I worked with her. It took several months to even get close to doing some of the techniques that I had done initially with the first client. Yet, in the long run both clients were able to avoid having surgery and returned to normal function. This situation illustrates that it is erroneous to speak of specific routines that can be used with clients having a particular condition because there are just too many variables. Each treatment should be unique and tailored for the specific needs of the client.

CHAPTER SUMMARY

In this chapter we have explored the theory and concepts of orthopedic massage. The greatest advantage of orthopedic massage is that it provides practitioners a comprehensive and systematic approach to pain and injury treatment. Unlike other modalities in this text, orthopedic massage is not really a technique, but rather an organized approach for treating these pathologies. As a comprehensive approach it is much more than a collection of techniques. In incorporates the need for proper assessment and evaluation, clinical decision-making, and a thorough understanding of the entire rehabilitative process in the field of orthopedics. In addition, it emphasizes the importance of being flexible and adapting to the particular needs of the client. This flexibility allows numerous treatment methods or techniques to be integrated into an orthopedic massage session or practice. Orthopedic massage offers practitioners a viable and effective approach to meeting clients' increased need for noninvasive solutions to musculoskeletal disorders.

CASE HISTORY

The client was referred for orthopedic massage treatment by an orthopedic physician, who he was still seeing for a serious knee injury. He was also currently in physical therapy for the injury. He was in his late 20s when I saw him. In his early 20s, the client was actively involved in bodybuilding. Due to competitive practices within the bodybuilding field at that time, he and many of his colleagues took anabolic steroids to enhance their muscle building. He gave up bodybuilding in his mid-20s but had recently had an injury that the orthopedist attributes to his former years of steroid use.

While walking down a set of stairs he slipped slightly and when catching his fall, put a sudden load on his right leg. He felt a sudden searing pain through his quadriceps region and his leg immediately gave way under him. He went to see the doctor after this injury, and the orthopedist diagnosed him with a torn quadriceps retinaculum. The connective tissue of the retinaculum had been weakened by years of steroid use. By the time he was referred for massage, the injury was over 4 weeks old. The scar tissue that had accumulated in the area of the retinacular tear had limited his ability to flex his knee to only about 45° of flexion. The orthopedic surgeon stated that surgery was an option, but a last resort because of the nature of this tissue tearing. The surgeon was hoping that with a combination of physical therapy and massage, the scar tissue could be mobilized and the knee motion could be improved.

For several weeks deep friction massage and active engagement lengthening techniques were applied to the quadriceps muscle group. The treatment was painful for the client, but he was highly motivated to get better and recognized the benefits of an aggressive approach to the therapy. Because the massage therapy and physical therapy were performed in the same office, he received stretching and range of motion exercises in physical therapy immediately after each massage treatment. Within 4 weeks he had gained almost complete and full range of knee flexion once again and was able to avoid the surgery.

SUGGESTED READINGS

Hendrickson T: *Massage for orthopedic conditions*, Baltimore, 2003, Lippincott Williams & Wilkins.

Lowe W: *Orthopedic assessment in massage therapy*, Sisters, Ore, 2006, Daviau-Scott.

Lowe W: *Orthopedic massage: theory and technique*, Edinburgh, 2003, Mosby.

RESOURCES

Benjamin, Ben
www.benbenjamin.net/

Boulder College of Massage Therapy
www.bcmt.org/

Lowe, Whitney
Orthopedic Massage Education & Research Institute (OMERI)
www.omeri.com

Port Townsend School of Massage
www.massageeducation.com

Waslaski, James
Center for Pain Management
www.orthomassage.net

REFERENCES

1. Cherkin DC, Sherman KJ, Deyo RA, Shekelle PG: A review of the evidence for the effectiveness, safety, and cost of acupuncture, massage therapy, and spinal manipulation for back pain, *Ann Intern Med* 138:898-906, 2003.
2. Eisenberg DM et al: Trends in alternative medicine use in the United States, 1990-1997: results of a follow-up national survey, *JAMA* 280:1569-1575, 1998.
3. Thomas C: *Taber's cyclopedic medical dictionary*, ed 15, Philadelphia, 1987, FA Davis.
4. Sherman KJ et al: A survey of training and practice patterns of massage therapists in two US states, *BMC Complement Altern Med* 5:13, 2005.
5. ABMP: *2007 National consumer survey*, Evergreen, CO, 2007, ABMP.
6. McCaig LF, Burt CW: National Hospital Ambulatory Medical Care Survey: 2001 emergency department summary, *Adv Data* 335:1-29, 2003.
7. Lowe W, *Orthopedic massage: theory and technique*, Edinburgh, 2003, Mosby.
8. Lowe W: *Orthopedic assessment in massage therapy*, Sisters, OR, 2006, Daviau-Scott.
9. Fritz S: *Mosby's fundamentals of therapeutic massage*, ed 2, St. Louis, 2000, Mosby.
10. McComas A: *Skeletal muscle: form and function*, Champaign, IL, 1996, Human Kinetics.
11. Simons D, Travell J, Simons L: *Myofascial pain and dysfunction: the trigger point manual*, vol 1, ed 2, Baltimore, 1999, Williams & Wilkins.
12. McPartland JM: Travell trigger points—molecular and osteopathic perspectives, *J Am Osteopath Assoc* 104:244-249, 2004.
13. Chaitow L: *Positional release techniques*, ed 3, New York, 2007, Churchill Livingstone.
14. D'Ambrogio K, Roth G: *Positional release therapy*, St. Louis, 2007, Mosby.
15. Sucher BM: Myofascial release of carpal tunnel syndrome, *J Am Osteopath Assoc* 93:92-94, 100-101, 1993.
16. Cook JL, Khan KM, Maffulli N, Purdam C: Overuse tendinosis, not tendinitis. Part 2: Applying the new approach to patellar tendinopathy, *Physician Sportsmed* 28:31, 2000.
17. Davidson CJ et al: Rat tendon morphologic and functional changes resulting from soft tissue mobilization, *Med Sci Sport Exercise* 29:313-319, 1997.
18. Gehlsen GM, Ganion LR, Helfst R: Fibroblast responses to variation in soft tissue mobilization pressure, *Med Sci Sport Exercise* 31:531-535, 1999.

MULTIPLE CHOICE TEST QUESTIONS

1) Orthopedic massage could best be described as:
   a) a massage technique that is only used on orthopedic surgery patients
   b) a specific technique for treating joint trauma
   c) a comprehensive rehabilitation approach in massage
   d) a treatment approach primarily for sports injuries

2) Which of the following is an accurate statement about musculoskeletal disorders (MSDs)?
   a) They are the second–most common reason for a patient to seek the care of a physician in the U.S.
   b) They are most likely to occur in the sports environment and don't affect the average person.
   c) Massage should not be used to treat these conditions unless the person has been diagnosed by a physician.
   d) Very few people with MSDs seek the care of anyone other than a physician.

3) Which of the following is the most accurate statement about orthopedic assessment as used by the massage therapist?
   a) Assessment should only be done while being supervised by a physician.
   b) The main purpose of assessment is to determine how many treatments a client should get.
   c) The primary reason for performing assessment is to determine if massage treatment is appropriate.
   d) Assessment only happens in the first treatment with a client.

4) Which of the following is a primary component of the rehabilitation protocol?
   a) orthopedic assessment
   b) deep friction massage
   c) engage in tissue immobilization
   d) normalize soft tissue dysfunction

5) Which of the following is **NOT** a component of orthopedic massage?
   a) taking an accurate client history
   b) performing the same massage routine with each client
   c) evaluating the physiology of a tissue injury
   d) modifying a treatment based on the client's age

6) Which is the most accurate statement about massage techniques in an orthopedic massage treatment?
   a) Orthopedic massage is usually painful.
   b) Techniques are performed the same way with each client.
   c) Techniques vary based on the client's needs.
   d) Deep friction is a part of every treatment.

7) Which of the following most accurately describes active engagement techniques used in orthopedic massage treatments?
   a) The practitioner uses the client's active muscle contraction to aid in the technique.
   b) The client actively moves the area and then immediately rests while the therapist performs massage.
   c) The therapist performs a massage technique and the client relaxes the target muscle the entire time.
   d) Deep friction massage is applied to the antagonist of the target muscle while the antagonist is actively contracting.

8) Which of the massage techniques listed below is used during variations of a pin and stretch technique?
   a) petrissage
   b) friction
   c) compression broadening
   d) deep longitudinal stripping

9) Which one of the items would be considered a relative contraindication for orthopedic massage?
   a) massage of a client with third degree burns
   b) massage of a client with a herniated lumbar intervertebral disk
   c) vigorous stretching of a region with a severe acute ligament sprain
   d) direct massage of a client with a contagious skin condition

10) An accurate statement about musculoskeletal disorders (MSDs) is:
   a) They are an infrequent cause of visits to physicians.
   b) They are a pervasive healthcare issue in the U.S.
   c) You are required to see a physician if you have an MSD.
   d) Only a few massage therapists see clients with MSDs.

11) If a client presents with a condition that you can't recognize or is beyond your scope of expertise, the most appropriate response is to:
   a) refer the client to another healthcare practitioner
   b) refuse to treat them without a diagnosis
   c) have them call their doctor to get clearance for massage
   d) go ahead and treat them with just light massage work

12) Determining that the client's condition involves myofascial trigger points and then using a treatment that applies static compression and stripping techniques is an example of:
   a) three different stages of the rehabilitation protocol
   b) emphasis on strengthening and conditioning for rehabilitation
   c) applying principles of correct referral for scope of practice
   d) matching the physiology of the tissue injury to the effects of treatment

13) Which of the following statements is **NOT** accurate?
   a) Diagnosis is the naming or labeling of a pathologic condition.
   b) Diagnosis is not within the scope of practice for massage therapists.
   c) Assessment is the same thing as diagnosis.
   d) A physician will use assessment to arrive at a diagnosis.

14) Which of the following statements about orthopedic massage is most accurate?
   a) You have to be certified to practice orthopedic massage.
   b) Only practitioners working for a physician can practice orthopedic massage.
   c) Techniques used in orthopedic massage are not harmful for a client.
   d) It requires detailed knowledge of anatomy, kinesiology, and pathology.

15) The term *orthopedic massage* was:
   a) first used in the early 1980s
   b) not used until the late 1990s
   c) invented by James Cyriax
   d) originally used to describe massage in hospitals

16) In a lengthening stroke, the target muscle being treated is:
   a) first placed in a lengthened position and then further lengthened while static compression is applied
   b) first placed in a shortened position and then lengthened while a deep stripping technique is applied
   c) first placed in a lengthened position and then a broadening stroke is applied during an eccentric contraction
   d) first placed in a shortened position and then a broadening stroke is applied during a concentric contraction

17) In which of the client scenarios listed below would orthopedic massage be the **LEAST** appropriate modality?
   The client:
   a) requests an appointment to address low back pain
   b) would like to address stiffness from an old ankle sprain
   c) describes shooting nerve pain in the hand from occupational stresses
   d) asks for a general stress reduction and relaxation massage session

18) An orthopedic massage approach to help improve dynamic function of extremity muscles might use some of the active engagement methods. To mimic the physiology of what occurs during muscle contraction, broadening techniques are applied:
   a) during a concentric contraction
   b) during an eccentric contraction
   c) immediately after an isometric contraction
   d) during passive elongation of the muscle

19) Which of the following applications of the rehabilitation protocol shows the most correct order and effective application?
   a) strengthening exercises performed first, following by stretching and massage methods when applied to a tendinosis condition
   b) postural changes and ergonomic corrections at work followed by massage and stretching with a client having chronic low back pain
   c) deep friction applied to an ankle sprain followed by flexibility training and eventual strengthening and conditioning
   d) strength training used to address a frozen shoulder, which is later followed up with stretching and massage treatment

20) A massage therapist should engage in assessment:
a) to accurately identify the nature of the client's problem and determine if massage is appropriate
b) only to confirm the diagnosis given by a physician that has referred the client
c) during the first session only, just to determine if there is any pain the client is currently experiencing
d) only if the client says he or she have not already been given a diagnosis by the physician

Polarity Therapy

Leslie E. Korn

12

KEY TERMS

Life energy
Marmas
Prana
Rajasic
Satvic
Tamasic
Triune function

Polarity therapy (PT) is synthesis of ancient theories and techniques of energy medicine that integrates four aspects: Polarity bodywork, energetic nutrition, exercise and stretching postures, and communication/facilitation. PT is rooted in concepts derived from Ayurvedic medicine and integrated with cranial osteopathic manipulative techniques and pressure point/meridian therapies. The theory of Polarity therapy suggests that all forms and processes arise from a universal source of **life energy** that is in constant motion and of polarized positive and negative actions and reactions around a neutral core.

HISTORY

Dr. Randolph Stone was the founder of Polarity therapy. A lifelong student of the healing arts, he published seven books between 1947 and 1954. He was born Rudolph Bautsch in Austria in 1890 and immigrated to the United States of America in 1898. He settled with his family in Wisconsin and then in Minnesota. In the 1920s, Dr. Stone completed his primary medical certification as a Doctor of Osteopathic Medicine (DO) and then received his Doctor of Chiropractic (DC) and a Doctor of Naturopathic Medicine (ND). He maintained his practice in Chicago working with patients considered incurable using techniques learned from many other healing systems. Stone studied yogic meditation in Beas, Punjab, India for personal development, and yoga and Ayurvedic medicine deeply influenced his thinking. His theories and techniques suggest that the principles of polarization are universal phenomena. These ideas were influenced by Dr. Albert Einstein's atomic theories of the early twentieth century. PT is not only a set of techniques but a principle, he proposed, that should guide all therapeutic applications including both assessment and energy balancing at the physical, emotional, mental, and spiritual levels of existence. Stone[1] delineated concepts of energetic, myofascial, and structural manipulation based on what he referred to as "wireless energy currents"—a concept that is linked to field theory explicated by physicist David Bohm. Bohm postulates a cosmic "ocean" of interrelatedness among all things, saying that "individuals are interconnected and energies interchanged in ordinary human interactions are modulated in (via) a universal field that permeates all matter."[2]

Whereas Stone wrote about the reciprocal effects of emotion on autonomic nervous system dysregulation, he did not emphasize the integrative psychosomatic processing that has evolved with Polarity into the process-oriented bodywork therapies of the early twenty-first century. Indeed, by all accounts, this deeply spiritual, gifted healer's no-nonsense approach to verbal processing consisted of no more than to give a "Dutch uncle talk" to his patients and to leave it at that.[1] Nevertheless, Stone encouraged the extension of his work, by leaving out critical details in his charts, he said, in order to stimulate new thinking and avoid clinical dogma. The many contributions by Polarity practitioners who have followed since his death include practitioners who are dually-trained in both Polarity and Western psychological counseling and emphasize the use of PT for somatoemotional health, the integrating of Polarity with massage therapy, the development of comprehensive Polarity dance, application of sound and tuning forks, and the amplification of Polarity diet based on Ayurvedic principles.

◼◼◼ IN MY EXPERIENCE

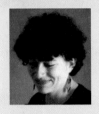

I learned Polarity therapy from Elizabeth Wagner, who was a model of spiritual integrity and an authentic healer. She taught that the essence of Polarity is in the quality of the relationship and that the techniques are the form through which energy and caring are facilitated. This philosophy has guided my work as a practitioner for over 30 years. When I began my study of Polarity, I had no idea it would become my lifelong career. I was living in the jungle, and I studied it for self-care and spiritual practice. However, I slowly began practicing and sharing it with the women in the village and over the next 2 years it blossomed into a professional practice. Polarity has provided me with a model to explore many aspects of spirituality and health, including energy fields and paranormal states of consciousness. Polarity is a form of meditation, and I have been fortunate to "meditate" for a living. Polarity has altered my own capacities to perceive beyond the normal range of empathy and sensory awareness into the realm of intuition, auric sound, and color. This is not unusual among many people who practice bioenergy field therapies over a long period of time. This enhanced capacity to perceive energy fields has enriched both my own spiritual life and my capacity to be of service to others. I have learned about how people store traumatic experiences energetically and of the myriad ways it is creatively processed and released. Polarity has made me very flexible, both physically and emotionally, as I have practiced the exercises and worked in both urban and jungle areas with a very diverse range of people. Polarity therapy has been a universal language of connection; it requires both the simultaneous merging of energy fields and the maintenance of emotional and physical boundaries in order to facilitate the "highest good" among and between people.

PRINCIPLES OF POLARITY THERAPY

The physical and subtle energies of the body and mind are reflected in both functional and structural relationships. A central precept of PT posits that a dynamic equilibrium is achieved by balancing the Positive, Neutral, and Negative reflexes in the body. These "polarities" are the basis of all action and change found in nature. The practitioner assesses, interprets, and responds therapeutically to these relationships.[3] In practice this requires manual contact with three reflex areas, or poles, when addressing an imbalance. For example, when treating a headache, the practitioner traces all the imbalances, which may include releasing reflexes in the head, neck, and shoulders; the gallbladder and liver; and particular points on the joints of the fingers and toes in the hands and feet.

THE LIFE FORCE

Polarity therapy is a dynamic system designed to balance the life force that animates all matter. The concept of the life force is a universal one found across all cultures and systems of medicine and healing. The Chinese refer to the life force as *Qi*, and the Indians call it **Prana.** A major tenet of PT is that health and healing are attributes of energy that flows in its natural and unobstructed state.[3] Artful touch, focused attention, intention—empathy and love—are the foundation of the practice.[4] Disease is considered to be an imbalance of this life force, and the Polarity practitioner provides bodywork, teaches specific exercises, and educates the client about healthy mental attitudes and nutritional methods that are both health building and detoxifying. Polarity is also a philosophy of life, providing insight into the role of action and reaction of one's behavior and lifestyle and its effects on one's health. Practitioners are encouraged to serve as a model of health and well-being for their clients and students. The goal of Polarity bodywork is to trace (by palpation) and release (by skilled touch) those energy blockages that manifest as pain or dysfunction.

To do this, the practitioner applies three depths of touch depending on whether the energy blockage reflects a **(Rajasic)** hyperactive, **(Tamasic)** hypoactive, or **(Satvic)** neutral state of activity. This application of the continuum of touch pressure within the energetic context makes Polarity unique among systems of biofield/touch therapies. A major emphasis includes understanding how poor nutritional habits and poor digestion lead to energy blockages that manifest as pain and discomfort. The practitioner acts as a guide and facilitator to support increased self-awareness as he or she educates the client to increase responsibility for lifestyle choices and activities that enhance well-being and bring about balance. Because PT has its roots in both chiropractic and cranial osteopathy, many practitioners work closely with practitioners licensed to perform manipulations and adjustments, which are made only after the energy underlying the imbalance is addressed.

In clinical practice, the dynamic concepts of positive and negative, attraction and repulsion manifest as structural compensatory strategies found in the geometric structures of the spine that support gravitational requirements, and in functional ways such as inhibition of respiratory processes and restriction of diaphragmatic function following emotional trauma. It is the practitioner's responsibility to "trace" these imbalances by conducting a thorough assessment and evaluation. This includes a refined proprioceptive sense of palpation to assess pulse, energy flow, and changes in temperature; history-taking; and skilled communication to support the helping and healing process. The practitioner helps the client achieve a state of balance through artful and specific strategies that allow the client's innate wisdom and the restorative capacities of the whole being to bring about improved health and well-being.

Reflexes may be functional, structural, mental, or emotional. Imbalances in one area (physical function) are reflected in imbalances in other reciprocal areas such as emotional or mental energy. These reflexes may be acute, chronic, or latent, consciously known, or unknown to the patient. A major set of reflexes found in the hands reflect acute response suggesting current imbalance whereas similar locations in the feet reflect chronic reflexes that may be old or latent, yet must be released lest they emerge as acute illness.

Touch pressure ranges from very light, (Satvic) (5 to 10 grams of pressure)—with palpation similar to methods like craniosacral therapy, healing touch, Reiki and therapeutic touch—to a moderate touch (Rajasic), to a deep, dispersing pressure (Tamasic). Moderate touch is where pressure meets tissue resistance, often the intersection where it may be tender but still feel good. Deep pressure incorporates manipulation through the myofascia similar to some of the techniques of Rolfing, as well as to techniques used by practitioners following in the tradition of Dr. Wilhelm Reich. This deep form of touch appears to resolve stagnation, crystalline deposits, scar tissue, and adhesions. Pressure on energy points, rocking, subtle bone manipulation, stretching, and rotation of joints are some of the methods used to help the patient achieve deep relaxation, improve digestive function, and gain greater self-awareness.

While a spiritual practice is not essential to the successful practice of PT, many practitioners and recipients alike bring a spiritual perspective to their healing practice. Indeed the deep relaxation and sense of well-being that accompany a PT session often lead to the higher order integrative experience of wholeness and interconnectedness called spirituality.

Healing is rooted in the rhythms of reconciliation: opposing forces that shift shapes as inner and outer, darker and lighter, hotter and colder, closer and farther. The autonomic nervous system is composed of two branches, the *sympathetic* and the *parasympathetic*. The reconciliation of these opposing forces is at the heart of Eastern and Western medical traditions alike. In Chinese tradition and in many tribal cultures, the rhythms of the body are considered one with the natural world. Disease or illness results when one becomes out of balance with these forces. Practitioners of traditional Chinese philosophy and medicine refer to these dynamic polarities as *yin* and *yang*. Ayurvedic medicine, the practice of Hindu culture in ancient India, refers to these concepts as the *ida* and the *pingala*. Both traditional Chinese and Ayurvedic healers refined the art of diagnosis by palpating the pulses considered to be the rhythms that were "witness of the soul." Assessment begins with pulse taking, postural assessment, and a detailed history. A pulse that is even in strength and beats and quality between the right and left sides of the body is considered balanced. The practitioner palpates the pulse in the wrist and the ankle in order to assess centrifugal or centripetal energy forces respectively. A stronger left pulse may signify excessive outgoing energy, which can lead to burnout or exhaustion. A stronger right pulse might suggest lack of outward expression, repression, or containment of energy.[5]

POLARITY BODYWORK

A major principle of Polarity posits that imbalances in one region are reflected in imbalances in other areas and pain or inflammation in one reflex area must be located and released in reciprocal areas. Stone called this **triune function** because each "pole" must be balanced with the others for lasting efficacy. The area of greatest pain or inflammation is the positive reflex site, and these reflexes may be traced to their neutral and negative poles, which in turn must also be balanced. This requires the placement of the hands in two different regions of the body simultaneously. Extensive charts delineating the structural and functional relationships based on gravity, the structure and function of the spine, as well as the wireless anatomy and energy currents provide a holographic approach to releasing tension and stress in the physical body via the energetic process. Stone writes: "Any tissue which is in a constant state of contraction or flaccidity reveals an energy block in its circuit of conduction or in the wireless pattern of energy flow."[1]

The core energy currents of PT move through the ultrasonic core, represented by the caduceus, the ancient symbol of healing. The upright staff represents the cerebrospinal energy. The two snakes represent the dual functions of the autonomic nervous system: the sympathetic and parasympathetic. Each serpent "represents part of the double chain of ganglion of the sympathetic nervous system descending on each side of the spinal column."[1] The right serpent is the sun essence, the heat, yang, or pingala; the left, the lunar essence, is the cooling yin or ida. The last open loop and the lower part of the staff are the *cauda equina*. The crossing over in the center denotes the nerve plexi, called chakras, in Hindu cosmology. These plexi, or nerve networks, link the cerebrospinal and central nervous system with the peripheral system.[1] The wings of the caduceus represent the two hemispheres of the brain. The knob at the center signifies the pineal gland, the most subtle endocrine gland of Western anatomy. The pineal gland is referred to as the crown chakra by the Hindus and together with the pituitary is considered the "third eye" (Figure 12-1).

THE FIVE ELEMENTS

The five elements—ether, air, fire, water, and earth— are specific frequencies that function along "wireless energy currents" (Table 12-1). Ether is made up of all the elements together. Stone linked the chakras and the regions of the body they refer to as five elements. Each of the five elements vibrates at a specific, energetic frequency and relates to a general quality, sense, function, and emotion. The elements flow through the body in electromagnetic waves, traveling from posi-

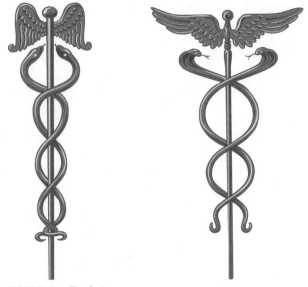

FIGURE 12-1 The Caduceus.

tive (+) through neutral (0) to negative (−) poles. This triune function suggests that each pole of an element must be balanced with itself and the other elements. For example the triad of earth includes the neck, the bowels, and the knees. The neck is the positive pole of the earth triad with corresponding reflexes in the colon and the knees. In assessing neck pain, structure and function, history, and ROM are evaluated. The contribution of (occupational) ergonomics, stress, and traumatic events is also evaluated. The neck has structural gravitational relationships to the lower spine and sacrum, and the effects of gravity on these relationships are assessed. Commonly neck pain reflects structural distortions in the sacrum, which must be addressed for complete recovery to occur in the neck. Yet chronic neck restrictions result also from the effects of poor digestion and elimination. Palpation and release of the small and large intestines and balancing of energy are explored with chronic neck pain. Reflexes in the knees are also released, and simultaneously contacting the knee points with the colon, or the colon and the neck, are part of the treatment plan. For people whose primary complaint involves the knees, energy tracing of the neck and the bowels fulfills the need to balance triune function.

Polarity practitioners touch **marmas,** special (Ayurvedic) energy centers, to balance both functional and structural balance. Marmas are like the acupuncture points but include larger areas

TABLE 12-1 The Elements

Element	Sense	Function	Qualities (Subelements)	Food Qualities	Taste	Color
▫◦☐▫● Ether▫▫	Hearing	Expression Space	• Grief • Desire • Anger • Attachment • Fear	Proper digestion requires a parasympathetic state, or relaxation. Choosing foods from the colors of the rainbow ensures balanced nutrition		Blue
▫✿☐▫● Air▫▫	Touching	Movement Diversity Expansion	• Speed • Lengthening • Shaking • Movement • Contraction	Fruits Nuts Oranges Apples Walnuts	Sour	Green
▫△☐▫● Fire▫▫	Seeing	Motivation Will Drive Upward Movement	• Hunger • Sleep • Thirst • Lustre • Laziness	Grains Legumes Rice-peas Corn Wheat Millet	Bitter	Yellow
▫②☐▫● Water▫▫	Tasting	Creativity Sexuality Downward Flow	• Semen • Saliva • Sweat • Urine • Blood	Tomatoes Melons Pineapple Sea vegetables Lettuce Rhubarb	Salty	Orange
▫☐☐▫▫ Earth ▫▫	Smelling	Structure Crystallization	• Bones • Hair • Skin • Blood Vessels • Flesh	Taro Beets Carrots Onions Potatoes Turnips	Sweet	Red

Adapted from Polarity Wellness Center, 1992.

of the body such as the abdomen or heart region. The marmas are linked to the chakras and reveal pathology via oscillations in temperature and other qualities and sensations palpable to the skilled practitioner. Energy flows down the right side of the body and up the left. To identify the direction at any point in the body, the practioner can place an imaginary spinning "crank" anywhere on the body. Turning it clockwise identifies the direction of chakra currents. Like meditation, PT helps the client focus attention and interoception, enhances sensory processing, and provides the opportunity to reframe and make meaning of somatopsychic experience.

COMMUNICATION/FACILITATION

PT emphasizes the importance of the practitioner's role in modeling a healthy lifestyle. A vital part of the theory of Polarity involves engaging clients to act positively on their own behalf and to assume a vital role in healing. The theory and practice of intention also play an important role, and many practitioners develop a meditation practice to focus the power of intention for healing and to release bioenergies. Understanding the personal meaning of physical and emotional imbalance or illness in one's life also increases awareness and efficacy of the treatment process. The role of love and compassion, or unconditional positive respect, coupled with the role of positive intention, facilitates the work of the practitioner with the client. The practitioner also encourages the client to think positively, release his/her negative emotions, and be cognizant of the effects of negative thinking on his health.

ENERGETIC NUTRITION

Energetic imbalances and disease processes can be traced to poor dietary habits and insufficient digestion. A major principle of PT is detoxification of the liver. Good quality fats (cold pressed olive oil, organic butter and ghee, flax seed oil) are rich in essential fatty acids essential for brain function and support healthy liver function. PT and detoxification derive from Ayurvedic nutrition, which is primarily vegetarian. It encourages live foods that are fresh and rich in enzymes (probiotics). There are two types of diets: one is called health building, and the second is the cleansing, or detoxification, diet. The health building diet is a vegetarian diet rich in vegetables, fruits and legumes, grains, fats, and enzyme-rich sprouts. The cleansing diet is designed for 3- to 10-day periods during which time only fruits and vegetables are consumed as part of an alkalinizing process. Foods also reflect different energetic qualities: for example "airy" foods such as fruits and nuts stimulate spirituality whereas the heavier "earthy" foods like cooked root vegetables are grounding and warming. During the cleansing process one also conducts a liver flush and drinks Polarity tea. Ayurvedic (subtropical) Indian healing traditions that are rooted in a vegetarian culture influenced Dr. Stone and thus the Polarity dietary concepts. However, subsequent practitioners who work with clients for whom vegetarianism is neither culturally nor genetically appropriate have applied the dietary principles of Polarity, without rigidly adhering to vegetarianism for specific individuals or communities (Boxes 12-1 and 12-2).

Note: Licorice use is contraindicated in people with high blood pressure or edema

---

BOX 12-1 Polarity Tea

1 oz. licorice root (pieces)
1 oz. fennel seed
1 oz. fenugreek seed
2 oz. flax seed
    Preparation: Mix the ingredients together while dry. Take 1 tablespoon of the mixture and simmer it in approximately 2 cups water. Strain and drink. The recommended dosage is 1-2 cups per day.

BOX 12-2 Liver Flush

Juice 6 oz. of fresh squeezed citrus juice (orange or grapefruit)
Juice 1 lemon
1 clove garlic (optional)
small piece of chopped fresh ginger
1-2 Tbsp Extra virgin organic cold-pressed olive oil
    Preparation: Mix all the ingredients together in a blender. Alternate 1 sip of the liver flush mixture with one sip of the Polarity tea in the morning. Wait 1 hour to eat breakfast.

POLARITY AND SOUND

The use of sound as a force for vibrational healing is an important adjunct to Polarity bodywork. Sound is applied in two ways: the voice or tuning forks. Both applications of sound balance the nervous system and facilitate relaxation of the whole organism.[6] Toning is defined as making a sound with an elongated vowel for an extended period. Toning frees up energy blocks and aligns the body's vibration. During a bodywork session, when pain is felt or an area is blocked, the practitioner asks the client to begin chanting a sound, like OM or another vowel sound, and to choose a tone associated with that area of the body. For example, the feet require the lowest tone and the head requires the highest tone. Once the tone is sounded, the practitioner joins in and matches the same sound, toning together as the bodywork continues.

Toning, humming, and Polarity bodywork can be used for any purpose but are especially useful when combined for the treatment of sinus congestion, earaches, colds, Meniere's disease (vertigo), and vertigo associated with fluid build-up in the inner ear.

During the session, the therapist sits at the head of the individual while placing her smallest fingers of the left and right hands gently inside the left and right ear respectively, and locates areas of tension in a 360° radius. During the palpation of each point, the client and practitioner hum together. The practitioner asks the client to find the hum quality, whether it is a high or low tone, that causes the most vibration at each one of the tender points. Once the client has found the tone, the practitioner matches that sound and they hum together for several rounds or breath cycles, usually for about 5 minutes, until the tenderness dissipates.

The second phase of this technique involves contacting and holding the ear and applying pressure to the many points along the length of the concha of the ear while stretching the whole ear gently in all directions. This technique does not involve massaging the ear but instead applies sustained pressure on specific points.

Tuning forks incorporate another mode of Polarity sound to balance the energy fields by producing pure musical intervals based on precise mathematical proportions, known as Pythagorean tuning. Dr. John Beaulieu, a registered Polarity practitioner, designed a process called BioSonic Repatterning that is used to align the chakras and the five elements. For example, creating 128 cycles per second intervals creates a deep earth tone that resonates the bones and relaxes the tissues. The fork is placed on the sternum, ribs, and upper spine to relieve back tension. The 64 cycles per second vibration is placed on the lower spine and is used for deep relaxation and is especially effective to relieve tension in the lower lumbar, sacrum, and coccyx area. The 32 cycles per second vibration is used to regenerate and stimulate nerves.[7]

STRETCHING POSTURES

Polarity yoga exercises are special yoga postures and movements designed to release and balance the vital energy. Polarity practitioners teach these exercises to clients for use at home between sessions to maintain and increase the benefits of the bodywork sessions (Figure 12-2).

BENEFITS OF POLARITY THERAPY

Individuals seek Polarity practitioners for a variety of reasons at different stages in their lives or during the course of their illness. Often people who feel "out of balance," fatigued, or experience low energy find that PT helps them reconnect to their deepest self. Others with chronic or acute pain, sports injuries and stress, or those who have not experienced success with conventional therapies are referred by a friend or relative who has benefited. Still others may be curious or may be seeking nonpharmaceutical alternatives for pain relief. Individuals may be referred by another practitioner

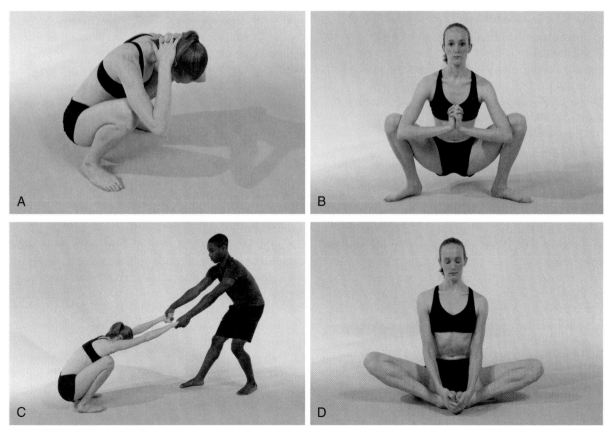

FIGURE 12-2 A, Squat Var. **B,** Squat Var. **C,** Assisted Squat. **D,** Relaxation pase.

for adjunctive work (for example, a psychotherapist may refer to a Polarity practitioner to support the somatic aspect of trauma resolution, or a surgeon may refer for preoperative relaxation or postoperative healing), or to assist in reducing the symptoms of withdrawal of pain medications or drug and alcohol detoxification.

There are numerous health conditions and disorders that result in referrals to Polarity therapists. Some of the conditions PT is useful for include:

- Somatization disorder
- Chronic and acute pain
- Temporomandibular joint pain
- Depression and anxiety
- Autism and Asperger's syndrome
- Chemotherapy-related fatigue
- Chronic fatigue and fibromyalgia
- Stress-related disorders, including organic dysfunction related to autonomic hyperarousal
- Migraines
- Asthma and allergies
- Irritable bowel syndrome
- General feelings of malaise
- Dementia agitation and dementia caregiver stress
- Pregnancy-related discomfort or general well-being
- Diabetes type II, including diabetic edema and neuropathy

PT has also been used for postsurgical recovery; to increase lymphatic (edema) and circulatory flow; and to treat sinusitis, asthma and allergies, osteoarthritis, and rheumatoid arthritis. Polarity treatment may be applied on the side-lying or seated positions during early, middle, and later stages of pregnancy; during delivery; and during postpartum care of mothers and infants. Digestive complaints, including irritable bowel, Crohn's disease, constipation, and poor peristalsis in adults and older adults, are common reasons for referral.

Specialized treatment approaches not common to other modalities include prostate drain and perineal treatment to release tissue congestion in the prostate and to release spasm or chronic contraction in the perineal area and anal sphincter. PT has been applied in cross-cultural settings for treatment of culture-bound syndromes such as *susto* (fright) and *mal de ojo* (evil eye). Because PT is rooted in touch, a nonverbal language that can be found in similar forms in most cultures, it can facilitate cross-cultural communication. Many cultures particularly North and South American

Indian cultures use touch therapies that do not involve disrobing, or extensive muscle manipulation, making Polarity an ideal approach for people whose cultural beliefs and/or modesty precludes disrobing. PT also helps attain optimal well-being and fosters optimal performance among athletes.

RESEARCH

Scientific research in bioelectromagnetics and bioenergy fields has proliferated significantly in the past 20 years. This research provides the foundation for understanding the effects of electromagnetic and subtle energy fields on human function and provides theoretic and conceptual links to Polarity and related biofieldtouch therapies fields.[8] Like other forms of biofield/touch therapies, PT facilitates responses associated with a reduction in sympathetic nerve activity. Direct contact of the vagus nerve occurs while touching areas on the neck and on the diaphragm. Pressure points on the concha provide direct access to vagus nerve fibers. PT stimulates circulatory, lymphatic, and immune response while regulating circadian rhythm[9] and the primary respiratory mechanism.[10] PT appears to facilitate a reduction in pain, anxiety, and depression and facilitates therapist-patient psychophysiologic entrainment.[9] Entrainment describes a state in which two or more of the body's oscillatory systems, such as respiration and heart rhythm patterns, become synchronous and operate at the same frequency. Entrainment occurs intraorganism and interorganisms, such as between therapist and patient and between individuals, groups, and cosmic rhythms.

During a treatment, PT commonly induces a state of consciousness termed reverie, associated with a predominance of theta brain waves that is known to support creativity. Theta states commonly occur just before falling asleep and often include imagery or problem-solving states. Axt[11] has conducted clinical research on the application of PT for the treatment of autism and of children with special developmental needs. Benford[12] undertook an experimental study on the mechanism of action of PT that showed statistically significant fluctuation in gamma radiation during treatment leading Benford to hypothesize that radiation hormesis, the beneficial physiologic effects derived from low dose LET (linear energy transfer) radiation, might underlie mechanism of action in PT. Roscoe et al[13] applied PT for the treatment of radiotherapy-related fatigue associated with cancer treatments and found significant improvement in the reduction of fatigue. Korn and Ryser[14] conducted a randomized controlled clinical research trial applying a standardized protocol of 21 points and manipulations on caregivers of family members with dementia. They found a statistically significant reduction in stress, depression, and pain and increased vitality and improvement in sleep.[16]

Polarity and Asthma

PT provides an integrated approach to treatment of and is used effectively to enhance respiration among people with asthma. Bodywork approaches include releasing constriction of the scalene and sternocleidomastoid muscles and diaphragm, and application of pressure on specific transverse processes of the thoracic vertebrae. Hydrotherapy, exercises, and nutrition enhance the treatment effect. Hydrotherapy includes the application of ice or a strong force of cold water to the upper thoracic vertebrae. This polarizes the tissue and drives blood deep into the spinal centers. Nutritional approaches include the elimination of inflammation-producing refined sugars and elimination of mucus-producing dairy products.

Asthma is but one condition that involves respiratory and diaphragmatic restriction. One of the common areas of complaint centers on the diaphragm, including inhibited respiration, hyperventilation, and pain, constriction, or numbing in the diaphragm. The diaphragm is the main and lower muscle governing respiration (Box 12-3).

Polarity and Emotional Health

Positive psychologic changes have been observed or reported by PT clients. These effects have a potential to decondition body memories, cognitive beliefs, and affective (emotional) states. PT facilitates sensory-motor biofeedback and awareness. The Polarity session also facilitates states of consciousness that decondition state-dependent memories held in body tissues. PT helps to define and improve body image by enhancing kinesthetic and proprioceptive recognition of boundaries. This response is therapeutic when working with people with body image–related disorders such as bulimia and anorexia or changes arising from loss of limb. PT has been hypothesized to help regulate complex neurobiologic rhythms within the body and between people, and it facilitates the capacity for attachment among healthy individuals and people suffering from attachment-related disorders.[8,9,15]

CONTRAINDICATIONS

There are no known contraindications to PT.

BOX 12-3 Exercise for Improved Respiration

Begin by either lying down or standing. Touch the tip of the breastbone, or sternum, called the xyphoid process, and begin to sense the tension there. Slowly trace the area underneath the ribs, pressing up underneath the ribs as you follow their outline. Stay close to the ribs themselves. The point at the end of the sternum is an "alarm point" in Chinese medicine, denoting a vital diagnostic area. Moving along the underside of the rib, begin to press in under the ribs contacting the diaphragm. It will be a little tighter on the right at the liver, but you will have a sense of the dull ache that denotes tension of this muscle. Note areas of tension and how you feel. Returning to the area of the sternum, find the area that was most painful. With the forefinger of the left hand, apply gentle pressure there and lay your hand, palm open, in the space between the pubic bone and the umbilicus. Focus attention on breathing deeply and rhythmically into the area of pain, allowing the warmth from your hand and the depth of your breath to release the tension. In Polarity, this is considered a grief point and may be held for a minute or two or until pain diminishes.

OVERVIEW OF A TREATMENT

The following are some basic contacts and holds that represent a variety of energy-balancing techniques. They may be done in the order presented. The right hand is considered positive and sends energy, and the left hand is negative and receives energy.

The cradle hold in PT is used to bring balance to the parasympathetic and sympathetic nervous systems (Figure 12-3). Structural contacts are the mastoid

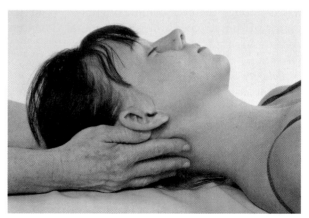

FIGURE 12-3 Cradle (Ether).

process and occipital condyle. Muscles involved include the auricularis posterior, sternocleidomastoid, and trapezius. Nerve contact is facilitated via the cervical plexus branches (C2-C4). Reflex points of contact are particularly related to the release of emotions.

Polarity Therapy

Hands cradle occipital bone at base of skull. Vital role in relationship of structural and motor forces in cerebrospinal fluid; via direct relation to sacral region; CNS balance.

Structural

Mastoid process occipital condyle

Muscles

Auricularis posterior, sternocleidomastoid, trapezius

Nerves

Dorsal rami cervical spinal and branches from cervical plexus: Greater occipital C2; third occipital C3; lesser occipital C2, 3; auricular C2, 3; transverse cervical; C2, 3; supraclavicular C3, 4

Fascia

Cervical sternocleidomastoid

(A)cupressure/(N)euro(L)ymphatic/(N)euro(V)ascular

A: Governing vessel 14, 15, 16 Longitudinal—large intestine, triple warmer, gallbladder, bladder, and governing vessel particularly with respect to release of emotions

NL: central

NV: kidney

Reflex zone

Dermatome: C2, 3L Longitudinal: 1 -5

In the second PT point, one brings balance to the parasympathetic and sympathetic nervous systems, while also facilitating alignment with the craniosacral system. The structural contact is the occipital condyle, while muscle contacts are sternocleidomastoid and trapezius. Vagus parasympathetic stimulation is facilitated through the neck contact (Figure 12-4). Reflex points of contact correspond with central functions and stress related functions. This point facilitates deep relaxation.

Polarity Therapy

Stimulating the vagus nerve brings cranial rhythm and nervous system rhythm together. Parasympathetic contact areas release blockages and balance the parasympathetic nervous system to enhance motility of brain, mobility of cranial sutures, transfer of reciprocal tension membranes, and to bring CNS to balance.

Structural

Occiput

Sides of neck

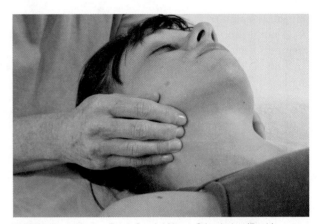

FIGURE 12-4 Neck—Tenth Cranial Nerve Stimulation (Earth).

Muscles

Sternocleidomastoid

Trapezius

Nerves

Celiac ganglion

Superior mesenteric ganglion

Inferior mesenteric ganglion

Parasympathetic stimulation according to Table 12-1.

Fascia

Cervical sternocleidomastoid

(A)cupressure

(N)euro(L)ymphatic

(N)euro(V)ascular

A: Bladder 10, small intestine 16, large intestine 16, triple warmer

NL: central

NV: stress

Reflex zone

Dermatome: C 3, 4 Longitudinal: 1-5

Music tone

Key of G

NERVE STIMULATION OF POLARITY PROTOCOL

Parasympathetic

Efferent

Afferent

Cardiac plexus

Pulmonary plexus

Inferior cervical cardiac branch

Thoracic cardiac branch

Left recurrent laryngeal nerves

Motor—muscles larynx (not cricothryroid)

Sensory—larynx and below vocal cords, esophageal plexus, anterior vagal trunk—gastric branch

Gallbladder and bile duct

Intestine—small, large accompanying superior mesenteric artery and branches as far as the left splenic flexure

Hepatic plexus

Efferent

Origin: dorsal vagus nucleus and nucleus ambiguus (motor to pharyngeal and laryngeal muscles)

Muscles:

Salpingopharyngeus, levator veli, palatinipalatogossus, superior pharyngeal constrictor,

Stylopharyngeus, middle

Pharyngeal constrictor, inferior

Pharyngeal constrictor

Cricothyroid esophagus—circular and longitudinal

Esophageal

Afferent

End: solitary tract nucleus

Visceral afferent including taste, spinal tract, and spinal tract nucleus of trigeminal nerve

Somatic afferent—auricular and meningeal branch

Visceral afferent and dorsal vagal nucleus

Pharynx, larynx

Pulmonary plexus

Cardiac plexus

Gastric, gallbladder, accessory mesenteric artery

The occipital condyle PT point focuses on balancing the central nervous system through the parasympathetic and alignment with the craniosacral rhythm. Structural contact on the occipital condyle is maintained, while incorporating the mastoid process. Muscle contact continues with the trapezius, sternocleidomastoid, and introduces the semispinalis capitis and splenius capitis. Nerve contact is the greater auricular and lesser occipital. Reflex points influence neck and head tension, along with regulatory and bridge channels.

Polarity Therapy

Parasympathetic stimulation. Also to open the foramen magnum and secondary positioning effect on temporal bone (abdominal reflex). Reflex to lumbar and sacral region. Pressure points release of neck and head tension, especially frontal headache, affects consciousness. According to Stone, "The effect is primarily in the energy field through the induced current in the meninges and their relaxation and balance, rather than purely physical."

Structural

Occipital condyle

Mastoid process

Muscles

Trapezius, semispinalis capitis, splenius capitis, sternocleidomastoid

Nerves

Greater auricular, lesser occipital

(A)cupressure

A: Gallbladder 20, 21, 22 Traditional association: important to regulatory and bridge channels

Reflex zone

Dermatome: C2

Longitudinal: 2-4

Music tone

Key of G and A

Applying pressure on the ears influences full body relaxation and stimulation of vitality centers in buttocks and breasts.

Polarity Therapy

The lobe is a major center of vitality. The size of the lobe signifies innate constitutional vitality. The vagus nerve comes to the surface in the middle of the concha.

Soft tissue

Contact is the concha of ear.

Nerves

Contacts are the trigeminal, facial, glossopharyngeal, and vagus nerves.

In the trapezius contact (Figure 12-5), pressure points are contacted to facilitate expansion of the chest and release of gas. Contact is made both with the trapezius fascia and muscle belly. Efferent nerve contact is through the external accessory nerve, while proprioceptive is via C3 and C4 nerves, with cutaneous through C4-C6. Reflex points influence neck and shoulder tension, personal, and cultural tension as well as respiratory functions. Both allopathic medicine and PT

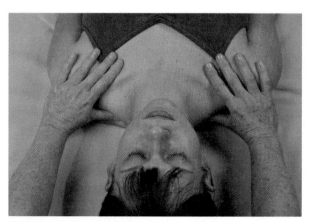

FIGURE 12-5 Trapezins (Air).

interpret pain in the upper shoulders (trapezius) or back as possibly due to gallbladder congestion.

Polarity Therapy
Superior positive pole of diaphragm. Respiratory reflexes flow into arms and down body (right side) and up arms and body (left side)— electromagnetic currents.

Structural
Trapezius fascia
Muscles
Trapezius

Nerves
Efferent—External branch accessory nerve. Proprioceptive via third and fouth spinal nerve
Cutaneous—medial branch C4-C6
(A)cupressure
A: Gallbladder 21. Traditional barometer of personal and cultural tension. Release neck and shoulder tension.Very important release for free passing of strange flow up the neck and through head.

Reflex zone
Dermatome: C4-C6
Longitudinal: 4.5

Music tone
Key of G and F

PT contact in the Belly Rock point is made with the left hand on the upper part of the body and the right hand in the central part of the body (Figure 12-6). This stimulates a general relaxation and balancing of the digestive, respiratory, and nervous systems. The left hand makes contact with the forehead (frontal bone, procerus and epicranius muscles, and trigeminal nerve), while the right hand lies across the abdomen and sympathetic abdominal nerves. Reflex points influence increases in blood and lymphatic circulation through the entire body.

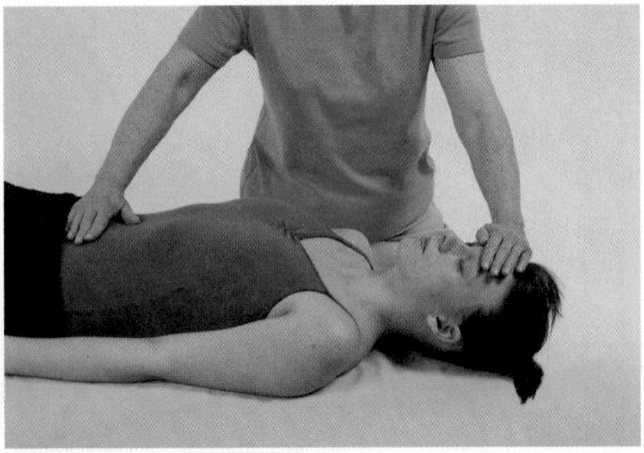

FIGURE 12-6 Belly Rock (Fire and Earth).

Left Hand Position, Forehead

Polarity Therapy
Relaxation by short rhythmic motion. Adjusting polarity of digestive system with respiratory and nervous systems. Right hand (RH) on forehead, left hand (LH) on abdomen.

Structural
Frontal bone, arteries and veins—supraorbital, supratrochlear

Muscles
Procerus, epicranius

Nerves
Ophthalmic division—trigeminal nerve, supraorbital and supratrochlear cutaneous, trigeminal
(N)euro(V)ascular
(N)euro(L)ymphatic
NV: Increases blood circulation through entire body. Holding assists blood from leaving forebrain under stress.

Reflex zone
Dermatome:
Longitudinal: midline, 1-3

Right Hand Position, Abdomen

Polarity Therapy
Structural
Hand placement: R and L lower quadrant midline and slightly out from midline, hypogastric region, interspinous plane, intertubercular plane.
Overlying: greater omentum, small intestine, ileum, sigmoid colon, rectum, ureters L5-S2/3
Depending on size of body—ascending colon, cecum
M)uscle
(L)igament
M: internal abdominal oblique, transverses abdominus, rectus dominus (lower)
L: medial umbilical ligament

Nerves
Iliohypogastric (T11)—lateral cutaneous branch, subcostal (T12)—anterior cutaneous branch, pelvic splanchnic, sacral plexus

Fascia
Linea alba (lower), rectus sheath, Scarpa's subcutaneous (membrane), camper's subcutaneous (fatty), umbilical
(A)cupressure
Conception vessel 4-6
Stomach 21-29
Kidney 12-18
(L)ymph
(N)eurolymphatic

L: Lumbar common iliac, external iliac, inferior epigastric, sacral

N: Triple warmer, kidney, bladder

Reflex zone

Dermatome: T10, 11, 12

Longitudinal: midline, 1-3

Music tone

Key of D

Kidney reflexes in the feet involve reflex stimulation on the feet (Figure 12-7). Stimulation of the kidneys and adrenals is facilitated, balancing the cerebrospinal nervous systems (both parasympathetic and sympathetic) structurally, the cuboid bone is contacted. Muscle contact is with the quadratus plantaris, interosseus, and lumbrical muscles, while tendon involves the flexor digitorum and longus tendon. The nerve contracts are medial and deep plantar nerve. The ankle is part of the air element (chest-shoulders/lungs, kidneys and ankles); both allopathic medicine and PT recognize the retention of fluid in the ankles as indicative of sluggish kidney function.

Polarity Therapy

Superior and inferior location of body ovals and their wireless circuits are found in the feet—as chronic, negative pole, symptomatic reflexes. Flows back to the invigorating center. When stimulating kidney also stimulating adrenals; indicative of balancing parasympathetic and sympathetic nervous systems.

Structural

Cuboid bone

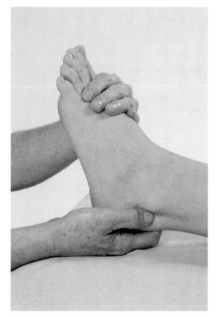

FIGURE 12-7 Kidney reflexes on the foot (Air).

(M)uscles

(T)endon

M: Quadratus plantaris, interosseus, lumbrical 2,3

T: Flexor digitorum longus tendon

Nerves

Medial and deep plantar

Reflex zone

Dermatome: L5, S1, L4

Longitudinal: 4-5

Music tone

Key of E

Reflex stimulation on the feet, particularly the large toe, continues in PT point 10 (Figure 12-8). This stimulation encourages general relaxation and releases the tension, especially to the shoulders and sinuses. Structural contact is made with the medial cuneiform and sesamoid bones. Tendon contact is with the flexor hallucis brevis and longus. The nerve contact occurs with the plantar digital nerve.

Polarity Therapy

Reflex for shoulder (relieving shoulder and neck tension) and sinus (to nose, tongue, speech, and hearing). Helpful with sciatica, circulation, congestion from smoking; hold for drainage.

Structural

Bones: Medial cuneiform, sesamoid

(M)uscles

(T)endon

T: Flexor hallucis brevis and longus

Nerves

Plantar digital

(A)cupressure

Spleen 2 and 3

Reflex zone

Dermatome: L5

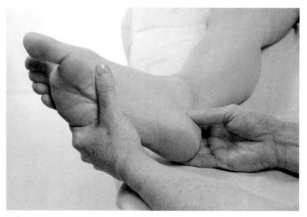

FIGURE 12-8 Ball of Large Toe (Fire).

Longitudinal: 1
Exercise
Scissors kick, squat with simultaneous supraorbital notch contact
Music tone
Key of G and C

Connection with the diaphragm balances the cerebrospinal system with the vital action centers of the ears, breasts, and buttocks (Figure 12-9). Structural connection is with the diaphragmatic pleura below the twelfth rib. Muscle contact is with the diaphragm. Ligament contact involves the medial and lateral arcuate ligaments. The nerve contact corresponds with the phrenicoabdominal nerve. Reflex points influence repressed internalized emotions, panic, anxiety, inhibited expression.

Polarity Therapy
Dense muscle release where center of muscle needs to be emptied to function freely, diaphragm is the functioning neuter pole of life, lifting and activating what is below. Distributes fine energy waves to reach cell tissue. Repolarizing effect and very soothing.

Structural
Below twelfth rib, diaphragmatic pleura
Arteries: phrenic, suprarenal, hemiazygos
Muscles
M: diaphragm
L: medial and lateral arcuate
Nerves
Phrenicoabdominal (branch of phrenic)
(A)cupressure
Repressed internalized emotions
Reflex zone
Dermatome: T8,T9
Longitudinal: 1-5

Exercise
HA breath, HA breath with woodchopper, squat
Music tone
Key of E

Shoulder Point and Hand Web

The PT point connects the upper body and extremities, balancing from the hands to the vital centers. Structurally contact is made in the posterior shoulder (long head of triceps, teres minor, teres major, and infraspinatus) as well as the deep and superficial palmar arch. Contact is made with branches of the brachial plexus (deep and superior lateral brachial, median and ulnar). Reflex points influence the shoulder, scapula, and neck as well as defense energy and regulation of resistance of the exterior regions of the body.

Polarity Therapy
Shoulder is release for arm, hand, and neck (same side). Together with hand web full release through upper body.
Reflexes are to liver, abdominal (digestive), and brachial areas.
Structural
Circumflex scapular artery
Muscles
Triceps—long head, teres minor, teres major, infraspinatus
Nerves
Superior lateral brachial, deep brachial (branches of brachial plexus)
(A)cupressure
Small intestine 10. Traditional association: influences entire shoulder, scapula, and neck. Facilitates the release of positive points of this area. (Figure 12-10)

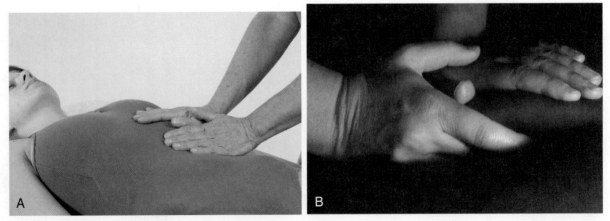

FIGURE 12-9 A. Starting point of diaphragm, B. placement of hands on body.

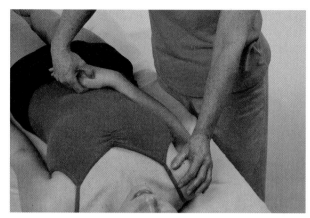

FIGURE 12-10 Shoulder point and hand web.

Indicative for hypertension. Gallbladder 23. Traditional association: "great regulator channel" connecting with stomach, gallbladder, and bladder. Controls the defense energy of the body and regulates resistance as well as exterior regions of the body.

Reflex zone
Dermatome: C4,C5
Longitudinal: 5

Hand

Polarity Therapy
Reflex for sound vibration of speech and hearing; throat, swallowing and touch, feeling, respiration, and circulation (heart and lungs). Hand is functional neutral pole and softtissue contact represents negative poles in thumbs. Invokes diaphragm-abdominal release. Reflexes organs situated laterally and also to negative poles of heels on outside.

Structural
Deep palmar arch
Superficial palmar arch

Nerves
Median ulnar
(branches of brachial plexus)
(A)cupressure
Large intestine 4. Traditional association: general tonic point; "Hegu"—the great eliminator

Reflex zone
Dermatome: C6, 8
Longitudinal: 1-2

Sacral/Perineal Rock

The perineal rock is an integral aspect of Polarity bodywork. Dr. Stone originally called his therapy perineal therapy because this technique was so essential to his theory of energy balancing. Of this treatment he says: "Our aim is to balance the two nervous systems in their bipolar effects with the circulation or the flow of 'prana' in the body."[1] As these two contacts are held changes will take place. The stomach or gallbladder, and sometimes both, will gurgle and drain freely. Vagus and superficial reflexes are released. The patient may sigh and yawn and relax. In clinical practice, the perineal technique may be used at any point in the session. It is also effective in emergency situations when a client is anxious or cannot sleep. It is used to induce parasympathetic dominance and releases both physical and emotional tension. This first phase involves contact on the sacrum and coccyx. The second phase, which is described in Dr. Stone's textbooks, involves direct contact on the perineum and underneath the coccyx. Therapists must be trained for the second phase advanced technique and must work only within their scope of practice. The client should give permission for this technique and feel comfortable with the intimate contact.

To begin the perineal rock, position the client on her left side supported by a small pillow for her head and between the knees. The practitioner sits or stands at her back and simultaneously places the left hand at the foramen magnum to release neck and general tension and the right hand at the sacrum.

Structural
At the upper body includes the foramen magnum and occipital bone. The lower body contacts are on the sacrum, coccyx, termination of the dural sac, and interior hypogastric plexus.

Muscles
Contacts at the upper body include the posterior atlanto-occipito membrane and ligamentum nuchae. The lower body soft tissue contacts include the supraspinal, sacrospinous, posterior sacroiliac, and the sacrococcygeal (lateral and posterior).

Nerves
Involvement includes the medulla oblongata, spinal root accessory at the upper body, the supraspinal, sacrospinous, posterior sacroliac, and the sacrococcygeal (lateral and posterior).

Side Perineals, Lower Contact

Structural
With the sacrum, coccyx termination of the dural sac and interior hypogastric plexus

Ligament
Contact involves the supraspinal, sacrispinous, posterior sacroiliac and the sacrococcygeal (lateral and posterior)

Nerve

Contact is the filum terminalis (internal and external) coccygeal, splanchnic (pelvic and sacral plexus)

Upper Contact: Foramen Magnum and Occipital Condyle

Polarity Therapy

Gentle, rhythmic unlocking of energy blocks. Particularly vital force of emotional locks and frustration. With contact of foramen magnum and occipital condyle releases neck and general tension and promotes relaxation.

Structural

Foramen magnum, occipital bone, meninges, vertebral artery, and meningeal branches of vertebral artery

(F)ascia

(L)igament

F: Posterior atlanto-occipito membrane

L: Ligamentum nuchae

Nerves

Medulla oblongata, spinal root accessory

(A)cupressure

Reflex zone

Music tone

Key of A and B

Lower Contact

Polarity Therapy

Structural

Sacrum, coccyx termination of dural sac, interior hypogastric plexus (artery and vein)

Muscle

(L)ligament

L: Supraspinal, sacrospinous, posterior sacroiliac, lateral and posterior sacrococcygeal

Nerves

Coccygeal, pelvic splanchnic, internal filum terminalis, external filum terminalis, sacral plexus (superior and inferior), gluteal, sciatic posterior, femoral cutaneous, pudenal, sacral splanchnic

Reflex zone

Dermatome: S1-5

Longitudinal: midline 1-3

Gluteal/Trapezius Contact (Fire and Air)

This contact continues the connections between the upper and lower body, facilitating the balance of the central nervous system (via sympathetic nervous system) with the thoracolumbar nervous system, for general relaxation. The upper anatomic contacts are as described previously. The lower structural contact is with the ischial tuberosity. Muscular contact is made with the gluteus maximus and semitendonous muscles, while ligament contact is through the sacrotuberous ligament. Both the sciatic nerve and posterior femoral (cutaneous division) nerves are contacted (Figure 12-11).

Polarity Therapy

The gluteal connections are a respiratory and autonomic sensory reflex for mental, emotional, and nervous tension release. This position balances active spinning chakras. The gentle impulse moves deep by polarizing and balancing of the superior and inferior or the within and without. It is used for balance of respiratory, emotional, and sensory energy current and is a gentle, relaxing technique by use of penetrating prana in breath, which may activate every cell. When applied to both sides it balances full body flow, and releases hip problems and back pain.

Structural

Ischial tuberosity

Muscle

(L)igament

M: Gluteus maximus, semitendonous

L: Sacrotuberous

Nerves

Sciatic, posterior femoral—cutaneous

Reflex zone

Dermatome: S2

Longitudinal: 3

Repeat all unilateral points and holds on the other side of the body.

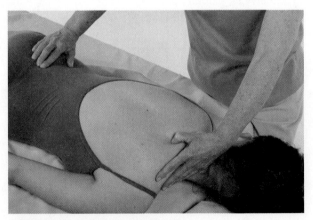

FIGURE 12-11 Gluteal/trapezins contact.

Brain Balance

The cranial hold completing the PT protocol facilitates full body and spinal relaxation, offering final release of tension in the head (Figure 12-12).

Structural

Contact is made with the bony plates of the skull (frontal, parietal, temporal, occipital, and outer wing of sphenoid).

Muscle

Contact is with the auricularis and epicranius (frontal and occipital muscles).

Fascia

Contact is with the galea aponeurotica and the temporalis fascia.

Nerve

Contact is with cranial nerves: trigeminal, occipital, and vagus.

CERTIFICATION REQUIREMENTS

The American Polarity Therapy Association (APTA) oversees the registration process for practitioners at two levels and also registers Polarity educators. Many massage therapy practitioners take elective PT seminars and continuing education classes in polarity therapy without undergoing the registration process. To become an Associate Polarity Practitioner (APP), you must meet the following criteria:

- Become a member of the American Polarity Therapy Association (APTA).
- Be at least 18 years of age by the date of application.
- Have completed at least 155 hours of study in an APTA-approved program that fulfills training

curriculum requirements for Associate Polarity Practitioner.

- A Registered Polarity Practitioner (RPP) must complete at least 675 hours of study in an APTA-approved program.

Areas of study required for Associate and Registered Polarity Practitioners include: theory and basic principles of Polarity, anatomy and physiology (including both the energy model and orthodox model of anatomy), energetic evaluation and integration, Polarity bodywork, communication and facilitation, energetic nutrition, stretching postures, personal Polarity experience sessions received and given with and without clinical supervision including guided feedback, business management, promotion, professional ethics of law, and electives. In order to become a Registered Polarity Educator (RPE), one must be a Registered Polarity Practitioner and receive recommendations from an RPE.

CHAPTER SUMMARY

PT provides a comprehensive approach to biofield touch therapies that incorporates touch, attitudinal healing, nutrition, and exercise. Polarity is a synthesis of the Ayurvedic system of assessment, pressure point therapies and the cranialosteopathic manipulative therapies. It provides three depths of touch making it suitable for people of all ages and degrees of "imbalance." Polarity does not diagnose but rather helps each individual find balance by releasing energy flow throughout the body. Polarity is a principle that understands the cyclical nature of change—of action and reaction—and requires self-care activities, fosters self-awareness, and encourages responsibility for one's health in order to achieve maximum benefit. Polarity is practiced as part of a massage practice or as a separate modality outside of a massage practice.

CASE HISTORIES

■ Case history 1

The client was referred for Polarity by both her psychologist and physician because she was insisting on many surgeries in spite of her physician's objections. Her physician felt that surgery may be a form of self-injury for her, and he referred her for assessment and therapy. She stated that she was considering gastric bypass surgery and then was planning plastic surgery to "tuck" the extra skin. She described chronic, severe bulimia and self-mutilation that led to repeated hospitalizations. She described severe pain in the region of her diaphragm. This pain had led her to several surgeries

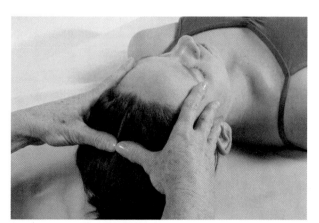

FIGURE 12-12 Brain balance.

including removal of the gallbladder, a portion of her intestines, and additional abdominal exploratory surgeries. She also experienced severe neck pain and had several spinal fusions.

Working as a member of the client's clinical team, I asked what she felt would be helpful and what her goals were for treatment. She requested that I work in the central area of her body to release the tension in her inner diaphragm, which was, she said, "tight as piano wires." I gently applied pressure under her rib cage directly into the area of pain as she breathed deeply. We applied the perineal rock at the start of every session and released tension throughout her shoulders and released those reflexes in the gluteal region. During these sessions, she experienced relaxation saying, "I haven't relaxed this much since I gave up recreational drugs. I didn't know it was possible."

After five 1-hour sessions, the client said that her physical pain had decreased by 50%. The next phase of our work included supporting her self-care capacity through Polarity exercise and nutrition. She was able to release a lot of physical pain. At our last session she said that she had "caught a glimpse into her future"—of reconnecting with her body, experiencing the pleasure of relaxation and deep breathing. She felt optimistic about the future and chose not to go ahead with surgery but to wait and explore her other options.

■ Case history 2

The client was a caregiver who had chronic pain and insomnia. Her baseline assessment revealed that she had frequent headaches, arthritis, heavy snoring, hemorrhoids, heartburn, heart palpitations, hiatus hernia, ulcers, and irritable bowel syndrome. She complained of limited mobility. She was considering her physician's suggestion that she undergo surgery to alleviate her back and shoulder pain. Her Polarity assessment showed significant imbalance in the air element, including anxiety, and inhibited respiration. The trapezius muscles (+ pole of air) were tight, the upper back was contracted, and she had shallow breathing. Chronic stress and exhausted adrenal glands (– pole of air) were confirmed by clinical lab tests, and she complained of stress and poor sleep. She also complained of pain in the ankles (– pole of air), which were also swollen. She had no previous experience receiving any form of massage or PT.

I began focusing on helping her to relax and trust the process. We included several minutes of diaphragmatic breathing at the start of every session. I included points that emphasized the triune pattern of Air element: of the shoulders, the diaphragm and kidneys, and the ankles (see protocol shown above). She received a 60-minute session weekly over the course of 8 weeks. At the end of every session I taught her a new Polarity exercises such as the "HA" breath and advised her to avoid foods that exacerbate stress such as sugar and coffee. During her last session I was able to lift and stretch underneath the scapula while she lay on her side. She stated that her level of pain was significantly better, that she felt less anxious, and that she could move her shoulders. She said she

had learned about the connection between her stress and her back pain and felt that now she had some tools to stay "balanced."

SUGGESTED READINGS

Burger B: *Esoteric anatomy*, Berkeley, Calif, 1998, North Atlantic Books.

Campbell M: *Quinta essentia, the five elements*, Cork, Republic of Ireland, 2003, Masterworks International.

Castellino R: *Polarity therapy paradigm regarding pre-conception, pre-natal and birth imprinting*, 1995, http://www.castellino-training.com/products/.

Chitty J, Muller ML: *Energy exercises*, Berkeley, Calif, 1998, North Atlantic Books.

Gordon R: *Your healing hands*, Berkeley, Calif, 2004, North Atlantic Books.

Korn L, Loytomaki S, Hinman T, Ryser R: Polarity therapy protocol for dementia caregivers—part 2, *Journal of Body work and Movement Therapies* 11:244, 2007.

Lipton E, Bryan AF: *The therapeutic art of polarity: an instructional manual for the associate polarity practitioner*.

Morningstar A: *Ayurvedic cooking for westerners*, Twin Lakes, Wis, 1995, Lotus Press.

Seidman M: *A guide to polarity therapy: the gentle art of hands on-healing*, Berkeley, Calif, 1999, North Atlantic Books.

Siegel A, *Polarity therapy—healing with life energy*, Great Britain, 2006, Masterworks International.

Stone R: *Health building: the conscious art of living well*, Sebastopol, Calif, 1986, CRCS Publications.

REFERENCES

1. Stone R: *Polarity therapy*, vols 1 and 2, new ed, Sebastopol, Calif, 1986, CRCS Publications.
2. Bohm D: *Wholeness and the implicate order*, Boston, 1980, Ark Paperbacks.
3. Association American Polarity Therapy Standards: http://www.polaritytherapy.org/.
4. Korn L: To touch the heart of (the) matter: polarity therapy, *Somatics*, (Spring, 1985) 30–34.
5. Morningstar A: *The ayurvedic guide to polarity therapy hands-on healing: a self-care guide*, Twin Lakes, Wis, 2001, Lotus Press.
6. Salamon E et al: Sound therapy induced relaxation down regulating stress process and pathologies, *Sci Mont* 9:116–121, 2003.
7. Beaulieu J: *Polarity therapy workbook*, High Falls, NY, 1994, BioSonic Enterprises.
8. Oschman JL: *Energy medicine: the scientific basis*, New York, 2000, Harcourt Publishers.
9. Korn L: *Somatic empathy*, Olympia, Wash, 1996, Day Keeper Press.
10. Sills F: *The polarity process*, Berkeley, Calif, 2002, North Atlantic Books.

11. Axt A: Alternative therapies and the pineal gland connection, *Journal of Alternative Therapies* 2:12, 1996.

12. Benford MS et al: Gamma radiation fluctuations during alternative healing therapy, *Alternative Therapies in Health and Medicine* 5:51, 1999.

13. Roscoe JA et al: Treatment of radiotherapy-induced fatigue through a nonpharmacological approach, *Integrative Cancer Therapies* 4:8–13, 2005.

14. Korn L, Ryser R: Designing a polarity therapy protocol: bridging holistic, cultural, and biomedical models of research, *Journal of Bodywork and Movement Therapies* 11:129, 2007.

15. Field T: Attachment as psychobiological attunement: being on the same wavelength. In Reite M, Fields T, editors: *The psychobiology of attachment and separation*, New York, 1985, Academic Press.

16. Korn, L. et al. A randomized trial of a CAM therapy for stress reduction in American Indian and Alaskan native family caregivers. In press. *The Gerontologist*.

MULTIPLE CHOICE TEST QUESTIONS

1) What techniques does Polarity therapy incorporate?
   a) pressure points, rocking
   b) breathing and sound therapy
   c) nutrition and light touch
   d) all of the above

2) Polarity is derived from:
   a) Chinese medicine
   b) hot stone therapy
   c) Ayurvedic medicine
   d) myofascial massage

3) Research on Polarity therapy suggests that it:
   a) doesn't work well on infants
   b) decreases depression
   c) should be used on elders with caution
   d) can aid in fertility

4) Polarity therapy emphasizes improving:
   a) circulation
   b) lymphatic flow
   c) energy flow
   d) diabetic neuropathy

5) How many elements are there in Polarity therapy?
   a) 3
   b) 4
   c) 5
   d) 6

6) Polarity contact with the vagus nerve occurs at the:
   a) sternum
   b) ear concha
   c) hallucis longus
   d) third metacarpal

7) In the Polarity model, the shoulders, kidneys, and ankles are part of the:
   a) air element
   b) fire element
   c) wood element
   d) water element

8) The cradle hold involves contact with the:
   a) occiput
   b) iliac crest
   c) perineum
   d) all of the above

9) When using Polarity to treat asthma, always use:
   a) both hot and cold packs
   b) cold packs only
   c) hot packs only
   d) no hydrotherapy

10) Sound therapy in Polarity uses:
   a) CDs
   b) tuning forks
   c) operatic vibrations
   d) whistles

11) Polarity therapy nutrition is:
   a) vegetarian
   b) paleo-diet
   c) metabolic typing
   d) blood type diet

12) In Polarity, "vitality centers" refer to:
   a) buttocks and breasts
   b) toes and fingers
   c) cranium and scalene
   d) bilateral "Hegu" points

13) Polarity therapy addresses the following:
   a) physical well-being
   b) emotional well-being
   c) spiritual and mental well-being
   d) all of the above

14) Polarity nutrition has two kinds of diets. They are:
   a) cleansing and purging
   b) purging and bone building
   c) health building and cleansing
   d) carnivorous and fasting

15) The sense associated with the water element is:
   a) smell
   b) taste
   c) sound
   d) touch

16) A satvic touch is used for:
    a) hyperactive state
    b) a neutral state
    c) a hypoactive state
    d) all of the above

17) When using the hands to send energy:
    a) the right hand receives and the left hands sends
    b) the left hand sends and the right hand sends
    c) the right hand sends and the left hand receives
    d) the right hand is negative and the left hand is positive

18) Triune function refers to:
    a) providing at least 3 Polarity sessions
    b) balancing positive, neutral, and negative poles
    c) applying pressure at least 3 times
    d) a breathing exercise taught in 3 steps

19) The trapezius is which pole of the diaphragm?
    a) positive
    b) negative
    c) neutral
    d) unrelated

20) How many types of pressure/depths of touch are there in Polarity?
    a) 2
    b) 3
    c) 4
    d) 7

Prenatal Massage

Elaine Stillerman

13

STUDENT OBJECTIVES

Upon completion of this chapter, students will be able to do the following:

- Understand the history of prenatal massage.
- Recognize the appropriate strokes and techniques associated with prenatal massage.
- Understand the physiologic, emotional, and psychologic changes that occur to the expectant mother.
- Learn how prenatal massage affects and benefits the major physiologic systems of the pregnant woman's body and its influence on the in utero environment.
- Understand the contraindications and precautions for prenatal massage and proper client positioning.
- Practice a basic prenatal massage routine.
- Know where to go to get more information, advanced training, and professional certification.

KEY TERMS

Abruptio placentae
Aortocaval compression
Braxton Hicks contractions
Clotting factor
Coagulating factors
Diastasis recti
Doulas
Ectopic pregnancy
Edema
Embryo
Emotional lability
Estrogen
Fetus
Fibrinogenic activity
Fundus
Gestation
Gravida
Homan check or Homan sign

Midwife (midwives, midwifery)
Operculum
Oxytocin
Placenta
Placenta previa
Preeclampsia
Pregnancy-induced hypotension
Progesterone
Relaxin
Stress
Supine hypotensive syndrome
Trimester

Prenatal massage is made up from a wide variety of appropriate massage techniques that treat the common discomforts of pregnancy, support the dynamic physiologic changes the expectant woman undergoes during each of the three **trimesters** of pregnancy, allay **stress,** and prepare the **gravida** (pregnant woman) for labor and childbirth. (Human **gestation,** pregnancy, takes approximately 280 days or 40 weeks, on average. This time frame is subdivided into three distinct phases, called trimesters.)

HISTORY

Massage and touch have a long and respected tradition in women's journey to motherhood. From ancient times to the eighteenth century, the responsibility of birth was the domain of **midwives,** who were poor and uneducated women but highly skilled in their craft. Within their practice, massage played a very important part to speed labor and turn breech presentation. During labor, if the baby was not in its preferred head-down or vertex position, the laboring woman would lie down on her side while the midwife pressed her abdomen with enough pressure to turn the baby.[1]

DVD To better understand concepts in this chapter, watch *Prenatal Massage* video on the **DVD** found at the back of this book.

241

The midwifery practice also included abdominal massage, massage of the legs and back, as well as massage to correct breech presentation.[1]

In some indigenous cultures, the role of the birth assistant was to physically hold and support the laboring woman and to massage her to speed delivery.

An English midwifery text written in the sixteenth century, *The Sloan Manuscript No. 2463*, instructs the midwife to "anoint her hands with the oil of white lilies and then gently stroke the mother's belly about the navel."[2]

In the United States during colonial times, doctors usually had no formal medical training while women, also without formal training, were the primary health care providers and prominent lay practitioners.[3-6] By the end of the eighteenth century, it was accepted that their lack of formal training proved that midwives had no intellectual capacity to learn the "modern" obstetric techniques. Wealthy families chose to go to physicians and hospitals to have their babies, whereas poor women stayed with the midwives. The practice of massage during birth all but disappeared as the status and work of midwives were overtaken by physicians.[7,8]

Starting in the late 1950s, a movement toward more maternal control took hold as the American College of Nurse-Midwives was established in 1955 and La Leche League was founded in 1956. During this time, Drs. Lamaze and Bradley offered women unique pain-relieving techniques for labor.[9]

During the 1960s through 1970s, obstetric technology was replacing the hands-on skills of doctors, but midwifery was enjoying a renaissance. The midwives continued to foster attitudes about maternal control during pregnancy and labor, and in 1980, a new movement reintroduced the time-honored tradition of prenatal massage to massage practitioners, childbirth educators, **doulas** ("hand maiden" or "servant" in Greek; a labor or postpartum support professional), and the obstetric community.[10] As evidence-based studies continue to validate and reinforce the beneficial effects of prenatal massage, pregnant women, as well as the once-reticent medical community, are embracing massage as an integral part of their prenatal care.[11]

APPROPRIATE STROKES AND TECHNIQUES FOR PRENATAL MASSAGE

Appropriate strokes and techniques for prenatal massage are those that respect and support the dynamic physiologic changes the pregnant woman undergoes. They also must recognize the specific precautions and contraindications that are based upon these physiologic adaptations.[11] Practitioners should review their techniques to determine if certain adjustments or substitutions have to be made to be safe during pregnancy. These changes may include positioning modifications, stroke elimination, or technique adaptations.

Since pregnant women should not lie flat on their backs after the first trimester, positioning modifications have to be made. Positioning the client on the treatment table in a recumbent or semisitting position with her torso at an angle at least 45° to 70° and her legs and feet elevated eliminates the dangers of **pregnancy-induced hypotension** (a decrease of maternal blood pressure cutting off blood and oxygen to the fetus).

Also essential to appropriate prenatal care is the understanding that all deep massage must be avoided on a woman's legs after the first trimester and up to 3 months postpartum to prevent dislodging blood clots. The most effective and safest modality to use on her legs is manual lymphatic drainage.

Here is a list of several techniques that are safe during pregnancy, although some may need to be refashioned to some extent while others that are not listed may be employed as long as they respect the anatomy and physiology of pregnancy and the contraindications and precautions listed in this chapter:

- Applied kinesiology evaluates the body function through dynamic muscle testing.[12]
- Craniosacral therapy is a gentle manipulation that locates and corrects imbalances in the craniosacral system, which is made up of the brain, spinal cord, cerebrospinal fluid, dural membrane, cranial bones, and sacrum. The effect of this system is realized to a large extent by the body's innate healing and self-correcting abilities. It was developed by Dr. John Upledger.[13] Side-lying is also a comfortable alternative for craniosacral therapy positioning.
- Energy work, such as Polarity therapy and Reiki, work with the human energy biofield to encourage balance.[13]
- Gravitational or positional release stretches tightened muscles by placing the affected limb in the position of the tension and relies upon the weight of the limb (or gravity) to lengthen the shortened muscle fibers.
- Joint mobilization takes each joint through its full range of motion to locate resistance

or tension. The joint is moved to a position opposing the tightness until there is a release.[13]

- Lomilomi is an ancient Hawaiian technique brought to westerners' attention most notably by Aunty Margaret K. Machado.[13]
- Manual lymphatic drainage is a specific form of physiotherapy used to empty and decongest lymph pathways.[13] This light stroking (10 to 30 grams of pressure) should always be used on a pregnant woman's legs (even during the first trimester as a safety precaution and for 3 months postpartum) to prevent dislodging blood clots and reduce edema of the legs. Manual lymph drainage can also be applied to a pregnant woman's arms and hands if she is experiencing carpal tunnel syndrome, de Quervain's syndrome, or swelling. Manual lymph drainage follows a specific protocol of emptying the proximal channels of a limb first, followed by the medial and distal. The light pressure is always toward the heart for maximum drainage.
- Myofascial release uses slow stretching movements to evaluate and release fascial restrictions.
- Passive and active exercises help relax and strengthen muscles and joints by activating stretch receptors. Passive movements are performed by the practitioner while the client relaxes; active exercises require the client's participation.
- Proprioceptive work helps balance and strengthen the muscles by relaxing hypertonic muscles and strengthening hypotonic muscles. Balance is achieved by working either the spindle cells found within the belly of the muscles or the Golgi tendon organs located in the tendons close to the musculotendinous junction.[13]
- Reflexology uses various methods of touch to stimulate specific points on the hands or feet that reflex to particular organs, to maintain optimum health and restore energy throughout the body.[13] Attention must be paid, however, to the amount of pressure used on the feet during pregnancy: 10 to 30 grams of pressure is the recommended pressure, but the points can be held longer to achieve treatment goals.
- Shiatsu and acupressure are ancient techniques of traditional Chinese medicine (traditional Oriental medicine) that press on particular points, called tsubos, along energy pathways, called meridians, to release stagnated energy thought to create "dis-ease." This type of

bodywork uses ischemic compression, which must be avoided on a pregnant woman's legs after the first trimester (I suggest avoiding it entirely) and for the first 3 months after the baby is born.
- Strain/counterstrain is a technique designed to relieve muscle dysfunction and pain. A position of relief is found and held for 90 seconds. This technique was developed by Dr. Lawrence Jones.[13]
- Swedish massage increases circulation, brings nutrition to muscles, speeds up waste absorption, and relieves pain and discomfort. The strokes of Swedish massage include effleurage, petrissage (kneading), friction, vibration, and tapotement. This technique was formalized by Dr. Per Henrik Ling. Swedish massage is contraindicated on a pregnant woman's legs after the first trimester and for the first 3 months postpartum.
- Tragerwork is a way of teaching movement reeducation and neuromuscular release. It was developed by Dr. Milton Trager, who espoused educating the client rather than treating her.[13]
- Trigger point release compresses the trigger points, which are highly sensitive areas within muscles, ligaments, tendons, and fascia that can cause referred pain elsewhere in the body. This technique was pioneered by Dr. Janet Travell and popularized by Bonnie Prudden.[13]
- Tui Na is an ancient Chinese system that uses a variety of techniques (grasping, rolling, pressing, rubbing, vibrating, etc.) to treat injuries of the soft and connective tissue and balance qi energy.

There are other bodywork modalities that may be appropriate for the pregnant woman. At all times, however, proper positioning is important to maintain, and techniques on the legs must be light-handed, superficial, and flow toward her heart.

PHYSIOLOGIC, EMOTIONAL, AND PSYCHOLOGIC CHANGES OF PREGNANCY

Physiologic Changes of Pregnancy

In order to provide the most appropriate and supportive bodywork for a pregnant client, it is important to understand the dynamic changes that occur during her (approximate) 40 weeks of pregnancy. For a more detailed examination and exploration of these changes, please refer to my book *Prenatal Massage: A Textbook* of *Pregnancy, Labor, and Postpartum Bodywork* (Mosby, 2008). Approximately 1 week after conception, the uterus starts to form a rudimentary **placenta** ("flat cake" in Latin), or afterbirth, that is a specialized organ for maternal-fetal gas and nutrient exchange. As this organ grows, increased levels of hCG (human chorionic gonadotropin) are released into the maternal blood supply and by the second week after conception, sufficient amounts can be detected in the mother's urine to confirm the pregnancy.

After 3 weeks, she notices that she missed her menstrual cycle and she might actually be aware of certain physiologic changes such as breast sensitivity or soreness and fatigue. Before the first 12 weeks of gestation the conceptus is called an **embryo.** After 3 months, the embryo is referred to as a **fetus.**

Musculoskeletal System

Dramatic changes occur to the pregnant woman's musculoskeletal system. These changes are mediated by an increase in steroid hormones that are initially secreted by her ovaries and subsequently by the placenta. In the early weeks and months of pregnancy, hormonal changes regulate her physical adaptations. As her pregnancy progresses, postural alterations and shifting result from the increased size and bulk of her uterus and by the relaxation of her joints.[14-16]

- As pregnancy progresses, her center of gravity shifts forward, creating an anterior pelvic tilt and increased lumbar spine compression. The natural lordotic curve is exaggerated because of **progesterone, relaxin** (hormones that support the pregnancy and soften connective tissue to make room for expanded uterine growth), and the weight of the gravid uterus on the intravertebral disks.[16]
- As she walks, she leans backwards to counterbalance her anterior shift in gravity. Walking in this position is often accompanied by lateral rotation of her shoulders. This further compresses the joints and muscles of the lumbar spine. Large breasts and stooped shoulders exacerbate lumbar, dorsal, and cervical spinal curves.[15] In this position, the supporting pelvic ligaments, particularly those of the lumbosacral, symphysis pubis, and sacroiliac joints, are overstressed. (When she sits or sleeps in a side-lying position, she medially rotates her shoulders creating myofascial restrictions in the chest.)
- Cervical protraction often contributes to weakness, numbness and/or tingling in the fingers and hands and carpal tunnel or de Quervain's syndromes (Figure 13-1).[15,17]

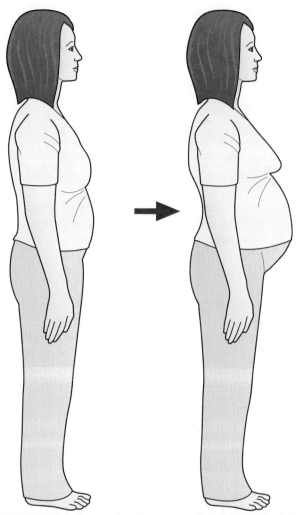

FIGURE 13-1 A, Posture of early pregnancy. **B,** Exaggerated lordotic curve in later pregnancy. (From Fraser D, Cooper M: *Myles' textbook for midwives,* Edinburgh, 2003, Churchill Livingstone.)

- To make room for the growing uterus and fetus, a pregnant woman's rib cage expands anteriorly and laterally as much as 2 to 3 inches.
- A pregnant woman's pelvis widens and her hips laterally rotate to accommodate her widening pelvis. To maintain an erect posture, and because of the hypertension in the hamstrings caused by their anterior pelvic tilt, women hyperextend their knees and their plantar vaults (medial arches) may flatten. Most women complain of backaches after the fifth month.[16]
- Leg cramps often occur in the second half of the pregnancy and are caused by maternal nutritional deficiencies (calcium, magnesium, potassium, and phosphorus) as well as postural adaptations. Nearly 10% of pregnant women experience restless

leg syndrome right after getting into bed at night. Although the reasons for this are not clear, it may be associated with anemia.[18]

- **Estrogen,** the female hormone formed in the ovaries, and relaxin affect the composition of cartilage and ligamentous structures, particularly the pelvis, allowing them to soften and loosen in preparation for labor and childbirth. However, this causes the pelvis to become hypermobile, resulting in additional lumbar instability and muscle and ligament strain and discomfort.[16]

- Another adaptation that has far-reaching effects on the pregnant woman's posture is the changes to her abdominal core muscles: the rectus abdominis, internal and external obliques, and the transverse abdominis muscles. As the uterus expands and becomes an abdominal organ, the pregnant woman's core muscles stretch, weaken, lose tone, and separate adding to lumbar instability and increased lower back pain. Stretching of the round ligaments (the pair is located at the sides of the uterus) may also add to lower backaches.[16] The separation along the linea alba of the rectus abdominis muscle is called a **diastasis recti.** During pregnancy, it helps if the pregnant client recruits the most intrinsic abdominal muscle, the transverse abdominis, when lifting heavy objects or during exercise to support the heavy uterus, minimize the diastasis recti, and thereby encourage a more aligned posture, stabilize the lower spine, reduce backaches, and facilitate labor (Box 13-1 and Figure 13-2).[19-23]

After reviewing the musculoskeletal changes and adaptations of pregnancy, it is fair to conclude that the majority of the musculature in the anterior of her body becomes hypotonic and weak as pregnancy progresses (except for the pectoralis muscles, which become hypertonic as a result of medial shoulder rotation) and the musculature in her back becomes hypertonic and constricted. The massage practitioner's goals, therefore, would be to improve the balance of the pregnant client's musculature by shortening and strengthening the intrinsic and extrinsic muscles in the front of her body (with the exception of the pectorals, which are already shortened and need to be elongated) and stretching and elongating the muscles on the back of her body.

Cardiovascular System

The dramatic changes that occur within the cardiovascular system (heart, veins, arteries, and blood) support

---

BOX 13-1 **Proper Prenatal Exercises**

Since all abdominal muscles have a common attachment in the linea alba of the rectus abdominis where the separation occurs, exercises that concentrate on recruiting the transverse abdominis, or the deepest abdominal muscle, will decrease the diastasis recti, encourage lower back stability, and minimize the common discomforts of pregnancy associated with poor posture. Some of these exercises include:

- Pelvic tilts done either lying down, standing, or kneeling. Tilt the pelvis backward to shorten the abdominal muscles and elongate the lumbar spine. Bring the transverse inwards by moving the umbilicus to the spine. The client should breathe normally while holding the stretch to 10 seconds. Repeat up to 10 times.

- Sit in a chair or crossed-legged on the floor. While breathing normally, bring the belly halfway back toward the spine. This is the starting position. From this position, contract the transverse all the way back to the spine and hold for a count of 25. Count out loud and breathe normally. That is one set. Relax only to the starting position after each count of 25 and repeat a total of 10 sets. Do this several times throughout the day.

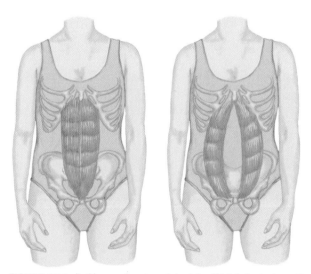

FIGURE 13-2 *(Left)* normal rectus abdominis; *(Right)* diastasis recti of pregnancy. (From McKinney ES: *Maternal-child nursing,* St. Louis, 2005, Saunders.)

---

normal maternal metabolism and the increased needs of the pregnancy, and provide for fetal growth.

- As the pregnancy progresses, the increase in blood volume is commensurate with the woman's weight, the number of previous pregnancies and births she has had, and whether this is a single or multiple birth.[24] Blood volume starts to increase as early as the sixth week of pregnancy and continues through the end, with an average increase of 30% to 50%. This amount will increase for a multiple pregnancy.[25]

- The extra blood volume is accommodated by a slightly larger heart. The cardiac muscle can increase in size as much as 12%, and the mother's heart is pushed upward and rotated toward the left as the diaphragm is compressed by the enlarged uterus.[15,24] These changes reverse after the pregnancy.
- All blood components increase as a result of the additional blood volume. This increase is comprised of additional serum protein, neutrophils, enzymes, plasma, platelets, **clotting factor** (to prevent excessive blood loss and hemorrhaging during and after labor—this is also known as **fibrinogenic activity**), albumin, and white and red blood cells. Since plasma levels increase earlier during pregnancy than do red blood cells, hemoglobin and hematocrit levels drop, sometimes resulting in iron-deficiency anemia.

- During pregnancy, maternal blood pressure, which generally lowers by 10%, can be affected by stress and the client's position.[19] Brachial pressure is highest when she is sitting and lowest when she is side-lying. Supine positioning can cause dangerous hypotension, called **supine hypotensive syndrome** or **aortocaval compression,** as the fetus and heavy uterus compress the vena cava.[14] After only 4 to 5 minutes lying on her back, a reflex bradycardia occurs and heart production is cut in half. Women feel faint, dizzy, short of breath, or nauseous. (This is why a pregnant woman should never be positioned on her back without appropriate elevation and support.) Turning her to her left side will usually decrease the symptoms and restore cardiac output to normal (Figure 13-3).

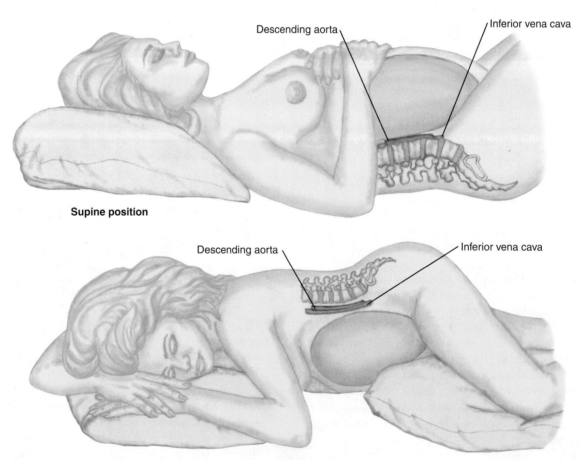

Descending aorta Inferior vena cava

Supine position

Descending aorta Inferior vena cava

Right lateral position

FIGURE 13-3 (Top) Supine hypotensive syndrome. The weight of the uterus compresses the inferior vena cava and descending aorta. (Bottom) A lateral recumbent position corrects supine hypotension. (From McKinney ES: *Maternal-child nursing*, St. Louis, 2005, Saunders.)

• As pregnancy progresses, blood flow to her lower extremities is slowed due to sluggish venous return, increased venous pressure, and the additional pressure in the veins of her legs, vulva, rectum, and pelvis.[26] This often leads to **edema,** or swelling, or varicose veins of the legs and vulva and hemorrhoids.[27]

• hCG and prolactin, the nursing hormone, suppress maternal immune response, which results in a decrease in the production of white blood cells' ability to fight infection, particularly viral infections. This decrease in immune function starts in the tenth week and remains at this level until the baby is born.[28]

• As a protective mechanism against excessive blood loss at birth and during early postpartum, there is an increase in **coagulating factors** (fibrinogenic activity) and fibrinogen with a decrease in anticoagulants, or fibrinolytics.[15,29,30] (This activity continues throughout the first few months of postpartum, thereby affecting the bodyworks you choose to employ.) The decrease in anticoagulants along with vasodilation contributes to a five- to six-fold increase in the risk of thromboembolism in pregnancy (and early postpartum).[29,31] Blood clots may also develop because of the weight of the uterus slowing femoral and iliac circulation, sluggish blood flow, greater blood volume, and higher levels of progesterone relaxing smooth muscle fibers. Blood clots may be present in any vein but are more prevalent in the deep veins, where blood flow is restricted and generally more stagnant. During pregnancy, the veins that might harbor these thromboemboli or deep vein thromboses are the iliac, femoral, and saphenous veins of the inner thigh and calf.[31]

If clots do aggregate within the deeper vessels, the client's legs might feel sore and achy, but these clots do not pose any major health treat. Illness and death during pregnancy from venous thromboembolism occur in 1 in 1000 to 1 in 2000 pregnant and postpartum women.[32,33] During pregnancy, the clots most frequently begin in the veins of the calf muscles or in the iliofemoral portion of the deeper venous system, with the left leg being most susceptible.[34-36]

The symptoms of thrombi are localized heat, swelling, reddening, muscle contraction over the site of the clot(s), increased edema of the limb, sensitive dermatome above the clot, and very painful legs. Thrombi are also often asymptomatic, which is another reason all deep strokes are avoided on the legs during pregnancy and up to 3 months postpartum.

The bodyworker must recognize the potential danger when massaging the legs of a pregnant woman (or new mother), even in her first trimester, and always assess the legs for clots before beginning the treatment and use appropriate, light lymphatic drainage at all times (Box 13-2).

By the third trimester, pregnant women have as much as 40% or more interstitial fluid resulting in more swelling in the lower extremities. Restricted femoral and iliac circulation, the weight of the uterus, myofascial restrictions of the pelvis, and gravity all work

---

BOX 13-2 **Pretreatment Evaluations for Blood Clots**

Prior to every treatment during pregnancy and for up to 3 months postpartum, two evaluations should be performed to check for the presence of any clots.

• Before placing any pillows between your client's legs in a side-lying position, gently move your hand down the back of both legs feeling for any localized heat, swelling, redness, muscle contraction, or sensitive skin.

• The other assessment involves her legs slightly flexing her legs and then passively dorsiflexing her feet to test for the presence of thrombi in her calves (the greater saphenous vein). This examination is called the **Homan check** or **Homan sign** (Figure 13-4).[15,37]

Those clients who are most at risk at developing thromboembolism are sedentary women or those confined to bed rest, women over 30, overweight women, those who suffer from autoimmune diseases such as lupus, and those having their fourth or more child.[38]

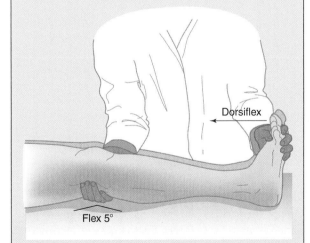

FIGURE 13-4 The Homan check or Homan sign to test for the presence of blood clots in the calf. (From Leifer G: *Maternity nursing: an introductory text,* ed 9, St. Louis, 2005, Saunders.)

against efficient lymph reabsorption. Although the swelling is generally not a health concern, the pregnant woman's legs feel stiff and achy from this fluid retention. However, for nearly 25%, this swelling can present a problem. Swelling during pregnancy is considered to be pitting edema if a small depression remains after finger pressure is applied to the swollen area.

An essential pretreatment evaluation tests for pitting edema and **preeclampsia,** a serious, often life-threatening hypertensive condition that occurs after the twentieth week of pregnancy. Symptoms may include a sudden spike in blood pressure, pitting edema or extreme swelling, headaches or migraines—often accompanied by "floaters"—and proteinuria in the urine. Preeclampsia and other hypertensive disorders of pregnancy are responsible for at least 76,000 maternal and infant deaths each year.[19] Pregnancies complicated by preeclampsia or eclampsia have high maternal and perinatal death rates[38] (Box 13-3).

Respiratory System

There are many adaptations during pregnancy to the respiratory system.

- The increased blood volume and cardiac output increase pulmonary blood flow.[39]
- Nasal congestion, nose bleeds, and enlarged vocal cords are all common during pregnancy.[40] Almost 70% of healthy women develop pregnancy-induced dyspnea, or shortness of breath, in their first or second trimesters.[39] To compensate, some women hyperventilate and become dizzy.
- As her uterus grows, the **fundus,** or the top of her uterus, compresses the respiratory diaphragm so that it is elevated from its normal position. The rib cage widens anteriorly and laterally 2 to 3 inches, often resulting in thoracic discomfort. Inspiration becomes deeper, allowing for 30% to 40% increase in tidal volume, and oxygen use increases by 15% to 20%.[14-16]
- By the third trimester, breathlessness is not unusual. As a result of her larger breasts and side-lying sleeping, shoulder medial rotation can create myofascial restrictions throughout the rib cage.

Gastrointestinal System

One of the earliest and most recognized signs of pregnancy is nausea, or morning sickness, affecting 50% to 90% of pregnant women. It generally goes away by the second trimester, although some women can suffer throughout their pregnancies, as levels of hCG decrease.

BOX 13-3 Pretreatment Evaluation for Pitting Edema

The test for pitting edema is performed on both legs prior to the treatment, before pillows are placed between the client's legs in a side-lying position. Press just above her ankle and slowly count to five. Remove your finger and wait 10 to 30 seconds. If the indentation does not fill in, or if the ischemic region has not become red again, do not proceed with the massage (Figure 13-5).

Preeclampsia can also be seen in the upper torso, hands, face, or entire body during the first or second trimester. The client's face may appear quite swollen, even bulbous, and the swelling may contribute to hand and arm edema preventing her from making a fist at any time during the day. If these symptoms are present, or if the client tests positive for pitting edema in either or both legs, massage is contraindicated and she should seek immediate medical attention.

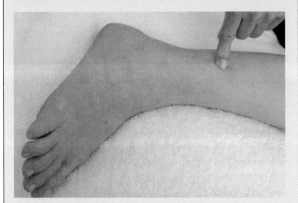

FIGURE 13-5 To test for pitting edema, press your finger above the client's ankle for a count of 5. If the impression does not disappear after 10 to 30 seconds, do not massage. (From Stillerman E: *Prenatal massage: a textbook of pregnancy, labor, and postpartum bodywork,* St. Louis, 2008, Mosby.)

- As the uterus continues to grow, her visceral organs are displaced and progesterone slows down the function of smooth muscle, affecting the gastrointestinal tract, uterus, ureters, and blood vessels.[24,41] This contributes to sluggish motility of the stomach contents and peristaltic action of the intestines. The results are heartburn and constipation.
- Other discomforts may include esophageal reflex and intestinal gas. Progesterone also causes the gallbladder to become more flaccid, increasing bile volume storage and and causing a slower emptying

time. Some women complain of itchy skin in late pregnancy, which may result from excessive amounts of bile salts.

Urinary (Renal) System

- Urination becomes very frequent during the first trimester because of the pressure of the uterus on the bladder. The urge to urinate lessens as the fundus rises out of the pelvis at the fourth month but returns in the last trimester as the enlarged uterus compresses the bladder and squeezes it against the symphysis pubis. As the fetus grows, the bladder is displaced upward and flattened.
- Even though more waste is excreted, the volume of urine remains the same, making the urinary system more efficient during pregnancy. The adaptations of the urinary system continue for about 6 weeks postpartum.

Reproductive System

- During pregnancy, ovulation and menstruation cease.
- The uterus undergoes dramatic changes during pregnancy. By term, this $7.5 \times 5 \times 2.5$ cm pear-shaped organ weighing 2 ounces expands to a $30 \times 22.5 \times 20$ cm housing for the fetus, placenta, amniotic sac, and amniotic fluid and weighs over 2 pounds.[14,43]
- The uterine lining thickens to support the pregnancy, and this muscle actively contracts throughout the pregnancy to help circulate the blood through the placenta and strengthen for labor. These contractions are called **Braxton Hicks contractions.** As the pregnancy progresses, the uterus displaces from the pelvis to the abdomen.
- The cervix, the opening of the uterus, stays closed during pregnancy and is filled with a mucous plug, the **operculum,** to protect the fetus against bacterial infections. This mucous plug is expelled as the cervix softens and effaces (shortens) for labor or during labor.[44]
- Blood flow to the vagina and vulva increases.

Endocrine System

The most dramatic adaptation of the endocrine system is the creation and growth of the placenta as an endocrine organ.

- The placenta synthesizes, elaborates, produces, and stores numerous hormones that regulate maternal and fetal development.[16] The increase in hormones is essential to the progress and continuation of the pregnancy. The corpus luteum of the ovaries initiates most of the hormonal production until the placenta assumes that vital role.
- The adrenal and pituitary glands increase in size and hormonal production.

Nervous System

- Sciatic nerve pain, numbness, or sensory changes in the lower extremities are caused mostly by compression of the pelvic nerves and venous stasis by the enlarged uterus rather than nerve damage.
- Carpal tunnel or de Quervain's syndrome may be caused by a protracted cervical spine, swelling involving peripheral nerves, and flexor/extensor retinaculum softening from the hormone relaxin.[45]
- Poor posture contributes to tingling of the hands, and neuromuscular conditions, such as leg and thigh cramps, or tetany, may result from insufficient maternal calcium, magnesium, and potassium stores.

Integumentary System

Among the earliest signs of a confirmed pregnancy are the changes to pigmentation.

- The nipples and areolae darken very early, and skin darkening is observed from the third month on in 90% of pregnant women.[43]
- Other skin changes may include itching, rashes, skin tags, hives, acne (improved or worsened), increased hair growth, angiomas (vascular spiders), palmar erythema (reddening of the palms of the hands or soles of the feet), the development of a linea nigra (a darkened line over the diastasis recti), the "mask of pregnancy," or chloasma, and stretch marks.

Emotional and Psychologic Changes During Pregnancy

The news of a pregnancy changes a woman's—a family's—life forever. It is rather common, however, for women to undergo a myriad of diverse and even conflicting emotions about their pregnancies, especially during the first weeks. **Emotional lability,** or uncontrollable, unpredictable mood swings, are part of the early experience.[15]

Stress can also have profound and long-lasting effects on the pregnancy. Some of the harmful effects might be low birthweight and premature labor, delayed infant neuromotor development, weakened effectiveness of **oxytocin** (the hormone of mother love, calmness, and uterine contractions), prolonged labor or a failure to progress, uterine vasoconstriction, increased labor pain, elevated maternal heart rate and blood pressure, higher incidences of miscarriage, obstetric complications, increased stress hormones, unhealthy lifestyle habits, and depression.[46,47]

The shocking number of clinically depressed pregnant women dispels the idea that all pregnancies are happy or wanted. On average, it is estimated that 10% to 20% of pregnant women are depressed and are at greater risk for postpartum depression.[48]

Other emotional issues that may come up for some pregnant women include her body image, the effects of the pregnancy on her partner and other family members, or if she is a survivor of childhood or domestic abuse. Pregnancy can be a defining experience for some women and it is important to recognize, affirm, and respect all that she is feeling.

BENEFICIAL EFFECTS OF PRENATAL MASSAGE

In addition to the numerous beneficial effects of massage on the pregnant woman's changing physiology, its stress-reducing benefits are of paramount importance to insure a healthy pregnancy and birth outcome. Massage has a powerful ability to sedate and restore the nervous system.[49] The relaxation provided by a therapeutic massage is further enhanced by the pain-reducing, or analgesic, effect it provides.[49] Beta-endorphins and serotonin, a neurotransmitter, are secreted during a massage and work together to inhibit the central nervous system and produced a relaxed, feel-good result.[49,50]

A study by the Touch Research Institute proved decreased anxiety levels, stress hormones, and obstetric complications in women who received massages regularly during their pregnancies.[51] When you consider the sequelae of stress during pregnancy, a nurturing massage can provide considerable benefit to the expectant mother and her baby.

Massage can also have a major impact on treating the common discomforts of pregnancy and supporting the numerous physiologic adaptations the pregnant woman's body makes.

- Massage can decrease chronic muscle tension, restore balance to overstretched muscles, release tension in contracted muscles, normalize joint range of motion, reduce pain, and support improved postural alignment.[49,52,53]
- Massage can speed up sluggish circulation, enhance lymph absorption, relieve congested vessels, normalize blood pressure, and ease varicose veins.[49,52,54]
- The deep relaxation of massage fosters deeper breathing and can often ease several of the respiratory conditions associated with pregnancy, such as dyspnea or shortness of breath.
- Massage can stimulate peristaltic activity of the intestines and relieve constipation and intestinal gas.
- Massage prepares the expectant woman physically, emotionally, and mentally for labor.
- Massage elevates mood and encourages loving maternal care.[11]

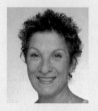

CONTRAINDICATIONS AND PRECAUTIONS OF PRENATAL MASSAGE

Practitioners must understand that it is equally important to know which bodywork modalities are appropriate to use during a client's pregnancy as well as when massage is contraindicated or when local precautions have to be exercised.

Massage should never be provided if your pregnant client exhibits any of the following:

- Uterine bleeding or staining
- Premature or preterm labor; labor between 20 to 37 weeks is considered preterm labor
- Pitting edema
- A sudden spike or elevation of blood pressure, or any hypertensive condition
- **Placenta previa,** a placenta that is attached to the lower segment of the uterus and occludes or encroaches on the margin of the cervix
- **Abruptio placentae,** separation of the placenta from the uterine wall
- **Ectopic pregnancy,** implantation of the embryo outside the uterine cavity
- Severe abdominal pain
- Throbbing or migraine headaches
- If she hasn't felt fetal movement in 8 to 10 hours[11]

Other precautions to be aware of include:

- Avoid use of electric heating blankets, pads, hot stones, or hydrocollators.
- Avoid all and any deep strokes on her legs throughout her pregnancy and for up to 3 months postpartum.

- Wait 1 week after (invasive) genetic testing (amniocentesis or chorionic villi sampling).
- Make sure your client is not hungry.
- Ask permission before massaging her abdomen or breasts.
- Never place a pregnant woman flat on her back. Make sure her upper torso is elevated from her hips at an angle between 45° and 70° and her legs are elevated (Figure 13-6).
- Don't hyperextend her joints.
- Make sure all pretreatment evaluations are performed before every massage.
- Clients who are prescribed bed rest may be able to receive a massage depending on the reasons they are confined to bed. If the condition is not a contraindicated one (see above), the massage should last ½ hour, she should be lying on her left side, and there is to be no leg or foot massage since incidence of blood clots increases appreciably.[11]

There are a number of acupuncture points where deep, protracted pressure must be avoided during pregnancy. In most instances, uterine contractions may result if pressure on these points is too deep or held too long. All the points are bilateral:

- Kidney 1, located on the soles of both feet midway across the ball of the feet down from the middle toe, draws energy downward (Figure 13-7*A*).
- Large intestine 4, located in the webbing of the thumbs and index fingers, may start uterine contractions (Figure 13-7*B*).
- Spleen 6, located approximately 3 finger-widths above the medial ankles under the tibias, may start the onset of uterine contractions (Figure 13-7*C*).

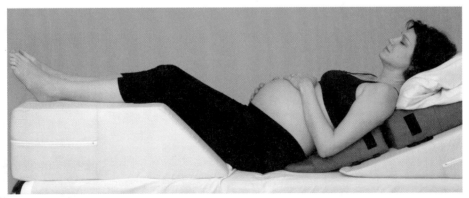

FIGURE 13-6 In a semisitting position, make sure your client's upper torso is elevated from her hips at an angle between 45° and 70° and her legs are elevated. (From Stillerman E: *Prenatal massage: a textbook of pregnancy, labor, and postpartum bodywork,* St. Louis, 2008, Mosby.)

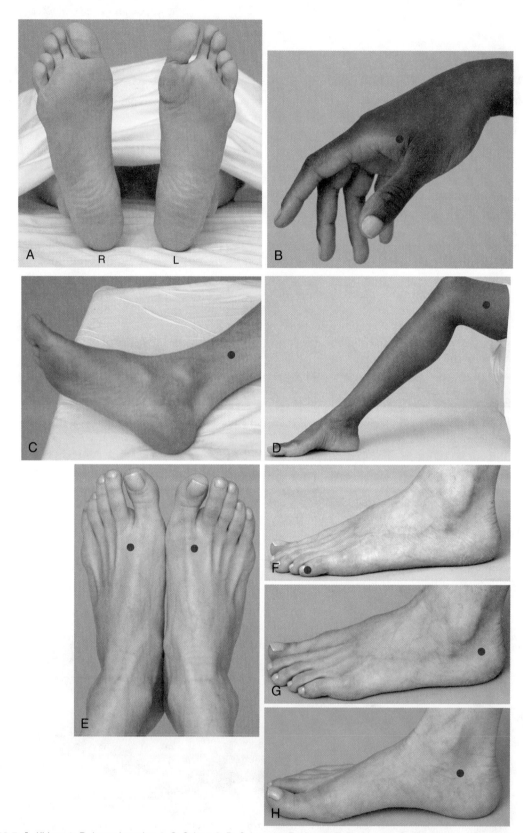

FIGURE 13-7 A, Kidney 1; **B,** Large intestine 4; **C,** Spleen 6; **D,** Spleen 10; **E,** Liver 3; **F,** Bladder 67; **G,** Ovary reflex; **H,** Uterus reflex; (From Stillerman E: *Prenatal massage: a textbook of pregnancy, labor, and postpartum bodywork,* St. Louis, 2008, Mosby.)

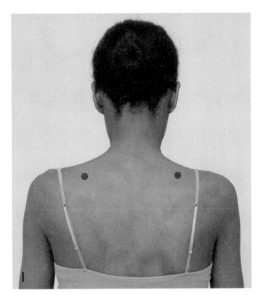

FIGURE 13-7 *cont'd* **I,** Gallbladder 21.

- Spleen 10, located approximately 2 inches above the patellae at the middle of the belly of the vastus medialis, may release the contents of the uterus and may stimulate uterine bleeding (Figure 13-7*D*).
- Liver 3, located between the first and second toes, 2 finger-widths proximal to the web, may encourage uterine bleeding, release excessive fluid, and begin the onset of labor (Figure 13-7*E*).
- Bladder 67, located at the lateral side of the tips of the small toes, turns fetal presentation and is used to speed up a difficult labor (Figure 13-7*F*).
- Ovary reflex or bladder 61, located midway between the lateral anklebones and heels, stimulates the ovaries (Figure 13-7*G*).
- Uterus reflex, or kidney 5, located midway between the medial anklebones and heels, stimulates the uterus (Figure 13-7*H*).
- Gallbladder 21, located on the highest points of the trapezius, slightly to the rear, may cause the secretion of prolactin (the nursing hormone) and oxytocin, thereby encouraging uterine contractions (Figure 13-7*I*).[11]

BASIC PRENATAL MASSAGE ROUTINE

Author's note: In order to provide the most effective and appropriate massage to your pregnant clients, it is important to take advanced training that deals specifically with the physiologic needs of this population. What follows is a simplified version of a basic massage routine.

After doing the pretreatment evaluations and then positioning your client comfortably on the massage table in a side-lying position, you are ready to begin your massage. Make sure that the pillows between her legs are high enough to keep her hip, knee, and ankle on the same horizontal level. Position other pillows under her neck, at the small of her back, under the abdomen, or in front of her chest as needed (Figure 13-8). The correct use of the body support system is also safe in prone and supine positions throughout the entire pregnancy, or as long as the client is comfortable.

Remember that the direction of your strokes is horizontal to encourage elongation of compressed muscles and joints. Use as much pressure as your client prefers except on her legs where the pressure remains a constant 10 to 30 grams.

- Start with a pelvic tilt. Place one hand over your client's sacrum and the other hand on her ASIS. Lean your body towards her feet as you pull her sacrum inferior and her ASIS toward her head. Hold the stretch for a count of 5 and release gently. Repeat a few more times. Massage her back and neck. Pay special attention to the trigger points around her scapulae and lower back.
- Massage her pelvis and hips. Start with your palms open and gradually get deeper with

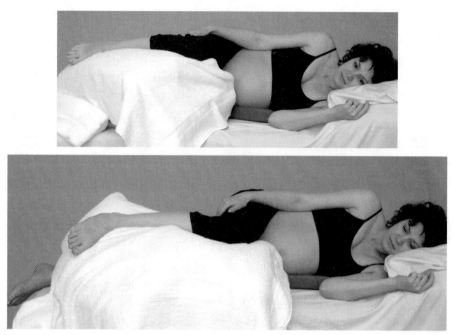

FIGURE 13-8 *(Top)* Pillows' placement with client's legs parallel. *(Bottom)* Some clients prefer to bring their top leg forward. This position is particularly comfortable when the baby is occiput posterior. Make sure her hip, knee, and ankle are always on the same horizontal plane to prevent pulling the sacroiliac joint. (From Stillerman E: *Prenatal massage: a textbook of pregnancy, labor, and postpartum bodywork*, St. Louis, 2008, Mosby.)

pressure from your fingertips or heel of hands (pisiform bone).

- Treat the trigger points in her pelvis and hips (Figure 13-9).
- Massage her neck and the occipital ridge.
- Have your client lean back slightly and turn her face upward. Massage her face and scalp, and then return her head to a neutral position and massage her neck again.
- Massage her arm, using her body to rest the limb. Start from her elbow and always stroke towards her heart.
- Ask permission before beginning abdominal massage. With your palms open, lightly effleurage in a clockwise direction (Figure 13-10).
- Bring the bottom half of the sheet between her legs and expose the top leg. Use very little lubrication, or just what is on your hands. To effectively address the lymph system, the skin should stretch under your hands. Starting at her hip, stretch her skin slowly and lightly—using 10 to 30 grams of pressure (the weight of a quarter)—and work your way down her entire leg to her foot, proximal to distal, with the direction and pressure of the stroke towards her heart. Repeat

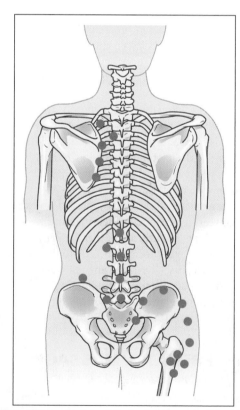

FIGURE 13-9 Trigger points of the back, hips, and pelvis. All points are bilateral. (From Stillerman E: *Prenatal massage: a textbook of pregnancy, labor, and postpartum bodywork*, St. Louis, 2008, Mosby.)

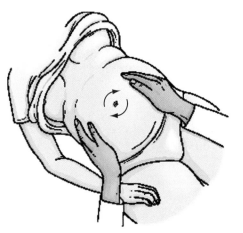

FIGURE 13-10 Always ask permission before massaging a pregnant woman's abdomen. Use an open palm and light pressure in a clockwise direction. (From Stillerman E: *Prenatal massage; a textbook of pregnancy, labor, and postpartum bodywork,* St. Louis, 2008, Mosby.)

the stroke from hip to foot 5 more times, working different aspects of the limb. The swelling this stroke relieves is found within the superficial skin lymph capillaries. The strokes must be light in order to reduce the swelling effectively. Use very little lubrication to introduce a stretching effect on the underlying skin.

- From her hip, do lymphatic compression (a gentle hold). You will be using the same 10 to 30 grams of steady pressure. Cup your hands around her thigh and hold each compression, from thigh to foot, for a count of 10. There will be approximately 6 compressions per limb.
- Effleurage her feet using the same 10 to 30 grams of pressure and rhythm. Stretch her toes and gently petrissage the sole of her foot.
- Wipe off the bottom of her foot.
- Remove the pillows and have your client turn *under* (on hands and knees) to the other side. Replace the pillows.
- Repeat the arm and leg massage. Wipe off the bottom of her feet.
- End your prenatal massage with a few more pelvic tilts and effleurages on her back.

Let her rest for a few minutes, and help her off the table if she needs help. (Make sure she recruits her transverse abdominis and doesn't "jack-knife" off the table.)[11]

CHAPTER SUMMARY

Massage and ritualistic touch have a long and honorable history during pregnancy. Midwives, who attended the majority of births in the United States until the 18th century, always used touch and massage to ease the pain of childbirth and keep the laboring woman calm and focused. Massage practitioners today have a myriad of appropriate techniques to support their pregnant clients and treat the common discomforts of pregnancy.

In order to provide the most supportive work, practitioners must understand the anatomy and physiology of pregnancy. Nearly every biologic system is affected by the pregnancy, and appropriate bodywork will support these physically pervasive changes. In addition, pregnancy often causes emotional issues that can be ameliorated by nurturing, respectful care. It is as important to understand the precautions and contraindications of massage as it is to learn what modalities are beneficial.

It is my strong belief that prenatal massage, like any hands-on modality, is best learned in a classroom situation with the onsite supervision of a trained professional.

CASE HISTORY

The client worked at a doctor's office and was 6 months pregnant with her first child when she started her prenatal massages with me. As usual, I took her medical history and explained what prenatal massage was going to be. I also cautioned her about certain warning signs, such as a spike in blood pressure, pitting edema, severe headaches or migraines, which would preclude treatment.

With the presence of any of these symptoms, a dangerous hypertensive condition known as preeclampsia (formerly referred to as *toxemia*) may result. Preeclampsia is a serious complication of pregnancy characterized by elevated maternal blood pressure, pitting edema or excessive edema in the upper torso, and/or proteinuria in the urine. When convulsions or coma are associated, it is called *eclampsia*. With these pathologic conditions, massage will introduce more waste products into a system that can no longer degrade the toxins. Maternal and/or fetal death can occur.

She was coming regularly for her massages up until her thirty-ninth week. Twenty minutes before her appointment, my phone rang. She said she wasn't feeling very well and had taken her blood pressure at work. It was dangerously high. Based upon what I had told her about the risks associated with elevated blood pressure, she cancelled her appointment and called her doctor.

Days later, she called. In the background I heard a baby's cry. Her blood pressure had suddenly spiked and she developed pre-eclampsia. Her doctor induced the labor, and her son was born strong and healthy. She too was feeling a lot better. She said had I not cautioned her about her blood pressure, she might have still come for the massage. I assured her that once she got to my office, I would have performed the pretreatment evaluations and asked her to call her doctor instead of massaging her. This just confirms the importance of explaining prenatal precautions with your clients.

SUGGESTED READINGS

Stillerman E: *MotherMassage: a handbook for relieving the discomforts of pregnancy*, New York, 1992, Dell.

Stillerman E: *Prenatal massage: a textbook of pregnancy, labor, and postpartum bodywork*, St. Louis, 2008, Mosby.

RESOURCES

PROFESSIONAL TRAINING
MotherMassage®: Massage during Pregnancy
Elaine Stillerman, LMT
PO Box 150337
Brooklyn, New York 11215-0337
(212)-533-3188
www.MotherMassage.Net

ASSOCIATIONS AND RESOURCES
Association of Labor Assistants and Childbirth Educators (ALACE)
www.ALACE.org

Childbirth Connection (formerly Maternity Center Association)
www.Childbirthconnection.org

Childbirth & Postpartum Professionals Association (CAPPA)
www.CAPPA.net

Diastasis Rehab
www.diastasisrehab.com

Doulas of North America (DONA)
www.DONA.org

International Childbirth Education Association (ICEA)
www.ICEA.org

Lamaze International
www.Lamaze.org

Midwives Alliance of North America (MANA)
www.MANA.org

Midwifery Today
www.Midwiferytoday.com

REFERENCES

1. Goldsmith J: *Childbirth wisdom*, New York, 1984, Congdon and Weed.
2. Brainin K: *Pregnancy and birth*, London, 2005, Active Birth Centre.
3. Feldhusen AE: The history of midwifery and childbirth in America: A time line, *Midwifery Today* 53:2000.
4. Rooks JP: *Midwifery and childbirth in America*, Philadelphia, 1998, Temple University Press.
5. Starr P: *The social transformation of American medicine*, New York, 1984, Basic Books.
6. Wertz R, Wertz DC: *Lying-in: a history of childbirth in America*, New Haven, Conn, 1989, Yale University Press.
7. Calvert R: *The history of massage: an illustrated survey from around the world*, Rochester, Vt, 2002, Healing Arts Press.
8. Sullivan N: A short history of midwifery, MidwifeInfo. Available at http://www.midwifeinfo.com/content/view/32/30. March 2002.
9. Feldhusen AE: The history of midwifery and childbirth in America: A time line, *Midwifery Today* 53:2000.
10. Stillerman E: *MotherMassage: a handbook for relieving the discomforts of pregnancy*, New York, 1992, Dell.
11. Stillerman E: *Prenatal massage: a textbook of pregnancy, labor, and postpartum bodywork*, St. Louis, 2008, Mosby.
12. Walther DS: *Applied kinesiology*, vol 1, Pueblo, Colo, 1981, Systems DC.
13. Stillerman E: *The encyclopedia of bodywork*, New York, 1996, Facts on File.
14. Leifer G: *Maternity nursing: an introductory text*, St. Louis, 2005, Saunders.
15. Lowdermilk DL, Perry SE: *Maternity & women's health care*, ed 8, St. Louis, 2004, Mosby.
16. Coad J: *Anatomy and physiology for midwives*, St. Louis, 2001, Mosby.
17. Fraser D, Cooper M: *Myles' textbook for midwives*, ed 14, Edinburgh, 2003, Churchill Livingstone.
18. Blackburn ST, Loper DL: *Maternal, fetal and neonatal physiology*, Blackwell, 1992, Oxford.
19. Gray H: *Anatomy: descriptive and surgical*, ed 15, New York, 1977, Bounty Books, Crown Publishing.
20. Tupler J: *Maternal fitness*, New York, 1996, Simon and Schuster.
21. Brill P: *The core program*, New York, 2001, Bantam Books.
22. Stillerman E: *MotherMassage: massage during pregnancy training manual*, 2004.
23. Sapsford RR et al: Co-activation of the abdominal and pelvic floor muscles during voluntary exercises, *Neurol Urodynam* 20:31-42, 2001.

24. DeCherney P, Nathan L: *Current obstetric & gynecologic diagnosis & treatment*, ed 10, New York, 2003, McGraw Hill.

25. Malone F, D'Alton M: Multiple gestation: Clinical characteristics and managements. In Creasy R, Resnik R, eds: *Maternal-fetal medicine*, ed 4, Philadelphia, 1999, Saunders.

26. deSweit M: The cardiovascular system. In Chamberlain G, Broughton-Pipkin F, eds: *Clinical physiology in obstetrics*, Oxford, 1998, Blackwell Science.

27. Cunningham FG et al: *Williams obstetrics*, ed 21, New York, 2001, McGraw Hill.

28. Girling JC: Physiology of pregnancy. In *Obstetrics, anaesthesia and intensive care medicine*, Abingdon, England, 2001, Medicine Publishing Company.

29. Symonds E, Symonds I: *Essential obstetrics and gynaecology*, ed 3, Edinburgh, 1998, Churchill Livingstone.

30. Coustan D: Maternal physiology. In Coustan D, Haning R, Singer D, eds: *Human reproduction—growth and development*, London, 1995, Little Brown.

31. Alexander D: Deep vein thromboembolism and its management in pregnancy, *Massage Ther J* 32:58, 1993.

32. deSweit M et al: Thromboembolism in pregnancy. In Jewell D, ed: *Advanced medicine*, London, 1981, Pitman Medical.

33. Rutherford S et al: Thromboembolic disease associated with pregnancy: an 11 year review, *Am J Obstet Gynecol* 164:286, 1991.

34. Bergqvist D, Hedner U: Pregnancy and venous thrombo-embolism, *Acta Obstet Gynecol Scand* 62: 449-453, 1983.

35. Bergqvist A, Bergqvist D, Hallbook T: Deep vein thrombosis during pregnancy: a prospective study, *Acta Obstet Gynecol Scand* 62:443-448, 1983.

36. Hull RD, Raskob GE, Carter CJ: Serial impedance plethysmography in pregnant patients with clinically suspected deep-vein thrombosis: clinical validity of negative findings, *Ann Intern Med* 112:663-667, 1990.

37. Jeffries WS, Bochner F: Thromboembolism and its management in pregnancy, *Med J Australia* 155:253, 1991.

38. Rath W, Fardi A, Dudenhausen JW: HELLP syndrome, *J Perinat Med* 28:249-260, 2000.

39. Campbell S, Lees C, eds: *Obstetrics by 10 teachers*, New York, 2000, Oxford University Press.

40. Steinfeld J, Wax J: *Maternal physiological adaptations to pregnancy*. In Seifer D, Samuels P, Kniss D, eds: Philadelphia, 2001, Lippincott Williams & Wilkins.

41. Hellman LM, Pritchard JA: *Williams obstetrics*, ed 14, New York, 1971, Appleton-Century-Crofts.

42. Hermida R, Ayala D, Iglesias M: Predictable blood pressure variability in health and complicated pregnancies, *Hypertension* 38:736-744, 2001.

43. Calder A: Normal labor. In Edmonds K, ed: *Dewhurst's textbook of obstetrics and gynaecology for postgraduates*, ed 6, Oxford, 1999, Blackwell Science.

44. Padua L et al: Symptoms and neurophysical picture of carpal tunnel syndrome in pregnancy, *Clin Neurophysiol* 112:1946-1951, 2001.

45. Depression during pregnancy, Pregnancy-info. Available at http://www.pregnancy-info.net/depression_during_pregnancy. html. Accessed on March, 2006.

46. Ascher H: Maternal anxiety in pregnancy and fetal homeostasis, *JOGN Nurs* 7:18-21, 1978.

47. March of Dimes: *Stress and pregnancy*, 2003.

48. Tarkin L: Dealing with depression and the perils of pregnancy, *New York Times*, p F5, January 13, 2004.

49. Fritz S, Grosenbach J: *Essential sciences for therapeutic massage*, ed 2, St. Louis, 2004, Mosby.

50. Ironson G et al: *Relaxation through massage is associated with decreased distress and increased serotonin levels*. Paper presented at the Academy of Psychosomatic medicine meeting, San Diego, 1992.

51. Field T et al: Pregnant women benefit from massage therapy, *J Psychosom Obstet Gynaecol* 290:31-38, 1999

52. Despard L: *Text-book of massage and remedial gymnastics*, ed 3, London, 1932, Oxford English Press.

53. Muller EA, Schulte am Esch J: Die wirkung der massage auf die leistungsfahigeit von muskeln, *Int Z Angew Physiol* 22, 1996.

54. Kellogg JH: *The art of massage*, Battle Creek, MI, 1929, Modern Medical Publishing.

55. Bennett HA, Einan TR: Depressive symptoms among pregnant women screened in obstetric settings, *J Women's Health* 13:1, 2004.

MULTIPLE CHOICE TEST QUESTIONS

1) What may cause pregnancy-induced hypotension?
   a) positioning your pregnant client semisitting
   b) positioning your client flat in a supine position
   c) positioning your client on her right side
   d) positioning your client on her left side

2) How much pressure is used in manual lymphatic drainage?
   a) to the client's comfort level
   b) as deep as you can go
   c) to 7 grams of light pressure
   d) to 30 grams of pressure

3) What is the function of the placenta?
   a) It is a specialized organ for maternal-fetal gas and nutrient exchange.
   b) It secretes hormones to sustain the pregnancy.
   c) It stores numerous hormones vital to the pregnancy.
   d) all of the above

4) Which is not a contributing factor in the increased lordotic curve in late pregnancy?
   a) diastasis recti
   b) secretion of progesterone and relaxin that relax the connective tissue
   c) the weight of the gravid uterus on the intravertebral disks
   d) posterior pelvic tilt

5) Which is not a postural adaptation of late pregnancy?
   a) Her cervical spine retracts.
   b) Her shoulders laterally rotate while she is standing up.
   c) Her pelvis widens and hips laterally rotate.
   d) Her knees hyperextend.

6) How do estrogen and relaxin affect a pregnant woman's connective tissue?
   a) They provide greater stability and support.
   b) They allow the tissues to relax and soften in preparation for labor and childbirth.

   c) They provide tighter connections to help support the heavy uterus.
   d) They have no effect during pregnancy.

7) What is an important goal for massage practitioners when treating the musculoskeletal system of a pregnant woman?
   a) elongate the anterior muscles of her body
   b) tighten the posterior muscles of her body
   c) improve the balance of her musculature by shortening the anterior muscles and elongating the posterior muscles
   d) avoid massaging her lower back and pelvis

8) How much additional blood volume does a pregnant woman have by the end of her pregnancy?
   a) 10% to 20%
   b) 20% to 30%
   c) 30% to 50%
   d) 40% to 60%

9) Edema in her lower extremities is caused by all of the following except:
   a) sluggish venous return
   b) increased venous pressure
   c) decreased venous pressure
   d) additional pressure in the veins of her legs, vulva, rectum, and pelvis

10) How much of an increased risk is thromboembolism during pregnancy?
    a) 2 to 3 times greater
    b) 3 to 4 times greater
    c) 4 to 5 times greater
    d) 5 to 6 times greater

11) The purpose of pretreatment evaluations is to:
    a) test for the presence of pitting edema and blood clots
    b) test for high blood pressure
    c) test for elevated heart rate
    d) test for increased respiration

12) What is the top of the uterus called?
    a) cervix
    b) vulva
    c) cornua
    d) fundus

13) What are Braxton Hicks contractions?
   a) prelabor or preparatory uterine contractions
   b) early labor contractions
   c) a rare reaction to the pregnancy
   d) a postpartum uterine contraction to dislodge the placenta

14) What hormone stimulates the onset of uterine contractions?
   a) prolactin
   b) oxytocin
   c) relaxin
   d) progesterone

15) Massage during pregnancy has all of the following benefits except:
   a) prepares the expectant mother emotionally, physically, and mentally for labor
   b) speeds up sluggish circulation
   c) decreases chronic muscle tension.
   d) elevates maternal blood pressure

16) Massage is contraindicated in all of the following instances except:
   a) abruptio placentae
   b) pitting edema
   c) gestational glucose intolerance
   d) ectopic pregnany

17) Which of the following is not a contraindicated acupuncture point for pregnancy?
   a) Spleen 3
   b) Spleen 6
   c) Spleen 10
   d) Bladder 67

18) A massage technique that decompresses the lumbar spine is:
   a) sacral lift
   b) anterior pelvic tilt
   c) posterior pelvic tilt
   d) abdominal lift

19) After permission is given, when is it safe to massage a pregnant woman's abdomen?
   a) never
   b) always
   c) only after the second trimester
   d) only during the third trimester

20) Which muscle should pregnant women recruit while getting on and off the massage table, turning over, and lifting any objects to provide lumbar stability?
   a) erector spinae muscles
   b) rectus abdominis
   c) external obliques
   d) transverse abdominis

Reflexology

Laura Norman

14

INTRODUCTION TO REFLEXOLOGY

Reflexology is a method for activating the healing powers of the body through the feet and hands. The technical definition recognized by The American Reflexology Certification Board **(ARCB)** is a bit more complex: "Foot and hand reflexology is a scientific art based on the premise that there are **zones** and **reflex areas** in the feet and hands which correspond to all the parts of the body. The physical act of applying pressure using thumb, finger and hand techniques result in stress reduction which causes a physiological change in the body." There are five imaginary vertical lines used to divide the body head to toe on each side ending in each foot, and similarly running down the arms into the tips of the fingers. Not only do these zones run lengthwise, but they pass through the body, so that a zone located on the front of the body can also be reached from behind. All organs and parts of the body lie along these zones.

Modern reflexology is both a science and an art. As a science, it requires careful study, faithful practice, a sound knowledge of the techniques, and skill. And yet as one of the healing arts, reflexology yields the best results when the reflexologist works with dedication, patience, focused intentions, and above all, loving care.[1]

DVD To better understand concepts in this chapter, watch *Reflexology* video on the **DVD** found at the back of this book.

Reflexology connects individuals through the intimate act of touch. Whether it is between practitioner and client, partners or friends, when we touch another person something happens between us. If we continue to reach out to each other, a relationship grows and it spreads to others. When you feel good, others respond positively.

Reflexology is about working with more than just the feet and reflex points that correspond to each organ, gland, and part of the body (Figure 14-1). It encompasses the whole person—physically, mentally, emotionally, and spiritually. The science of reflexology considers the feet to be minimaps of the human body with areas linked to a corresponding area or point on the foot. By targeting a certain area or point, reflexology encourages relief to the corresponding part of the body.

Reflexology is easy to learn and yet so powerful. It has grown so popular in recent years that surgeons and other medical doctors, chiropractors, podiatrists, dentists, nurses, midwives, physical therapists, occupational therapists, and massage therapists use it as a complementary modality. For example, Dr. Mehmet Oz, a prominent cardiovascular surgeon, formed a complementary cardiac care unit at Columbia-Presbyterian

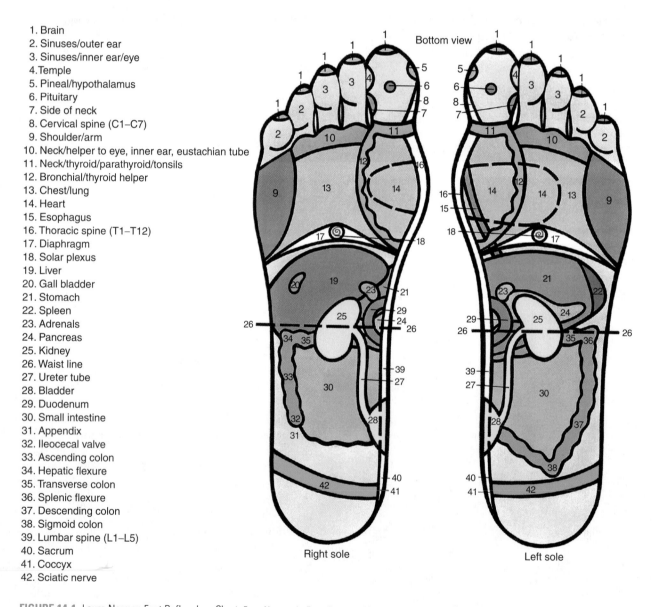

1. Brain
2. Sinuses/outer ear
3. Sinuses/inner ear/eye
4. Temple
5. Pineal/hypothalamus
6. Pituitary
7. Side of neck
8. Cervical spine (C1–C7)
9. Shoulder/arm
10. Neck/helper to eye, inner ear, eustachian tube
11. Neck/thyroid/parathyroid/tonsils
12. Bronchial/thyroid helper
13. Chest/lung
14. Heart
15. Esophagus
16. Thoracic spine (T1–T12)
17. Diaphragm
18. Solar plexus
19. Liver
20. Gall bladder
21. Stomach
22. Spleen
23. Adrenals
24. Pancreas
25. Kidney
26. Waist line
27. Ureter tube
28. Bladder
29. Duodenum
30. Small intestine
31. Appendix
32. Ileocecal valve
33. Ascending colon
34. Hepatic flexure
35. Transverse colon
36. Splenic flexure
37. Descending colon
38. Sigmoid colon
39. Lumbar spine (L1–L5)
40. Sacrum
41. Coccyx
42. Sciatic nerve

Bottom view

Right sole

Left sole

FIGURE 14-1 Laura Norman Foot Reflexology Chart. From Norman L: *Feet first: a guide to foot reflexology,* New York, 1998, Simon & Schuster.

◧◨◨ IN MY EXPERIENCE

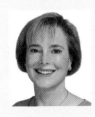

When I work with my clients, I work with more than their feet, hands, and ears. I also work with them as a whole person, i.e., holistically—physically, mentally, emotionally, and spiritually. I coach them to connect with their greatness and to embrace their heart's desires.

Marion, a stressed-out executive, came to see me because she was unhappy with her job … and with her life. We talked about her personal and professional goals and about how to focus on her choices during the session. Marion responded very well to the reflexology—as she said afterward, "I went somewhere else, somewhere very peaceful" during her session.

She experienced such amazing results from her reflexology sessions with me that she took my introductory reflexology Workshop and went on to complete my Reflexology Certification Training Program. Today Marion lives far from the corporate world—she is a nationally certified reflexologist, massage therapist, and physical therapist. She is happy, fulfilled, and at peace within herself.

Medical Center in New York City. He integrates reflexology into his pre- and post-surgery protocols for his heart patients, as detailed in his book, *Healing from the heart* (Dutton Publishing 1995, Boston).

Many interested lay people also choose to learn reflexology to help reduce stress in their everyday lives and as a way of connecting in a loving way with partners, friends, and family members. With reflexology, you and your clients will not only reap the benefits of stress reduction, relaxation, pain management, and improved body function, you will also discover powerful techniques for living a happier and healthier life.

HISTORY OF REFLEXOLOGY

Reflexology is both old and new. From ancient texts, illustrations, and artifacts, we know that the early Chinese, Japanese, and Egyptians worked on the feet to promote good health. Discovered in Egypt, a pictograph from the Physician's Tomb (c. 2300 BC) may be some of the earliest evidence of reflexology being applied (Figure 14-2).

The use of healing pressure applied to the feet has been practiced by North American Native Americans for generations. One theory claims that this form of reflex therapy was passed down to them by the Incas.

Jenny Wallace, a Cherokee Indian from the Bear Clan, practices as a foot therapist in America today. According to her: "In my tribe, working on the feet is a very important healing art and is part of a sacred ceremony that you don't have to be ill to take part in. The feet walk upon the earth and through this your spirit is connected to the universe. Our feet are our contact with the earth and the energies that flow through it."[2]

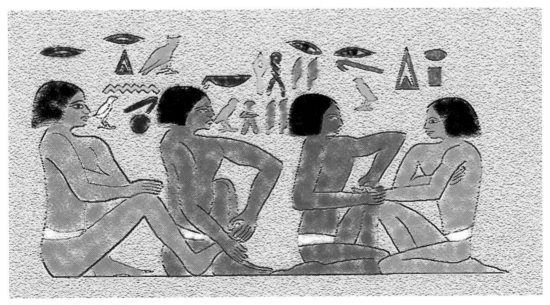

FIGURE 14-2 Physician's Tomb pictograph.

What joins the ancients with moderns is the desire to solve the mysteries of the human body. The first recorded scientific reference to reflexology—in 1890—was by knighted research scientist and medical doctor Sir Henry Head. He demonstrated that a neurologic relationship exists between the skin and the internal organs.

Nobel prizewinner in medicine Sir Charles Sherrington proved that the entire nervous system and body adjust to a stimulus when it is applied to any part of the body. Around the same time in Germany, Dr. Alfons Cornelius observed that pressure to certain spots on the body triggered muscle contractions, changes in blood pressure, variation in warmth and moisture in the body, as well as directly affecting the "psychic processes," or mental state of the patient. The Russians, beginning with Drs. Ivan Pavlov and Vladimir Bekhterev, explored reflex responses in the body for nearly a century.[3]

In 1917, Dr. William Fitzgerald, an American, published *Zone therapy, or relieving pain at home*. In it he describes his success with relieving pain through use of various devices on the hands and fingers. A reporter wrote an article detailing the events of a dinner party where Dr. Fitzgerald demonstrated his theories. The party was attended by a well-known concert singer who had announced that the upper register tones of her voice had gone flat. Throat specialists had been unable to discover the cause of this affliction. Dr. Fitzgerald, according to the newspaper article, asked to examine the fingers and toes of the singer. After his examination, he told her that the cause of the loss of her upper tones was attributed to a callus on her right great toe. After applying pressure to the corresponding part in the same zone for a few minutes, the patient remarked that the pain in her toe had disappeared, "whereupon the doctor asked her to try the tones of the upper register. Miraculously, it seemed to us the singer reached two notes higher than she had ever sung before."[4]

Dr. Fitzgerald's "zone therapy" intrigued one physician, Dr. Joseph Riley, who discussed it with his staff therapist, Eunice Ingham. Eunice began to use zone therapy in her work with patients. She concluded that since the zones ran throughout the body and could be accessed anywhere, some areas might be more accessible and effective than others.

Eunice discovered that the feet were the most responsive areas for working the zones because they were extremely sensitive. Eventually, she mapped the entire body onto the feet and discovered that an alternating pressure on the various points had therapeutic effects far beyond the previously limited use of zone therapy for pain reduction. And so modern reflexology was born.

In 1991 the first scientific research study regarding the efficacy of reflexology began. The study applied strict scientific protocols to evaluating the effect, if any, of reflexology on PMS (premenstrual syndrome). Under the direction of the American Academy of Reflexology and Bill Flocco, the study showed a statistically significant reduction in PMS symptoms beyond what could be attributed to chance or the placebo effect. This reflexology study has the distinction of being the first published in a scientific peer review medical journal, *The Journal of Obstetrics and Gynecology*.

Thanks to the passion of Eunice Ingham and those who followed in her path, reflexology continued to grow throughout the United States and has achieved worldwide acceptance today. In China, reflexology is accepted by the central government as a means of preventing and curing diseases and preserving health. In over 300 research studies, covering over 18,000 cases involving 64 different illnesses, the Chinese have shown that reflexology provides some improvement 95% of the time.

In Japan and Denmark, reflexology has been incorporated into the employee health programs of several large corporations, saving each company many thousands of dollars annually in paid sick leave benefits. In Thailand and India foot reflexology clinics abound, with high concentrations in tourist areas. According to statistics from the reflexology Association of Canada, Thailand leads the world in demand for Reflexology, with about 65% of its population using reflexology in one form or another each year.[5]

WHY THE FEET?

As you can see from Figure 14-3 the feet are a perfect microcosm or minimap of the whole body. All the organs, glands, and parts of the body represented in the feet are laid out in the same arrangement as in the body. Even the inside curve of the foot corresponds to the natural curves in the spine. The toes are like little heads. The ridge beneath the toes on the top part of the ball of the foot is a natural shoulder or neck line.[2]

Other parts of the body exhibit these same correspondences, though less obviously. The hand, the ear, even the iris of the eye each contain reflex points for the entire body. But these points are better defined in the feet, and because they are more spread out and accessible, they are easier to work with.[2] Later in this

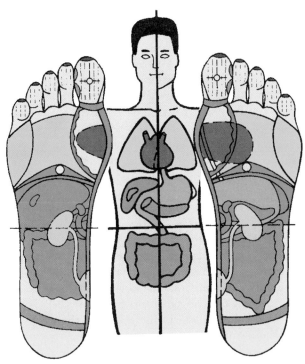

FIGURE 14-3 Feet as minimap of body. From Norman L: *Feet first: a guide to foot reflexology*, New York, 1998, Simon & Schuster.

chapter we will explore the divisions of the feet and areas of the body to which they correspond.

PERSONAL PREFERENCES IN REFLEXOLOGY

Persons not used to having someone else touch their bodies or who are uncomfortable about getting undressed may not seek help from some complementary modalities. The head, heart, chest, and trunk areas of the human body seem more private than the extremities. The feet are distant enough from the torso that most people are not threatened by someone working on them, which may help them feel more safe and secure. Clients also save time with reflexology by not needing to get undressed and dressed again. They can just take off their shoes and socks and relax.

ANATOMIC REASONS FOR REFLEXOLOGY

Feet are farthest from the heart, where circulation tends to stagnate. It is not uncommon for people with chronically poor circulation to have tender or swollen hands and feet. It is good to stimulate and encourage blood

flow to these extremities. Gravity pulls toxins downward and inorganic waste material such as uric acid and other **deposits** can build up in the bottoms of the feet. An experienced reflexologist can actually feel these deposits with his or her hands and clear them, improving circulation throughout the entire body.[2]

OTHER REASONS FOR REFLEXOLOGY

We abuse and neglect our feet when we ought to do something good for them. Of all the parts of the body, feet take a real beating. Between bearing our weight, hard surfaces, inappropriate shoes, and poor postural habits, the muscles and joints of the modern foot receive little nurturing. In fact, 4 out of every 5 people experience daily pain in their feet, but tune it out of their conscious awareness and become inured to it through a neurologic process known as **adaptation.**

Even without awareness, constant pain takes its toll in muscle tension elsewhere in the body, especially in the back, neck, and shoulders. Without realizing it, as people try to adapt to pain, it increases their fatigue and irritability. Adaptation to stress is noted through what you observe visibly and with your sense of touch. Examples include puffiness, calluses, corns, unusually high or low arches.[1] **Stress cues** in the feet provide a road map for the reflexologist to apply pressure techniques to target the indicated stresses. These stress cues are "any part of the foot that shows adaptation to stress. Adaptation to stress is noted through what you observe visibly and with your sense of touch."[1] Clients often express amazement at the variety of improvements they feel and about how little they had realized they needed reflexology.

ADDITIONAL HYPOTHESES OF REFLEXOLOGY

Although nearly all experts agree that reflexology does work, there are many hypotheses as to *how* it works. Here are several interesting hypotheses formerly listed on the American Reflexology Certification Board website.

The Energy Hypothesis

Inside the organism, communication between organs is incessant. It is maintained through the complex system of blood circulating and energy linking the cells. This communication is happening thanks to an electromagnetic field and to vibrating exchanges between body and spirit. This vital energy of the life force is well known in oriental medicine. It circulates rhythmically among all organs, touching all living cells. Sometimes blocks happen on the pathways of this energy, and reflexology helps the energy to recirculate.

The Lactic Acid Hypothesis

According to the hypothesis, lactic acid is sometimes transformed into microcrystals deposited in the hands and feet. These deposits stop or disturb the flow of life energy. Reflexology allows these microdeposits to be crushed and recycled, allowing the energy to circulate again.

Hypothesis of the Proprioceptive Nervous Receptors

According to some researchers, there may be direct and unknown connections between certain parts of the feet and hands and organs of the body. Therefore, reflexing the feet and hands directly affects the different organs of the body.

Hypothesis of the Relaxing Effect

Many physical problems have to do with persistent tension and stress. Reflexology relaxes the patient. The foot is covered with joint kinesthetic receptors. Manual manipulation of these receptors affects postural integrity. The proprioceptor mechanism (i.e., the process by which the body knows where it is in space through movement, position, and weight) feeds postural information into the central nervous system. Proprioception can respond through chemical or electrical stimulation. It can happen that so much information is fed into the system that pain is blocked and/or ignored (i.e., pain gate theory), which in turn produces relief of pain and allows **homeostasis,** a dynamic state of balance, and relaxation to occur.

    Reflex zone therapy works on the constitutional rather than on the symptomatic level. It deals with the person and not the illness. It detoxifies the body. Energy cannot flow along the sheath of the human nervous system when there is tension in the nerves and the muscular structure through which those nerves travel. Reflexology relaxes stress and tension.

REFLEXOLOGY WORKS ON THREE LEVELS

The view of the body having paths of energy and coordinated reflex points has existed for literally thousands of years. Up to now, no one has been able to explain in precise scientific terms why reflexology works, but recent studies and experience with acupuncture and related therapies are revealing findings that are helpful in bringing a fuller explanation to reflexology. Reflexology works on three levels; the physical, the mental, and the spiritual. At the physical level reflexology works by affecting organs and circulation by reestablishing, unblocking, and stimulating blood, oxygen, nutritional, and energy pathways. Tension is released, nerve activity is balanced, and congestion and other deposits (a buildup of acidic crystals, also known as lactic acid) are thrown off. On the mental level, the act of touching another human being is an effective therapy in itself. Lastly, from the spiritual aspect, a healing force from the universe is called upon and used by both the client and the practitioner.

Electrical Impulses

When pressure is applied on a tender reflex, there is an electrical impulse triggered and a subtle energy flow brings the remarkable return of vitality, even in the midst of receiving treatment. It is my belief that the electrical impulse acts on the body in the same way that the stimulus of light acts on the retina of the eye. It has been proven that the action of the full spectrum of light on the retina of the eyes, in which are embedded the endings of the optic nerve, produces an electrical impulse that is carried to the hypothalamus. From there it is passed down to the pituitary gland, which passes down to the lesser glands, thereby activating all the functions of the body. It is my belief that stimulating the reflexes produces similar results.

Autonomic Impulses

Reflexology is based on the knowledge of how to accurately manipulate the body's intricate stimulus-response mechanism. Compression massage deals with subcutaneous receptors located deeper than the skin—i.e., not in the skin, but reaching them through the skin. Working on the feet, we deal almost exclusively with autonomic reflexes. Pressure applied to a nerve ending constitutes a "stimulus." This stimulus sets in motion a "nerve impulse" and electrochemical impulses that effect a change in nervous processes. Pressing (stimulating) points on the feet evokes polarity reflexes in all organs in a particular zone. Massaging reflex points in the various zones benefits one's health because of the resultant polarizing and balancing of vital energies.[7]

WHAT REFLEXOLOGY IS NOT

There has been a lot of misinformation about reflexology, as there is about many of the nontraditional methods of healing. Reflexology is not foot massage.

Although many states require a nationally certified reflexologist to also have a massage license, Reflexology differs from massage in several important ways. Massage works through the musculature, using methods of stroking to restore metabolic balance within the soft tissue. Reflexology is the application of specific thumb and finger walking techniques to reflex points in the hands and feet that correspond to all parts of the body. Reflexology works through the nervous system and subtle energy pathways to improve the function of organs and glands, and all systems of the body. And only footwear comes off, as only the feet and hands are touched. Even though many clients present specific ailments and extra time may be spent working a particular area, reflexology is not considered a cure.

Reflexology is effective because it coaxes the body to heal itself. The reflexologist acts as a conduit for healing. Although some practitioners prefer to use tools, most use their hands exclusively. Reflexology works with subtle energy flows, revitalizing the body so that the natural internal healing mechanisms of the body can do their own work. People attest to better health, more energy, less stress and, in some instances, a marked reduction in or disappearance of a specific ailment. But it was not the reflexologist nor the session that caused these changes. The body is capable of healing itself when it has been returned to a balanced state.[2]

BENEFITS OF REFLEXOLOGY

Since ancient times, healers have employed various methodologies to strengthen and balance energy flow. Many of these systems, including acupuncture, shiatsu, and reflexology, are based on how energy flows in zones or meridians throughout the body.[6]

Reduces Stress

The word "stress" is derived from the Latin word *stringere,* which means "to draw tight." The descriptive "uptight" in current slang paints a fairly accurate picture. The body's original hormonal and chemical defense mechanisms, the so-called "fight-or-flight" responses, still function today. We, however, have little opportunity to release the powerful energy these mechanisms create, resulting in stress and anxiety. Reflexology alleviates the effects of stress by inducing deep relaxation, allowing rebalancing of the nervous system.

Improves Circulation

One of Eunice Ingham's favorite sayings was "Circulation is life. Stagnation is death."[8] We all know how important it is for blood to flow freely through the body, carrying oxygen and nutrients to every cell that makes up the tissues of the body and removing the waste products of metabolism and other toxins. Stress and tension constrict the cardiovascular system and restrict blood flow, making circulation sluggish. Reflexology reduces stress and tension, allowing the miles of cardiovascular vessels to conduct the flow of blood naturally and easily.

Cleanses the Body

The body has built-in mechanisms for cleansing itself, including the **lymphatic system,** a complex network of lymphoid organs and lymph vessels that produce and transport lymph fluid from tissues to the circulatory system, **excretory system,** the bodily process of discharging wastes (i.e., kidneys and colon), and **integumentary system** (i.e., the skin). When these become blocked or function improperly, toxins and waste matter build up. A healthy body is like a healthy home: you have to take the garbage out regularly. By deepening relaxation, reflexology causes all the systems of the body to function more efficiently, including those that eliminate waste products.[2]

Helps Nature Achieve Homeostasis

The term *homeostasis* means being in a dynamic state of balance. The body's primary job is survival. For the body to be healthy, everything must work together. We are made up of thousands of parts, each functioning according to its own rules and purposes. To keep our body running harmoniously, a tune-up is often needed. As after a motor tune-up, the end result is a machine that runs smoothly, with all its parts contributing synergistically.

Revitalizes Energy

We each experience energy in our own unique way. You know when you are lethargic or full of vim and vigor. But one thing everyone agrees on—energy flows. According to Polarity theory, energy must flow unimpeded between the negative and positive poles that every atom and cell contains. By relaxing and opening up energy pathways, reflexology revitalizes the body and supplies it with energy on all levels.[2]

Provides Preventive Health Care

Preventive health care is becoming more important as we recognize the health-threatening dangers in our environment: stress, fatigue, chemical additives in food, polluted water supplies, radioactivity, and poor air quality to name only a few. The added strain on everyone's immune system today should warn us to find time to unwind and relax, because the immune system only functions at its peak when we successfully manage the effect of the stressful situations in our daily lives. Our immune system also responds synergistically, relying on other bodily processes to maintain its own lines of defense. Only when our body is well balanced are we in the proper shape to stay healthy.[7]

Rewards the Practitioner

Body workers and healers will tell you that their work is rewarding. It's natural because we help others to feel good and enjoy better health. A little known "secret" of body workers is that because we act as a channel for healing energy during sessions, the circuit completes itself by bringing health and well-being to us, too. As the client relaxes, we also become more grounded and centered. After a session the reflexologist feels a great sense of satisfaction and receives "strokes" of another kind in the gratitude lavished by the client.[2]

CONTRAINDICATIONS

Although reflexology is safe, there are times when it might be wise to:

a) use caution and avoid working certain parts of the foot
b) get a physician's permission
c) decline to perform a session

When to use caution and avoid working certain parts of the foot:

- Cuts, bruises
- **Bone spur** (a bony growth formed on normal bone)
- If toenails appear ingrown or corns are tender or sensitive
- Diabetic wounds
- Warts

When to get physician's permission and release signed:

- Unstable blood pressure
- **Peripheral neuropathy** (numbness or pain in legs or feet)
- Immediately after surgery requiring hospital stay
- After an organ transplant
- During early stages of induced labor to prevent precipitous labor (a labor that is too fast)

When to decline to perform a session:

- Varicose veins that are dilated and knotty, and irregular-shaped veins with incompetent valves
- **Phlebitis** (inflammation of a vein)
- History of blood clots
- Severe or pitting **edema,** which is an abnormal swelling caused by an accumulation of fluid. It can also be associated with cardiac and kidney disease and with protein deficiency. *Refer the client to a physician immediately.*
- Current fractures, recent foot surgeries, severe sprains of the foot or ankle
- Athlete's foot or other contagious or infectious diseases or anything that appears as such on the client's foot
- Lacerations, ulcers, open wounds and/or sores that are oozing fluids on the feet
- Gout
- Infection in the bone, osteomyelitis, or bony tuberculosis

Other Contraindications

Pregnancy conditions in which reflexology should be used with extreme caution, be avoided, or doctor's permission be obtained:

- History of repeated spontaneous abortions

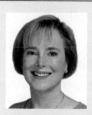 ■■■ IN MY EXPERIENCE

One of my favorite populations to work with is women choosing to conceive and who are pregnant. Working the nervous system through the feet helps women to deeply relax. Working their endocrine system helps balance their hormonal levels and glandular function. In this relaxed, balanced state they are more receptive to conceive. Performing reflexology during pregnancy, labor, and delivery allows us to reach internal organs and glands to strengthen the body's systems, promote profound relaxation, and ease the discomfort.

Leslie came to me after 3 years of trying to conceive. Six weeks later, after her eleventh reflexology session with me, Leslie came in screaming with joy that she was pregnant. I worked on her throughout her pregnancy, easing her morning sickness, alleviating body aches and water retention, and helping her to maintain regular bowel movements.

I continued giving Reflexology to Leslie throughout her labor and delivery. After Leslie gave birth to a beautiful little girl, I gave the baby her first reflexology session and then did the same for the new father, who needed it more than anyone!

- First trimester of pregnancy (avoid reproductive areas)
- Preterm labor or spontaneous membrane rupture in this or previous pregnancy
- Antepartum hemorrhage in this or a previous pregnancy
- Preeclampsia, eclampsia, or severe preexisting essential hypertension
- Multiple pregnancy due to the concern of preterm labor
- Breech presentation, transverse presentation
- Medical conditions exacerbated by pregnancy—e.g. cardiac disease, gestational glucose intolerance (formerly called gestational diabetes)

Guidelines for children, babies, elderly, or sick

- Less time
- Less pressure
- More often

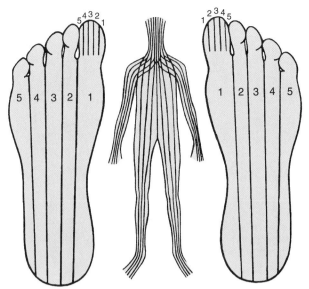

FIGURE 14-4 The body's energy zones. From Norman L: *Feet first: a guide to foot reflexology*, New York, 1998, Simon & Schuster.

SESSION OVERVIEW

Very few people give much thought to their feet until they hurt. Then each step can be a painful reminder of their importance. To a reflexologist's eye, your feet reveal a complex map of all the organs and systems of your body. Understanding and using this map, the practitioner can address discomfort or blocked energy in each part of the body by stimulating the appropriate points on the feet.

Reading the Map

The feet are actually a mirror of the entire body, with each foot representing one half of the body, the left and right feet corresponding to the left and right side of the body (see Figure 14-1).

Zones

Reflexology was originally called "zone therapy" because it is based on the 10 energy zones that run the length of the body from head to toe.

Each zone can be considered a channel for the intangible life energy or life force called *ch'i*, *qi*, or *prana* in Eastern medicine and martial arts. Stimulating or "working" these energy pathways in the foot by applying pressure with the thumbs and fingers affects the entire zone throughout the body.[2] If you think about a gingerbread man cookie sliced lengthwise in 10 equal parts you'll start to get a clearer picture of the zones (Figure 14-4).

GUIDELINES

In addition to the zones, there are **guidelines,** 4 horizontal divisions on the feet that differentiate the divisions of the foot and the areas of the body to which they refer (Figure 14-5):

- Shoulder/neck line
- Diaphragm line
- Waist line
- Pelvic line

Using these guidelines and the five zones on each foot as a grid, you can locate any area of the body on the foot. A reflex point is a specific area or point on the foot that corresponds to another part of the body. When a reflex point is stimulated by the thumbs or fingers, there is a response to the stimulus in the corresponding part of the body.

In a reflexology course you will learn more specifics regarding which parts of each foot correspond to which organs and glands and how best to work them.

PREPARING THE ENVIRONMENT

Presession preparation is important. As we mentioned earlier, a reflexology session is much more than just working on the feet. When two people come together for the benefit of one or the other, the energy circuit they create is profoundly enriching to both on a physical, emotional, mental, and spiritual level. The work itself helps the one who gives as well as the one who receives.

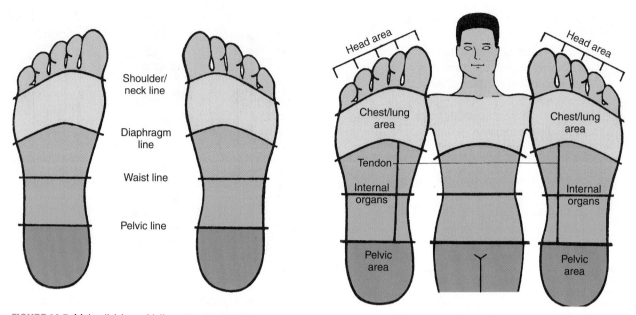

FIGURE 14-5 Major division guidelines. From Norman L: *Feet first: a guide to foot reflexology,* New York, 1998, Simon & Schuster.

Your attitude and the environment of the room where the session will take place will begin the relaxation process. A clean, comfortable, quiet environment is essential, free from the distractions of daily life, such as ringing phones and loud children.

Professionals may use a massage table; a recliner or even a bed. The lighting should be adjustable, and a light blanket should be within reach. Some people enjoy soothing music or environmental CDs with natural sounds. Reflexologists I train often incorporate the principles of **feng shui,** the ancient Chinese practice of placement and arrangement of space to achieve harmony with the environment, when setting up their session room to harmonize the external elements of the environment.

Practitioners should prepare before each session by making sure they have used a specialized disinfectant soap such as "*Tea tree*" and cleaned under their nails. It is important to feel peaceful and centered before beginning in order for your client to feel relaxed and ready.

The client also needs to be prepared ahead of time, being advised not to use or consume caffeine, cigarettes, drugs, alcohol, or a heavy meal for at least 2 hours before the session. Always ask about the new client's health history and find out if there is any history of blood clots, present diagnosis of diabetes, or pregnancy.

Do a visual examination of both feet prior to touching them to assess them for any contraindications. Check the condition of the feet looking for corns, cuts, or bruises. You have to avoid working on those areas. Many reflexologists wrap their client's feet in wet, hot towels to let the heat soak through, freshen the feet, and soften the tissues to gain easier access to the points before beginning the session. Applying the hot towels is also deeply relaxing and nurturing.[2]

DURING THE SESSION

A session varies from 30 to 60 minutes, perhaps a little longer for new reflexologists. Regularity is the key to effective reflexology. It's beneficial to plan a series of 6 to 10 frequent sessions to assess how the body is responding before creating a maintenance plan. It is safe enough to have full-hour sessions three times a week if necessary. After completing a series, suggest weekly, biweekly, or monthly maintenance sessions.

Tenderness in the Feet

When the session begins, the reflexologist might find tension, lack of flexibility, or tender areas. Tenderness in the feet doesn't necessarily indicate that there are health issues in the corresponding body areas. Tenderness might be due to local conditions of the foot such as bunions, plantar warts, corns, calluses, hammertoes (drawn up) or claw toes (unable to straighten out), or ingrown toe nails.

Note: Encourage your clients to let you know when they experience tenderness and/or discomfort. Watch their body language and facial expressions as nonverbal cues.

What the Client May Experience

Reflexology experience varies for each client. Some are able to relax more quickly, some may take longer to relax, and some actually fall asleep. Due to "energy movement," a naturally occurring phenomenon in the body, the client may experience tingling, or an "electrical" type sensation throughout the body or in a specific corresponding area. Some clients experience light-headedness, dizziness, fatigue, or the need to urinate.

Clients with lots of toxins resulting from poor health choices or chronic stress may experience a "healing response" after the session (see Box 14-1). Symptoms may include diarrhea, sneezing, nausea, or headaches, lasting 24 to 48 hours. It is always wise to use a lighter pressure and spend less time when working on this type of client. Also, explain to them before their first session that the healing response is a possibility but a positive step toward better health.

REFLEXOLOGY TECHNIQUES

The ARCB believes that students who plan to use reflexology professionally should learn these techniques with supervised, hands-on instruction.

How to Hold the Foot

The foot must be held firmly, gently, and correctly so the reflex points and areas are reached and stimulated properly. Always hold the foot with both hands. One of the hands holds the foot while the other is working and stimulating the reflex areas and points. The **holding hand** holds the foot, opposite and parallel to the **working hand.** The holding hand provides support, stability, and leverage to give strength and endurance for working the points effectively. The holding hand may be moving (traveling) with the working hand or may be stationary, in a firm but gentle fixed position, nurturing and caressing. The working hand applies compression, stimulation, and/or moving (traveling).

Relaxation Techniques

There are many wonderful and creative relaxation techniques. The relaxation portion of the session shows the client or your partner that it's going to be fun and enjoyable. It's a time to build trust and help them relax and enjoy the session.

Relaxation and reflexology techniques are done on bare feet, not through socks or stockings. Each of these techniques is performed on each foot. In a session, the practitioner will perform all the techniques on one foot before moving on to the other foot.[2]

Apply a small amount of a nongreasy cream to the feet for the relaxation session. Clients find it soothing and comforting, and it makes skin soft and flexible. Ideally, the cream should be absorbed by the time the actual reflexology work begins, so you don't slide over the reflex areas and points or find the feet too slippery to apply sufficient pressure to them. If the feet seem too greasy when you begin to work the reflex areas and points, apply a little powder or cornstarch to absorb the excess or wipe with a towel.

ARCB recommends six basic **relaxation techniques**—special techniques that soothe and calm— designed to promote relaxation. These techniques are also used for working the relative reflex areas to help improve circulation. In addition to the basic six relaxation techniques, reflexologists use their creativity and expand their repertoire to include many other relaxation techniques. Here are the six ARCB relaxation techniques:

1. Relaxing the foot: This is a rapid back and forth movement of the foot as the hands are loosely held against the **medial,** the inside or great toe side of the foot, and **lateral,** the outside or fifth digit side of the foot, sides of the foot. Use light pressure and do not squeeze the foot (Figure 14-6).
2. Loosening the ankle: Place the heel of each hand under the ankle bones using a firm pressure. Do not rub the skin. Perform the same back and forth motion as above (Figure 14-7).

BOX 14-1 Healing Response

Clients with a lot of congestion and toxins in their bodies may experience a "healing response," which can begin during the Reflexology session or shortly afterward. Typical reactions in a healing response are headache, diarrhea, coldness, nausea, and sinus congestion. While it may be temporarily unpleasant, the healing response often indicates the reflexology is working! Healing responses usually pass within 24 hours. As the body rids itself of toxins and impurities, it is less likely to occur the next time.

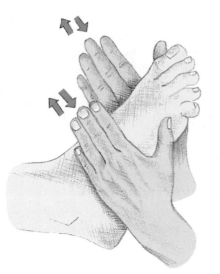

FIGURE 14-6 Relaxing the foot. From Norman L: *Feet first: a guide to foot reflexology,* New York, 1998, Simon & Schuster.

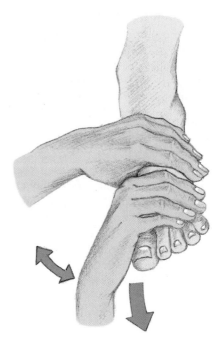

FIGURE 14-8 Spinal twist. From Norman L: *Feet first: a guide to foot reflexology,* New York, 1998, Simon & Schuster.

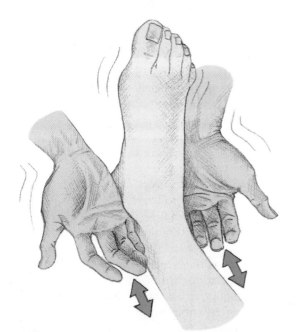

FIGURE 14-7 Loosening the ankle. From Norman L: *Feet first: a guide to foot reflexology,* New York, 1998, Simon & Schuster.

3. Spinal twist: Stand up if your client is lying on a bed; kneel if your client is lying on the floor. With the hand closest to the leg hold the foot stationary at the arch of the foot as close to the ankle bone as possible. The webbing of your hand should be on the inside edge of the foot. Place the second hand on the foot beside the first, in a similar manner keeping the index fingers next to each other on top of the foot and the thumbs next to each other under the foot. Twist gently back and forth with the second hand (the one closer to the toes). The higher hand holding the foot stationary does not move when the other hand twists. Keep your arms straight and elbows locked for better pressure. Repeat several times and then move both hands (still touching each other as described above) toward the toes, repeating as necessary until you have "twisted" the entire foot up to the base of the toes (Figure 14-8).[2]

4. **Metatarsal** kneading: Grasp the top of the foot just beneath the toes with one hand and make a fist with the other. Press the back of the fingers of the first (not the knuckles) into the fleshy area on the ball of the foot (which corresponds to the lungs and chest). As you release the press, but still maintaining contact, gently squeeze the toes themselves with the other hand. Keep both hands in place on the foot even in the release. Do this several times. Alternately press, then release and squeeze in a rhythmic movement (Figure 14-9).[8]

5. Relaxing the toes using the holding hand: Grasp the metatarsal head of the toe being rotated by placing the thumb on the **plantar** (bottom) surface and the index and middle fingers on the **dorsal** (top of the foot or back of the hand) surface. Then

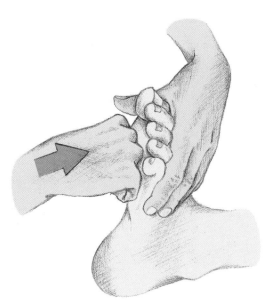

FIGURE 14-9 Metatarsal kneading. From Norman L: *Feet first: a guide to foot reflexology,* New York, 1998, Simon & Schuster.

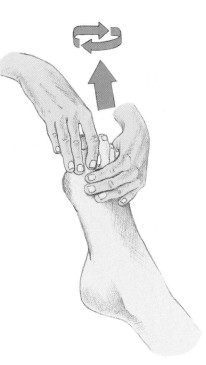

FIGURE 14-10 Relaxing the toes. From Norman L: *Feet first: a guide to foot reflexology,* New York, 1998, Simon & Schuster.

with the working hand place the thumb along the shaft of the toe to the base on the plantar surface. The rest of the fingers grasp the dorsal surface down to the base of the toe. Lifting gently, rotate in a curricular motion both clockwise and counterclockwise (Figure 14-10).

6. Relaxing the area beneath the head of the metatarsals: The thumb of the working hand is placed on the plantar aspect at the diaphragm line, with the fingers on the dorsal aspect. Hold firmly. The thumb of the holding hand is placed on the plantar aspect on the ball of the foot. The fingers are opposite on the dorsal surface. Hold firmly, lifting up the ball of the foot and pulling the foot over the top of the thumb. Start with the thumb at the medial edge of the diaphragm line and move along in small increments to the lateral edge of the foot (Figure 14-11).[2]

Once the client and his or her feet are relaxed, the reflexologist begins the systematic, manual stimulation of the reflex point/areas using the thumbs and fingers.

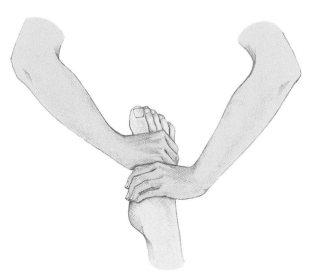

FIGURE 14-11 Wringing the foot. From Norman L: *Feet first: a guide to foot reflexology,* New York, 1998, Simon & Schuster.

BASIC REFLEXOLOGY TECHNIQUES

ARCB recommends four basic reflexology techniques. There are also additional Reflexology techniques used to work the areas and points. Here are the six techniques to work the reflex areas:

1. Basic thumb technique—thumb walking: The basic thumb technique is applied by bending the thumb at the first joint (at a 45-degree angle) while using the medial edge of the thumb. The remaining four fingers provide support and leverage. Used on a large fleshy area on the sole or plantar aspect in a steady, even caterpillar-like forward motion—never backward (Figure 14-12).

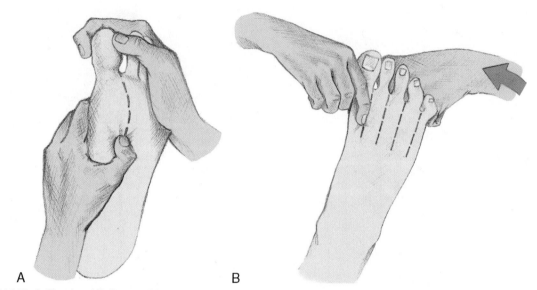

FIGURE 14-12 **A,** Thumb and **B,** finger walking. From Norman L: *Feet first: a guide to foot reflexology,* New York, 1998, Simon & Schuster.

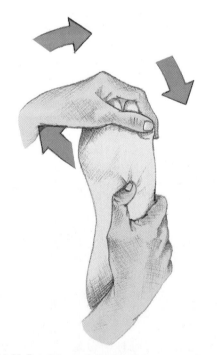

FIGURE 14-13 Rotation on a point. From Norman L: *Feet first: a guide to foot reflexology,* New York, 1998, Simon & Schuster.

2. Basic finger technique—finger walking: The basic finger technique is applied by working with the medial edge of the finger, while bending the first joint of that finger and applying pressure in a steady, even caterpillar-like forward motion—never backward. The thumb provides support and leverage. Used on bony, thin-skinned areas, e.g., dorsal, lateral, and medial surfaces (Figure 14-12).

3. Rotation on a point—pinpoint rotations: Press the thumb into the point you want to work; the fingers support the thumb by being opposite and parallel to it. The holding hand (hand that supports) lifts the foot up, flexes it down, and rotates the foot in a circular motion onto the thumb so it presses firmly into the point. Use on tender reflexes, e.g., spinal reflex, diaphragm, adrenals, spleen, gallbladder (Figure 14-13).

4. Pivot on a point: An alternative to the rotation on a point is the pivot technique. Basically it is a thumb walking while the other hand presses the foot straight back and pivots it away from you onto the thumb. To do this, grasp the foot with the holding hand, fingers resting over the top of the foot. Thumb walk with the other hand on a diagonal across the area to be worked. As you thumb walk, use the holding hand to pivot or twist the foot away from you on and off the thumb in a smooth, rhythmical fashion (only from the inside of the foot to the outside).

5. Flexing on a point: This is the same procedure as pivoting on a point, except the holding hand moves the foot backward and forward on the thumb instead of pivoting or twisting away.

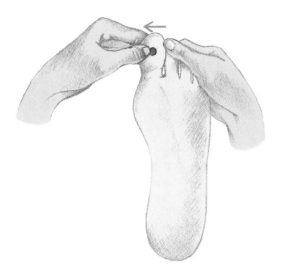

FIGURE 14-14 Hook and back-up. From Norman L: *Feet first: a guide to foot reflexology,* New York, 1998, Simon & Schuster.

BOX 14-2 Reflexology and Visualization

Our brain is like a computer. We can program anything. When we envision our goals in our mind and embrace them in our hearts, they can manifest. When we are in a deeply relaxed state like we experience during a Reflexology session (from soothing the over 14,000 nerves in our feet), we are open and receptive to suggestions we give ourselves.

As a matter of fact my clients report they feel like they are in such a profound state of relaxation that they feel like they are in a deep trance during their Reflexology sessions. (Because of the concentration of nerves in such a small area, Reflexology provides the ideal internal environment to receive.) Being in this powerful, relaxed, and receptive place allows us to create our desired outcomes. What we put our attention on grows stronger in our life. Focusing on what we'd like to have happen from a relaxed, open space encourages what we put our attention on to happen more easily.

---

6. Hook-in and back-up: A more advanced technique, which is the act of pushing in and pulling the thumb back toward the hand to apply pressure. Used on specific pinpoint reflexes that are deep and harder to reach, e.g., pituitary gland, sigmoid colon, and ileocecal valve (Figure 14-14).

THE POWER OF USING VISUALIZATION WITH REFLEXOLOGY

We are only beginning to understand the power of the mind. Whatever the brain thinks about, whether it is real or not, is how the body will respond (Box 14-2).

Here are some guidelines to follow: First, relax and breathe deeply. Let your mind go blank as far as you are able. Choose a visualization for general relaxation or one that is specific to the part of your body that needs healing. You may want to imagine healing energy flowing to that part of the body and "see" it as a special color or as light. Others visualize pain or discomfort in a graphic or symbolic way, such as a knot in a rope or a blazing fire. In the visualization they untie the rope or throw water on the fire. Another approach is seeing yourself well and feeling wonderful, doing activities that will be easy for you once the healing is complete. Visualizations are personal, and there is no right or wrong way to do them.

While you enjoy the visualization you created, continue it for as long as you like during the session, maintaining it for a minimum of 2 or 3 minutes.

CERTIFICATION REQUIREMENTS

A revolution is underway. More and more, complementary therapies are being used by, and in conjunction with, the traditional health care professions. The demand for qualified reflexologists by the public and the health care industry continues to grow. With acceptance of Reflexology as a valuable and noninvasive therapy comes the responsibility for the profession to provide qualified practitioners who meet established national standards. In response to this demand, I and other leaders in reflexology created the American Reflexology Certification Board (ARCB) in 1991.

American Reflexology Certification Board

The American Reflexology Certification Board (ARCB) is a nonprofit corporation. As an independent testing agency, it offers a national certification program for reflexologists. Its primary aim is to certify the competency of those reflexologists who practice on a professional basis and wish to be recognized as meeting national standards. Your involvement with ARCB and national certification are the next step after you have completed a course of study in reflexology and have further developed your hands-on skills by working on clients. ARCB is an independent testing agency, not a membership organization. It is not affiliated with any association, training program, or instructor. Nor does it accredit teachers or curricula. The ARCB program does not interfere with, nor negate, certification programs offered by different schools. ARCB encourages each school to test its students before awarding a diploma or certification of completion. ARCB certification is an important step offering increased credibility for both the practitioner and the field of Reflexology.

The goal of national certification is to promote reflexology through the recognition of competent professional practitioners. Reflexologists who successfully pass the national certification process promote higher standards of education, ensure public safety, and demonstrate their commitment to the profession through self-improvement. Creation of national standards and identification of nationally certified practitioners build consumer confidence in the quality of services offered.[4]

To maintain your national certification you must pay dues and enroll in ARCB-sanctioned education courses each year.

National Certification Testing Prerequisites

1. Be 18 years of age or older
2. Have a high school diploma or the equivalent
3. Have completed a "hands-on" Reflexology course through certification providing a minimum of 110 hours
4. The documentation of 90 postgraduate sessions on ARCB forms

You can obtain more information about certification and educational requirements by visiting the resources at the end of the chapter.

CHAPTER SUMMARY

"Let me remind you that reflexology is a means of equalizing the circulation. We all know circulation is life. Stagnation is death. Everything around us that is alive is in motion, nothing stands still. Our vitality is either increasing or decreasing according to the quality and circulation of our bloodstream."[8]

To those such as Eunice Ingham and others who dedicated their lives to the study and promotion of Reflexology, we owe a great debt. Through their work, millions of people across the globe can enjoy the outstanding health benefits of this modality.

Reflexology:

- Is a science and an art that is based on the principle that there are reflex areas and points in the feet and hands that correspond to each organ, gland, and part of the body.
- Connects individuals through the intimate act of touch on the hands and feet.
- Saves clients time and the self-consciousness about getting undressed.
- Removes inorganic waste material such as uric acid and other deposits that can build up in the bottoms of the feet.
- Reduces stress and tension, allowing the miles of cardiovascular vessels to conduct the flow of blood naturally and easily.
- Relaxes and opens up energy pathways, so the body is revitalized and energy is supplied on all levels.
- Works through the nervous system and subtle energy pathways to improve the function of organs and glands, and all systems of the body.

For those who wish to pursue the field of reflexology this chapter has given you a glimpse into its history, benefits, contraindications, and techniques, in addition to the personal satisfaction and health benefits for you as the practitioner. My hope is that you will join us in our passion and pursuit to bring about a healthier, happier world.

CASE HISTORIES

■ Case history 1

Like all good health practitioners, Reflexologists keep comprehensive records of each session, checking responses, as well as changes in general health. Sometimes these histories are dramatic and add to the overwhelming evidence of the benefits of Reflexology.

A 59-year-old woman came to consultation in October 1999 for a uterine polyp detected accidentally in an ecographic control.[8] The polyp was 8mm. The treatment began by stimulating uterus and abdominal lymphatic ganglia (according to localizations presented in my book, *Principles of Reflexology*). The sessions were conducted twice a week for 3 months. Later I decreased the sessions to one per week for 3 months more, and I continued with one session every 2 weeks until ecographic studies showed that the uterine polyp had disappeared. The duration of the sessions was 10 minutes in each foot and for each hemiuterus and another 10 minutes for abdominal lymph nodes.

Comments: the palpation in the first consultation, one could feel with clarity a mobile, soft, and very painful "deposit" in both feet (in the report 1, the polyp is located in anterior uterus face, in and of itself the palpation detects deposits in both feet). After six sessions the deposit began to fragment and progressively disappeared.[9]

▪ Case history 2

A client of mine was in the hospital suffering from a kidney stone and was in tremendous pain.[2] He was scheduled for surgery the next morning. His wife called me, and I came to the hospital that evening to relax him. In addition to working on his feet to reduce his stress, I had him visualize the kidney stones breaking up and dissolving. During our session he was so relaxed he fell asleep. When the nurse woke him in the morning for surgery, she found he had passed the kidney stone in his sleep. It was in a strainer the nurse had placed on him the previous night. His doctor cancelled the surgery and sent him home.

A couple of years later, the same client had a goiter on his neck that was getting bigger each day. I gave him a full session and continued working on him every other day. Within a few weeks the goiter was entirely gone.

SUGGESTED READINGS

Byers D: *Better health with foot reflexology*, Saint Petersburg, Fla, 2001, Ingham Publishing.

Issel C: *Reflexology, art science, history*, Sacramento, Calif, 1990, New Frontier Publishing.

Kunz K, Kunz B: *The complete guide to foot reflexology*, Upper Saddle River, NJ, 1986, Prentice Hall Press.

Kunz K, Kunz B: *My reflexologist says feet don't lie*, 2001, Reflexology Research Project Press.

Manzanares J: *Principles of reflexology 1 & 2*, Barcelona, Spain, 2000, Property Intellectual Registrar: www.reflexologic.com DR.JMC@teleline.es.

Marquardt H: *Reflexotherapy for the feet*, New York, 2000, Thieme Publishing.

Norman L: *Feet first: a guide to foot reflexology*, New York, 1988, Simon & Schuster.

Voner V: *The everything reflexology book*, Avon, Mass, 2003, Adams Media.

For a more complete list of books on reflexology visit: **Larkin's Reflexology Booklist:** *http://homepage.eircom.net/~footman/booklst.html.*

RESOURCES

The Laura Norman Method of Reflexology[SM]
Beginner to Certification Training Programs
New York City

212-532-4404
Delray Beach, Florida
561-272-1220
New England
413-854-2615
email: classes@lauranorman.com
www.lauranorman.com

CERTIFICATION
ACARET
American Commission for Accreditation of Reflexology Education and Training
PO Box 19384
Seattle, WA 98109-9384
email: acaret@acaret.org
Phone: 206-856-8165
Fax: 727-319-6911
http://www.acaret.org/

American Reflexology Certification Board
http://www.arcb.net/history.htm
Certification and licensing requirements vary from state to state. Here is a complete list of the state-by-state requirements: http://www.reflexology-research.com/LAWS_1.html

ASSOCIATIONS
International Council of Reflexologists
PO Box 78060
Westcliffe Postal Outlet
Hamilton, ON L9C 7N5
Canada
+1 (905) 387-8449
www.icr-reflexology.org

International Reflexology Association
25 South Fourth Street
PO Drawer 421
Warrenton, Virginia 20188
540-351-0800
http://www.internationalreflexologyassociation.com

The Reflexology Association of America
4012 Rainbow Ste. K-PMB#585
Las Vegas, NV 89103-2059
978-779-0255
http://www.reflexology-usa.org/
For a list of state and national reflexology associations visit: http://www.holisticwebworks.com/reflexology-Associations.htm

REFERENCES

1. Kunz K, Kunz B: *The complete guide to reflexology (revised)*, Upper Saddle River, NJ, 1986, Prentice Hall Press.
2. Norman L: *Feet first: a guide to foot reflexology*, New York, 1988, Simon & Schuster.
3. Dougans I, Ellis S: *The art of reflexology*, 1992, Element Books.
4. American Reflexology Certification Board Website: *A brief history of reflexology*, http://www.arcb.net/history.htm.
5. Byers D: *Better health with foot reflexology*, rev ed, St. Petersburg, Fla, 1987, Ingham Publishing.
6. International Reflexology Association website: http://www.internationalreflexologyassociation.com/home/index.php?site_config_id=10&page_selection=67.
7. American Reflexology Certification Board website http://www.arcb.net.
8. Ingham E: *Stories the feet can tell thru reflexology*, St. Petersburg, Fla, 1984, Ingham Publishing, Inc.
9. Manzanares J: *Principles of reflexology 1 & 2*, Barcelona, Spain, 2000, Property Intellectual Registrar.

MULTIPLE CHOICE TEST QUESTIONS

1) Complete this sentence from the definition of reflexology recognized by ARCB: Foot and hand reflexology is a scientific art based on the premise that there are:
   a) meridians running in parallel paths laterally throughout the body
   b) zones and reflex areas in the feet and hands which correspond to all the parts of the body
   c) ten zones or guidelines acting as reflexive points that mirror the body
   d) ch'i energy zones running medially in the body

2) Complete this sentence from the definition of reflexology recognized by ARCB: The physical act of applying pressures using thumb, finger, and hand techniques results in:
   a) stress reduction which causes a physiologic change in the body
   b) energy flow through longitudinal pathways resulting in improved health
   c) the stimulation and balance of the corresponding organ resulting in stress reduction
   d) curing disease by applying deep pressure

3) The science of reflexology considers the feet to be minimaps of the human body with areas:
   a) corresponding to lateral and postlateral zones throughout the body
   b) linked to a corresponding area or point in the foot
   c) divided into ten zones and four divisions
   d) corresponding to medial and postmedial zones throughout the body

4) The first recorded scientific reference to reflexology was in:
   a) 1742 by Dr. Riley Moorehead
   b) 1890 by Sir Henry Head
   c) 1902 by Lord Phillip Fitzgerald
   d) 1918 by Eunice Ingham

5) Which one of these individuals DID NOT contribute in some way to the development of Modern Reflexology:
   a) Dr. William Fitzgerald
   b) Dr. Joseph Riley
   c) Lord William T. Riley
   d) Eunice Ingham

6) Massage works through the musculature, using methods of stroking to restore metabolic balance within the soft tissue. Reflexology works through:
   a) the nervous system and subtle energy pathways
   b) stress reduction through relaxation to promote self-healing
   c) harmonizing the body's systems naturally
   d) all of the above

7) From a reflexologist's point of view, _____ is the key factor in the human experience which contributes to disease. The missing phrase is:
   a) toxins
   b) muscle strain
   c) stress
   d) environment pollution

8) Which country tops the world in reflexology practice, with about 65% of its population using it in one form or another?
   a) Thailand
   b) India
   c) USA
   d) Denmark

9) Many people experience daily pain in their feet and tune it out of their conscious awareness with a neurologic process known as:
   a) adaptation
   b) tarsal inversion
   c) proximal distancing
   d) pain referral

10) In addition to the zones, there are _____, creating 4 horizontal divisions on the feet. Using these and the zones as a grid you can locate any area of the body on the foot.
   a) guidelines
   b) meridians
   c) flex points
   d) response points

11) Which is NOT a benefit of reflexology?
   a) reduces stress
   b) improves circulation
   c) diagnosis of illnesses
   d) revitalizes energy

12) There are times when it might be wise or necessary to avoid working certain parts of the foot or get permission from a doctor. Which of these is NOT considered a contraindication?
a) unstable blood pressure
b) varicose veins
c) obesity
d) severe edema

13) Which of these statements is false?
a) Reflexologists do not diagnose illness.
b) Reflexologists can diagnose diseases through developing sensitive touch techniques.
c) Reflexology is not considered a cure; it helps the body heal itself.
d) The Reflexologist is a channel for healing.

14) The body has built-in mechanisms for cleansing itself. Which term is NOT associated with a mechanism for cleansing?
a) lymphatic
b) excretory
c) integumentary
d) interlymphatory

15) Which word pertains to a particular area of the foot?
a) dorsal
b) lateral
c) plantar
d) all of the above

16) The immune system also responds _____, relying on other bodily processes to maintain its own lines of defense. What is the missing word or phrase?
a) reflexively
b) synergistically
c) in kind
d) automatically

17) Finish this sentence: reflexologists specify that there are 10 energy zones that:
a) run the length of the body
b) run counterclockwise, and pass through the body
c) are found in each of the feet
d) correspond with 10 reflex points in the feet

18) ARCB recommends six basic relaxation techniques. Which one of these terms is NOT one of them?
a) relaxing the foot
b) loosening the ankle
c) hook-in and back-up
d) relaxing the toes

19. Which method is considered a basic reflexology technique?
a) the caterpillar crawl
b) push and pull
c) finger tapping
d) thumb walking

20. The goal of the American Reflexology Certification Board (ARCB) is to promote Reflexology: Which one is false?
a) through the recognition of competent professional practitioners
b) through local and international certification
c) by promoting higher standards of education
d) by ensuring public safety

Shiatsu

Sandra K. Anderson

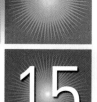

15

STUDENT OBJECTIVES

Upon completion of this chapter, students will be able to do the following:

- Explain what shiatsu is, describe how a shiatsu treatment is performed, and discuss what a typical treatment session is like.
- Discuss the benefits, contraindications, and precautions for receiving shiatsu.
- Trace the history of shiatsu.
- Describe the different major types of shiatsu.
- Briefly explain traditional Chinese medicine and the five elements in relation to shiatsu, including what qi (ki) is and what channels are.
- Describe basic shiatsu techniques.
- Discuss the roles connection, touch sensitivity, and intuition play in performing shiatsu.
- Outline the four methods of assessment.
- Explain common imbalance patterns in each of the five elements.
- Discuss shiatsu training and licensing requirements.

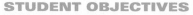

KEY TERMS

Acupressure
Anma (Amma)
Anmo
Ashiatsu
Channels (meridians)
Dragon's (tiger's) mouth
Earth
Fire
Five Element shiatsu
Four Methods of Assessment
Hara
Ki
Macrobiotic (barefoot) shiatsu
Metal
Namikoshi shiatsu
Ohashiatsu
Palming
Qi
Seiza
Traditional Chinese medicine
Tsubo therapy
Water
Watsu
Wood
Yin/Yang
Zen shiatsu

Shiatsu is a Japanese type of bodywork. It combines art and science, theory and practice, strength and softness, intellect and intuition. It is about supporting and it is about letting go and knowing when to do which.

In Japanese, *shi* means finger and *atsu* means pressure, so shiatsu is literally "finger pressure." However, this definition is overly simplistic. The implication is that all a practitioner needs to do to perform shiatsu is press her fingers onto another person's body, which is not the case.

Shiatsu is based on the same principles as is acupuncture, which is part of **traditional Chinese medicine.** Traditional Chinese medicine views the entire human being as body, mind, and spirit. Every living thing is part of the greater continuum of its environment, the Earth, and the universe. **Qi** (pronounced "chee") is the Chinese term for the energy or force that gives and maintains life. Qi is also the body's "energy," which can be thought of vitality or vigor. Optimally, Qi flows within living creatures in a balanced, harmonious way, sustaining health. If Qi is not flowing properly, disharmony and lack of balance result in pain, discomfort, or other disorders.[1]

To better understand concepts in this chapter, watch *Shiatsu* video on the **DVD** found at the back of this book.

281

Qi flows in specific streams in the body called **channels,** or **meridians.** These channels are connected to the organs of the body and share the names of the organs. Examples are the Lung Channel, Large Intestine Channel, Stomach Channel, and Spleen Channel. (In keeping with the convention of traditional Chinese medicine texts, the names of the organs and their associated channels are capitalized when discussed from this point of view. When organs are discussed from the Western medical view, they are not capitalized.) The organs and channels have certain physical, mental, psychologic, emotional, and spiritual functions in the body, and the balanced flow of Qi in the channels sustains these functions[2] (Figure 15-1).

Along the channels are points where the Qi is accessed easily. When the flow of Qi is disrupted for any of many possible reasons, it can be brought back

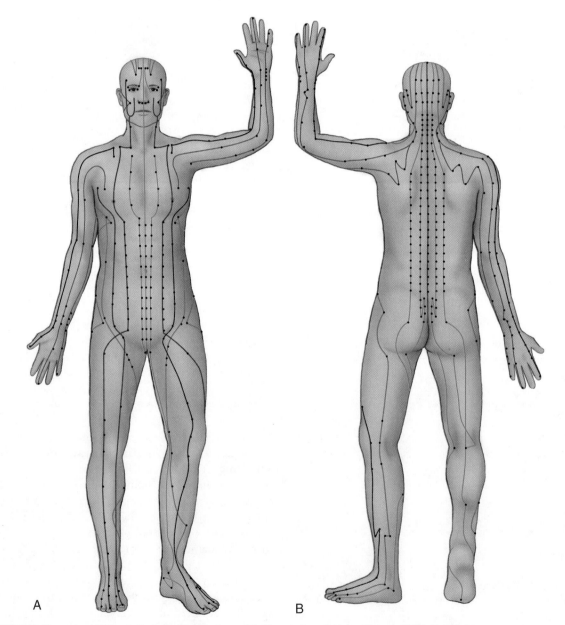

A   B

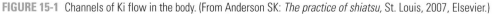

FIGURE 15-1 Channels of Ki flow in the body. (From Anderson SK: *The practice of shiatsu*, St. Louis, 2007, Elsevier.)

into equilibrium by affecting the Qi at the points. Acupuncturists insert needles into the points to balance Qi. Shiatsu practitioners, however, use their own Qi to support and stabilize their client's Qi. Some types of shiatsu mainly focus on addressing points; other types address the entire channel.

The goal of shiatsu is to help rebalance the client's energy and alleviate discomfort. Shiatsu typically is performed on a futon (mat) on the floor, covered by a single sheet. Small pillows or bolsters can be used to prop the client comfortably. Shiatsu can also be performed on a massage table or with the client sitting in a chair. Soothing music can be played to help the client relax. Hand cleaner, such as witch hazel or diluted alcohol, and a hand towel can also be placed within easy reach. The cleaner can be used to freshen up the client's feet or for the practitioner to clean her hands before working on the client's face.

■□□■ IN MY EXPERIENCE

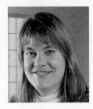

While everyone seems to have heard of massage, shiatsu may be new to many people. Because it does not sound like massage, I have found that sometimes clients are hesitant to try it. However, when I talk about the benefits of shiatsu, and that clients remain fully clothed, they usually become more interested. What have been the best selling points are all the stretches and how good they can make clients feel, and that when the treatment is over, they will most likely feel rested and calm, but not groggy they way clients sometimes feel after a massage.

Because of the nature of techniques performed, such as stretches and joint range of motion, both the practitioner and client need to wear comfortable, loose-fitting shirts and pants. Draw-string or elastic waist pants work the best. Shiatsu can be done in bare feet as long as the feet are clean or in clean socks. No lubricants are used. The shiatsu practitioner uses palpation, physical manipulation techniques, stretches, and range of motion movements to balance the client's Qi, and to assist in moving it more evenly throughout the client's body. In addition to finger pressure the shiatsu practitioner can use pressure from his thumbs, palms, forearms, elbows, knees, and feet during the course of the treatment. The shiatsu practitioner's strength comes from the center of her body (belly and hips) and is transmitted outward through her extremities. However, the physical movements a practitioner uses are guided by her foundational knowledge, perceptions, and insight gained through trusting her intuition (Figure 15-2).

WHO CAN RECEIVE SHIATSU?

Shiatsu can be appealing to many different persons. It can be performed on the old and the young, those in excellent health and those in fragile health, those who are experienced in receiving many different types of bodywork and those who have never received any type of bodywork at all. It may be especially attractive to

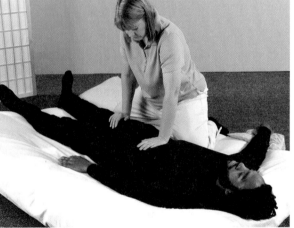

FIGURE 15-2 Shiatsu being performed. (From Anderson SK: *The practice of shiatsu*, St. Louis, 2008, Elsevier.)

those who feel uncomfortable removing their clothes for a massage treatment.

People can receive shiatsu for relaxation or to help them with specific conditions. In particular, shiatsu can help alleviate insomnia, anxiety, depression, headaches, muscular tension, digestive tract issues, and sinus congestion. In some cases it can also help increase local circulation and the movement of lymph.

Sometimes conditions that are contraindicated for massage therapy are not contraindicated for shiatsu. For example, the flare-up stages of autoimmune diseases such as lupus and rheumatoid arthritis are contraindications for massage therapy because massage techniques can stimulate the production of histamine, which would worsen the inflammation that occurs during flare-up stage. Also, the massage techniques may simply be too painful for the person to receive. Instead, shiatsu could be performed with clearance from the client's health care provider. Stretches and range of motion techniques would be contraindicated. However, the simple act of the shiatsu practitioner placing her hands on the client to support his Qi may help the client feel better. If the client cannot tolerate touch, shiatsu can be performed energetically above the person.

Certain conditions call for caution in receiving shiatsu. For clients who have debilitating conditions such as osteoporosis, or those undergoing chemotherapy, only the lightest pressure or energetic work above the body should be performed. The application of shiatsu techniques also has local contraindications such as varicose veins, wounds, bone fractures, recent scars, and areas of inflammation. Inflamed, painful joints, including arthritic joints, are contraindications for range of motion techniques. Also, any vertebral column issues, such as a herniated disk or ankylosing spondylitis, are contraindications for certain range of motion techniques and across-the-body stretches.

Performing shiatsu on pregnant clients involves special considerations. The client may not be able to get down on the futon, so the treatment may need to be done on a massage table. If the client is 4 or more months pregnant, she should be propped in a semi-reclining position when supine with her upper torso (from her hips) at an angle between 45 and 70 degrees and her legs elevated. Once she is no longer able to lie prone, side position can be used to work on her back and posterior legs. Beacause ischemic compression on the legs is contraindicated during pregnancy, especially during the first three months, all palming, thumbing, and finger pressure work should be done lightly on the lower extremities. There are also certain points along certain channels that should not be worked as they have a strong "down bearing" effect on Qi. If a pregnant woman is past her due date, then working these points may be useful in stimulating the downward flow of Qi and possibly starting labor and delivery.[3]

HISTORY OF SHIATSU

Shiatsu as practiced today is a relatively young bodywork practice. Its roots, however, extend deep into millennia of traditional Chinese medicine. Its techniques come from systems developed by ordinary people, imperial physicians, blind practitioners, and physicians for the samurai.

One of the oldest forms of body treatments in Asia, An Wu, developed in China more than 5000 years ago. An Wu resembled Western massage. It consisted of pressing, gliding, stretching, and percussing the body. The practitioner used his thumbs, fingers, forearms, elbows, knees, and feet on the points along the channels of Qi flow.

At the same time, traditional Chinese medicine concepts were being developed. In brief, the ancient Chinese viewed themselves as part of nature and the universe around them, with Qi as a unifying factor. Because their view of health and disease was that both are on a continuum of Qi flow, An Wu and traditional Chinese medicine naturally developed together. As ancient practitioners worked with Chinese medicine and physical manipulation techniques on the body, they became their culture's physicians. Gradually, An Wu came to be known as **Anmo,** which began to become popular as a medical treatment.

By the fifth century AD, Anmo had developed into a more sophisticated system of theory, diagnosis, and treatment. During this time Anmo spread to other Asian countries such as Korea, Japan, and India. Throughout the ages, as more and more physicians palpated and massaged patients, they pinpointed the effects of pressing certain locations on Qi channels. They also discovered that more specific pressure on these more specific locations had greater effect. These locations on Qi channels were narrowed down into points. Over time, pressure on these points became more and more precise, until needles were finally inserted into the points, giving birth to acupuncture. The points were named, numbered, and classified in the system that is still used today. This system is common to both acupuncture and shiatsu.

Acupuncture gradually took over in China as the primary form of medicine. However, palpatory and massage techniques remained important foundational techniques. Physicians had to master bodywork before they were allowed to progress to using needles. Even though acupuncture became the primary form of healing, massaging (as in rubbing and pressing the channels and points) remained quite popular.

The theory of Qi and traditional Chinese medicine traveled throughout Asia, and so did hands-on physical manipulation. Because of geographic proximity, Japanese culture and Chinese culture have had a close relationship. During the sixth century AD, monks from China traveling to Japan brought combinations of Chinese philosophies that included Buddhism, Taoism, and Confucianism. They also brought knowledge of Chinese medicine. Trading between China and Japan opened up more communication between the two countries, and Japanese students were sent to China to learn more about Chinese culture and medicine.

Acupuncture and Anmo were readily infused into Japanese culture. As the years progressed, acupuncture remained relatively the same as when it arrived in Japan. However, Anmo was modified and refined to fit Japanese culture and gradually evolved into **Anma,** or **Amma.** Japan's early history was marked by many warring states and no unified central government. By 1185, these states were known as shogunates, and their leaders were called shoguns. They had highly trained, armed men called samurai to fight their battles. The fighting techniques the samurai used are the origins of modern Japanese martial arts. The medical practitioners in Japan were expected to keep these men healthy and fit. Anma became a mixture of the original Anmo techniques imported from China and techniques specifically developed for samurai needs.

During the Edo period (1602-1868) Anma reached its height of popularity. New Anma techniques and methods were developed, schools were established, and texts were written to teach Anma. The shogunates had been organized into a functioning country ruled by one shogun appointed by Japan's emperor. Along the way, the samurai lost most of their importance. Over time, their fighting techniques meshed more with Buddhist, Taoist, and Confucian philosophies than with actual combat, and modern martial arts were born.

Not many professions were open to the visually impaired during this period. Anma was available to them, however, with the reasoning that the blind must have greater touch sensitivity. It was also seen as a form of welfare. Soon Anma was being practiced mostly by blind practitioners, and because being visually impaired limited the education these practitioners were able to receive throughout this period, much technical and clinical wisdom was lost, and Anma became known as being useful only for relaxation.

During the mid-1800s, the power of the shoguns fell and imperialism rose. The Meiji period of Japan (1868-1912) saw an overhaul of the Japanese government. It was re-created in a Western framework, and changes were instigated to make Japanese society more like Western society. Western medicine dominated, and traditional medicine was relegated to the realm of folk medicine. The therapeutic value of Anma and Asian medicine was rejected, although segments of the population were still attached to these practices and Anma remained an occupation for the blind. Also during this time Western massage therapy was introduced to Japan.

By the beginning of the 1900s, Anma had lost so much credibility that it was considered shady employment. The practitioners of the true art of Anma sought a way to distinguish themselves from charlatans and "body shampooers." A new name was needed, and in 1919, Tamai Tempaku published a book called *Shiatsu Ho,* which translates to "finger pressure method." This text united Anma and Western anatomy and physiology and used concepts from Ampuku (a type of abdominal massage) and Do-In (self massage).

Shiatsu began to develop a different look from the established techniques and principles used in authentic Anma. Shiatsu practitioners started merging Western bodywork techniques from chiropractic medicine and massage therapy with conventional Anma methods. Western medicine concepts such as anatomy, physiology, and psychology were used along with traditional Chinese medicine theory.

In 1925 the Shiatsu Therapists Association was formed to promote shiatsu as a legitimate profession and to distinguish it from Anma. Also in 1925 Tokujiro Namikoshi (1905-2000) founded the Clinic of Pressure Therapy in Hokkaido, Japan. As a child, Namikoshi discovered his gift for manual therapy by helping alleviate his mother's rheumatoid arthritis symptoms. He went on to study Anma and Western massage therapy. Because he studied both subjects, his focus was to practice shiatsu within a Western structure. He did not emphasize the study of channels. Instead, he concentrated on knowledge of the physical structure of the body and the nervous system and stressed the anatomic locations of points. The **Namikoshi** style of **shiatsu** involves applying methodical patterns of pressure along the points. In successive years, both the conventional and Western (Namikoshi) styles of shiatsu were taught and practiced. In 1940 Namikoshi opened the Japan Shiatsu Institute in Tokyo, which helped further awareness of shiatsu as a valid profession.

In 1955 the Japanese government officially recognized shiatsu as a part of Anma. This was the first legal sanction of shiatsu. In 1957 Namikoshi's Japan Shiatsu Institute was officially licensed as the Japan Shiatsu School by the Minister of Health and Welfare. The school proved to be enormously popular, and Namikoshi's son, Toru, went on to teach shiatsu in Europe and the United States, thus helping spread shiatsu beyond Japan's borders.[1,3,4]

Because shiatsu is a mixture of traditional and modern concepts and techniques, evolution is inherent in this type of bodywork. The nature of shiatsu is innovation. Many modern derivatives exist; following is a brief explanation of the most common types of

---

BOX 15-1 Types of Shiatsu

As previously discussed, Namikoshi shiatsu, also called Nippon shiatsu, was developed by Namikoshi and is quite common in Japan. It involves a whole-body routine that incorporates stretches, but the emphasis is more on points than channels. It tends to be a vigorous treatment.

The Japanese word for a point on a channel is *tsubo*. Katsusuke Serizawa proved their existence scientifically by measuring their electrical activity on the skin. He developed **tsubo therapy,** which emphasizes stimulating tsubo, whether through moxibustion (herbal heat therapy), acupuncture, or finger pressure. **Acupressure** is the Western derivative of tsubo therapy, which involves working the tsubo by pressing with the fingers.

Zen shiatsu was developed by Shizuto Masunaga (1925-1981) and also is popular in Japan. Masunaga discovered, through palpation and personal insight, the existence of extensions of the classic channels that zen shiatsu makes use of. Because of this, treatment emphasis is more on the channels than the tsubo. The practitioner's intuition and connection with the client's Ki are vital. The treatment can be either gentle or vigorous.

Ohashiatsu was developed by Wataru Ohashi, who opened the Shiatsu Institute in New York City in 1974. Ohashiatsu focuses less on finger pressure along the channels and more on stretching and physically manipulating the client's body to achieve Ki balance.

Five Element shiatsu focuses on patterns of disharmony in the Five Element Cycle (discussed shortly) as an assessment tool. The treatment plan uses techniques to balance the client's Ki and restore the harmony of the Five Element Cycle.

Macrobiotic, or **barefoot, shiatsu** was developed by Shizuko Yamamoto and combines macrobiotic nutritional principles with shiatsu techniques to assist clients in their health and healing processes. This style of shiatsu combines pressure on tsubo with stretches and physical manipulation. It is also called barefoot shiatsu because practitioners originally used their bare feet to apply many techniques. Currently barefoot shiatsu means techniques specifically applied with the feet, whether they are bare or have socks on them. **Ashiatsu** is an offshoot of barefoot shiatsu. In Japanese, "ashi" means foot and "atsu" means pressure. The client may lie on a futon on the floor or on a massage table. The practitioner supports herself with wooden bars suspended from the ceiling while performing different foot techniques along the client's body. While the practitioner mainly uses her feet, she may also use her knees, elbows, palms, and fingers.[1,4]

Watsu is a type of shiatsu performed in water. "Wa" comes from "water," and "atsu" comes from "shiatsu." It was developed in the 1980s by Harold Dull, who combined zen shiatsu techniques he had learned with the weightlessness of water. The practitioner continually supports the client in the water while rocking and gently stretching him to open channels and allow increased Ki flow. Being in the water allows the client to relax more fully tissues.

---

shiatsu currently practiced. All styles of shiatsu involve working with Qi in some way to effect harmony in the client's body. The Japanese word for Qi is **Ki** (pronounced "kee"). Throughout the rest of this chapter, Qi will be used in relation to traditional Chinese medicine, and Ki will be used in discussions about shiatsu, but it is important to note that Qi and Ki mean the same thing (Box 15-1).

THEORY AND PRACTICE

Practice involves learning techniques and proper mechanics. By learning from a skilled instructor, the shiatsu practitioner knows a variety of techniques to use for any area of the client's body and any of a variety of disorders the client may be experiencing. Practice also means honing skills through consistently working on a range of clients—different ages, levels of vitality, body shapes and sizes, and so on. Over time, applying shiatsu methods to many clients develops a practitioner's awareness, connection, and intuition, which are crucial to the work of shiatsu. Without these, performing shiatsu becomes a series of procedures done to the client, not the therapeutic experience that results when practitioner and client work together.

The cultivation of intuition, connection, and awareness is only part of the picture. Another necessary component is knowledge gained from the study of Western anatomy, physiology, and pathology. The shiatsu practitioner should have knowledge of Western anatomy, physiology, and pathology to understand the physical structure and functioning of the human body, and to understand disorders and disease from the Western perspective. Asian bodywork assessment techniques, discussed later in this chapter, give the practitioner information she can use to tailor the shiatsu treatments to the client's needs. Yet another foundation of Asian bodywork is traditional Chinese medicine.

The ancient Chinese were an agricultural people. Their survival depended on understanding and living with the cycles of the weather, the seasons, and lunar and solar cycles. One season flows into the next, the moon waxes and wanes, clouds build into a summer storm, rain falls, and blue sky reappears. Over thousands of years the people grew to understand the universe, the earth, nature, and themselves as all interconnected, and that every living creature's life cycle is a microcosm of a large cycle involving the heavens and the earth. Traditional Chinese medicine has its origins in these natural processes.

YIN AND YANG

Lao Tzu, who lived in the sixth century BC, wrote about the Tao in a book entitled the *Tao Te Ching. Tao* has been translated to mean "road, path, way, means, doctrine, God, the universe, nature," and "that which is." Most refer to the Tao as meaning "the way" or "the path." In the text, he describes how everything in the universe formed from the "great ultimate source." Outside of this was only emptiness. The Tao is the primary law of the universe, the law that is the genesis for all other laws and principles of the workings of the universe and the world. In a real sense, the Tao cannot be known, understood, or defined. From this concept arose the two prime principles of **Yin and Yang.** The Tao is manifested through the actions and interactions of Yin and Yang, through which all of creation is organized.

Yin and Yang are represented by a classic symbol (Figure 15-3). They are pivotal to the traditional philosophy, science, and culture in China and Japan and are essential to understanding traditional Chinese medicine. To truly understand Yin and Yang, two apparently opposing thoughts must be held at the same time: in lightness there is dark, and in darkness there is light. In the Yin/Yang symbol, the dark area has a seed of light, and the light area has a seed of dark. The light and dark areas in the Yin/Yang symbol are not static; one flows into the other. The concepts of Yin and Yang are not fixed; they are

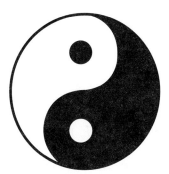

FIGURE 15-3 Yin/Yang symbol. (From Anderson SK: *The practice of shiatsu,* St. Louis, 2008, Elsevier.)

in constant movement, always transforming each other. They are the natural limits for each other; Yin can only go so far before it becomes Yang; Yang can only go so far before it becomes Yin. For example, the coldness and darkness of winter (Yin) only last for so long until the warmth and light of spring (Yang). So Yin and Yang should not be thought of as absolutes, such as everything dark is Yin and everything light is Yang. Instead, there is a continuum, a relationship.

When Yin and Yang came together, Qi was released. The Qi created the Five Elements, and from the Five Elements, everything else was created.

QI, ORGANS, AND CHANNELS

Long before Western science had an understanding of the structure and function of the human body, the ancient Chinese had developed insight into the interrelations of Qi and the organs. They were prohibited from cutting into bodies to see how they function, so by using manual therapy techniques and intuition, they came to view the human body as functioning due to the flow of Qi in a system of channels. Qi in the channels is connected to organs of the body and is the living force that causes the organs to function. In traditional Chinese medicine, the organs have specific physiologic functions that are remarkably similar to the functions of organs in Western science, as well as emotional and spiritual correlations.

The organs in traditional Chinese medicine are: Lung, Large Intestine, Stomach, Spleen, Heart, Small Intestine, Kidneys, Urinary Bladder, Liver, Gallbladder, Triple Heater (also called Triple Warmer, Triple Burner, and its Chinese name *san jiao*), and Heart Protector (also called Heart Constrictor or Pericardium). The channels connected to the organs have the same names: Lung Channel, Large Intestine Channel, and so forth. Triple Heater and Heart Protector, however, are a little different. Triple Heater is named for the three "heaters" (burners or warmers) of the body. The Upper Heater is associated with the functions of the Lungs and Heart, and combines air with food. Qi, the Middle Heater is where food is processed into food Qi by the functions of the Spleen and Stomach. The Lower Heater includes the functions of the Large Intestine, Small Intestine, Urinary Bladder and Kidneys. It also serves to separate the pure from the impure and eliminate waste. Triple Heater is associated with the lymphatic and immune systems. Heart Protector provides an energetic buffer zone around the heart and defends the emotional core of a person; it is also related to blood vessels and circulation.

TABLE 15-1 Yin Yang Organ Channels and their Corresponding Element

Yin Organ	Yang Organ	Element
Lung	Large Intestine	Metal
Kidney	Urinary Bladder	Water
Spleen	Stomach	Earth
Liver	Gallbladder	Wood
Heart	Small Intestine	Fire
Heart Protector	Triple Heater	Assisted Fire

From Anderson SK: *The practice of shiatsu*, St. Louis, 2008, Elsevier.

All the organs and channels are divided into Yin and Yang pairs. Each pair belongs to one of the Five Elements (Table 15-1). There are two additional strong currents of energy that are related to the body's core and support the body's Qi. They are not considered part of the 12 organ channels; instead they belong to a group called the Eight Extraordinary Vessels. Conception (Directing) Vessel, known by its Chinese name *Ren Mai*, travels up the anterior midline. It serves to stabilize and descend the body's Qi. It also plays a role in the conception of a baby, and maintaining the pregnancy. Governing Vessel, known by its Chinese name *Du Mai*, travels up the posterior midline. It serves to sustain and raise Qi.

In a perfect world, all living beings would have Yin and Yang in balance and smooth flow of Ki. Ideally, most human beings are born with a full and equal amount of both. Various experiences in life such as emotional upset, physical trauma, illness, childbearing, and stress, to name a few, can cause blockages in the even flow of Qi. Asian bodywork therapies are designed to balance the flow of Qi. Specifically, shiatsu works by balancing the flow of Qi (Ki) in the organ channels.

FIVE ELEMENTS

In traditional Chinese medicine, natural phenomena were systemized into Five Elements (also known as "Phases"): **Metal, Water, Earth, Wood,** and **Fire.** Seasons, foods, flavors, colors, and sounds were categorized into each of the elements. The Five Elements were seen as a part of a cycle. The cause and progression of illnesses and disorders were perceived to be based on patterns of transformation within the cycle. Lack of health was seen to be caused by a lack of harmony among certain elements. Ancient medicine expanded the Five Element theory to include aspects of the body: organs, sense organs, tissues, emotions, and behavioral attributes. Everything categorized under the Five Elements is referred to as correspondences; these correspondences were used, and still are used today, as a reference for traditional Chinese medicine physicians in their practice of diagnosis and treatment. Many shiatsu practitioners, depending on the type of shiatsu they practice, also use the Five Elements as a reference in designing treatment sessions (Table 15-2).[2,3,5]

BASIC SHIATSU TECHNIQUES

Since shiatsu is traditionally performed on a futon on the floor, the practitioner needs to be comfortable squatting, sitting, and lunging as she moves around the client. In order to be stable and grounded, the shiatsu practitioner needs to have a solid connection with the earth, keep her back straight, and lower her center of gravity into her **hara** (the Japanese word for belly).

Her hara is the source of her Ki and strength and provides direction for the treatment. The practitioner keeps her hara facing toward the area of the client's body. This helps direct Ki flow from the practitioner to the client and Ki flow within the client. Ki travels from the practitioner's hara out through her arms and legs to make contact and connect with the client in an effort to move, change, support, and balance the client's Ki.

Every shiatsu practitioner feels the connection to her client's Ki differently. For some, it feels like a merging with the client's Ki; for others, it might feel like a current of electricity flowing between themselves and their client. Others still may feel an energetic surge or, perhaps, an energetic drain. Still others may feel it subtly with the thought of just knowing they have made the connection.

To support her hara and give effective treatments, the practitioner must have a secure stance. One way the practitioner does this is by sitting in a wide *seiza* position. **Seiza** is a kneeling position in which the gluteals rest on the heels. A wide seiza is one in which the practitioner's legs are open at least 45 degrees (Figure 15-4). This position allows smooth pivoting so the practitioner can keep her hara aimed at the area being worked on. To reduce chance of injury to herself or the client, the practitioner should never twist or apply techniques at an awkward angle.

TABLE 15-2	**Five Element Correspondences**				
	Metal	**Water**	**Earth**	**Wood**	**Fire**
Season	Autumn	Winter	Late Summer	Spring	Summer
Direction	West	North	Center	East	South
Color	White	Black, Blue	Yellow, Brown	Green	Red
Taste	Pungent	Salty	Sweet	Sour	Bitter
Odor	Rotten	Putrid	Fragrant	Rancid	Burnt
Climate	Dryness	Cold	Dampness	Wind	Heat
Development Stage	Harvest	Storage	Transformation	Birth	Growth
State	Quieting	Slumber	Transition	Awakening	Wakefulness
Spiritual Quality	Po (Corporeal Soul; Body; Material)	Zhu (Ambition; Will)	Thought and Ideas	Hun (Ethereal Soul; Immaterial)	Shen (Spirit; Awareness)
Yin Organ/Time of Day	Lungs 3-5 am	Kidneys 5-7 pm	Spleen 9-11 am	Liver 1-3 am	Heart 11 am-1 pm
Yang Organ/Time of Day	Large Intestine 5-7 am	Urinary Bladder 3-5 pm	Stomach 7-9 am	Gallbladder 11pm-1am	Small Intestine 1-3 pm
Sense Organ	Nose	Ears	Mouth	Eyes	Tongue
Tissue	Skin and Body Hair	Bones	Muscles	Sinews	Vessels
Emotion	Sadness; Grief	Fear	Pensiveness	Anger	Joy
Sound	Crying	Groaning	Singing	Shouting	Laughing

From Anderson SK: *The practice of shiatsu*, St. Louis, 2008, Elsevier.

From this position, the practitioner rises up to apply more pressure. This allows the strength for application of pressure and Ki connection to continue coming from her hara instead of just using muscle strength from her

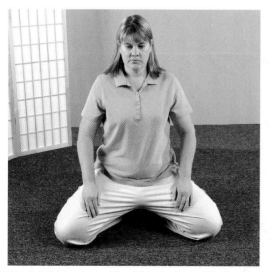

FIGURE 15-4 Wide seiza position. (From Anderson SK: *The practice of shiatsu*, St. Louis, 2008, Elsevier.)

shoulders or knees, which can put the practitioner at risk for injury and may hurt the client. The practitioner's shoulders, arms, hips, and legs should remain relaxed throughout the treatment.

It is easy to move from seiza into squatting and lunging positions. Practitioners should practice shifting through these stances until they are able to move around the client smoothly. An ideal shiatsu treatment is one that is performed fluidly, like a dance.

Remembering to breathe, and breathe efficiently, is also important when performing shiatsu. It helps the practitioner have clear, focused thought and also helps to ground, or stabilize, the practitioner. Since shiatsu treatments are generally an hour long, the treatment is fundamentally an hour-long workout. The practitioner has to able to breathe smoothly and evenly throughout the treatment to ensure enough oxygen to do the work. Running out of breath during the treatment or breathing shallowly can be an indication that she does not have a secure connection to the ground.[2,3]

The shiatsu practitioner uses most of her own body to perform techniques during a treatment. The hands are used for palming, thumbing, and fingertip work. Also used are elbows, knees, feet, and forearms.

Palming is a technique in which the practitioner uses the palm of her hand to apply pressure to the client's body. It is a way for the practitioner to assess the client's Ki flow in his body. Palming can also warm up the client's tissues by increasing blood flow to the area and increasing Ki flow. This can be especially helpful to warm up tissues before stretches and joint ranges of motion are performed.

Pressure is distributed evenly through the palm, and the fingers are relaxed. Only enough pressure is applied to make contact and connect with the client's Ki. The pressure of palming, thumbing, and fingertip work (described next) comes from leverage, not muscle strength. The practitioner leans, not presses (Figure 15-5). Palming is applied smoothly and evenly, and with the idea of sensing how the Ki is flowing in the channels beneath the practitioner's palm. The pressure should be applied with the palm perpendicular to the client's body, or in towards the center of the client's body. This way the pressure is able to penetrate into the channels more directly. The practitioner exhales with the client when applying pressure, then releases the pressure gradually when the client inhales. Varying amounts of pressure may be used depending on the depth needed to contact the client's Ki. When the practitioner's Ki and the client's Ki connect, they can support each other and the practitioner has the opportunity to bring about necessary change in the client's Ki flow.

The thumbs and fingertips are used to work more specifically on the channels and tsubo. Pressure is applied with the ball of the thumb and the pads of the fingertips. As with palming, leverage for pressure should come from the practitioner's hips, and the pressure is directed at a 90-degree angle into the bone until Ki contact is made (Figure 15-6).

Fingertips are used to work areas of channels that may be too awkward to reach with the thumbs. The practitioner should not strain or hyperextend her fingertips or wrists while working (Figure 15-7).

The **"dragon's mouth,"** also called the **"tiger's mouth,"** is formed between the index finger, the thumb, and the web between the index finger and thumb when

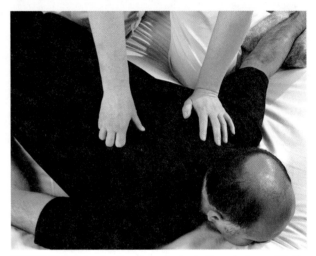

FIGURE 15-6 Using the thumbs on the back. (From Anderson SK: *The practice of shiatsu*, St. Louis, 2008, Elsevier.)

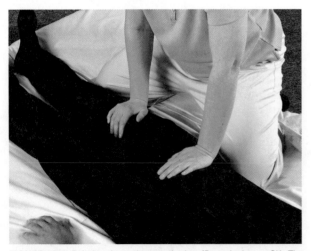

FIGURE 15-5 Palming down the anterior leg. (From Anderson SK: *The practice of shiatsu*, St. Louis, 2008, Elsevier.)

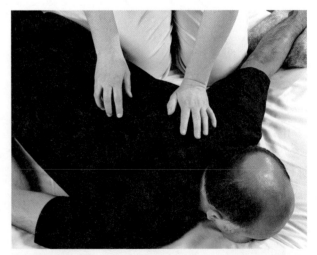

FIGURE 15-7 Fingertip work on the back. (From Anderson SK: *The practice of shiatsu*, St. Louis, 2008, Elsevier.)

the thumb is abducted. Pressure applied with dragon's mouth is particularly useful for addressing the lateral sides of the client's torso, the upper trapezius, and the lateral side of the client's neck. Again, the angle of pressure applied is 90 degrees into the client's body in order to connect with the client's Ki. When using dragon's mouth along the client's torso, the practitioner may rise up on her knees so that leverage for pressure comes from the practitioner's hips (Figure 15-8).

Forearms can be used by the practitioner to address a larger area than palming can cover. They can be used on the client's legs, arms, and back. Again, the intent is to provide enough pressure at a 90-degree angle to make contact and interact with the client's Ki (Figure 15-9).

Elbows are used to provide a more penetrating pressure than from thumbing or fingertip work. Elbows can be used on the client's legs and back.

Like the elbows, the knees can be used to provide a deeper pressure than thumbing or fingertip work. The knees also cover a broader area than palming. Knees can be used on channels located on the client's legs, and sometimes the back and arms, if the client's arms are large enough to bear the pressure (Figure 15-10).

The feet are used in much the same way as the palms. They are applied in several ways, such as on the client's hamstrings, posterior legs, and back. When standing and using feet on the client's back, the practitioner makes sure she is stable and grounded so as to not lose balance during these techniques (Figure 15-11).

Stretches help elongate muscles and increase the Ki flow in them. Stretches can also bring the channels closer to the surface of the body. The client's tissues are warmed by palming before the stretch is performed. The practitioner performs the stretch while breathing with the client, inhaling while bringing the limb into position and increasing the stretch as the client exhales.

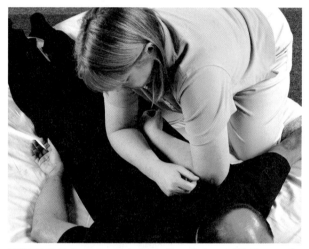

FIGURE 15-9 Forearms on the back. (From Anderson SK: *The practice of shiatsu*, St. Louis, 2008, Elsevier.)

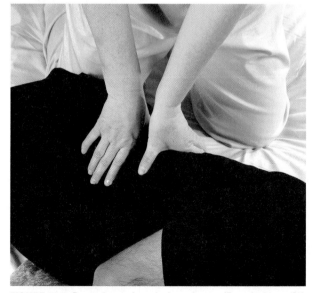

FIGURE 15-8 Dragon's mouth on the lateral torso. (From Anderson SK: *The practice of shiatsu,* St. Louis, 2008, Elsevier.)

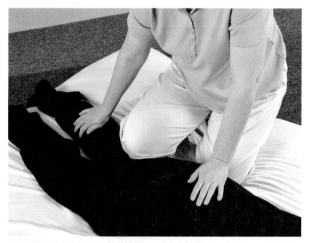

FIGURE 15-10 Knee on the posterior leg. (From Anderson SK: *The practice of shiatsu*, St. Louis, 2008, Elsevier.)

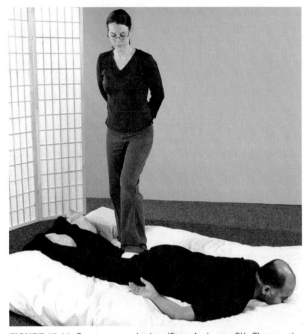

FIGURE 15-11 Foot on posterior leg. (From Anderson SK: *The practice of shiatsu*, St. Louis, 2008, Elsevier.)

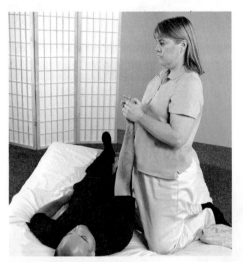

FIGURE 15-12 Basic arm Stretch

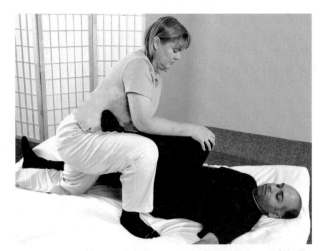

FIGURE 15-13 Knee-to-chest leg stretch. (From Anderson SK: *The practice of shiatsu*, St. Louis, 2008, Elsevier.)

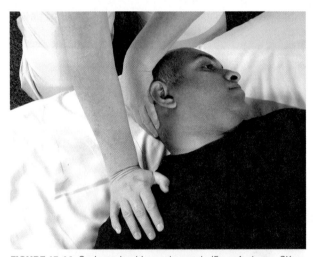

FIGURE 15-14 Occiput: shoulder neck stretch. (From Anderson SK: *The practice of shiatsu*, St. Louis, 2008, Elsevier.)

Ki tends to collect and become stagnant in certain places of the body such as the joints. Signs of Ki stagnation are joint stiffness, pain, and limited range of motion. Performing joint range of motion movements warms and loosens joints, brings blood to the area, increases nutrition within the joint by moving the synovial fluid within the joint, and increases Ki flow. Many range of motion techniques can be incorporated into a shiatsu treatment. When performing joint range of motion techniques, the practitioner makes sure she has a wide base and is quite stable to prevent injury to herself or the client.

Many different stretches are used in shiatsu. A basic arm stretch involves the practitioner kneeling beside the supine client and gently pulling his arm straight up (Figure 15-12). For the legs, a knee-to-chest stretch can be performed (Figure 15-13). A basic stretch for the neck involves the practitioner gently pulling on the client's occiput and pushing his shoulder at the same time (Figure 15-14).

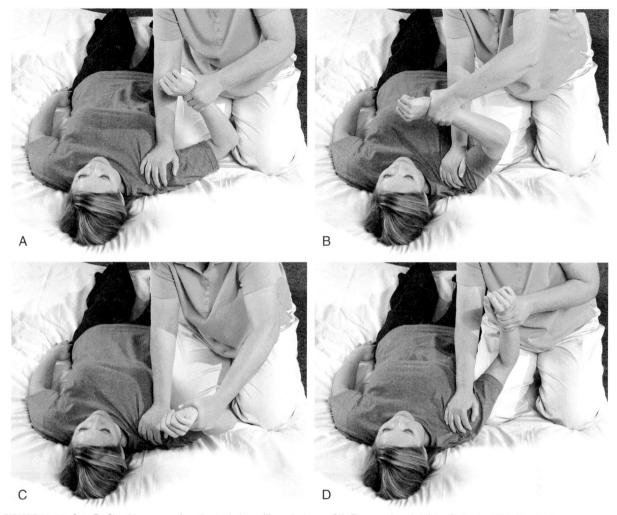

FIGURE 15-15 A to **D,** Shoulder range of motion technique. (From Anderson SK: *The practice of shiatsu,* St. Louis, 2008, Elsevier.)

One shoulder range of motion technique involves the practitioner kneeling next to the client, facing his head. While keeping the client's elbow flexed at 90 degrees, she move his arm clockwise several times in a wide range of motion (within the client's tolerance), then moves the arm counterclockwise several times in a wide range of motion (within the client's tolerance) (Figure 15-15).

A hip range of motion technique involves the practitioner half-kneeling by the client's legs. She guides his leg clockwise several times in a wide range of motion (within the client's tolerance), then moves his leg counterclockwise several times in a wide range of motion (within the client's tolerance)[2,3] (Figure 15-16).

PREPARATION TO PERFORM SHIATSU

Besides techniques, there are several other factors involved in performing effective shiatsu treatments. These include connection, touch sensitivity, and intuition. They can make the difference between a treatment in which the client feels like the practitioner is working with him and his needs, and a treatment in which the practitioner is merely performing techniques on him.

The foremost aspect of any shiatsu treatment is the practitioner's connection with the client. It is the single most contributory factor to restoring balance and effecting healing change in any therapeutic treatment. When

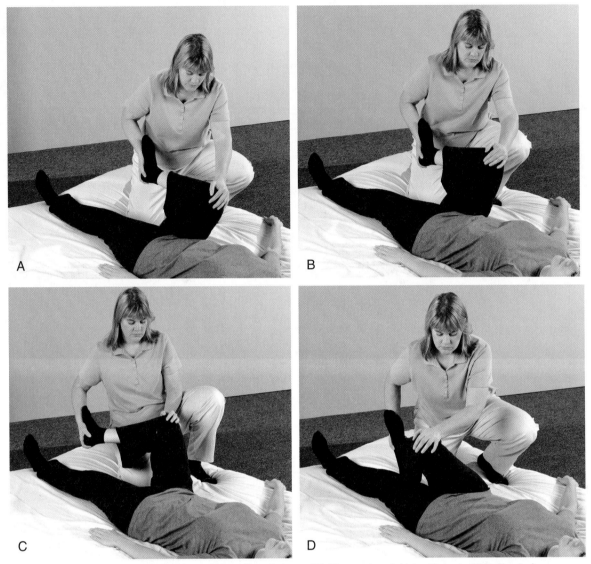

FIGURE 15-16 A to **D,** Hip range of motion technique. (From Anderson SK: *The practice of shiatsu,* St. Louis, 2008, Elsevier.)

the practitioner is centered, relaxed, and has attained an open, receptive mind that is free from distractions, her Ki is able to flow freely to connect with the client's Ki. As mentioned before, Ki connection feels different to every shiatsu practitioner, such as a feeling of merging with the client's Ki, a current of electricity, an energetic surge or drain, or as a thought of just knowing the connection has been made. When the practitioner feels this connection, she will then have a sense of readiness to begin the treatment.

The Ki connection allows the practitioner to facilitate reharmonizing of Ki imbalances within the client. The connection is readily transmitted through

the practitioner's touch and is palpable to both the practitioner and the client. The tactile techniques that are part of shiatsu are then transformed from simple human-to-human contact to therapeutic treatment.

The beauty of shiatsu is in its simplicity. Although a client can present with any of a variety of signs and symptoms, sometimes a simple touch of good intention is enough to balance disharmonies of Ki. Through touch sensitivity the practitioner is able to feel the quality of the client's Ki in various parts of his body. She can discern his Ki flow and uses that information to customize the treatment session to his needs. Developing touch sensitivity starts on the first day of shiatsu (or any bodywork) study and continues throughout the practitioner's lifetime.

Along with touch sensitivity and connection is the development of the practitioner's intuition. Touch sensitivity and intuition are the shiatsu practitioner's most powerful tools. They enable the practitioner to determine the best way to work with the client. Although it may seem mysterious to some, everyone has intuition. Sometimes intuition is referred to as a having a hunch or gut instinct.

The dictionary defines intuition as "quick and ready insight" and "the power or faculty of attaining direct knowledge or cognition without evident rational thought and inference." The key words are "evident rational thought." In the most-uncomplicated explanation, intuition possibly comes from simply piecing together many small bits of information until a complete picture is formed. On the surface it may appear as if no process occurred in how the information about the client's physical and energetic states came together for the practitioner. However, with knowledge and practice the practitioner is able to formulate a "picture" of the client and the client's needs seemingly without effort.

THE FOUR METHODS OF ASSESSMENT

Shiatsu techniques can be learned, and protocols can be followed. The same treatment can be given over and over without much thought given to the theoretic basis of Asian bodywork. However, doing the same routine by rote, or with minimal variety, serves neither clients nor the practitioner well. The most effective and interesting treatments are those that are customized for each client's needs.

The **Four Methods of Assessment** are used in traditional Chinese medicine. These methods integrate theory and practice, and are ways the practitioner is able to determine what will serve the client best. The methods are listening, observing, palpating, and asking. Although using one of these methods to determine the design of the client's treatment may be effective, the shiatsu practitioner benefits by using two, three, or all four methods. One assessment may indicate a particular imbalance that other assessments could support or contradict. When using all Four Methods, at least three of them generally will point toward the element imbalance or discomfort pattern that the shiatsu practitioner should address during treatment.

During the listening assessment, the practitioner listens to what the client is saying, how he is saying it, and perhaps what the client is not saying. Although listening to what the client is saying is important, the practitioner can also open her awareness to the tone of the client's voice. For example, if the client's voice is weepy, that can indicate an imbalance in the Metal channels (Lung and Large Intestine). If the client is laughing while describing a sad event, that can indicate a Fire imbalance (Heart and Small Intestine Channels). If the client seems to leave something out when recounting events that might be relevant to his current state, this omission can be a clue to his emotional state. Some things may be too painful or sad for the client to talk about, or perhaps he has a lot of anger. The practitioner needs to be sensitive to the client's state, and if there is something the client seems to be unwilling to say, should not press him for more information. Instead, the practitioner should make a mental note to see if something shows up in other assessments of the client.

The observing assessment is just what it sounds like: assessing the client for visual clues in his posture, body movements, demeanor, and body energy patterns: all of these illustrate the client's Ki. A person who has excess Ki generally has bold movements and a loud voice, whereas someone who is deficient in Ki can be slower moving and have a weak voice. Someone whose Ki is relatively in balance stands up straight yet is relaxed.

Ki patterns can manifest several ways. If the Ki is more in the upper half of his body, then the treatment session should begin with work on the lower half of the client's body to draw Ki downward and balance his upper and lower body. If the Ki is more in the lower half of his body, than the treatment session should begin with work on the upper half of the client's body to draw Ki upward and balance his upper and lower body. If the client's Ki appears weaker on one side of his body, the practitioner should begin the treatment session on that side. By drawing Ki to that side, the two sides balance out.

Palpation means to assess by touch. By making contact through mindful touch, or palpation, with the intent of connecting practitioner Ki with client Ki, areas of focus can be determined for the treatment session. Although the other assessments—listening, seeing, and asking—help complete the picture of the client, the palpating assessment gives the most complete view of the client and the client's needs for the immediate treatment session. In fact, even if no other assessment is performed, the palpating assessment is enough to give the practitioner all the information needed to formulate and carry out a client-centered treatment. By being relaxed and centered and opening her awareness, the shiatsu practitioner can get a good sense of Ki flow and blockages in the client's body. Palms and fingertips are initially used by the practitioner, and, as she gains expertise, she may use her forearms, knees, and soles of her feet as well. Palpation assessments are used in two main ways. One is as an initial assessment to design a treatment focused on the client's Ki patterns. The other is an ongoing assessment throughout the treatment to feel when the client's Ki flow has changed.

The asking assessment can consist of two parts: an intake form (also known as a pretreatment form or health history form) and the pretreatment session interview. The asking assessment serves two purposes: (1) to get information about the client's state and any conditions he may have that could influence the design of treatment, and (2) to establish a connection with the client. The shiatsu practitioner can learn about the client and have an interchange that can establish trust. This is important; a shiatsu treatment, as in any body-

work treatment, is only effective if the client trusts the practitioner.

The dynamic of the asking assessment therefore is significant. It begins with the shiatsu practitioner greeting the client and introducing herself. A firm handshake and good eye contact are essential. The simple question, "How are you today?" begins the asking assessment. The shiatsu practitioner should listen to the client attentively. As the client gives information about himself, the practitioner should restate anything she is unsure of to clarify the information (Box 15-2 and see Table 15-2).[3]

Imbalances in the Five Elements

The majority of discomforts people experience present themselves in a surprisingly small number of common imbalance patterns. While every client is unique, it is likely the shiatsu practitioner will encounter

---

BOX 15-2 Pretreatment Questions

The following is a list of questions the client may be asked in order for the practitioner to get as complete a picture of the client as possible, and to have a good framework for designing the treatment session. Many of these questions may be asked on an intake form.

- How do you feel right now?
- Do you have any areas of discomfort, such as pain, tightness, stiffness, or limited joint movement? Please describe the location and quality of the discomfort. (The answers can be clues to the quality of the client's Ki.)
- How long have you had this discomfort? (Chronic conditions present Ki patterns differently than acute conditions.)
- Do you know what caused the discomfort? If so, what was it?
- What have you done so far to relieve this discomfort? What have the results been?
- Have you had any major illnesses recently? (This can be a clue to the client's overall Ki strength, vulnerability of a particular element, or any physical limitations the client has.)
- Have you had any accidents recently? This can be a clue to the client's overall Ki strength, vulnerability of a particular element, or any physical limitations the client has.)
- Have you had any surgeries recently? This can be a clue to the client's overall Ki strength, vulnerability of a particular element, or any physical limitations the client has.)
- Are you taking any medications? If so, what are the effects and side effects? (This is important to know in case the client is taking a medication, such as an analgesic, that can interfere with his ability to sense pressure.)
- Are you prone to any illnesses? (These can indicate imbalances in particular elements.)

- Does your body tend to run hot or cold? (This could be an indicator of robust or deficient Ki.)
- What type of exercise do you do, and how often do you do it? (This can give an overall view of whether the client keeps his Ki moving or if it is stagnant. It can also indicate certain elements that may need to be addressed. For example, if the client exercises excessively, Wood channels—Liver and Gallbladder—could be imbalanced; if the client does not exercise, Earth channels—Stomach and Spleen—could be imbalanced.)
- How much fluid do you drink each day? (If the client has a low fluid intake, the Water element—Bladder and Kidney Channels—could be affected.)
- How is your diet? (Whether the client has a balanced diet can have direct effects. For example, a diet high in fat, dairy, and sugar can show up in irregularities of Ki flow in the Stomach and Spleen channels.)
- Do you crave particular types of food? (These are indicators of element imbalances. For example, craving sugar is an Earth element indicator, craving salty foods is a Water element indicator, and craving sour foods is a Wood element indicator.)
- How is your digestion? (If the client's digestive processes are not regular, that can indicate a Metal element issue and show up in the Large Intestine channel.)
- How are your sleep patterns? (If the client has trouble falling asleep, staying asleep, or waking up repeatedly throughout the night, Heart and Heart Protector channels may need to be addressed.)
- What are your energy patterns throughout the day? Is your energy up at certain times and down at other times? (These times can indicate imbalances in certain channels.)

characteristic symptoms of imbalances in particular elements and channels. These characteristic symptoms can provide a starting point for the practitioner to design individualized, client-centered treatments.

When the Metal element is out of balance, symptoms may include respiratory problems, constipation, and skin disorders. A person may have frequent colds, nasal congestion, and a sore or tickly throat. Chronic skin conditions such as psoriasis or eczema tend to relate to the Lungs, whereas acne or boils are eliminative and therefore are symptoms of a Large Intestine imbalance. Dryness is the climate for Metal, and dry skin, or even a lack of sweating, indicates a Metal imbalance.

The emotion associated with the Metal element is grief. When a person cannot stop grieving, or is unable to grieve at all, the Metal element should be addressed. Metal is also associated with structure and the ability to be detail oriented. Imbalances may be indicated by either the overwhelming need to have everything in its place or the inability to keep things neat and orderly. As with any of the psychologic effects of an imbalance, either too much or not enough indicates disharmony. Another symptom when Metal is out of balance is that the person may have difficulty relating to others, and feelings of isolation or depression may result.

When Water is out of balance a wide variety of symptoms may be present. Any sort of kidney or urinary disorder is indicative of a water imbalance, such as kidney stones or urinary tract infections. Hormones of all types provide the body's cells with impetus to carry out their functions, and any hormone disorders are related to a Water imbalance. Bone issues such as arthritis and osteoporosis may be present. A Water imbalance may also cause tooth problems; teeth are part of the bones. The lower back, particularly near the kidneys, may be sore or painful. The ears are the sense organ of water, and hearing problems and ringing in the ears are considered Water issues.

The emotion for the Water element is fear. A certain amount of fear is natural and healthy because it helps keep a person safe. In a Water imbalance this may show up as anxiety, tension, or phobias. The water connection to the backbone relates to a person's willpower and determination. When Water is out of balance, the person may be unable to initiate action. He may want to get something done but does not have the drive to get up and do it. Fatigue is commonly associated with water, as is susceptibility to stress.

Just as important as excessive fear is a lack of fear. With this type of Water imbalance, someone may be drawn to activities such as extreme sports, racing cars, and horror movies. Another symptom when water is out of balance is that the person may want to "pool" his resources by spending quiet time alone. Conversely, a person may have difficulty being alone and strive to spend all his time surrounded by others to avoid the depths of the self.

When Wood is out of balance, the liver and gall bladder organs may have disorders, and detoxification of the body may be compromised. Even if the gall bladder has been removed, the Gallbladder channel is still present and should be addressed. Vision problems and eye problems, such as blurred vision or dry or painful eyes, relate to the Wood element. In women Liver relates to certain aspects of the menstrual cycle, and a Liver imbalance may be noted by scanty or no menstruation. Tendon issues such as repetitive motion injuries may occur with a Wood disharmony, and a lack of flexibility or stiffness in the muscles may also be present. Because the Gallbladder channel is on the sides of the body, the right and left sides of the body may look different in the case of a Wood imbalance. Pain may exist in the neck and shoulders, the sides of the body, or the hips. Migraine headaches are often associated with a Wood imbalance because they usually affect only one side of the head and/or vision.

The Wood element governs the smooth flow of Ki, including the emotions. The Wood element is particularly affected by the repression of any emotions. Anger is the emotion of Wood, and it can be especially toxic when held in and not expressed. When Wood is out of balance the person may seem to get angry quite easily or may never be able to get angry at all. Another symptom of a Wood imbalance is that the person may have difficulty creating effective plans and decisions for the long term (a Liver channel imbalance) or short term (a Gallbladder channel imbalance). Too much planning or the inability to make plans can lead to no action being taken at all.

When Fire is out of balance, obvious symptoms may include problems with the heart organ or the small intestine. Blood pressure issues, atherosclerosis, and other circulatory disorders may be present. The person may have difficulty with temperature regulation, often feel too warm or too cold, or have cold hands and feet, or sweat excessively. Triple Heater relates to the lymphatic and immune systems. An imbalance may lead the person to be prone to edema or to get sick often. Small Intestine is said to separate the pure from the impure and therefore has an important role in the digestive process. If a person has difficulty assimilating nutrients, the Small Intestine may be out of balance.

Heart is connected to the tongue, and through this, speech; as such, Fire is associated with communication. Speech impediments such as stuttering may indicate a Heart imbalance.

The condition of the Heart is easily seen in a person's complexion. It should have a healthy pinkness, and the eyes should be bright and expressive. If the face is overly red or too pale, a Fire imbalance may be present. The emotion for Fire is joy or contentment. If someone is always laughing or giggling, especially at inappropriate times, this indicates a Fire disharmony. Likewise, a Fire imbalance also may be present if a person almost never laughs. Insomnia is also linked to Heart channel imbalances.

Small Intestine controls assimilation, which applies to concepts and emotions as well as nutrients and other substances. To learn something new or process an event that has taken place, a person must assimilate it into his being. Part of that experience must become that person; in other words, he must own it. Small Intestine is often involved when a person experiences symptoms long after a traumatic event. A person may be unable to assimilate an experience at the time it occurred because of being in shock. Also, if a person is able to take in new information but unable to remember it clearly, or put it to use, the Small Intestine Channel may need to be addressed. Fire relates to connection, both with the self and others. If a Fire imbalance is present the person may have few trusted, close friends because of excessive emotional barriers. The opposite may also be true, as with people who wear their hearts on their sleeves.

The physical manifestations of an Earth imbalance may include any sort of digestive disorder, such as acid reflux, bloating, or loose stools. A person may have a loss of appetite or pain in the abdomen. Fatigue sometimes occurs, and women may have symptoms such as scanty menstruation or dizziness. The female reproductive hormones are connected with the Earth element, and issues with fertility are considered an Earth imbalance. When Earth is out of balance, muscles may be achy and the person may not want to exercise.

Spleen provides the sense of taste and the enjoyment of food; when it is out of balance various eating disorders may occur. A person may overeat, want to eat all the time, eat too quickly, or have no appetite. The flavor for the Earth element is sweet: craving sweets or eating a lot of sweet things indicates an Earth imbalance. Spleen is also said to house thought and is responsible for processing new ideas as well as food. If a person thinks too much or constantly worries, the appetite is affected because Spleen cannot keep up. When a person eats while obsessively worrying, digestion often is poor.

Stomach, which accepts food, is responsible for all aspects of acceptance in life. If a person has difficulty accepting nourishment in the form of emotional support from others, the Earth element is involved. Eating disorders are often related to the inability to accept nourishment on other levels. Also, Stomach is located at the front of the body and is related to the "front" that a person puts out to others. When an Earth imbalance is present, often this front is overly nurturing toward others or tries to please everyone else.[3,6]

THE TREATMENT SESSION

How the treatment session is designed makes the difference between the shiatsu practitioner helping the client create needed change and the session not being useful to the client. Thoughtfulness on the part of the practitioner and attention to detail can make the client's experience positive as well as therapeutic. The treatment itself can be simple or complex; it can encompass only a few techniques or a myriad of skills; it can be short or it can take a few hours, although shiatsu treatments are usually an hour long. No matter how a shiatsu treatment is performed, each and every shiatsu treatment must have the practitioner's undivided attention on the client and the intention for therapeutic change.

The treatment session begins when the practitioner greets the client. She should greet him with good eye contact and a firm handshake. As she is doing this, she is already starting to use one or more of the Four Methods of Assessment. Without obviously looking, she is visually assessing the client's Ki and postural patterns.

The client may be asked to fill out an intake form, or the practitioner may go right into a pretreatment interview; both of these are part of the asking and listening methods. When talking to the client, the practitioner should use reflective listening; the client needs to know that she is taking an active interest in his needs. The practitioner is listening to what the client is saying, how he is saying it, and what the client is not saying.

If the client has not received a shiatsu treatment before, the practitioner would explain how the treatment is performed, and what the client can expect to experience. For example, she might say something like, "You will remain fully clothed, and the treatment is given on a futon on the floor. I will be checking your channels of Ki, or energy, for disruptions in the flow. These disruptions can cause pain and discomfort. I will be using my palms, fingers, thumb, forearms, elbows, knees, and feet to apply pressure along the channels. My intent is to use my Ki to support your Ki and balance its flow. Some areas may feel tender so let me know if I'm using too much pressure. I will also be performing stretches and range of motion techniques to help smooth out your Ki flow. Let me know if you feel any discomfort as I am doing these. You won't need to help me do any of these techniques; your job is to just lie down and let go. Afterwards, you may feel very relaxed and centered. Many times people feel rested and have a clear mind." The practitioner should also invite the client to ask any questions he has before, during, and after the treatment.

Based on the assessments the practitioner has performed, she has information about the client's current physical, emotional, and energetic states that help her design the treatment, particularly which of the client's channels need addressing. As she is palpating and connecting with the client's Ki throughout the treatment, she is constantly reassessing the client's Ki flow and so she may change the treatment plan depending on what she finds.

The treatment may begin with the client supine, prone, or in side position. If, for example, the client's Ki is more in the upper half of his body, the practitioner might have the client start supine and work on his feet first to draw Ki downward. If the client is having back pain, the practitioner may have the client start in prone position so she can assess and address the Ki in the channels that run through the client's back first. If the client is experiencing symptoms related to Gallbladder channel, then having the client start in side position may make the most sense since this channel is by and large on the lateral sides of the body. Once the client is lying down, the practitioner will prop him with small pillows to make him comfortable. The pillows can be placed under his knees or head, for example.

The practitioner starts by placing one or both hands on the client with a light to moderate pressure. The intent is for the practitioner's Ki to connect with the client's Ki. The practitioner waits for the client's Ki to rise up to meet her Ki; this may happen instantly or may take from a few seconds to a few minutes, depending on the quality of the client's Ki. Once the client's Ki meets the practitioner's, she assesses it and determines what techniques will be the most effective for the client.

The practitioner will move the client into a position that makes accessing the channels she will work on easier. She will use the small pillows to prop the client as needed to ensure his comfort. Generally, the practitioner will palm down a channel first. She may then work more specifically on the channel using her thumbs, fingertips, elbows, and perhaps her toes. As she works, she continually assesses any distortions in the client's Ki and works to rebalance them. She may also perform stretches and joint range of motion techniques on the body area where the channels she is working on are located. As she is working on a particular area of the body, she may notice that the Ki in channels other than the one she started working on needs rebalancing and so would work on those other channels as well.

Once the Ki in the channel is flowing smoothly again, the practitioner would move to another part of the client's body to work. She would again start by resting her hands on the client in this new area and wait for his Ki to rise up and meet hers. Then she would palm down the channel, work it more specifically, and perform stretches and range of motion techniques if needed.

Usually the practitioner gradually moves around the client's entire body until all areas feel complete and balanced. She would have the client move from supine to prone, and prone to supine, and assist him in moving into side position if the treatment calls for it. Sometimes, however, specific areas of the client's body may need so much attention that the entire treatment is focused on them. In this case, a full body treatment would not be performed.

At the end of the treatment, the practitioner closes by resting her hands lightly on the client's body, usually on his back (if he is prone) or his stomach (if he is supine). She lets them rise up and down as the client inhales and exhales. After a few moments, as he inhales, she brings his hands up and off his body.

The client is allowed to rest for a little while after the treatment. The practitioner then offers him water and asks how he is feeling. Listening to feedback about how he feels and what techniques worked or did not work for him is vital to the practitioner. She can use this information for future treatment sessions with the client. She can discuss what she discovered during the course of the treatment and also make suggestions, within the scope of practice of shiatsu, that can help the client continue to make progress. The following are examples of suggestions for each of the Five Elements.

Metal (Lung and Large Intestine channels) imbalances: perform breathing exercises; organize a closet or drawer; get rid of clothes that aren't being worn; perform gentle, regular exercise; have a good cry; and avoid smoke and polluted air.

Water (Kidney and Urinary Bladder channels) imbalances: take a bath, especially with Epsom salts; write in a journal; meditate; avoid caffeine and other stimulants; and spend time near bodies of water, such as the ocean or a lake.

Wood (Liver and Gallbladder channels) imbalances: spend time in nature, particularly in the woods; write down a goal and plans to achieve that goal; exercise regularly; find healthy ways to express anger; and avoid excesses of things such as food, drink, and exercise.

Fire (Heart, Small Intestine, Triple Heater, and Heart Protector Channels) imbalances: have a long conversation with a good friend; watch a funny movie and laugh out loud; meditate; go to a party; and avoid caffeine and other stimulants.

Earth (Spleen and Stomach channels) imbalances: get regular exercise; do something nice for yourself; cook a healthy meal and enjoy each bite; sing; avoid sweet foods and cold or frozen foods.

It is also important that the practitioner document every treatment session she performs. The documentation should include the client's name and age; date of treatment; results of the pretreatment interview with the client; results from the Four Methods of Assessment; what channels were addressed and the techniques used; how the client responded to the techniques; pertinent information from the posttreatment discussion with the client; and any suggestions the practitioner gave the client.[6]

TRAINING

To become a professional shiatsu practitioner, students learn this modality through a formalized program of study. This can involve becoming apprenticed to an experienced practitioner or attending a school in which shiatsu is taught. There are no national standards regarding shiatsu education. Programs can vary widely, from less than 100 hours of training up to 2 or 3 years. There are also many different styles of shiatsu, and each school presents its unique version. It is recommended that prospective students do careful research to determine which school is best for them. The curriculum should include, at the very least, not only shiatsu techniques, but also traditional Chinese medicine, Western anatomy and physiology, and a clinical component so that students can practice what they are learning while being supervised by an experienced practitioner. The American Organization for Bodywork Therapies of Asia (AOBTA) is a good source for finding shiatsu schools and programs.

Currently certification requirements for professional shiatsu practitioners vary widely throughout the country. In some instances, practitioners need to be licensed by the state in which they live or, if there is no state licensure, by their county, city, or town. In other instances, shiatsu practitioners need to study massage therapy and be licensed as a massage therapist in order to practice shiatsu. In yet other cases, practitioners may not need to be licensed at all. There may be specific education requirements, such as graduation from an accredited school with a certain number of hours of study. Passing a licensing examination may also be required. It is best that those interested in pursuing shiatsu as a career check with all their local and state licensing bodies to find out what is necessary in the region in which they want to practice.

CHAPTER SUMMARY

Shiatsu is a Japanese form of bodywork. Based on the same principles as acupuncture, it is performed on a fully clothed client on a futon on the floor. Instead of using needles to change Ki flow in the client's channels to alleviate pain and other discomforts, shiatsu practitioners use their palms, fingers, thumbs, forearms, elbows, knees, and feet to apply pressure. Shiatsu has a long and interesting history. Today, many different forms of shiatsu are practiced.

Western anatomy, physiology, and pathology are important foundational concepts to the study of shiatsu. Equally important is traditional Chinese medicine, which includes Yin and Yang, Qi, and the Five Elements. The channels the Qi flows through are connected to organs of the body, and most of them are named for these organs. The channels are in Yin and Yang pairs, and each pair of channels corresponds to one of the Five Elements.

There are many different techniques performed as part of shiatsu. Basic ones include palming, thumbing, fingertip work, dragon's mouth, simple stretches, and range of motion techniques for the joints. The Four Methods of Assessment are methods the practitioner uses to determine what the client needs. During the course of the treatment session, the practitioner uses her Ki connection with the client, touch sensitivity, and intuition to know what techniques to apply along which channels to make the treatment customized for each individual client.

CASE HISTORIES

■ Case history 1

The client is 44 years old and has almost completed massage therapy school. When she came for a treatment, she was in the middle of finishing several projects, including writing a paper for one of her classes. She drove 2 hours to see me, and, after the treatment needed to drive the 2 hours back home because she had student clinic the next day. Upon using the Four Methods of Assessment, I determined that she had been doing quite a bit of organization of information lately, and that she was concerned about getting sick since she was depleting herself (as can happen during school) and did not have the time to rest adequately. She also said she was mildly constipated. She was a little sad because she had not been socializing as much as she would have liked. Foods she had been craving included pungent ones, like strong cheeses, and she had been putting hot sauce on a lot of her meals lately. Her postural patterns indicated that Ki was stagnant in her pelvic area.

I worked mainly on her Large Intestine and Triple Heater channels. The Ki in her Triple Heater seemed to be pulsing strongly outward. As I worked, I got warmer and the client got colder, to the point of needing a blanket. It took quite a bit of time and support to balance out her Triple Heater channel. I performed quite a few leg stretches and hip range of motion techniques to help loosen her pelvic area. Her back needed extra work as well, so I supported the Ki in her back with palming, thumbing, and resting my forearms on the muscles on either side of her spine. After the treatment, I suggested she spend a little less time organizing and some more time with her friends.

During the treatment, she said she was wide awake and relaxed at the same time, quite a different experience for her. A few days after the treatment, I followed up with her and she said that after she had driven home, she was very tired and went to bed right away. The next day she had clinic in which she had to perform five massages. She said she felt very energized, happy, and able to do all her treatments seemingly without effort. Normally afterwards she said she would just want to go home and relax, but she felt so good she went over to a friend's house and ended up doing two more chair massages. She also said that the next two days she had several bowel movements, which made her very happy.

■ Case history 2

The client is 52 years old and has been a legal assistant for 20 years. For about 7 years she has been receiving shiatsu treatments from me every other week. She also regularly receives other forms of bodywork such as massage therapy, reflexology, and hot stone therapy.

She has a moderately sized extended family that has been a source of concern, tension, and turmoil. Her job is also stressful at times. Deadlines for court dates are sometimes short, and client crises can arise out of the blue. She has found that her most frantic times of the week are Mondays and Fridays, and so schedules her treatments on the weekends. Recently she had her house renovated, a process that took many months.

Because of the strains placed on her by her family, her job, and house remodeling, the client has struggled with daily headaches, insomnia, tight joints, and aching muscles at various times in her life. Since she is a long-term client of mine, all of her channels have needed addressing at one time or another. However, the two elements that have most consistently needed balancing are Wood and Earth. Liver and Gallbladder channels are affected by her obligation to make many short-term and long-term planning decisions. Stomach and Spleen channels are affected by her family situation.

During shiatsu treatments with her, I focus on balancing the channels that need the most work, as well as incorporating many stretches and range of motion techniques. I spend extra time addressing channels in her head and neck to help release tension that can cause headaches. Point work on her feet is designed to help keep her grounded.

She states that after a shiatsu treatment she feels buoyed, then later feels sleepy because she is so relaxed. Her mind and her thoughts are clearer. In the years since she started receiving shiatsu and other forms of bodywork regularly, her headaches have decreased to almost none. Her joints feel looser, and her muscles feel less tense. She still has insomnia off and on, but the night after a shiatsu treatment she is able to sleep quite well. She considers shiatsu and bodywork part of her health maintenance program.

SUGGESTED READINGS

Anderson SK: *The practice of shiatsu*, St. Louis, 2007, Elsevier.

Beinfield H, Korngold E: *Between heaven and earth*, New York, 1991, Ballantine Books.

Beresford-Cooke C: *Shiatsu theory and practice*, ed 2, St. Louis, 2003, Churchill Livingstone.

Dull H: *Watsu: freeing the body in the water*, ed 3, Victoria, BC, Canada, 2004, Trafford Publishing.

Jarney C, Mojay G: *Shiatsu, the complete guide*, London, 1999, Thorsons.

Kaptchuk TJ: *The web that has no weaver*, Chicago, 2000, Contemporary Books.

Liechti E: *The complete illustrated guide to shiatsu*, Boston, 1998, Element Books.

Lundberg P: *The book of shiatsu*, New York, 2003, Fireside.

Namikoshi T: *The complete book of shiatsu therapy*, New York, 1981, Japan Publications.

Reichstein G: *Wood becomes water, Chinese medicine in everyday life*, New York, 1998, Kodansha International.

Somma C: *Shiatsu*, Upper Saddle River, NJ, 2007, Pearson.

RESOURCES

American Massage Therapy Association
www.amtamassage.org

American Organization for Bodywork Therapies of Asia
www.aobta.org

National Certification Board for Therapeutic Massage and Bodywork
www.ncbtmb.com

Shiatsu Society of the UK
www.shiatsusociety.org/public/index.shtml

Shiatsu Therapy Association of Australia
www.staa.org.au

Shiatsu Therapy Association of Ontario
www.shiatsuassociation.com

REFERENCES

1. Liechti E: *The complete illustrated guide to shiatsu*, Boston, 1998, Element Books.
2. Lundberg P: *The book of shiatsu*, New York, 2003, Fireside.
3. Beresford-Cooke C: *Shiatsu theory and practice*, ed 2, St. Louis, 2003, Churchill Livingstone.
4. Somma C: *Shiatsu*, Upper Saddle River, NJ, 2007, Pearson.
5. Reichstein G: *Wood becomes water, Chinese medicine in everyday life*, New York, 1998, Kodansha International.
6. Anderson SK: *The practice of shiatsu*, St. Louis, 2007, Elsevier.

MULTIPLE CHOICE TEST QUESTIONS

1) Which of the following is a characteristic of a shiatsu treatment?
   a) Lubricant is applied to the client.
   b) Client is unclothed and draped with sheets.
   c) Focus is on balancing the client's Ki.
   d) It involves techniques to elongate fascia around muscles.

2) The shiatsu practitioner's strength comes from here:
   a) hands
   b) head
   c) knees
   d) abdomen

3) Which of the following concepts is the basis of shiatsu?
   a) Pain, discomfort, and other disorders are caused by an imbalance in the client's Ki.
   b) Discomfort is alleviated through the use of medications.
   c) Western anatomy, physiology, and kinesiology are the primary areas of knowledge.
   d) Body, mind, and spirit are viewed as separate from the physical body.

4) The energy or force that gives and maintains life is called:
   a) acupuncture
   b) Anmo
   c) Ki
   d) tsubo

5) Which of the following conditions is massage therapy contraindicated for and shiatsu possibly indicated for?
   a) flare-up stage of lupus
   b) osteoporosis
   c) cancer
   d) chronic insomnia

6) Which of the following is a local contraindication for shiatsu?
   a) headaches
   b) muscular tension
   c) constipation
   d) varicose veins

7) Why was the term *shiatsu* coined?
   a) True practitioners of Anma wanted to distinguish themselves from charlatans.
   b) An easier name for the bodywork practice was needed.
   c) Anma was no longer a valid bodywork modality.
   d) Few practitioners of traditional techniques existed.

8) Namikoshi's significance in the development of shiatsu is that he:
   a) founded the Japan Shiatsu Institute, which helped further awareness of shiatsu as a valid profession
   b) eliminated any use of Western science and bodywork techniques from the practice of shiatsu
   c) incorporated the use of needles in shiatsu treatments
   d) focused strictly on Western bodywork techniques

9) A description of the relationship of Yin and Yang is that they are:
   a) absolutes
   b) always transforming each other
   c) in opposition of each other
   d) the same thing

10) In the body, Ki flows through an organized system of:
    a) blood vessels
    b) tsubo
    c) channels
    d) nerve pathways

11) Which of the following is a Yin organ?
    a) Lung
    b) Small intestine
    c) Gallbladder
    d) Triple Heater

12) Blue is associated with what element?
    a) Metal
    b) Water
    c) Earth
    d) Wood

13) What emotion is associated with Fire?
   a) fear
   b) sadness
   c) anger
   d) joy

14) What sound is associated with Earth?
   a) singing
   b) shouting
   c) laughing
   d) crying

15) What part of the body is the hara?
   a) chest
   b) low back
   c) abdomen
   d) neck

16) Which of the following describes proper shiatsu body mechanics?
   a) locked knees
   b) wide stance
   c) straight arms
   d) elevated shoulders

17) Which of the following may indicate a Metal imbalance?
   a) chronic skin conditions
   b) blurred vision
   c) high blood pressure
   d) acid reflux

18) A Metal imbalance may be indicated in a client who:
   a) needs to spend a lot of time alone
   b) is incapable of connecting with others
   c) is unable to stop grieving over a sad event
   d) constantly worries

19) Which of the following is a self-care recommendation for a client with a Wood imbalance?
   a) avoid excessive intake of food, drink, and exercise
   b) take a bath, especially with salt
   c) have a long conversation with a good friend
   d) do something nice for yourself

20) Which of the following is a self-care recommendation for a client with a Fire imbalance?
   a) do something nice for yourself
   b) go to a party
   c) avoid smoke and polluted air
   d) take a bath

Sports and Fitness Massage

Sandy Fritz

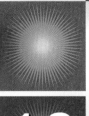

16

STUDENT OBJECTIVES

Upon completion of this chapter, students will be able to do the following:

- Describe therapeutic massage application for athletes and those with physical activity–related concerns.
- Identify indications and contraindications for massage common for this population.
- Develop basic massage treatment plans supportive of physical performance activities.
- Adapt massage therapy applications based on performance-related outcomes.

KEY TERMS

Athlete
Maintenance massage
Medical massage
Orthopedic massage
Peak performance
Performance
Post-event massage
Pre-event massage
Promotional (event) massage
Recovery massage
Remedial massage
Traumatic injury

INTRODUCTION

Sports massage receives its name from the population it treats, not from the techniques that are performed. In other words, sports massage is massage that is done when working with athletes.

An **athlete** is a person who participates in sports in either an amateur or in a professional capacity. As a result of the physical and mental demands of his or her activities, the athlete requires precise use of his or her body. The nervous system and muscles are trained to perform in a specific way. Often the activity involves repetitive use of one group of muscles more than others, which may result in hypertrophy, changes in strength, movement patterns, connective tissue formation, and compensation patterns in the rest of the body. These factors contribute to the soft tissue difficulties that often develop in athletes. Using this definition, many people can develop similar conditions, not just those involved in sports-related activity.

Fitness is part of a healthy lifestyle and includes body, mind, and spirit focus. One aspect of fitness is physical fitness, which requires the physical activity necessary to support optimal well-being. This chapter targets common issues regarding physical movement and **performance** for the professional and amateur athletes, as well as for those people who enjoy recreational activities or anyone involved in physical fitness programs. In addition, individuals who are entertainers, such as musicians and dancers, share similar issues with those whose occupation involves physical activity, such as construction workers and mechanics. When accumulated strain develops for any reason, the fitness/wellness balance is upset resulting in illness and/or injury. For competing athletes, a major stress factor is the demand of performance. Often performance exceeds an athlete's fitness level resulting in a decrease in overall fitness. Performance demand requires increased energy expenditure, which in turn strains adaptive mechanisms and increases recovery time.

The content of this chapter is also appropriate for those receiving physical therapy. It does not address specific rehabilitation, but rather the discomfort that can occur because of the rehabilitation activities.

Peak performance is the ultimate level activity achievable by an individual but it is a short-term event. Peak performance cannot be sustained for extensive periods of time. Fitness must be achieved before performance, and fitness must be supported to endure the ongoing strain of peak-performance activity. Attempts to continue to perform at peak typically result in injury or illness.

Traumatic injury is an unexpected event that damages the body. Accidents are a common cause of traumatic injury. Rehabilitation from this type of injury often requires physical training. Although persons receiving such therapy may not be athletes, they often experience the same aftermath—postactivity soreness, fatigue, joint pain, etc. During rehabilitation, restoration of function is a primary goal.

Appropriate treatment plan development and massage application are necessary to prevent injuries. Athletes at peak performance are particularly fragile. This means that any demands to adapt, including those made by massage, need to be assessed in light of the athlete's adaptive capacity. A lack of understanding about the scope of demands placed on athletes often leads to inappropriate massage care.

Massage can be very beneficial for athletes if the professional performing the massage understands the biomechanics required by the sport. In the absence of such understanding, however, massage can impair optimal function. Any type of massage before a competition must be given carefully. If a massage professional plans to work with an athlete on a continuing basis, it is important that the practitioner come to know the athlete and become an integral part of the entire training experience.[1]

With athletes, the psychologic state is crucial to performance: often the competition is won in the mind. Although massage therapists are not the sport psychologist, athletes often look to us for support, continuity, and feedback. Many athletes are very ritualistic about precompetition readiness. If massage has become part of that ritual and the massage professional is inconsistent in maintaining appointment schedules, the athletes' performance can be adversely affected.

The experts for athletes are sports medicine physicians, physical therapists, athletic trainers, exercise physiologists, and sports psychologists. It is especially important for athletes to work under the direction of these professionals to ensure proper sport form and training protocols. Obviously, professional athletes or educational athletes (high schools or colleges) are more likely to have access to these professionals than the amateur or recreational athlete. Childhood sports and fitness programs such as softball and soccer should be supervised by professionally trained coaches and trainers. However, because these programs are often staffed by volunteers, training in fitness conditioning and performance skills varies. Those involved in physical rehabilitation are supervised by the physical therapist or other health professional, such as an exercise physiologist. People engaged in basic physical fitness may consult trainers but generally exercise without supervision and then may become hurt because of inappropriate physical activity. These individuals may need to be referred for appropriate training in physical fitness to prevent further injury.

The assumption is that athletes are strong, healthy, and robust individuals, but this is not always true. In actuality, they may be fatigued, injured, in pain, immune suppressed, emotionally and physically stressed, and truly unable to adapt to one more stimulus in their life. When these conditions are not observed or understood, athletes often receive inappropriate massage that includes invasive methods that can be fatiguing at the least and result in tissue damage at the worst. Individuals involved in physical fitness and physical rehabilitation programs are especially sensitive to adaptive strain injuries. Often the best massage approach is the general, nonspecific massage that feels good, calms, and supports sleep. In physiologic terms, this produces parasympathetic dominance in the autonomic nervous system, which supports homeostasis, or self-healing.

CATEGORIES OF SPORTS MASSAGE

In the past, massage for athletes used to be categorized by when it was given and the reasons for the bodywork. These categories included **pre-event,** intercompetition, **recovery massage, post-event, maintenance massage,** remedial, **medical, orthopedic massage,** and **promotional** or **event massage.**[2] However, if you are using outcome-based goals, these categories become irrelevant. If massage is being used to assist preexercise warm-up, it should be focused on those goals. Thus, to categorize massage as "pre-event" or "post-event" can be misleading. But since the reader may still encounter sports massage presented in these categories (remember, there is no such thing as sports massage per se), it is important to describe each category.

Pre-Event Massage

Pre-event massage is a stimulating, superficial, fast-paced, rhythmic massage that lasts 10 to 15 minutes. The emphasis is on the muscles used in the sporting event, and it can be given as early as 3 days before the event or right before the event. Massage techniques that require recovery time, such as deep transverse friction, or those that are painful are strictly contraindicated. Focus should be on improving circulation and not overworking any area.

Intercompetition Massage

Intercompetition massage, given during breaks in the event, concentrates on those muscles being used or about to be used. The strokes are short, light, and focused. For a better outcome, massage therapists familiar with a particular athlete and his or her event should provide intercompetition massage.

Recovery Massage, Post-Event, or Maintenance Massage

Recovery massage, post-event, or maintenance massage focuses primarily on athletes who want to recover from a strenuous workout or competition when no injury is present. The method is similar to a generally focused, full-body massage using any and all methods to support a return to homeostasis.

Remedial, Rehabilitation, Medical, or Orthopedic Massage

Remedial, rehabilitation, medical, and orthopedic massage are interrelated terms and refer to the same procedures. However, the term **remedial massage** is sometimes used to describe application for minor-to-moderate injuries while rehabilitation massage is used for more severe injuries or as part of the postsurgical intervention plan. If the injury or surgery is related to bones, joints, and surrounding soft tissue it can be considered orthopedic massage. The methods of massage used in rehabilitation vary. Immediately after injury or surgery, the massage techniques are often nonspecific, offer general stress reduction, and promote healing. Attention is given to the entire body while the area of injury or surgery heals. Any immobility, use of crutches, or changes in posture or gait during recovery will likely set up compensation patterns. Massage can manage these compensation patterns while the physician, physical therapist, and trainer focus on the injured area. During active rehabilitation, massage can become part of the recovery process, supervised by an appropriately qualified professional, as part of a total treatment plan.[3]

Promotional or Event Massage

Promotional massage is usually given at events for amateur athletes. The massages are offered as a public service to provide educational information about massage. It is important to receive written documentation

of informed consent from each person receiving a massage at these events. One way to do this is to develop an informed consent statement on the top of a sign-in sheet and have each participant read and sign it before receiving the massage. A short brochure or pamphlet explaining the benefits, contraindications, and precautions of sports massage is given to each participant. With permission from the organizer of the event, the brochure could include contact information to allow participating athletes to contact the massage professional at a later date.

The sports event massage lasts about 15 minutes and is quick paced. It is important for massage providers to follow a sports massage routine at these types of events. The use of lubricants is optional, and massage practitioners may choose not to use them because of the risk of allergic reaction, staining of an athlete's uniform, or other unforeseen factors.

During these events, it is important to watch for any swelling that may indicate a sprain, strain, or stress fracture. If these symptoms appear, providers should refer the athlete to the medical team for immediate evaluation. It is also important to watch for evidence of thermoregulatory disruption, such as symptoms of hypothermia or hyperthermia, and refer the individual immediately for medical attention if these are noted. Refrain from using any diagnostic terms (since it is out of our scope of practice to make diagnoses) or alarming the individual.

If a massage professional is doing promotional work at sports massage events and is working with many unfamiliar athletes, it is best to do post-event massage since the effects of any neurologic disorganization caused by the massage are not significant to the event. Avoid using connective tissue work, intense stretching, trigger point work, or other invasive work at these sporting events. Instead, the massage should be superficial, supportive, and focused more on enhancing general circulation.

Often a group of massage professionals and supervised massage students work at an event as a team. A team leader who is familiar with the sport is placed in charge. All the massage practitioners follow a similar routine that is specific to the event while keeping in mind the importance of ethical and professional behavior.

SPORTS, FITNESS, AND REHABILITATION OUTCOMES

The main outcomes of massage for sports and fitness are: increased body stamina, stability (joint stability and general body control), mobility, flexibility, agility, reduced soft tissue tension and binding (feeling of being stiff and stuck), normalized fluid (blood and lymph) movement, management of pain and reduced suffering, support of healing mechanisms, improved mood, increased physical and mental performance, and experiences of pleasure.

These outcomes can be classified as four major goals for sport and fitness performance:

- Performance enhancement and recovery
- Condition management
- Rehabilitation/therapeutic change
- Palliative care

Performance Enhancement/Recovery

As previously discussed, fitness and performance are not the same. Optimal performance is most often achieved once fitness is reached first. Competition often motivates athletes to push their bodies to activity levels beyond their fitness capabilities. Performance, therefore, becomes a strain to the system. Balancing fitness and performance is tricky with athletes. It is also important for those whose goals are fitness oriented not to exceed the beneficial physical outcomes by overdoing it and becoming injured.

Continuous performance demands often interfere with fitness and compromise health. Normal function and performance are not the same. A person learning to walk again after an accident may exert the same amount of effort and can have the same physical manifestations and demands on his or her body as an athlete training to decrease a 40-yard dash time. However, one is seeking to regain normal function and the other is striving for peak performance. Therefore, performance demands more of the athlete than normal function. The massage therapist needs to consider how the massage application supports the goals for physical activity in the following ways:

- Achieving normal function through conditioning
- Maintaining fitness
- Supporting performance that places demand on the body beyond normal function that could damage the body over time

All people who engage in exercise strive for performance at some level. For instance, the elderly person beginning a cardiac rehabilitation program, the professional athlete striving for success in competition, the child beginning to walk, or any others using their bodies in precise ways are all concerned about their ability to carry out an action in an accomplished way. The motivations may be varied, but the outcome is increased proficiency when performing the activity.

Physical performance involves training, practice, and demand on the body. When desired performance levels are achieved and practiced they become automatic.

Enhancing performance requires increasing demand on the body through practice. Maintaining performance involves paying attention to the demands on the body and continuous reinforcement. Recovery is necessary to restore depleted energy and regenerate damaged soft tissue. Most athletes train at levels below peak performance with the outcome of reaching peak during competition. This process is compromised if ongoing competition is extended over a period of time. Therefore, athletes involved in a protracted season, such as baseball and basketball players, can experience difficulty maintaining peak performance because of the duration of the activity. Massage application can support performance by facilitating recovery and removing impediments to training.[4]

Condition Management

A massage that is given to maintain an athlete's condition can be used to manage an ongoing strain that is not going to improve or get worse. Examples include inherent joint laxity, previous injury, emotional demands, and playing schedule. This category of care is perhaps the most important and also the most difficult. Massage application needs to support and maximize function without straining adaptive mechanisms. The elements of all four categories—performance, enhancement, rehabilitation, and palliative care—are combined to support function and performance in the short term, such as assisting the athlete to play the next game. The goal here differs from the goal of a massage that focuses exclusively on rehabilitation, which is targeted to reversing the strain and returning to norm.

Rehabilitation/Therapeutic Change

Injury is a common result of physical activity. Anyone who has worked with the competing athlete knows the importance of injury prevention and effective, accelerated injury recovery. Most athletes practice or compete when injured at one time or another. When injury is involved, performance is compromised because it takes more energy, accommodation, and compensation to perform when injured. Rehabilitation returns the individual to normal function, and for the athlete this means return to peak performance or the ability to function above normal. Massage for rehabilitation and therapeutic change is complex and requires the most training.[5]

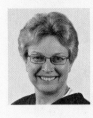

I have worked with professional athletes for many years, primarily football and basketball players. The interplay between fitness, performance, and peak performance is very hard to balance. The pressure during the season is to win championships, and the competition within the team to maintain playing position continues to push the athletes into performance/peak performance that exceeds fitness. The problem is that the more athletes push, the more potential they have for injury. I have supported both a Superbowl championship and a national basketball championship. Playoff games to win championships are at the END of a long season. Massage becomes a very important aspect of the athlete being able to sustain performance.

Palliative Care

Comforting, supporting, nurturing, and providing pleasure are essential elements in the palliative care of the athlete (Figure 16-1). Attention to a warm environment, the atmosphere, and ambience are part of this experience. Patience, flexibility, and commitment are part of the process. Competing athletes are tired, disappointed, and in pain much of the time. Periods of exhilaration or disappointment occur within complex life experiences. The losing athlete needs more support than the winning one. Most often the older athlete needs more care than the younger one. When exercising for fitness, weight loss, and rehabilitation, similar conditions exist. Reducing suffering and offering pleasurable sensations are invaluable in reducing the psychological and physical responses to these stresses.

It is inevitable that athletes will reach plateaus during both training and rehabilitation. Once the satisfaction of seeing ongoing changes is diminished, palliative care may be able to support the individual through these frustrating times. Diminished performance resulting from fatigue and other pressures can be assuaged temporarily by a massage practitioner's nurturing touch. Sometimes the athlete is enduring too much pain and palliative massage offers the best treatment.[6]

However, it is important to remember that touch is a multidimensional experience that encompasses the client's and therapist's body/mind/spirit experience and their interplay within the therapeutic relationship. Although massage can be explained in terms of stimuli and forces, these do not define the integrated experience. Practitioners should not overlook the power of nurturing, compassionate, and respectful care. While research has identified most of the physiologic mechanisms of massage's effects, the unquantifiable mysteries of the unknown still have to be honored.

Maintenance Care

For athletes, regular massage allows the body to function with fewer restrictions and accelerated recovery time. Most athletes require varying depths of pressure, from light to very deep; therefore it is essential that the massage practitioner use effective body mechanics (Figure 16-2). Working with athletes can be very demanding. Their schedules may be erratic, and their bodies change almost daily in response to training, competition, or injury. Athletes can become dependent on massage and the professional relationships they develop with their therapists; therefore commitment by massage professionals is necessary.

Knowledge and Skills

Any massage professional working with this population should be able to recognize common sports injuries and, when an injury is detected, refer the athlete to the appropriate medical professional. Once a diagnosis has been made (by an appropriate expert) and the rehabilitation plan developed, the massage professional can support

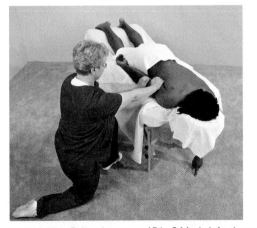

FIGURE 16-1 Relaxed massage. (*Fritz S:* Mosby's fundamentals of therapeutic massage, *ed 4, St. Louis, 2009, Mosby.*)

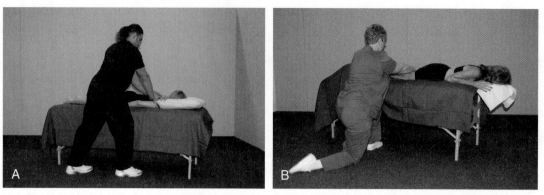

FIGURE 16-2 Proper positioning for body mechanics. **A,** Perpendicularity: staking the joints. Keep the back straight. **B,** Alternate view, kneeling. (*Fritz S:* Sports and excercise massage: comprehensive care in athletics, fitness, and rehabilitation, *St. Louis, 2005, Mosby.*)

the athlete with general or medical (orthopedic) massage applications and appropriate methods to enhance the healing process.

Many factors contribute to mechanical injuries or trauma in sports. Trauma is defined as a physical injury or wound sustained in sports that was produced by an external or internal force. Healing mechanisms manifest because of the inflammatory response and resolution of the inflammatory response. Different tissues heal at different rates. For example, skin heals quickly, whereas ligaments heal slowly. Stress can influence healing by slowing the repair process. Sleep and proper nutrition are necessary for proper healing.

Typically, posttrauma massage is focused on circulation enhancement and lymphatic drainage to reduce swelling. Contraindications may exist for deep transverse friction, focused, intense myofascial release, and extensive trigger point work. Medication use, particularly analgesics for pain and antiinflammatory drugs, is common, and their effects must be considered (Box 16-1). Pain medication reduces pain perception, so athletes often return to their game before healing is complete. This interferes with successful healing. Antiinflammatory drugs may slow the healing process, particularly connective tissue healing, since productive inflammation is necessary for tissue healing to occur.

Thus, the outcome of massage application is to influence the adaptive, restorative, and healing capacities of the body. Anatomic and physiologic outcomes are as follows:

- Local tissue repair, such as a sprain or contusion
- Connective tissue normalization that affects elasticity, stiffness, and strength, such as increased pliability of scar tissue or overall flexibility
- Shifts in pressure gradients to influence body fluid movement

- Neuromuscular function interfacing with muscle tension-length relationship; force couples (groups of muscles that work together to stabilize and move joints); tone of muscles; concentric, eccentric, and isometric muscle action patterns of muscles working together to support efficient movement
- Mood and pain modulation through shifts in autonomic nervous system function yielding neurochemical and neuroendocrine responses
- Increased immune response to support systemic health and healing

Each of these desired outcomes for massage supports rehabilitation, fitness, and performance recovery.

Application

In general massage and bodywork are described in terms of methods and modalities instead of the physiologic response they elicit. To better understand the relationship of massage application to sports performance, it is necessary to move beyond the classic description of massage in terms of effleurage or gliding strokes, petrissage or kneading, compression, friction, vibration, rocking, shaking (oscillation), tapotement or percussion, joint movement, etc. Instead, massage application needs to be described by the stimulus used on a specific receptor or the force applied to affect specific tissues or physiologic functions. Variations in depth of pressure, drag on the tissue, speed of application, direction of movement, frequency of application, duration of application, and rhythm allow for extensive application options based on treatment plan outcomes (Figure 16-3).

The effects of massage are determined by reflexive and mechanical actions or some combination of both. Reflexive responses result from stimulus to the nervous system that activates feedback loops with the therapeutic intent of adjustment in neuromuscular, neurotransmitter, endocrine, or autonomic nervous

---

BOX 16-1 Anabolic-Androgenic Steroids

Anabolic-androgenic steroids are man-made substances related to male sex hormones. "Anabolic" refers to muscle-building, and "androgenic" refers to increased masculine characteristics. "Steroids" refer to the class of drugs. These drugs are available legally only by prescription, to treat conditions that occur when the body produces abnormally low amounts of testosterone, such as in cases of delayed puberty and some types of impotence. They are also prescribed to treat body wasting in patients with AIDS and other diseases that result in loss of lean muscle mass. Abuse of anabolic steroids, however, can lead to serious health problems, some irreversible.

Today, athletes and others abuse anabolic steroids to enhance performance and also to improve physical appearance. Anabolic steroids are taken orally or injected, typically in cycles of weeks or months (referred to as "cycling"), rather than continuously. Cycling involves taking multiple doses of steroids over a specific period of time, stopping for a period, and starting again. In addition, users often combine several different types of steroids to maximize their effectiveness while minimizing negative effects (referred to as "stacking").

Health Hazards

The major side effects from abusing anabolic steroids can include liver tumors and cancer, jaundice (yellowish pigmentation of skin, tissues, and body fluids), fluid retention, high blood pressure, increases in LDL (bad cholesterol), and decreases in HDL (good cholesterol). Other side effects include kidney tumors, severe acne, and trembling. In addition, there are some gender-specific side effects:

- For men—shrinking of the testicles, reduced sperm count, infertility, baldness, development of breasts, increased risk for prostate cancer.
- For women—growth of facial hair, male-pattern baldness, changes in or cessation of the menstrual cycle, enlargement of the clitoris, deepened voice.
- For adolescents—growth halted prematurely through premature skeletal maturation and accelerated puberty changes. This means that adolescents risk remaining short for the remainder of their lives if they take anabolic steroids before the typical adolescent growth spurt.

In addition, people who inject anabolic steroids run the added risk of contracting or transmitting HIV/AIDS or hepatitis, which causes serious damage to the liver.

Scientific research also shows that aggression and other psychiatric side effects may result from abuse of anabolic steroids including extreme mood swings, paranoid jealousy, extreme irritability, delusions, impaired judgment, and manic-like symptoms leading to violence. Depression often is seen when the drugs are stopped and may contribute to dependence on anabolic steroids.

The National Institute on Drug Abuse (NIDA) is part of the National Institutes of Health (NIH), a component of the U.S. Department of Health and Human Services. Unless otherwise specified, NIDA's products are in the public domain and can be copied as a whole without seeking permission from NIDA. Also, text selections and graphics that do not have source citations listed beside, above, or below them can be used without permission. If the person or organization using such material wishes to cite the document or text, standard citation formats relating to publications and web sites should be followed.

---

system homeostatic mechanisms. For example, light stimulus of the skin usually results in a tickle or itching that is arousing and stimulating. Mechanical methods impose various forces such as tension, compression, rotation or torsion, bending, shearing, and the combination of these forces to change body structure or function.

Muscle tone is a mixture of tension in the connective tissue elements of the muscle and the intermuscular fluid pressure. An example of muscle tone dysfunction is delayed onset muscle soreness after exercise. Muscle tone is influenced more by the mechanical massage actions previously discussed. Motor tone is produced by the motor neuron excitability and influenced by reflexive massage application that inhibits motor neuron activity. The most common reason for increases in motor tone is an increase in sympathetic arousal and sustained sympathetic dominance. Another cause is proactive muscle

guarding after injury and nervous system damage.[6] Both situations are common in athletes.

INDICATIONS FOR MASSAGE

Massage can support the restorative process to help athletes maintain peak performance longer. However, the most beneficial effects of massage are to help people to stay within the healthy range of physical functioning and to support those who wish to achieve fitness.

Therapeutic massage is indicated for both illness and injury with caution and supervision by the appropriate health care professional, such as the athletic trainer. Massage techniques for illness involve very general application of massage to support the body's healing responses (e.g., stress management, pain control, and restorative sleep). This type of massage, sometimes

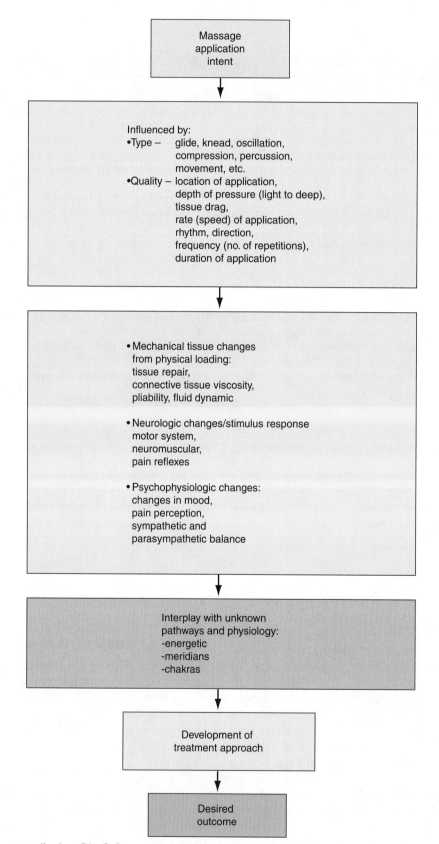

FIGURE 16-3 Massage application. *Fritz S:* Sports and excercise massage: comprehensive care in athletics, fitness, and rehabilitation, *St. Louis, 2005, Mosby.*

called general constitutional application, reduces the stress load so that the body can heal more efficiently.

Massage for injury incorporates aspects of general constitutional massage, because healing is necessary for tissue repair. In addition, the more mechanical application of lymphatic drainage is used to control edema. Gliding methods are used to approximate (bring close together) the ends of some types of tissue injury, such as minor muscle strains and ligament sprains (Figure 16-4). Hyperstimulation analgesia and counterirritation reduce acute pain. Methods to increase circulation to the area support new tissue formation. Connective tissue applications are used to manage scar tissue formation.

In general, massage is indicated for:
• Relaxation and pleasure
• Anxiety reduction
• Mild depression management
• Enhanced immune function
• Efficient circulation of body fluids
• Effective digestion and elimination
• Enhanced growth, development, and regeneration of soft tissue
• Treating soft tissue dysfunction
• To relieve nerve impingement syndrome
• Exercise recovery and performance
• Inflammation management (Table 16-1)
• Pain management
• Mood management

CONTRAINDICATIONS

(Sports) massage is contraindicated in some instances, and when these conditions are present, it may be necessary to adjust or avoid certain techniques. Where contraindications exist and massage is indicated, the

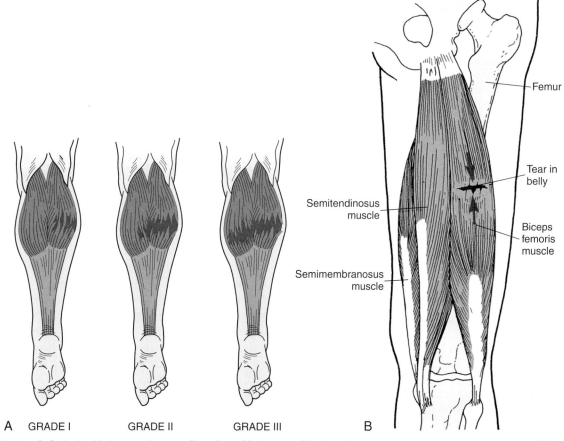

A   GRADE I   GRADE II   GRADE III   B

FIGURE 16-4 A, Calf pull with degrees of severity. (From Salvo SG, Anderson SK: *Mosby's pathology for massage therapists,* St Louis, 2004, Mosby.) **B,** Muscle strain. This muscle strain is located in the biceps femoris muscle of the hamstring group (in this case, a tear in the midportion of the belly of the muscles). Arrows show direction of the massage stroke. (From Thibodeau GA, Patton KT: *The human body in health and disease,* ed 2, St Louis, 1997, Mosby.)

TABLE 16-1 Stages of Tissue Healing and Massage Interventions

STAGE 1: ACUTE INFLAMMATORY REACTION	STAGE 2: SUBACUTE REPAIR AND HEALING	STAGE 3: MATURATION AND REMODELING
Characteristics Vascular changes Inflammatory exudates Clot formation Phagocytosis, neutralization of irritants Early fibroblastic activity	Growth of capillary beds into area Collagen formation Granulation tissue; caution necessary Fragile, easily injured tissue	Maturation and remodeling of scar Contracture of scar tissue Alignment of collagen along lines of stress forces
Clinical Signs Inflammation Pain prior to tissue resistance	Decreased inflammation Pain during tissue resistance	Absence of inflammation Pain after tissue resistance
Massage Intervention Protection Control and support of effects of inflammation (PRICE)* Passive movement mid-range General massage and lymphatic drainage with caution; support rest with full-body massage (3 to 7 days)	Controlled motion Promoting development of mobile scar Cautious and controlled soft tissue mobilization of scar tissue along fiber direction toward injury. Active and passive, open- and closed-chain range or motion, mid-range. Support healing with full-body massage (14 to 21 days)	Return to function Increase in strength and alignment of scar tissue Cross-fiber friction of scar tissue coupled with directional stroking along the lines of tension away from injury Progressive stretching and active and resisted range of motion; full-range. Support rehabilitation activities with full-body massage (3 to 12 months)

*Protection, rest, ice, compression, elevation.
From Fritz S: *Mosby's fundamentals of therapeutic massage,* ed. 4, St. Louis, 2004, Mosby.

interaction should be monitored by a healthcare professional such as a physician, nurse, physical therapist, or athletic trainer. For professional athletes, particularly in team sports, there is an athletic training department in charge of health maintenance and injury rehabilitation. Their recommendations are valuable when determining appropriate massage application. When this type of professional support is not available, as is the case with the amateur athlete, the treatment decisions become more difficult and complicated. With athletes, a general recommendation is to be cautious and not to take risks. The closer to competition, the more important it is to follows these basic rules.

Conditions that may present contraindications requiring avoidance or alteration in application are:

- Acute injuries
- Systemic infections
- Contagious conditions
- Loss of sensation
- Loss of voluntary movement
- Acute or severe cardiac, liver, and kidney diseases

- Use of sensation-altering substance, both prescribed, such as pain medication, and recreational, such as alcohol
- Use of medications that thin blood (anticoagulants), nonprescribed medications such as aspirin, or prescribed medications, such as Coumadin (Warfarin)

Clients with any vague or unexplainable symptoms of fatigue, muscle weakness, and general aches and pains should be immediately referred to a physician. Many disease processes share these symptoms. This recommendation may seem overly cautious, but in the early stages of some very serious illnesses, the symptoms are not well defined. If the physician is able to detect a disease process early in its development, there is often a more successful outcome. A specific diagnosis is essential for effective treatment. Massage should be avoided in all instances of infectious diseases suggested by fever, nausea, and lethargy until a diagnosis has been made and recommendations from a physician can be followed.

Specific conditions that present contraindications and precautions for the athletic and physical rehabilitation population include the following:

Acute Local Soft Tissue Inflammation

To test for acute inflammation, apply enough pressure to the area to cause mild discomfort. Maintain this fixed pressure for up to 10 seconds. If the discomfort increases, this suggests that the tissues are in an acute state; if it decreases, it is safe to apply massage being careful not to disturb healing tissue.

Bone and Joint Injuries

With fractures pain and tenderness tend to increase around the injury site with any movement or weight-bearing activity. Stress fractures are very difficult to diagnose. Be especially concerned if the pain persists and is coupled with swelling and bruising in the injured area. Massage in the acute stage of these conditions is obviously contraindicated, as it would cause further damage.

Deep Vein Thrombosis (DVT)

During the application of massage a thrombosis (blood clot) can form in a vein and be dislodged, or a fragment (embolus) may break off. The veins usually affected are those in the calf and hamstring areas (greater saphenous, iliac, and femoral veins). Practitioners must take note that the acute pain and hard swelling felt when minimal pressure is applied might be misinterpreted as an acute muscle strain. There may be some general swelling and discoloration to the distal part of the limb, due to restricted circulation. If a DVT is suspected, the client should be referred to the doctor or hospital immediately. Pain during dorsiflexion of the foot (Homan sign) may also indicate the presence of a thrombosis.

Fungal Infections

Ringworm and athlete's foot are the most common fungal infections athletes experience. They can affect warm, moist areas, such as the areas between the toes, the armpits, or under the breasts. The affected area may appear red, with white, flaky skin. Although massage does not worsen the problem, it can cause irritation and could be transmitted to the therapist's hands. For these reasons, treatment of the affected areas is avoided and the practitioner can wear gloves as an added precaution.

Bacterial Infections

Boils are superficial abscesses that appear as a localized swelling on the skin. They eventually rupture and discharge pus. Folliculitis, which looks like a rash of very small blisters, is a condition when the hair follicles become inflamed. Massage can break the blisters, leaving the skin open to further infection. These areas present local contraindications for massage.

Lymphangitis

Bacteria can invade the lymphatic system through open wounds. The local area around the wound, which may itself be very minor, will appear red and swollen. A dark line can sometimes be seen running up the limb toward the lymph nodes, which may also be swollen and tender. Massage could spread the infection, and immediate medical treatment is required.

Myositis Ossificans

When a hematoma (a clot of blood) occurs from an untreated deep bruise, it sometimes ossifies and forms into small pieces of bone material within the soft tissues. This is more likely to happen when a fracture has also been involved because osteoblasts move into the tissues and can be the catalyst for the calcification. Massage on the area could cause the pieces of bone to damage the surrounding soft tissues.

Effects of Medications

The massage professional should be able to assess the effects of medications and should be aware of the ways massage may influence the athlete's reactions. Massage practitioners need to be specifically knowledgeable about antiinflammatory drugs, muscle relaxants, anticoagulants (blood thinners), analgesics (pain modulators), and other medications that alter sensation, muscle tone, normal reflex reactions, cardiovascular function, kidney or liver function, or personality. They also should be aware of the effects of over-the-counter medications, herbs, and vitamins as well. If a client is taking medication, it is important to have the physician confirm the advisability of therapeutic massage.

ASSESSMENT AND DOCUMENTATION

Massage therapists working with athletes, providing physical rehabilitation, or involved with fitness have an expanded assessment responsibility. Assessment identifies which structures need to be treated, creates a clear intention about the treatment goals, provides a baseline of objective information to measure the effectiveness of the treatment, and helps identify conditions that are contraindicated. When working with a client who is striving for optimal performance or has pain, dysfunction, or disability, massage therapists need to gather information about long- and short-term treatment goals, relevant data about activities and training activity, as well as information about pain or decreased function.

Information from athletic trainers, coaches, or other professionals is also important. Massage therapists must understand and apply assessment information provided by these trainers. If at any time you do not understand, ask these sports experts for clarification. Information gathered by massage therapists should be shared with the athletic trainers or other appropriate members of the sports and/or medical team in a concise and intelligent manner.

A plan based on efficient biomechanical movement would focus on reestablishing or supporting effective movement patterns. Biomechanically efficient movement is smooth, bilaterally symmetric, and coordinated,

with an easy, effortless use of the body. Functional assessment measures the efficiency of coordinated movement. During assessment, noticeable variations need to be considered (Figure 16-5).

SPECIFIC HISTORY

Targeting this information to the athlete or person in physical rehabilitation is the focus of this chapter. In addition to the general history, anyone who is working with an athlete or a person in physical rehabilitation needs information about the following for each client:

- Surgery or medical procedures
- Medications and supplements
- Use of hydrotherapy
- Electrostimulation

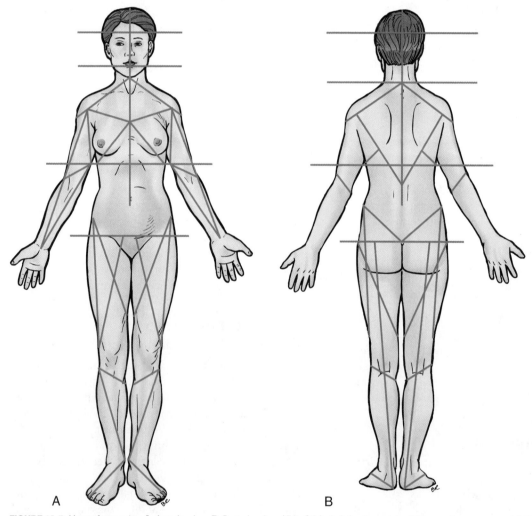

A   B

FIGURE 16-5 Lines of symmetry. **A,** Anterior view. **B,** Posterior view. (*Fritz S:* Mosby's fundamentals of therapeutic massage, *ed 4, St. Louis, 2009, Mosby.*)

- Therapeutic exercise activities
- Physical therapy interventions
- Nutrition
- Training protocols
- Training types such as strength and conditioning, agility, etc.
- Sleep patterns
- Breathing patterns
- Moods
- Cognitive loads (how much mental training required)

- Competition schedules
- Practice and training schedules
- Previous massage experiences
- Alternative therapies used (essential oils, magnets, etc.)
- Injury history
- Specific symptoms including pain levels and type, reduced function, fatigue
- Relieving factors (makes it better) and exacerbating factors (makes it worse)

■■□□ IN MY EXPERIENCE

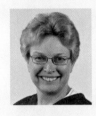

Massage therapists (and most people) assume athletes are physically fit—not necessarily true. I have heard many stories from athletes and coaches about how massage was too aggressive. Instead of feeling better, the next day they were really sore. In a couple of instances performance was really affected and there were serious repercussions. In one instance an athlete lost his starting position partly due to poor performance after an inappropriately given massage. This case proves that massage practitioners need to be trained to work with these individuals.

DOCUMENTATION

Documentation of the massage sessions varies depending on the environment in which massage is performed. Some of the more professional practices in massage require qualified and quantifiable goals written into the treatment plans, ongoing session charting such as SOAP notes, and periodic reevaluations for any revisions of the treatment plans.

APPLICATIONS

The methods of massage described introduce one or a combination of forces for therapeutic benefits. This process is influenced by the qualities of the applications: depth of pressure, drag, direction, duration, speed, rhythm, and frequency. Appropriate use of mechanical force and pressure is necessary. If insufficient intensity is used, the application will not be effective; conversely, excessive use of mechanical force can cause tissue damage.

The mechanical forces created by massage are tension loading, compression loading, bending loading, shear loading, rotation or torsion loading, and combined loading.

Tension Loading

Tissues elongate under tension loading with the intent of lengthening shortened tissues (Figure 16-6). Tension force is created by methods such as gliding and stroking with tissue drag, traction, and longitudinal stretching.

Compression Loading

Tissues will shorten and widen because compression loading increases the pressure within the tissues and affects fluid flow (Figure 16-7). Obviously, compression massage methods create compression loading.

Bending Loading

The therapist applies combined forces of tension on the convex side of the tissue and compression on the concave side of the tissue. Massage techniques such as kneading and compression

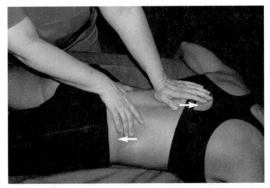

FIGURE 16-6 Tension loading. *Fritz S: Sports and excercise massage: comprehensive care in athletics, fitness, and rehabilitation, St. Louis, 2005, Mosby.*

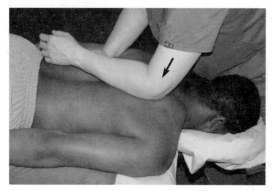

FIGURE 16-7 Compression loading. *Fritz S:* Sports and excercise massage: comprehensive care in athletics, fitness, and rehabilitation, *St. Louis, 2005, Mosby.*

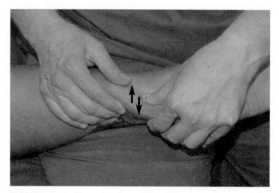

FIGURE 16-9 Shear loading. *Fritz S:* Sports and excercise massage: comprehensive care in athletics, fitness, and rehabilitation, *St. Louis, 2005, Mosby.*

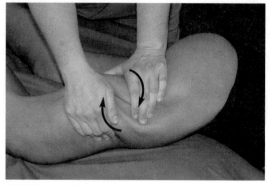

FIGURE 16-10 Rotation or torsion loading. *Fritz S:* Sports and excercise massage: comprehensive care in athletics, fitness, and rehabilitation, *St. Louis, 2005, Mosby.*

have an aspect of bending loading (Figure 16-8). Bending is used where combined effects of lengthening, shortening, and an increase in pliability are desired.

Shear Loading

Massage practitioners move the tissues back and forth creating a combined pattern of compression and elongation. Friction is a massage method that creates shear loading and is particularly effective in controlling inflammation and to ensure that tissue layers slide over one another instead of adhering to underlying layers, creating bind (Figure 16-9).

Rotation or Torsion Loading

Rotation or torsion loading is a type of force that combines compression and wringing resulting in elongation of tissue along the axis of rotation (Figure 16-10). It is used where a combined effect of improving fluid dynamics and connective tissue pliability is desired. Kneading creates torsion loading.

Combined Loading

Combining two or more forces is possible (Figure 16-11). The more forces applied to tissue the more intense the response. Tension and compression underlie all the different modes of loading; therefore, any form of massage manipulation is either tension, compression, or a combination of the two. Tension is important in conditions where tissue needs to be elongated, and compression is necessary where fluid flow needs to be affected. Oscillation of tissue can be considered combined loading. For example, shaking, a form of oscillation, provides shearing and torsion force.

JOINT MOVEMENT AND MUSCLE ENERGY METHODS

A client can assist with joint movements and muscle energy methods. Joint movements are effective because they provide a means of controlled stimulation to the joint mechanoreceptors.

Joint movements also encourage lubrication of the joints and contribute an important enhancement to the lymphatic and venous circulation systems. Much of

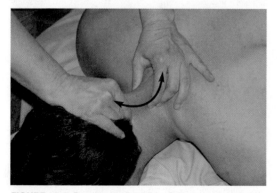

FIGURE 16-8 Bending loading. *Fritz S:* Sports and excercise massage: comprehensive care in athletics, fitness, and rehabilitation, *St. Louis, 2005, Mosby.*

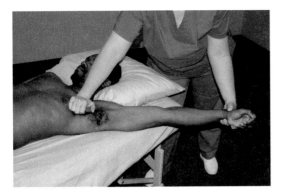

FIGURE 16-11 Combined loading. *Fritz S: Sports and excercise massage: comprehensive care in athletics, fitness, and rehabilitation, St. Louis, 2005, Mosby.*

the pumping action that moves these fluids in the vessels results from compression against the lymph and blood vessels during joint movements and muscle contractions. The tendons, ligaments, and joint capsules are warmed from the movements. This mechanical effect helps keep these tissues pliable.

Joint Movement Methods

Joint movements involve moving the jointed areas within the limits of the client's physiologic range of motion. The two types of joint movements are active and passive.

Active joint movements allow the client to move the joints by active contraction of muscle groups. The two variations of active joint movements are as follows:
1. Active assisted movements, which occur when both the client and the massage practitioner move the area
2. Active resistive movements, which occur when the client actively moves the joint against a resistance provided by the massage practitioner

Passive joint movements occur when the client's muscles stay relaxed and the massage practitioner moves the joint with no assistance from the client. When doing passive joint movements, feel for the soft or hard end feel of the joint range of motion. This is an important evaluation, and a hard end feel often indicates joint dysfunction requiring referral to a doctor. Joint oscillation is a passive joint movement.

Joint movements become part of the application of muscle energy techniques to lengthen muscles and part of stretching methods to elongate connective tissues. Because of this, massage professionals should concentrate on developing the ability to use joint movements efficiently and effectively.

Muscle energy techniques involve a voluntary contraction of the client's muscles in a specific and controlled direction, at varying levels of intensity, and against a specific counterforce applied by the massage

therapist. Muscle energy procedures have a variety of applications and are considered active techniques in which the client contributes the corrective force. The amount of effort may vary from a small muscle twitch to a maximal muscle contraction. The duration may be a fraction of a second to several seconds. All contractions begin and end slowly, gradually building to the desired intensity.

Counterpressure is the force applied to an area that is designed to oppose or match the effort or force exactly (isometric) or partially (isotonic). Muscle energy techniques usually do not use the full contraction strength of the client. With most isometric work, the contraction should start at about 25% of the strength of the muscle. Subsequent contractions can involve progressively greater degrees of effort, but never more than 50% of the available strength.

Many experts use only about 10% of the available strength in muscles being treated in this way and find that they can increase effectiveness by using longer periods of contraction. Pulsed contractions (a rapid series of repetitions) using minimal strength are also effective.

STRETCHING

Stretching is a mechanical method of introducing various forces into connective tissue to elongate areas of connective tissue shortening (Figure 16-12). Technically, stretching targets connective tissue. Muscle fibers shorten as a result of a chemical response. The application of a tension force restores normal resting length. Stretching affects the fibrous component of connective tissue by elongating the fibers beyond their normal resistance so they can enter the plastic range past the existing bind. Stretching also affects the ground substance of connective tissue (a gel-like material), warming and softening it and thereby increasing pliability. Stretching introduces forces of bend, torsion, and tension that mechanically affect connective tissue.

Developing good stretching techniques is perhaps as much an art as it is a science since there are so many variables. An individual muscle needs to be carefully isolated through specific positioning and stabilizing so that the stretch is focused. With the muscles that cross one joint only, this is usually quite simple. With two-joint muscles, the stretch becomes more complicated. One joint needs to be fixed so that it prestretches the muscle, while the other joint is moved to increase the stretch. This means that there may be two different techniques for the same muscle to focus the stretch at either end (Figure 16-13).

The muscle must be fully relaxed and non–weight bearing or it will not stretch fully, even though the client

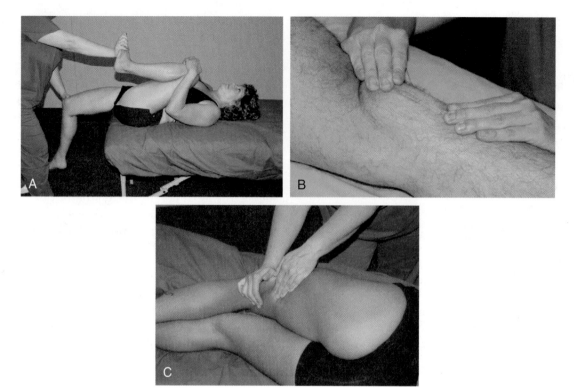

FIGURE 16-12 Stretching. **A,** Longitudinal joint. **B,** Direct—longitudinal. **C,** Direct—cross directional. *Fritz S:* Sports and excercise massage: comprehensive care in athletics, fitness, and rehabilitation, *St. Louis, 2005, Mosby.*

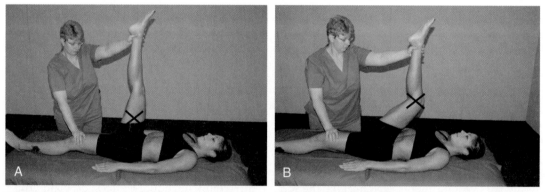

FIGURE 16-13 Stretching two-jointed muscles. **A,** Stretch position 1—proximal fibers. **B,** Stretch position 2—distal fibers. *Fritz S:* Sports and excercise massage: comprehensive care in athletics, fitness, and rehabilitation, *St. Louis, 2005, Mosby.*

may still feel a stretching sensation. When stretching a muscle, start by moving it slowly to the point where the client feels a mild discomfort. Hold it firmly but comfortably in that position. There should be no sensation of pain, tearing, or burning, as this would suggest that the fibers are being overstretched and possibly torn. Once the tissues begin to relax, the stretch can be gently increased. There are many differing opinions as to how long a stretch should be held, but it is generally accepted that the length of time is more significant than the intensity of the stretch.

FLUID DYNAMICS, LYMPHATIC DRAINAGE, AND CIRCULATION ENHANCEMENT

Fluid tension in the body is called hydrostatic pressure. Body fluid is considered extracellular (outside the cell) and intercellular (within the cell). About one third of the body fluid is extracellular and located in two areas of the body:

- The blood circulatory system, including the arteries and veins, and
- The interstitial anatomical space around cells and the lymphatic vessels

Fluids also move across these regions by diffusion from areas of higher salt concentration to lower salt concentration. The rate and volume of fluid movement will be determined by pumping mechanisms, such as heartbeat, muscle contraction and relaxation, rhythmic compression of fascial structure during movement, and respiration. Also influencing fluid movement is the viscosity of the fluid, the permeability of the membranes, and the size of the various vessels the fluid travels through. Massage that addresses the extracellular fluid can mechanically support the movement of fluid within these regions by stimulating hydrokinetics (transport of fluid) along pressure gradients from higher pressure to lower pressure. Vasodilators and vasoconstrictors of the circulatory system would therefore influence the movement of body fluid. The mechanical pumping and oscillation applications of massage, the reflexive release of vasodilators (primarily histamine) produced during massage, and either the vasodilatation or vasoconstriction response of hydrotherapy would interplay in various ways to influence the outcome of the treatment. Proper hydration (drinking water) is especially important to maintain fluid function.

In terms of methodical application, massage outcomes can target each main fluid area: arterial, venous, and lymphatic functions. All of these areas are strained during exercise. In general, massage targeted to increase arterial flow is part of the warm-up. Venous congestion and increased interstitial fluid can occur postexercise, indicating the need for lymphatic drainage. Methods to address venous return can also decrease interstitial fluid by moving it into the lymphatic system.

Recovery involves normalizing all fluid movement. Injury rehabilitation involves managing swelling and encouraging effective circulation to the injured area to support healing.

Specific situations involving focused massage techniques are: injury swelling, sprains, strains, contusions, postsurgical swelling, delayed onset muscle soreness, or chronic joint swelling. Strain, sprains, contusions, and surgery require specific treatments. These local first and second degree (mild and moderate) injuries benefit from both local and systemic lymphatic drainage. It is important to decongest the entire drainage area affecting the injured area—for example, a sprained ankle requires draining of the entire leg into the trunk.

PRICE (protection, rest, ice, compression, elevation) treatment should be used with injury for the first 24 hours. Movement of fluid from superficial tissues can begin after the acute stage begins to diminish. Proper medical care needs to be provided, and medical team orders must be followed.

Treatment for delayed onset muscle soreness (DOMS) can begin immediately after activity as a preventive measure. Part of the process of DOMS is inflammation with increased capillary permeability. Increased sympathetic autonomic nervous system influences on blood pressure also result in more fluid movement from the capillary beds into the space between tissue cells. This increases interstitial fluid and hydrostatic pressure within the tissue. Pressure from the fluid accumulation restricts lymphatic capillaries making it difficult to drain the area, which results in an increase in congestion. This puts more pressure on the pain-sensitive receptors eliciting aches and pains.

Chronic swelling usually occurs around injured joints, tendons, and bursae. A portion of the treatment of these conditions involves decreasing blood and lymph at the site of the injury. Edema acts as a protective mechanism to reduce the problem causing the inflammation and to restrict movement, preventing further injury. The goal of the massage is to reduce the edema and increase function, but not to interfere with the protective process and increased stability provided by the hydrostatic pressure.

With contusions, the entire area around the contusion needs to be drained of excess edema. However, caution is necessary because the capillaries have been damaged and the massage must not interfere with the healing process. Blood in the interstitial fluid increases the protein content of the fluid, which in turn increases the potential for fibrotic tissue to form. This is why it is essential to encourage lymphatic drainage to remove the interstitial fluid containing blood.

Circulation Methods

All massage stimulates the circulation and lymph movement. Lymph circulation involves two steps:

1. Interstitial fluid flows into the lymphatic capillaries. Plasma is forced out of blood capillaries into the spaces around the cell walls. As fluid pressure increases between the cells, cells move apart, pulling on the microfilaments that connect the endothelial cells of the lymph capillaries to tissue cells. The pull on the microfilaments causes the lymph capillaries to open like flaps, allowing fluid to enter the lymph capillaries.
2. Lymph moves through the network of contractile lymphatic vessels, although the lymphatic system does not have a central pump as the heart. In lieu of a pump, other factors assist in the transport of lymph through the lymph vessels.

The "lymphatic pump" of the body is the spontaneous contraction of lymphatic vessels as a result of the increase in pressure of lymphatic fluid. These contractions usually start in the lymphangions adjacent to the terminal end of the lymph capillaries and spread progressively from one lymphangion to the next, toward the thoracic duct or the right lymphatic duct. The contractions are similar to abdominal peristalsis and are stimulated by increases in pressure inside lymphatic vessels. Contractions of the lymphatic vessels are not coordinated with the heart or breath rate. If the pressure inside the lymphatic vessels exceeds or falls below certain levels, lymphatic contractions cease.

During breath inhalation the thoracic duct is squeezed, pushing fluid forward and creating a vacuum in the duct. During exhalation, fluid is pulled from the lymphatics into the thoracic duct to fill the partial vacuum.

The pressure provided by lymphatic drainage massage mimics the drag and compressive forces of movement and respiration and can move the skin to open the lymph capillaries. The pressure gradient from high pressure to low pressure is supported by creating low-pressure areas in the vessels proximal to the area to be drained (Figure 16-14).

The depth of pressure, speed and frequency, direction, rhythm, duration, and drag are all adjusted to support the lymphatic system and encourage efficient lymph absorption. The pressure is just enough pressure to move the skin in and out of bind (10 to 30 mm Hg). Lymphatic vessels, particularly those in the superficial tissues or outer 0.3 mm of the skin where surface edema occurs, are most affected by lymphatic massage. Moving the skin moves the lymph. Stretching the lymph vessels longitudinally, horizontally, and diagonally stimulates them to contract. Even simple muscle tension puts sufficient pressure on the lymph vessels to block them, interfering with efficient drainage. Only the light, slow strokes of lymphatic drainage allow the lymph vessels to open and drain.

There is an open, continuing discussion about the intensity of the pressure used in lymphatic drainage. Some schools of thought recommend very light pressure, such as that described by Dr. Vodder, which suggests using approximately 30 mm Hg of pressure, or about the weight of a quarter. Other methods, such as the technique described by Lederman, use a deeper pressure. Lederman holds that the stronger the compression, the larger the increase in the flow rate of lymph. Light pressure is used initially and then methodically increased as the area is drained.

The more fluid there is in the tissue, the slower the massage movements. Massage strokes are repeated slowly, at a rate of approximately 10 per minute in an area, which is approximately the rate at which the peripheral lymphatic vessels contract.

Begin by moving the lymph toward the closest cluster of lymph nodes located either in the neck, axilla, or groin areas. Gently massage the closest nodes first, then slowly move the fluid toward them, working proximally from the swollen area toward the nodes. Massage the unaffected side first, then the obstructed side. For instance, if the right arm is swollen, massage the left arm first.

The approach for lymphatic drainage is a rhythmic slow repetition of specific massage movements. Full-body lymph drainage massage lasts about 45 minutes. Focus on local areas about 5 to 15 minutes.

The purpose of circulatory massage is to encourage the efficient flow of blood through the body. This type of massage tends to normalize blood pressure, tone the cardiovascular system, and rid the body of the negative effects of occasional stress. It is an excellent massage approach to use with athletes and anyone else after exercise. Circulatory massage also supports the inactive client by increasing the blood movement mechanically; however, it in no way replaces exercise. Both the circulatory and lymphatic types of massage are very beneficial for the client who is unable to walk or exercise aerobically.

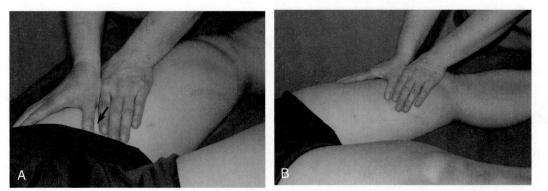

FIGURE 16-14 Procedure for swelling of an individual joint area or knee. **A,** Start skin drag; **B,** continue drag method toward the trunk, down the limb. *Fritz S:* Sports and excercise massage: comprehensive care in athletics, fitness, and rehabilitation, *St. Louis, 2005, Mosby.*

Compression is applied over the main arteries, beginning close to the heart (proximal), and systematically moves distally to the tips of the fingers or toes (Figure 16-15). These compressions are done with a pumping action at a rhythm of approximately 60 beats per minute or whatever the client's resting heart rate is. Compressive force changes the internal pressure in the arteries, stimulates the intrinsic contraction of arteries, and encourages the movement of blood out to the distal areas of the body. Compression also begins to empty venous vessels and forms an arterial-venous pressure gradient, encouraging arterial blood flow.

Rhythmic, gentle contraction and relaxation of the muscles support arterial blood flow. Both active and passive joint movement supports the transport of arterial blood.

The next step is to assist venous return flow (Figure 16-16). This process is similar to lymphatic massage as a similar combination of short and long gliding strokes is used in conjunction with movement. The difference is that lymphatic massage is done over the entire body and the movements are usually passive. With venous return flow, the gliding strokes move distal to proximal (from the fingers and toes to the heart) over the major veins. The gliding stroke is short, about 3 inches long. This enables the blood to move from valve to valve. Long gliding strokes carry the blood through the entire vein. Both passive and active joint movements encourage venous circulation. Placing the limbs above the heart allows gravity to work to an advantage.

The actual massage is a weaving of palpation and movement assessments with treatment followed by a

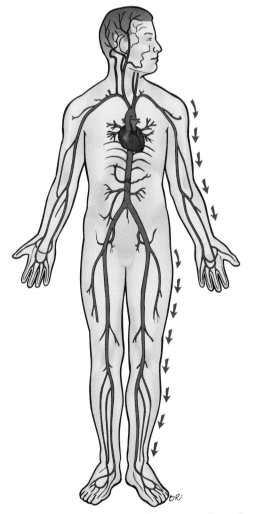

FIGURE 16-15 Direction of compression over arteries to increase arterial flow. (*Fritz S:* Mosby's fundamentals of therapeutic massage, *ed 4, St. Louis, 2009, Mosby.*)

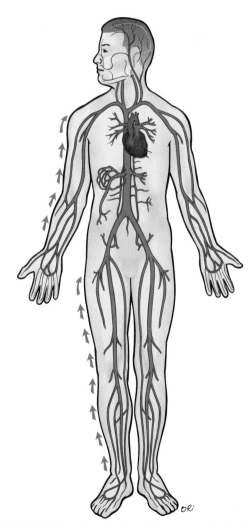

FIGURE 16-16 Direction of gliding/effleurage strokes to facilitate venous flow. (*Fritz S:* Mosby's fundamentals of therapeutic massage, *ed 4, St. Louis, 2009, Mosby.*)

postassessment. Gliding is palpation that can first discern surface edema and then move the fluid. Kneading is an assessment to identify any connective tissue bind and the stroke that reduces it. Active and passive joint movements are range of motion assessments that may become a muscle energy technique to lengthen and stretch an area of restricted movement. The postassessment again involves active and passive joint movements to see how the tissue has stretched. Circulatory massage follows a continuum of initial assessment, treatment, and posttreatment assessment.

General Approach for Massage Application

A general pattern is used during the massage session that consists of assessing each area, then addressing the outcome goals with appropriate massage methods.

The sequence of areas assessed and treated is as follows:

1. Skin, superficial fascia, and edema reduction
2. Deeper fascial structures, muscle layers, circulation, and edema reduction
3. Tissue density, ground substance, and fluid
4. Joint motion
5. Motor tone
6. Reflex mechanisms
7. Flexibility

The massage assessment/treatment protocol takes anywhere from 60 to 90 minutes but can take up to 2 hours if the athlete is large or the condition is complex. While it is appropriate to use some isolated spot work on areas that are problematic, the response is improved when this localized work is incorporated into the full body treatment. Ideally, during an active rehabilitation phase, the athlete would have a full body massage every other day incorporating the specific applications for rehabilitation. On alternate days, focus is on isolated applications to the injured area. If the athlete gets massages frequently, the massage duration can be shorter. If the client only comes in once a week, then the longer 2-hour massage may be required. If the client has two massage sessions a week, then 90 minutes may be sufficient, and for three massage sessions a week, 1 hour each is adequate.

JUSTIFICATION FOR PRACTICE

What does the research say? There has been a lot of research about DOMS.[7-12] The outcome of the studies varies, but a majority found massage administered immediately after or at 24 or 48 hours after exercise resulted in a reduction in DOMS. When the massage was administered 2 hours postexercise, the best results were achieved, implying that timing is a factor. Although a scientific rationale has not been identified for these results, Russian sports therapists advocated that restorative massage be administered 1 to 3 hours after exercise.

Studies have shown that massage aimed at muscle relaxation can result in an increased range of motion in a joint. Muscles span joints, and if the individual muscles and/or groups of muscles are encouraged to relax, this has a direct effect in extending the limit to which the affected joint or joints can move. Kneading has been shown to decrease neuromuscular excitability, but only during the actual massage, and the effects are confined to the muscle(s) being massaged.

During warm-up protocols, stretching exercises produce the greatest flexibility in connective tissue around the joints, although massage has a significant beneficial effect as well. Research has found that massage prior to activity could actually reduce the ability to generate force from muscle action. A different research study showed that maximal muscle power output during leg extension was significantly increased when the athletes received massage beforehand. Until this issue is resolved, the determining factor would be the athlete's responses.

Performance experts strongly discourage athletes from receiving their first massage close to an important competition. When in doubt about the advisability of massage, wait until after the performance. It is also important that massage be carefully integrated into the athlete's entire training and competition program. Random massages from multiple practitioners are less effective and could disrupt performance.

The effects of massage on lymph flow have been scientifically proven. There is a consensus within the literature demonstrating an increase in lymphatic flow as a result of lymphatic drainage massage. This data has implications for restorative massage outcomes and management of delayed onset muscle soreness. Lymph flow only increased with kneading and gliding massage, and active or passive exercise. Other studies, comparing massage with passive movement and electrical stimulation, also acknowledged lymph flow to be greatest following massage.[2,5]

Massage produces short-term analgesia by activating the gate-control mechanism by creating counterirritation and hyperstimulation analgesia. Cutaneous mechanoreceptors are stimulated by touch and rapidly transmit information within large myelinated nerve fibers to the spinal cord. These impulses block the passage of painful stimuli entering the same spinal segment. Other physical therapies acting upon this mechanism include thermal and electrical treatments and joint manipulation. Massage is a potent mechanical stimulus and a particularly effective trigger for the gate-control process.

Massage produces a heating effect on the tissue, and this in turn provides many important therapeutic effects. A mild degree of heating is effective in relieving pain because of heat's sedative effect on the sensory nerves. By virtue of relieving pain, associated muscle spasms and tensions are also relieved. Heating also increases the blood flow by dilating the capillaries and arterioles. Heating the tissues also causes an increase in muscle and ligament extensibility and ground substance pliability, enhancing stretching and facilitating muscle contractility.

CERTIFICATION

National Athletic Trainers Association Board of Certification (NATABOC) certifies athletic trainers and identifies quality healthcare professionals through a system of certification, adjudication, standards of practice, and continuing competency programs.

Six performance domains, based on the 1999 Role Delineation Study, have been established by the NATABOC:
- Prevention of athletic injuries
- Recognition, evaluation, and assessment of injuries
- Immediate care of injuries
- Treatment, rehabilitation, and reconditioning of athletic injuries
- Healthcare administration
- Professional development and responsibility

Education competencies established by the Education Council include:
- Acute care of injury and illness
- Assessment and evaluation
- General medical conditions and disabilities
- Healthcare administration
- Nutritional aspects of injury and illness
- Pharmacologic aspects of injury and illnesses
- Professional development and responsibility
- Psychosocial intervention and referral
- Risk management and injury prevention
- Therapeutic exercise
- Therapeutic modalities

CHAPTER SUMMARY

Many researchers maintain that the recuperative benefits from massage may be more psychologic than physiologic. Massage promotes a feeling of well-being

and even euphoria. The psychologic benefits of massage include controlled arousal before competition or training with positive mood states. Physical relaxation can improve blood flow and reduce muscle tone and tension in connective tissue. Studies on fascia in humans using electron photomicroscopy found smooth muscle cells widely embedded within the collagen fibers and concluded that these intrafascial smooth muscle cells enable the autonomic nervous system to regulate a fascial pretension, independent of muscular tonus.

When comparing the various research in sports massage, one finds some areas of consensus along with the opposing and contradictory opinions. Ongoing research will continue to clarify physiologic mechanisms that underpin the various therapeutic effects. The future will depend on this research and its continued collaboration with medicine, physical therapy, and sport performance. The focus of this chapter has been to describe the underlying theme of all of the methods and the relationship to sport and fitness goals, measurable outcomes, and physiologic pleasurable mechanisms even if research has not totally proven the response correlation.

CASE HISTORIES

■ Case history 1

A female client, 19 years old, is participating in collegiate volleyball championship. The game has been very intense, and the client is stiff and sore in the morning. When she receives massage, deep and focused work is very uncomfortable. Massage application that targets fluid movement combined with rhythmic joint movement helps the most. This client appears to be experiencing postexercise soreness, fluid retention, and mild inflammation in the tissues, which is characteristic of delayed onset muscle soreness. Massage that targets fluid movement will encourage the reduction of fluid and assist the circulation that supports the healing process.

■ Case history 2

A male golfer has been receiving chiropractic care for low back pain related to the rotation movements involved in the sport. The chiropractor has also identified hamstring shortening, which limits knee extension. He indicates to the massage therapist that during light massage application the hamstrings need to be lengthened so that full knee extension is possible. Using joint movements and palpation, the massage therapist is able to assess that the major tissue change occurs in the hamstring from the midbelly toward the knee. He also notes that the hamstring function isolated to the hip is within normal range. Massage application involves increasing tissue pliability and reducing motor tone in the hamstring muscle group, as well as using gliding and kneading to introduce tension and torsion forces. The muscles are gradually lengthened using muscle energy methods and connective tissue stretching.

SUGGESTED READINGS

Johnson J: *The healing art of sports massage*, Emmaus, Pa, 1995, Rodale Press.

Paine T: *The complete guide to sports massage*, London, 2000, A&C Black.

RESOURCES

Fritz S. Sports and Excercise Massage
www.amtamassage.org

REFERENCES

1. Cafarelli E, Flint F: The role of massage in preparation for and recovery from exercise, *Physiotherapy in Sport* 16:17-20, 1993.
2. Cook G: *Athletic body in balance*, Champaign, Ill, 2003, Human Kinetics.
3. Fritz S: *Fundamentals of therapeutic massage*, ed 4, St. Louis, 2007, Elsevier.
4. Clews W: Making muscles malleable, *Sport Health* 14:32-33, 1996.
5. Clews W: Where does massage draw the line? *Sport Health* 11:1-21, 1996.
6. Knost B et al: Learned maintenance of pain: muscle tension reduces central nervous system processing of painful stimulation in chronic and subchronic pain patients, *Psychophysiology* 36:755-764, 1999.
7. Gulick DT, Kimura IF: Delayed onset muscle soreness: what is it and how do we treat it? *Journal of Sport Rehabilitation* 5:234-243, 1996.
8. Weber MD, Servedio FJ, Woodall WR: The effects of three modalities on delayed onset muscle soreness, *Journal of Orthopaedic and Sports Physical Therapy* 20:236-242, 1994.
9. Hastreite D: Regional variations in certain cellular characteristics in human lumbar intervertebral discs, including the presence of smooth muscle actin, *Journal of Orthopaedic Research* 19:597-604, 2001.
10. Hodges P, Heinjnen I, Gandevia S: Postural activity of the diaphragm is reduced in humans when respiratory demand increases, *Journal of Physiology* 537:999-1008, 2001.
11. Lee J et al: Trunk muscle imbalance as a risk factor of the incidence of low back pain: a five year prospective study, *Journal of the Neuromuscular System* 7:97-101, 1999.
12. Wittink H, Michel T: 2002 *Chronic pain management for physical therapists*, ed 2, Boston, 2002, Butterworth Heinemann.

MULTIPLE CHOICE TEST QUESTIONS

1) Massage application to support athletic performance can be considered _____.
   a) nontherapeutic
   b) outcome based
   c) a unique modality
   d) primarily palliative

2) Which of the following statements is most correct?
   a) Fitness interferes with peak performance injury.
   b) Adaptive mechanisms cause repetitive use.
   c) Performance demand exceeds energy output used to maintain fitness.
   d) Peak performance is the ultimate outcome of fitness training.

3) The difference between repetitive injury and traumatic injury is
   a) the unexpected event for trauma
   b) the inflammation-healing mechanisms
   c) overuse event for traumatic injury
   d) rest and recuperation to support sleep

4) Which of the following statements is most true?
   a) The best massage approach for the athlete prior to competition requiring peak performance is connective tissue stretching and specific focus such as friction and point compression.
   b) Athletes at midseason tend to be less fragile and prone to illness than during fitness conditioning prior to the start of the playing season.
   c) Athletes at peak performance will exhibit both maximum achievement and increased injury potential.
   d) Recovery massage is provided when a specific outcome is required relating to rehabilitation from injury.

5) A client uses massage between tennis matches and days off. Which of the following best categorizes the approach?
   a) maintenance
   b) promotional
   c) rehabilitation
   d) intercompetition

6) Which of the following outcomes for massage targeted to athletes is most appropriate regardless of the situation?
   a) performance enhanced
   b) condition
   c) rehabilitation
   d) palliative care

7) Which of the following best describes regaining normal function as opposed to increasing performance?
   a) physical therapy after knee surgery
   b) agility training to walk a balance beam
   c) stretching to support long jump during track and field
   d) practicing a golf swing at a driving range

8) Which of the following is an important factor in the healing of sport injury?
   a) sustained edema
   b) normal inflammatory response
   c) appropriate application of traumatic force
   d) sustained use of muscle relaxer medication

9) A client experienced a mild ankle sprain 3 days ago. Which massage method should NOT be used at this stage of the healing process?
   a) lymphatic drainage
   b) circulation enhancement
   c) deep transverse friction
   d) general palliative massage

10) A client's mental focus is better at practice after a massage. Which of the following best explains this response?
    a) fluid movements
    b) mood modulation ANS response
    c) PRICE care
    d) connective tissue changes

11) A client received a large bruise on her calf during soccer practice. Which of the following needs to be most adjusted in the bruise area to prevent further trauma?
    a) rhythm
    b) direction
    c) depth of pressure
    d) speed

12) Which of the following mechanical forces best relates to gliding application?
   a) tension
   b) duration
   c) shear
   d) compression

13) Increased muscle tissue density and decreased pliability related to intermuscular pressure is
   a) motor tone
   b) motor neuron driven
   c) sympathetic ANS arousal
   d) muscle tone

14) During the subacute healing stage, which of the following is contraindicated (should not be used)?
   a) lymphatic drainage
   b) general circulation massage
   c) aggressive stretch
   d) rhythmic rocking (oscillation)

15) A client fell 6 months ago during a bike race and developed scarring on the shin from the injury. Which of the following is most effective in increasing pliability of the scar tissue?
   a) PRICE care
   b) lymphatic drainage
   c) arterial circulation support
   d) connective tissue method

16) A client who is on three bowling leagues indicates that she is experiencing some numbness and tingling in her right hand. What is the appropriate action to take?
   a) general massage/local contraindication area—refer for diagnosis (loss of sensation)
   b) refer for diagnosis—contagious condition
   c) general massage, ice, and stretching—no need for referral
   d) immediate referral to the emergency room—cardiac symptoms

17) Which of the following presents the most life-threatening condition?
   a) fungal infection
   b) stress fracture
   c) deep vein thrombosis
   d) myositis ossificans

18) Which of the following assessment categories is most unique to the athlete population?
   a) surgery or medical procedures
   b) medication and supplements
   c) sleep pattern
   d) training protocols

19) Which of the following is an aspect of PRICE care?
   a) antiinflammatory medication
   b) hydrotherapy
   c) rehabilitative exercise
   d) heat application

20) In the suggested sequence for massage application, which of the following occurs first?
   a) skin superficial fascia edema
   b) motor tone
   c) flexibility
   d) deeper fascial layers

Structural Integration

Peter Schwind

INTRODUCTION

Structural Integration is a highly specific manual treatment of the connective tissue network. The main goals of structural integration are alignment of the human body within the field of gravity, harmonious tone of the body's tissues, and well-coordinated movement. Structural Integration also makes use of movement education and perceptual exercises to achieve its goals. It is applied to people of all ages including infants and elderly people.

HISTORY

Structural Integration was developed by Ida Pauline Rolf (1896-1979). She received her PhD in biochemistry and physiology from Columbia University in 1920. As a scientist she worked at the Rockefeller Institute in the departments of chemotherapy and biochemistry. Dr. Rolf also had a widespread interest in alternative ways of working with the human organism. She explored yoga and its value for the body and the mind, and she studied the principles underlying osteopathy and homeopathy.

While working as a scientist she taught yoga.[1] And as an attempt to improve the efficiency of her teaching, she gradually began to apply a more intense contact to her students' bodies. She did not use oil on her hands, and she was not doing massage. What she discovered herself to be doing was to help her students, literally, to shape their own bodies while practicing yoga. This was Ida Rolf's first step toward a new way of working with the human body. From here we could say that she started a modality that focused on one specific type of tissue usually overlooked by other methods: the **connective tissue** and especially its muscle-related form—the **fascia.**

Connective tissue envelops all aspects of the internal organs and groups them in fascial containers. Fascia is a dense sort of connective tissue of the muscles, and it envelops these and all their subcompartments. Fascia is found in many other places in the body: containing, supporting, making bridges and links. It may be found quite superficially under the skin as well as very deeply.

After Ida Rolf stopped teaching, she began to develop Structural Integration as its own discipline. She had already taught her method to some osteopaths and chiropractors who tried to apply this approach within the medical field. However, this medical application was not her main focus. Her main goal was not the relief of symptoms but rather a general and meaningful improvement of the human potential.

In 1972, after more than 40 years of practice, Ida Rolf established the Rolf Institute of Structural Integration in Boulder, Colorado. In 1979, at the end of her life, training centers for the development of her work were emerging in Europe, South America, and Australia.

STRUCTURAL INTEGRATION MODALITY AND THE NATURE OF TOUCH

There are four important key terms that need to be grasped in order to understand Ida Rolf's concept: **structure, segmentation of the body, gravity,** and **plasticity of the fascial system.** According to Ida Rolf structure of the human body does not only mean the muscles and bones but also a sort of a spatial order of all the elements of the organism. "Every time you use the word structure with respect to a living body, you are talking about relationship between parts as they fit together to make the aggregate that we call the man."[1]

Traditional medical anatomy subdivides the human body into three systems: the musculoskeletal system, the system of organs or visceral system (and this includes the vascular and other "transport" systems), and the nervous system. And out of these three systems they derived a systematic system of body functions. There is, however, a fourth system that contains, enfolds, divides, and subdivides the other systems. This is the connective tissue with all its different manifestations as fascia, as membranes, and as ligaments. The founder of osteopathy, Andrew Tailor Still, had started to recognize these tissue types and their significance for physical dysfunctions. Ida Rolf tried to guide Still's observations into a very specific direction by recognizing that fascia plays an important role for the upright posture of man.

"Fascia is the organ of posture. Nobody ever says this, all the talk is about muscles. Yet this is a very important concept, and because this is so important, we as Rolfers [graduates of the Rolf Institute of Structural

Integration are called "Rolfers"] must understand both the anatomy and physiology, but especially the anatomy of fascia. The body is a web of fascia."[1]

In her teaching, she was always pointing out that the connective tissue acts like an envelope around the different elements of the body: the connective tissue that envelops bone is the periosteum; myofascia is the connective tissue envelope of muscles, and organs have variously named envelopes also built of connective tissue. All units of the organism down to the individual cells have their connective tissue support around them. Her extraordinary insight is only now being corroborated by research on fascia. It is that the main segments of the body are in permanent spatial communication and that this communication can only happen through fascia. Fascia is the medium of communication between all the different systems of the body, and it is the most important type of tissue for erect posture. In fact she called fascia "the organ of support."[2]

She went on to observe that fascia is in a permanent state of change during our lives because, as the "organ of support," it is constantly responding to the physical realities of a body in gravity. If a muscle is repeatedly used in a certain way its fascial envelope will develop stronger collagen fibers to support and protect the muscle's activity. However, the organism seems to have no regulatory system for this process. This means that, because of postural and gestural habits that cause individuals to use a group of muscles repeatedly, their system of fascial envelopes gets stronger and may finally inhibit proper flexion and extension function. Because all the fascial layers are connected like an **endless web,**[3] fascial strain may literally go from one segment of the body into others: tension around the right hip may travel to the left shoulder; ligamentous disorder of the left ankle may affect the knee, the hip, and the whole back way up to the neck. All the segments of the body are permanently communicating with each other through the fascial system.

Ida Rolf's revolutionary contribution was to relate the inner tensions existing within the body to a force that acts from outside on the body: this force is gravity. The earth is surrounded by its gravitational field. This field exerts an attractive force on the human body as long as the body is present within the gravitational field. While other manual methods were observing how forces act within the human body, Ida Rolf was widening their perspective. Looking at the findings of paleoanthropology, she made some far-reaching conclusions. She observed that as soon as the human being started to stand and walk on two feet millions of years ago, gravity had a more significant impact on the body. As soon as humans start to walk on two feet and free their hands for activity, any motion, any displacement of a body part for this has to happen in relationship to gravity. If, for example, a shoulder is pulled up permanently on one side, the body has to respond all the way down to the heels with a counterbalancing shift in weight to maintain balance within the field of gravity; otherwise the person would fall to the side. Whenever one body segment is out of line there will be compensations in all other segments of the body as they search for equilibrium. Figure 17-1 shows the Rolf Institute's logo.

Ida Rolf observed that better alignment leads to better coordination of movement and that when repetitive coordinative movements like breathing and walking are well organized they help maintain better alignment. She also saw that all segments of the human organism should be aligned around a central inner line using as little muscle tension as possible. Structural Integration meant, for her, to shape the body in such a way that inner alignment occurs easily and that movement flowing out from alignment is graceful (Figure 17-2).

To arrive at inner alignment, Ida Rolf developed the **recipe** for a series **of ten** manual treatment **sessions.** Each one of the 10 sessions has clearly formulated goals. The practitioner of Structural Integration will work toward these goals during the treatment hours tailoring his or her work to the needs of each individual client. Structural Integration is not a collection of scheme-like strokes, but a highly differentiated treatment that tries to pay tribute to the demands of the individual.

We have been describing the key terms structure, segmentation, and gravity. But if we really want to understand what actually happens during a treatment of this kind, we have to look closely at the fourth key term of Ida Rolf's concept, the plasticity of the fascial system. After observations in practice, Ida Rolf assumed that connective tissue can be literally shaped by the hand of a practitioner. Today research has taught us that this process of shaping connective tissue is much more complex than originally considered. Certainly there is some mechanically induced viscoelastic "deformation" happening under the practitioner's hands. However, there is also a stimulation of the mechanoreceptors going on in the fascial system. A good deal of the new research is just at its beginning, but there are enough new insights encouraging us to take a new look on plasticity. The old definition—"shaping the tissue"—may be seen as a metaphor for a process happening between the connective tissue system and the nervous system.

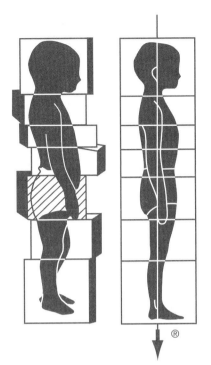

FIGURE 17-1 The logo of the Rolf Institute showing the contours of a young boy before (left) and after (right) treatment with Structural Integration illustrates alignment along a central vertical line. (Courtesy of the Rolf Institute of Structural Integration®.)

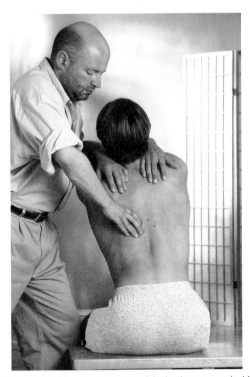

FIGURE 17-2 The deep fascial layers of the back are treated while the client is sitting on a bench.

BOX 17-1 Structural Integration and Fluid Exchange

As part of the natural process of aging, the connective tissue loses more and more fluid components. The organism builds up a larger percentage of collagen fibers while those components that contain fluid elements—for example, elastin—are reduced. Elastin is a protein that makes up elastic fibers. An older person tends to lose flexibility, and true upright sitting and walking become more difficult. The manual techniques used in Structural Integration help to restore a better balance between the different parts of the connective tissue system and allow a more efficient fluid exchange within the tissues. Better fluid exchange within the lymphatic and vascular systems will also help the organism to have better oxygen supply and a better metabolic process in general.

The connective tissue system has two main components, very dense **collagen fibers** and **ground substance.** Collagen fibers are built by protein structures with little fluid content; ground substance contains more fluid elements (Box 17-1). Collagen fibers can only be stretched up to 5 percent of their length,[4] but the ground substance responds significantly to pressure from the practitioner's hands. In this sense, plasticity allows the human body to be modified like a sculpture. After a session a person will find they have a higher level of flexibility and a more even tone throughout their body. Sometimes this will include drastic changes of a client's curvatures of the back and better alignment of the segments of the legs, for example. Some practitioners of Structural Integration take photos before and after the treatment as a record for themselves or as part of their therapeutic dialogue with their client.

With recent findings in research on the properties of fascia we now know that Ida Rolf's view of plasticity would only tell part of the story. Apart from the material properties of fascia, its capacity to respond to pressure and pulling forces, there are also bridges to the nervous system that influence the tension of the tissue in a particular area. Researchers are beginning to recognize that plasticity of the connective tissue is a process that includes activity of the brain. Robert Schleip, a German practitioner of Structural Integration, has published a substantial body of recognized work on this.[5]

STARTING POINT: VISUAL ANALYSIS—THE ART OF SEEING

In Structural Integration it is essential to observe the client's body, in underwear or wearing a bathing suit, prone, supine, sitting, and in various functions especially walking and breathing. This **visual analysis** is vital to a successful and efficient strategizing of the session and relating it to the daily life of the client. If, for example, a person works in front of a computer screen all day long, this will show up in their body. Because their eyes are fixed to a small area of the flat computer screen and their hands and arms are being carried in front of the trunk while they stare at the screen, the whole body simply collapses forwards. If this goes on for hours on end, tension will develop in certain areas. At first there will be a higher tension in certain muscles. If this tension becomes chronic, the tone of fascia will become denser as well, especially in those areas where the muscles have to work too hard. This typically happens at the transition between the back and the neck and at the transition between the neck and the head and also around the eyes. But symptoms might show up far away from the primary tensional areas; for example, within the lower back, especially where the last segment of the lumbar spine meets the sacrum. Nerve irritations may arise not only in those areas typical to repetitive strain from computer work, around the neck and within the forearms and hands, but also in the lower extremities, where the sciatic nerve, coming from the sacrum, travels down the legs.

People who work at the computer are certainly among the groups suffering the most from symptoms caused by muscle tension and fascial strain. But there are plenty of others who experience similar problems. Musicians, for example, who spend their lives holding a musical instrument in a particular way all day long; and, last but not least, bodyworkers can suffer from considerable strain as they bend forward over their tables while working with clients.

The visual analysis we have been talking about therefore also seeks to recognize the imprint of the profession on the client's body and to investigate how the professional life has shaped this person. In addition, the practitioner will also carefully include the client's general physical and emotional health history. This kind of analysis will focus on dominant emotional patterns that show in a person's preferred posture. Frequently this may include a careful observation of the signs of **physical and emotional trauma** which may have left their imprint in the body, posture, and gesture: Is there a tendency to collapse? Does the chest sink down most of the time? Does the breathing motion tend to be caught in an exhale pattern? Or does our client like to present a blown up chest most of the time, as if caught in inhalation? These and other questions will be kept in mind during this initial analysis.

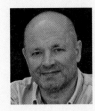

When people experience Structural Integration they sometimes undergo drastic postural changes. When they get up from the treatment table, they spontaneously move from a bent state to a much more upright way of standing. Some clients have a hard time adjusting to this. They sense that they might fall backward, and they actually feel like they are leaning backward while they are in fact almost perfectly aligned. In these cases it helps to allow the person to explore the old pattern of standing and have them compare it with the new one. A mirror can be a help to find out about the two physical realities and open a door for improved physical awareness. (Photo by David Hoptam.)

After this visual analysis a practitioner will want to look even more closely inside the physical structure. Our body is held upright by the actions of our muscles. If we were to switch off our muscle tone we would collapse immediately. However, it is not only muscle activity that makes our upright posture possible. There are other forces that come into play, forces that are not directly related to muscles and their activity. Inside our trunk we find cavities resting on each other: the pelvic and abdominal cavity, the chest cavity, and the cavity inside our head. Each one of these cavities is wrapped by connective tissue holding it together like a box or container. To allow us to stand and walk upright on our feet, there has to be a certain balance of forces acting between these individual containers. Pulling forces and forces of pressure act constantly inside these containers and between them helping the different visceral elements to form a "**column of organs**" in front of our vertebral spine. This reality goes back to the early stages of embryonic development. While humans spend their first months of life inside their mother's womb, the cavities of the fetus develop by the growth of the enveloping membranes. The organs have to slowly find their proper place inside the cavities, and the cavities have to align themselves in relation to each other. There is little space inside the mother's womb for all this. For this reason the shape of the young embryo will be exposed to extraordinary pressure. And yet within this small space and within all this pressure the essence of the shape of that person's body will emerge to be present to them their whole adult life.

The most challenging part of our visual analysis is to recognize a pattern inside a body that goes back all the way to the first months of the development of the embryo. This, undoubtedly, requires a lot of practical experience and knowledge of embryologic development on the part of the practitioner. For some clients this type of analysis will reveal the key to the deepest and oldest roots.

To confirm the findings of visual analysis the practitioner will add another mode of exploration: investigate the tissues by **palpation.** Palpation is characterized by a light and sensitive use of the practitioner's hands. Is the tissue tight or fibrous? Does it show appropriate span, or is there an overall lack of tone? Some people have a well-balanced "container." The muscles and bones act well together in movement. But they might still have restrictions inside this container within its contents or around the connective tissues forming the envelopes and ligaments that hold the organs in place. These kinds of restrictions require a well-trained eye, and they can only be verified by manual investigation using a sensitive hand. There is a method that deals specifically with this aspect of bodywork. This approach is called **visceral manipulation.** It has been developed by the French osteopath Jean-Pierre Barral. Visceral manipulation is a highly efficient treatment system that restores the organs' natural capacity of movement inside the body's cavities. Many practitioners of Structural Integration train in visceral manipulation and add this method to their way of working.

Other clients show the opposite pattern: their organs may be free of restrictions while all the tension is present within the muscles and their related fascia. There is certainly a "muscle type" or "container type" of tension and an "organ type" or "content type" of tension. And there are, of course, many variations of "mixed types" showing abnormal tension straddling the musculoskeletal and the organ systems simultaneously. Whatever the practitioner may have found by doing visual and palpative analysis, there is still one point missing. The client has been standing still or sitting on a chair or resting on a table for analysis, but what happens with his organism if he/she starts moving around? We have to complete our analysis by watching the client in motion. The client walks up and down the room, and the practitioner observes how this person touches the ground, pushes off the ground, and finds orientation in space using the eyes.*

---

*My colleague Hubert Godard (France) has developed a sophisticated system of tests for this.

This kind of observation is the starting point of the more detailed investigation of the client's everyday activity we have mentioned before. Is he/she moving around all day long, sitting on a chair in front of a computer screen, sitting or standing playing an instrument, using his/her body as a dancer or professional athlete? We have to find a conclusion for this individual organism and unique person. Based on that conclusion we can start with the hands-on work.

HANDS-ON WORK: IDA ROLF'S CLASSIC RECIPE OF TEN SESSIONS

Through decades of practical work, Ida Rolf developed her series of 10 treatment sessions as a type of journey through all the important layers of the fascial network of the body. Each session is initiated by the kind of analysis previously described. Most of the treatment is done while the client is resting on a table. Part of the work, especially deep work at the layers of the back, is done while the client is sitting on a bench (Figure 17-2). Some of the treatment, especially concerning the feet and legs, is done while the client is standing.

The goal of the first session is to create enough space between the main segments of the body for a more resilient breath. The practitioner works to eliminate compression between the thorax and the pelvis, between the thorax and the shoulders, and between the shoulders and the arms. This "separation" between the trunk's units will ultimately allow a freer breathing motion. And better breathing function is indeed one of the main goals not only of the first hour but of all 10 sessions. Ideally all elements of the torso have to slide on each other while we inhale and exhale (Figure 17-3). This can only happen if the fascia of the superficial layers of the trunk offers enough space for the inner breathing motion. While the diaphragm is contracting and the lungs fill with air, the thorax widens and all the spinal curves extend a little bit more. The whole body will be a little bit more upright during inhalation than during exhalation. Ida Rolf's students report that she used to say: "You don't finish a first treatment of structural integration unless you arrived at changing the pattern of breathing to the better."

An additional goal of the first treatment is the improvement of movement around the hip joints.

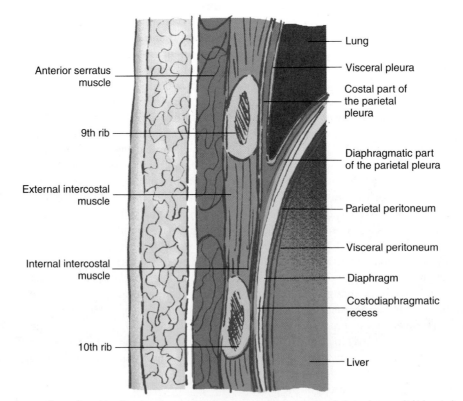

FIGURE 17-3 To arrive at a better breathing function the practitioner has to find the main restriction wherever it is located within the different layers of the thoracic wall. (*From Schwind P:* Faszien-und Membrantechnik, *Munich, 2003, Urban and Fischer.*)

By sitting on chairs most people lose mobility around this area and develop shortness in the back of their legs. During the first hour, all the connective tissue layers around the greater trochanter are intensively worked on.

The second session deals mainly with the feet and legs and how they relate to the back and the neck. One goal of the session is a better distribution of weight between the arches of each foot to allow a contact with the floor that is both flexible and secure (Figure 17-4). A second goal is to establish as much proper hinge function at the ankles, knees, and hips as possible. A third goal is to improve the mobility of the back in the area of the thorax. That means that the client is able to bend forward and backward more freely. A fourth goal is to create more flexibility in the outer and middle layers of the neck.

Before starting the third session, the practitioner observes the client's profile from each side while he or she stands and walks. The goal of this session is to allow better alignment around this lateral line. What this means is that the shoulder girdle and the thorax support each other as best they can, are aligned above the pelvis, and the head balances on top of the spinal curves. Ida Rolf always pointed out that the area between the twelfth rib and the pelvis is very important if one is to arrive at the balance of the whole body around a lateral line. At the end of the third hour this area below the twelfth rib should show significant inner motion while the client is resting on his or her side breathing. This **inner motion** shows that the kidneys are sliding along the two psoas muscles during inhalation and exhalation. Work on the neck, begun during the second session, is continued especially around its lateral layers.

Starting with the fourth hour, the pelvis and its relationship to the legs become the theme for the next three sessions. Sessions four, five, and six all deal with pelvic structures evaluated from a different point of view. These sessions (along with the seventh session) are the

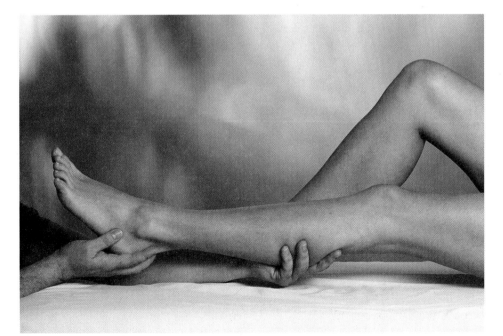

FIGURE 17-4 The deep layers of the lower leg are treated most successfully if the practitioner has the client move the foot while his/her hands receive the weight of the lower low leg.

so-called "**core sessions**" of Structural Integration. They aim at inner alignment and deal with the deep fascial and membrane layers of the organism.

The fourth session continues the work at the feet and legs that began in session two. While sessions one to three treated mainly the surface of the body and only occasionally reached deeper into inner bridges of the fascial system, another process starts with session four. This time the work on the feet and legs is carried from the ankle all the way up to the pelvic floor. And this time important ligaments are part of the game: those which regulate the stability of the ankle and knee and those that build a deep connection between the legs and the inner construction of the entire pelvic basin (Figure 17-5). The goal is to allow a gait characterized by legs that can swing freely under the hips while the shoulder girdle and pelvis show contralateral motion.

Also as a continuation of session two, the capacity of the back to bend forward and backward will be reevaluated. In session four the practitioner will address the deeper layers of the back and the neck.

During the fifth session, the client's walking patterns will be evaluated in relationship to the psoas muscle. The psoas muscle originates from the lateral lumbar spine and ends at the inside of the legs at the lesser trochanter (Figure 17-6). Because this muscle lies deep inside the body some sophistication is required to activate it properly. During the pioneer days of Structural Integration practitioners tried to activate this muscle by direct touch. Recently, more and more movement techniques using the client's active participation are employed to arrive at more elegant solutions for this. Another essential goal of the fifth hour is to work with the different fascial layers of the abdominal

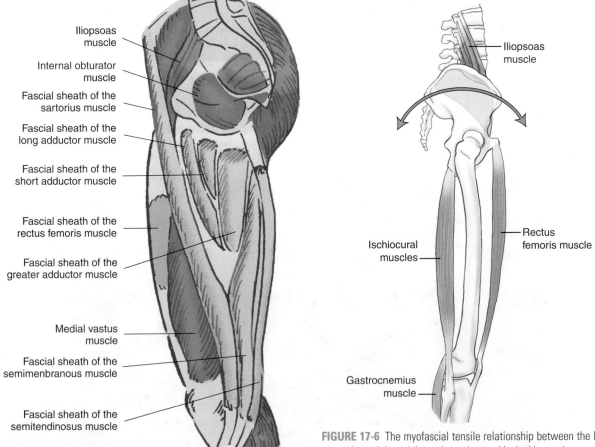

FIGURE 17-5 The fascial tubes at the inside of the leg show the interrelatedness between the inner static system of the thigh and the inner dynamics of the pelvis. (Drawing according to Benninghoff. *From Schwind P:* Faszien-und Membrantechnik, Munich, 2003, *Urban and Fischer.*)

FIGURE 17-6 The myofascial tensile relationship between the lower extremity and the pelvis can be understood by looking at the psoas and the leg muscles. The interaction of the different muscle groups and their related fasciae results in a forward or backward tilt around the hip axis. (*From Schwind P:* Faszien-und Membrantechnik, Munich, 2003, *Urban and Fischer.*)

and pelvic cavity to offer enough space for the organs and to support proper alignment of the column of organs in relation to the spinal column. In a way, the fifth hour continues the theme of contralateral walking, the theme of session four. But now, in session five, it is not only the contralateral swing between the shoulders and hips; it is the "inner motion" of the spine that has to be activated. The final goal is that all the vertebrae of the lumbar spine learn to side bend and rotate freely while walking.

The sixth session deals with the posterior of the pelvis. The goal is to get the legs well organized under the pelvis. In a way the sixth session completes the work that began during sessions two and four. This time the connection between the back of the legs and their fascial connections to the pelvis via the sacrotuberous and sacrospinous ligaments is important. The goal of this session is to balance the pelvic bones within the bed that the ligaments and fascia offer to them. Balance will show especially around the sacrum. This will be a wavelike motion of the sacral bone during breathing: when the client rests in prone position, the sacral base will move significantly. The better movement potential in the pelvic area will transmit all the way through the back up to the neck and head. For this reason it is important to include a profound treatment of the deep fascial layers of the neck into session six. In most cases the practitioner has to work on the fascia around the scalene muscles and the prevertebral fascia. This concluding work around the inner structures of the neck prepares the transition for the seventh hour and its emphasis on the head and neck area.

The seventh hour seeks to provide a better orientation of the whole person in space. So the head has to be balanced well on top of all the spinal curvatures. Ida Rolf called this "putting the head on." The practitioner observes how the client finds orientation through his or her eyes while walking. He palpates the inner mobility of the neck while the client rests on the table and incrementally works through all the lamina of the neck and the fascial layers of the head and jaw (Figure 17-7).

Within Ida Rolf's classical approach, the detailed treatment of the joint between the mandible and the head (temporomandibular joint) is a highlight. It aims for free movement of the jaw and frequently releases deep tensions in the client's neck. The seventh hour concludes the client's journey with the practitioner through all the main fascial and membranous layers of the body (Figure 17-8).

The main goal of sessions eight and nine is to balance the two girdles of the body, the shoulder girdle and the pelvic girdle, at a more meaningful level. The success of these sessions depends on the client's willingness to participate in **movement and perception explorations.** Only part of the work will be done manually as the client rests on the table. Much of the session might take place while the client sits, stands, or walks. This other part, which is called movement work,

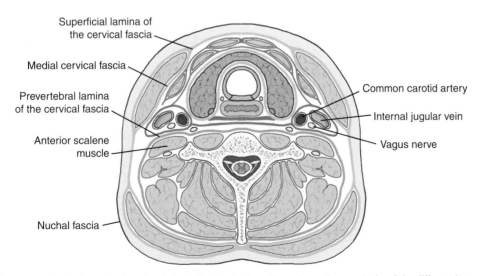

FIGURE 17-7 A cross-section of the neck at the level of the first tracheal cartilage shows the complexity of the different layers of fascia of the human neck. (*From Schwind P: Faszien-und Membrantechnik, Munich, 2003, Urban and Fischer.*)

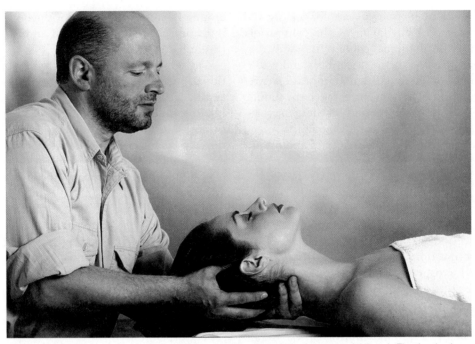

FIGURE 17-8 There are so many elements vital for our well-being travelling through the front part of the neck. That is why the practitioner's hands have to act with special care in this area.

opens a long avenue for the practitioner's creativity. Movement and perception explorations are communicated through verbal instruction, by guided imaging, and by subtle touch.*

When looking at the standard theories of Structural Integration, it becomes obvious that this cycle of sessions goes back and forth between the **upper pole of the body and its lower pole.** The upper pole stands for orientation in space and breathing as the engine of inner motion; the lower pole stands for tactile orientation by the feet, for "grounding" and contact with the earth. It makes sense that the last session of the cycle, session ten, usually starts around the ankle area and finishes at the junction of the neck with the head. This last session requires the capacity to make the right choices and stop at the right moment without doing too much.

Part of the essence of Ida Rolf's 10-session recipe is that the treatment starts with the superficial layers during the first hour. Gradually, session by session, the practitioner reaches the deeper layers. This happens particularly during sessions four, five, six, and seven, the so-called "core sessions." The Structural Integrator

will organize the whole body around a vertical line by freeing the tissues from unnecessary strain. Then during sessions eight, nine, and ten the practitioner will help to integrate the changes accomplished during the previous sessions. Integration, to the practitioner, means that the new structure will need to find its new harmony and that the client will want to learn how to use the new structure well. This exploration in gravity through the new structure means reeducation of movement and visual and tactile orientation in daily life.

An important aspect of the 10-series recipe is that it is a limited number of treatments. Session ten is a closure of the process. After a certain time—maybe half a year or a year later—additional sessions may be appropriate, a single tune-up session, or an advanced series of three or five to continue and deepen what was started in the original process of the 10 sessions.

MODES OF TOUCH IN STRUCTURAL INTEGRATION

The practitioners of Structural Integration use a large variety of tactile contact with the client's body. This kind of work has been known for its intensity. But it also has subtle and "microtactile" dimensions. For a practitioner of Structural Integration it is most important to respect that there are many different

---

*Some schools of Structural Integration, such as The Rolf Institute of Structural Integration, offer a special Movement Training.

tissue types in people's organisms. The muscle-bound athlete requires a different approach than the hypermobile, flexible, and slim body. Remember that within a single person the connective tissue system is not at all homogenous. Slim, flexible people frequently show great elasticity at the surface layer and at the large muscle units. But deep inside they tend to have tight restrictions within the smaller muscles and the ligaments. In my own practice I have found this to be true even in the bodies of professional acrobats. In such cases the practitioner has to find a subtle way to the deep layers without stretching the surface layers too much.

We learned earlier that it is typical for Structural Integration to be done without oil. Lubricants may be helpful in small amounts, but only if they do not lead to sliding. All parts of the practitioner's arms and hands are used for working: the fingertips, the flats of the hands, the first phalanges of the fingers, and occasionally the elbows (Figure 17-9). For some layers of the fascia very intense contact is required. In such cases the practitioner has to use the weight of his or her whole body in a well-coordinated manner to be successful. Videos of Ida Rolf at work show that it was not so much the active force she applied while working that made her touch so effective and efficient but the intensity of contact and her ability to communicate through touch.

We have already mentioned that how we use **touch in Structural Integration** is highly individual. The quality of our touch differs from practitioner to practitioner like our handwriting. However, there are certain established rules for contacting different types of tissue and different layers of the organism through different qualities of rhythm, direction, and by using different "tools"—hands, elbows, and so on. Observing these rules may help to make each of our individual styles more efficient:

- Overly tense myofascial layers of the musculoskeletal system require direct lengthening; this lengthening is performed as parallel as possible to the muscle fiber and transverse to the primary fiber direction of the fascia.
- Slack myofascial layers of the musculoskeletal system are treated carefully and in a slowly sliding manner; the contact is broad and superficial; linear contact and point loading are to be avoided.

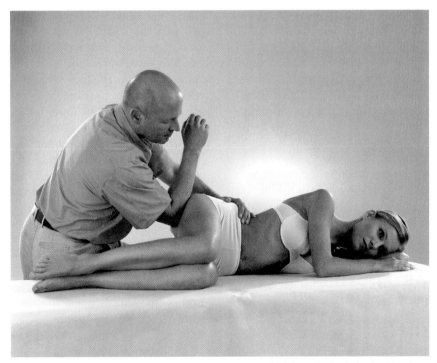

FIGURE 17-9 While using the elbow the practitioner has to be absolutely aware which layer he is aiming for. The photo shows an intervention directed to fascial layers around the greater trochanter.

- Band structures that create connections between bones respond well to so-called indirect techniques: the origin and connection of the band are brought closer together until a motion impulse is sensed at the origination and insertion surface of the bone. In the case of large bands, e.g., in the region of the pelvis, an alternative strategy may be used: the therapist initiates a slow-acting impulse by contacting the middle section of the band while observing the reaction of the bone structures held by the band by "listening." It is important to avoid overstraining the band fibers.

- Interosseous membranes and deep septae respond best to subtle contact: therapy is performed indirectly here as well. It follows the dominant fiber paths, allows the bones to slide more strongly into their fixations, provides a gentle impulse to reinforce the fixation, and at the moment of strongest fixation then follows the releasing countermotion by "listening."

- Envelopes and ligamentous structures of organs must be treated carefully. These layers of tissue require a sensitive contact that takes into account the so-called turgor effect, the inner pressure dynamics of the organ, and its fluid dynamics. In the course of one treatment session, the applications must be limited to two or a maximum of three organ complexes in order to allow the organ system sufficient range for self-regulation.

- Elements of the craniosacral system may be treated with very different contact quality. In adult clients, it must be appreciated that each technique begins indirectly, that the structures affected are initially moved into a stronger fixation and only then— with constant "listening"—is a minimally corrective impulse applied with the aid of the momentum of the craniosacral system. This procedure—first indirect and then carefully direct—must also be observed in treating the exterior layers of the cranium such as the galea aponeurosis and the temporal fascia.[4]

BENEFITS OF STRUCTURAL INTEGRATION

Some of the outcomes of Structural Integration have value for everybody who wants to improve general well-being and vital function of their organism. Certain pathologic conditions make manual techniques to the connective tissues contraindicated.

People of all professions and ages who received the 10-session series developed by Ida Rolf report a higher level of vitality and flexibility on a physical and emotional level. Young adults will enjoy the results of a course of Structural Integration by finding an easy way of being fluidly upright that has nothing to do with the traditional "sit up straight" advice. More mature people appreciate this work very much especially when they start to lose the integrity of their alignment if their systems are becoming less mobile. This happens quite frequently after their sixtieth or, for the more lucky ones, after their seventieth birthday. This moment when the tissue starts to lose elasticity; when the upper part of the back starts to curve and the whole person seems to bend forward; is the right time to help the tissue rediscover its vitality.

But what kind of treatment should young people receive? Children are not just smaller adults. Younger bodies, through early childhood to puberty, follow a different law. There are exceptions but usually these bodies will not show the tightness of the "armored" muscle fascia so typical of the adult person. That is why the practitioner will be well advised not to apply the 10-session recipe until after puberty is finished. Structural Integration for children and small infants has to work with a minimum of precise interventions over clearly spaced intervals. And the practitioner must be able to distinguish the many phases of growth with their particular patterns of development that should not be corrected by manual treatment. For example, all babies have flat feet and a heel that extends laterally under the lower leg. This will change step by step as soon as they start to stand on their own feet and activate the muscles of the lower leg and by that causing the arches within the feet to develop. Of course, if this process does not become apparent by the fourth year a few precise interventions may be appropriate. Such interventions may have to accompany the child over quite a long period of its development since the legs, for example, continue to develop and grow up to the age of eight. But this has to happen in a way that the child is not overwhelmed by a lot of manual interventions and can enjoy the treatments and their results (Figure 17-10). The rule is: the younger the child, the shorter the session should be. Thirty minutes is an absolute maximum for a 10-year-old, and for small infants 10 minutes are enough.

We need to be aware that the young child's body maintains this abnormal tension—deep inside the membranes and close to the joints within small tissue units. The larger muscles do not show the tightness

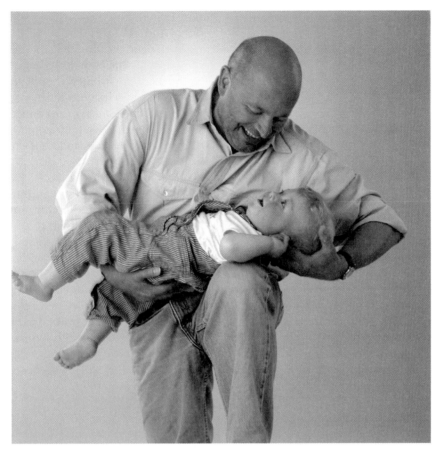

FIGURE 17-10 Working with children is one of the big challenges in Structural Integration. The practitioner has to work from knowledge, act with precision, and be capable of good communication with the child.

that is more typical for the adult. For this reason the practitioner has to work with a high level of precision with children and infants. When a practitioner is able to combine caution with precision, remarkable results can be achieved. This is also true for more serious growth disturbances. A good example is with cases of **scoliosis.** In this condition the whole vertebral spine curves into an S-shape within three-dimensional space, meaning that the curve is side-bending and rotating at the same time. Obviously it is not only the spinal column that shows this pattern; the twist will be present in the way the organs are situated inside the trunk and how they move during inhalation and exhalation. And the curves may also be palpated inside the membranes of the cranium and the pelvis. Scoliosis is present at the spatial arrangement of all the units of the organism and in the way the connective tissue builds bridges between these units. By working for greater elasticity of these bridges, we have a good chance to help the child suffering from

scoliosis to find what they are seeking: better alignment along a vertical line and more harmonious curvatures of the vertebral column.

Athletes will experience better performance within their chosen sport after the Structural Integration process. This can be better understood when we recognize what the intense treatment of the fascia means for muscle activity. Muscle and fascia are one unit: they always act together. Since fascia is a tight envelope around the muscle, the muscle can only act within the frame of this envelope. This is why a well-toned fascial envelope will help the muscle work more effectively. Flexor and extensor groups of muscles can work more efficiently as soon as the inhibiting strain is removed from the fascial envelope around them.[4]

As agonist and antagonistic become better balanced in their respective functions those sport activities which require highly sophisticated coordination alongside bursts of immense energy will blossom. The Oriental disciplines of martial arts are excellent examples of this: Aikido, Judo, Karate, and Shaolin are disciplines based on fast, fluent movement that carries motion into the smallest units of the muscular system. And Eastern disciplines that are closer to meditation, like the various styles of Tai Chi, the so-called "inner martial arts," and Yoga, can be practiced with more harmony after Structural Integration (Box 17-3). The act of paying attention during meditation becomes simpler since sitting upright with ready ease is the outward sign of the inner act of attention.

The application of Structural Integration for musicians and singers is a specialized field in itself. The many hours of practice required for the mastering of a musical instrument puts a whole world of strains on the musician's body. This is true for artists who play string instruments, wind instruments, keyboards, and percussion. Each instrument will put a certain imprint into the musician's body, an imprint that might be visible even when the instrument has not been played any more for years. It happens very

often that the instrument is played with too much effort. And some of their training does not take into sufficient account that the main instrument to make music is the body itself, not the guitar, the violin, the piano, or whatever. So it happens frequently that certain muscles tend to be overused while others remain inactive, causing the connective tissue system to become unbalanced and therefore no longer at the service of the musician and their external instrument. See Ida Rolf's very detailed discussion of the antagonism of flexors and extensors.

The 10 sessions of Structural Integration work very efficiently as preventive care for musicians (Box 17-4). Even receiving just the first three treatments of the series may be helpful, since these beginning sessions give much more freedom to the breath. This is especially helpful for singers.

While discussing musicians, we should not forget another group of artists who have helped to make Ida Rolf's work known. It was Marlene Dietrich, Greta Garbo, and Cary Grant who went to see Ida Rolf and received the series of Structural Integration. And indeed actresses and actors will always benefit from this work. Better alignment implies freedom from tension, and it permits a more graceful use of the body. This leads to a better expressive capacity of the artist, making any step, any gesture more authentic. Lee Strasberg, the teacher of so many successful Hollywood stars and founder of the famous Actors' Studio, asked his students to do the 10 sessions of Structural Integration when they started studying at his school.

The benefits of Structural Integration for artists may have to do with the nonphysical aspects of the work. This approach is certainly not psychotherapy but, as Ida Rolf stated: "The seat of the soul is physiological."[2]

Positive impact has been observed at the level of the **autonomic nervous system.** This system is essential for our life by ruling the activities of our organs and by balancing the somatic base of our emotions. The autonomic nervous system makes it possible to move into a very active state and return to calmness and relaxation. While the practitioner gives a stimulus to overstrained tissues, the autonomic nervous system will react with arousal and discharge. In doing so, the whole body is trained to explore its capacity for stress release.[7]

CONTRAINDICATIONS

We have already stated that the kind of touch used in Structural Integration varies from very subtle to very intense. Any serious medical conditions should be checked prior to treatment. There are some conditions that need special care and others where treatment with Structural Integration should be avoided.[8]

- **Aneurysm,** which is the bulging of the arterial wall, is found sometimes at the aorta and also at the arteries within the axilla. To localize this condition, an ultrasound scan is recommended. Any intervention that would put the critical area under pressure is to be avoided.
- **Arteriosclerosis** is characterized by a buildup of plaque within the arterial walls. An angiologist needs to evaluate the client's condition for potential risks posed by manual treatment. Working on the connective tissue system is not advisable in advanced stages of arteriosclerosis.
- **Autoimmune diseases** (lupus, rheumatoid arthritis, scleroderma, and ankylosing spondylitis) can be characterized by inflammatory processes. The immune system aggressively works against the body's tissues. Given these conditions, it is not advisable to work during acute phases of the condition.
- **Bipolar disorder (manic-depressive)**: during manic phases intense work on the tissues is not recommended. The manual treatment might precipitate further extreme emotional states.
- **Borderline personality disorder**: Structural Integration can be applied, but with great caution, and it is helpful for the practitioner to have psychologic training to back up the therapeutic relationship.
- **Cancer**: in case of tumors, the connective tissue frequently builds a sort of a shell around the cancerous cells as a way to prevent metastasis. For

that reason deep manual treatment of the connective tissue and membrane system has to be done very carefully and only after a physician has examined the client.

- **Cerebral palsy**: a serious condition of this kind should not receive treatment with Structural Integration; moderate cases may benefit if the practitioner chooses a very careful and creative approach.
- **Connective tissue diseases**: there are several conditions that do not react well to intense touch; one is fasciitis, which simply does not respond to manual treatment of the fascia; others are osteomyelitis, lupus, and scleroderma.
- **Diabetes**: avoid working on the area of recent insulin injections; a manual treatment might accelerate insulin uptake. Respect the motion restriction around thoracic vertebrae 8 and 9 (in relation to the pancreas), which will disappear after insulin injection.*
- **Embolism** or **thrombus**: intense work on the connective tissue might dislodge a thrombus. Deep tissue work is not recommended.
- **Feverish clients**: the cause of the fever has to be diagnosed first to ascertain any contraindications; in general, any intervention stimulating the tissues is not recommended.
- **Fractures of bones**: these are usually a contraindication for Structural Integration. However, membrane techniques may be used to reposition the parts of the bone. The practitioner may need a medical license for this.
- **Headaches**: if the headaches are caused by tension, there will be a positive reaction after Structural Integration in many cases. However, the situation is different with migraines (see Migraine below).
- **Hemangioma**: a sort of congenital benign tumor made up of newly formed blood vessels. Deep work at the connective level is to be avoided within the affected areas because of danger of internal bleeding. This is especially to be respected at the level of organs.
- **Hernia**: hernia of the abdominal wall does not allow deep work around the abdomen and pelvis. Minor cases of hernia may be treated using specific techniques that attempt to retract the hernia.

---

*This clinical observation was made by J-P Barral, D.O. (Grenoble, France).

- **High blood pressure**: the client should be controlled with medical supervision between the manual treatment sessions. Avoid low positioning of the client's head during treatment.
- **Intervertebral disk problems**: there are many different stages of this condition. Working with acute cases requires a high degree of precision and much practical experience. In situations like that, any manual treatment has to be done in close cooperation with a radiologist and a neurologist. Treatment of a chronic disk situation usually has a much more positive perspective.
- **Intrauterine device**: if a woman uses an IUD for birth control, manual intervention at the level of the abdomen, above the pubic symphysis, and the pelvic floor might displace the IUD and lead to serious complications.
- **Menstruation**: be careful around the pelvic area. Be aware that the tension around the abdominal wall and the thighs is connected with the inner space of the pelvis. The treatment might cause a very strong bleeding, so it may be preferable to postpone the session. Practical observations have shown that working at the connective tissue layers and ligaments of the pelvis shows excellent results, especially during the days immediately after completion of the menstruation.
- **Migraine**: is not to be treated during acute phases. Some migraines do not respond well to treatment of the connective tissue. Those that are tension based usually respond well.
- **Nose work**: be extremely cautious with people who have had cosmetic surgery. Clients who take drugs nasally, like cocaine, may have irregular conditions of their arteries within the nasal passages. Manual treatment may cause severe bleeding.
- **Osteoporosis**: this condition requires a very subtle approach. Deep work has to be avoided. Be aware that men and people taking steroid medication over a long period of time may also get osteoporosis.
- **Pain medication**: be aware that reduced sensitivity shuts off the client's control system to a certain degree. You may have to talk to the prescribing physician to find out whether the medication can be stopped on the days of manual treatment.
- **Pregnancy**: there is certainly danger of a spontaneous abortion (miscarriage), especially during the first 3 months of pregnancy. During later pregnancy the risk is not as high. You have to be aware of potential complications and stay in contact with the client's physician. Because of necessary hormonal changes during pregnancy, the woman's tissues are in a special, more elastic condition. This is also true for the months after delivery, when a special approach is also advisable.[4]
- **Skin disorders**: infected areas should not be touched. This is especially true for herpes and any open lesions.
- **Whiplash**: Structural Integration techniques are successful if the practitioner is able to find the "root" of the whiplash deep inside the organism. Avoid working at the most symptomatic areas, especially at the neck area when the client reports pain around the cervical spine. In practice there is a better prognosis when we start to work no earlier than 4 to 6 weeks after the accident to avoid irritations.

NEW DEVELOPMENTS IN STRUCTURAL INTEGRATION

When Ida Rolf developed her system of the basic "ten series" her main focus was to create a well-balanced body free of unnecessary stress. She was aiming for good alignment and graceful movement. However, this work does not intend to diagnose or cure any medical conditions. It clearly belongs to the field of integrative and preventive health care by improving human potential in all dimensions of life. The students of Ida Rolf have been following this trail since she died in 1979. When Ida Rolf died, the question of how to follow up the 10 basic treatments was left unanswered. She had been experimenting with a series of four advanced sessions that later developed into a series of five advanced sessions. And some of the teachers she had trained started to explore a fairly free mode of advanced work following what was later called "a nonformulistic approach." Currently, this advanced work unfolds in different directions.

Also within the traditional basic 10 sessions practitioners started to become open to new perspectives. At the time when Ida Rolf taught her first classes in the late 1960s, Judith Aston, one of her first students, entered a whole new world by exploring movement work. This more functional approach has become a main focus for various schools of Structural Integration ever since, and new territories have been explored over the last

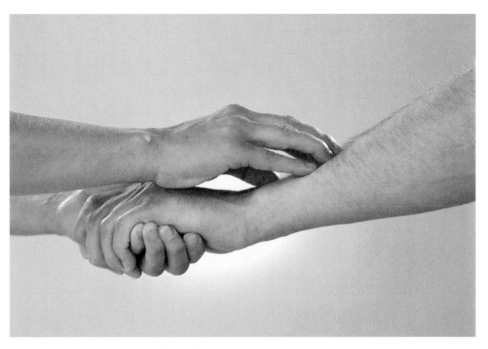

FIGURE 17-11 In terms of surgery, hand surgery is a field of its own. When working on the fascial layers of the forearm and hand, we have to be aware how well the human hand is represented within the human brain. Working at tissue layers of hand and forearm means much more than just working on tissue.

15 years. Eventually Movement or Functional work started to stand on its own feet and has now become a fully integrated and enriching part of the original manual or structural work.

And some practitioners of Structural Integration began to recognize the value of this work for specific clinical application. They started to carry it into the direction of clear diagnostics and the treatment of dysfunction.[4] They also realized that the work Ida Rolf did mainly on muscle fascia could be successfully applied to all sorts of connective tissue such as ligaments directly related to joints and membranes shaping the inner cavities and subcavities of the body. Through this, some of her followers entered into the field of **therapeutic applications:** they recognized that their work could achieve successful results for restrictions of joints, nerve irritations such as sciatica, brachyalgia, and carpal tunnel syndrome (Figure 17-11), the so-called "frozen shoulder" syndrome (Figure 17-12), and even for highly complex conditions such as whiplash. Following this new trail, Structural Integration is finding its place within the leading disciplines of manual medicine.

CERTIFICATION

There are various schools teaching Structural Integration. They have their own different entrance and certification requirements. For more information please refer to the institutions listed at the end of this chapter.

CHAPTER SUMMARY

Structural Integration, a manual approach originated by Ida P. Rolf, is characterized by a large range of possible applications. It was originally designed by its founder as a global manual treatment for preventive healthcare and well-being. In this sense, it can be applied successfully to people searching for better physical function, especially for postural improvement, and general reduction of strain. On a more psychological level, it has proven to be helpful in reducing stress. By eliminating unnecessary muscle tension, Structural Integration allows greater postural ease and enhanced coordination. Also for certain situations, Structural Integration can be an effective aid to the different schools of psychotherapy.

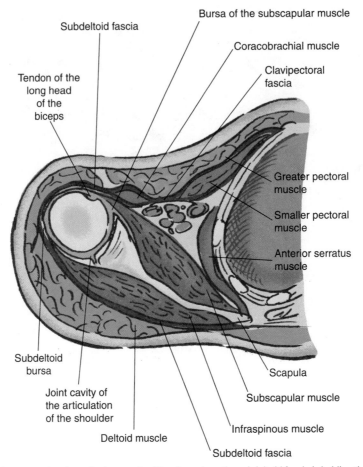

Subdeltoid fascia

Bursa of the subscapular muscle

Coracobrachial muscle

Clavipectoral fascia

Tendon of the long head of the biceps

Greater pectoral muscle

Smaller pectoral muscle

Anterior serratus muscle

Subdeltoid bursa

Scapula

Joint cavity of the articulation of the shoulder

Subscapular muscle

Infraspinous muscle

Deltoid muscle

Subdeltoid fascia

FIGURE 17-12 This horizontal cross-section through a human shoulder shows how the subdeltoid fascia is holding the shoulder together. The treatment of this very special sort of fascia is one of the keys to resolving frozen shoulder syndrome. (*From Schwind P:* Faszien-und Membrantechnik, Munich, 2003, *Urban and Fischer.*)

The classic method of Structural Integration is a comprehensive manual treatment of the fascial system of the human body consisting of 10 sessions, each one lasting approximately an hour. Aside from this traditional method, which has been applied for more than 50 years now, new insights and strategies for intervention are being developed. The practitioners of this form of bodywork have also refined the manual treatment strategies for the connective tissue system and found numerous possibilities for clinical applications. Some have been opening their mode of work toward movement education and the combination of movement education and manual work.

Today Structural Integration is taught worldwide by several schools. Most of the instructors who have been certified by the founder Ida P. Rolf are still actively teaching while generations of new instructors are contributing as practitioners, teachers, and researchers.

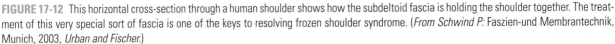

CASE HISTORIES

■ Case history 1

People wearing a cast after a fracture frequently develop serious motion restrictions around the joint next to the fracture. A client, an orthopedic physician himself, was looking for help after a fracture of the tibia he had suffered after receiving a kick during a soccer match several years ago. Ever since that accident, he was unable to move the ankle joint. He was also suffering from all sorts of compensations in other parts of his body. By the time he showed up for the first treatment, he had become very poorly aligned. While receiving the 10 basic sessions of Structural Integration, he regained his alignment and recovered his sense of an inner line. Mobility of his ankle joint improved step by step after the basic work was done on his feet and legs during the second, fourth, and sixth hour. After completion of the 10 sessions, the joint regained full normal mobility during both active and passive motion. Using some awareness exercises, he soon began walking the way he did prior to the accident. After this experience, he wrote a very positive report about Structural Integration for one of the leading German journals for orthopedic doctors.

■ Case history 2

In my practice I occasionally get clients with TMJ disorders, referred to me by dentists. They come to me with varying difficulties such as pain to the joint, irregular bite, and difficulty moving the jaw. In the cases of cramped or locking jaw, muscle tone and fascial strain have built up to such a degree that opening the mouth only half an inch is already a problem. I remember a case that was particularly severe. The dentist couldn't do any intraoral work, so preparatory work for the inlay was out of the question. The patient was only able to open his jaw on one side less than half an inch, while there was almost no opening possible on the other side. The dentist had already considered opening the joint by surgical intervention. Since he knew about the possibilities inherent in Structural Integration, he recommended opening the joint by working on the connective tissues around the head and jaw. After the practitioner applied the treatment of Ida Rolf's seventh hour of Structural Integration the client was able to open his mouth. What is interesting about this case is that the patient's wife called the practitioner's office 2 weeks after the treatment and complained about a change in the behavior of her husband. When asked what she meant she stated, "He's talking back all the time."[9]

SUGGESTED READINGS

Bond M, Miller St P: *The new rules of posture—How to sit, stand, and move in the modern world*, Rochester, VT, 2006, Inner Traditions.

Findley WT, Schleip R, eds: *Fascia research*, Munich, 2007, Urban & Fischer.

Maitland J: *Spacious body—Explorations in somatic ontology*, Berkeley, 1995, North Atlantic Books.

McHose C, Frank K: *How life moves—Explorations in meaning and body awareness*, Berkeley, 2006, North Atlantic Books.

Myers TW: *Anatomy trains—Myofascial meridians for manual and movement therapists*, Edinburgh, 2001, Churchill Livingstone.

Rolf IP: *Rolfing—Reestablishing the natural alignment and structural integration of the human body for vitality and well-being*, Rochester, Vt, 1989, Healing Arts Press.

Schulz L, Feitis R: *The endless web—Fascial anatomy and physical reality*, Berkeley, Calif, 1996, North Atlantic Books.

Schwind P: *Fascial and membrane technique*, Edinburgh, 2006, Churchill Livingstone.

Smith J: *Structural bodywork*, Edinburgh, 2005, Churchill Livingstone.

Stanborough M: *Direct release myofascial technique—An illustrated guide for practitioners*, Edinburgh, 2004, Churchill Livingstone.

RESOURCES

The Rolf Institute
205 Canyon Boulevard
Boulder, CO 80302
303-449-5903
800-530-8875
303-449-5978 Fax
info@rolf.org
www.rolf.org

European Rolfing Association
Nymphenburger Str. 86
80636 München, Germany
Tel.: 0049 (0)89-54 37 09 40
Fax: 0049 (0)89-54 37 09 42
info@rolfing.org
www.rolfing.org

Brazilian Rolfing® Association
Alameda Casa Branca, 600
01408-000 Sao Paulo SP
0055-11 3887-0670 phone & fax
rolfing@dialdata.com.br
www.rolfing.org.br

The Guild for Structural Integration
P.O. Box 1559
Boulder, CO 80306
303-447-0122
800-447-0150
303-447-0108 (fax)
www.rolfguild.org

Munich-Group/Muenchner Gruppe
Koenigin Str. 35A
80539 Muenchen, Germany
0049-(0)89-26 62 09
0049-(0)89-201 15 47 (fax)
info@muenchnergruppe.de
www.munich-group.com

The International Association of Structural Integrators
P.O. Box 8664
Missoula, MT, U.S.A. 59807
406-543-4856
877-843-4274
info@theiasi.org
www.theiasi.org

The Barral Institute
4521 PGA Boulevard #245
Palm Beach Gardens, FL 33418
866-522-7725 (toll-free U.S. phone)
561 686-5941 (standard phone line)
561 691-2029 (fax)
www.barralinstitute.com
info@barralinstitute.com

REFERENCES

1. Feitis R, Rolf IP: *Talks about rolfing and physical reality*, New York, 1978, Harper & Row.
2. Rolf IP: *Rolfing—Reestablishing the natural alignment and structural integration of the human body for vitality and well-being*, Rochester, Vt, 1989, Healing Arts Press.
3. Schulz L, Feitis R: *The endless web—Fascial anatomy and physical reality*, Berkeley, Calif, 1996, North Atlantic Books.
4. Schwind P: *Fascial and membrane technique*, Edinburgh, 2006, Churchill Livingston.
5. Schleip R, Klingler W, Lehmann-Horn F: Fascia is able to contract in a smooth muscle-like manner and thereby influence musculoskeletal mechanics, In Liepsch D, ed: *Proceedings of the 5th world congress of biomechanics*, Munich, Germany, 2006, Medimont International Proceedings.
6. Barral JP, Mercier P: *Visceral manipulation I*, Seattle, 1988, Eastland Press.
7. Rolf I: Structural Integration: a contribution to the understanding of stress, *Conf Psych* 16: 1973.
8. Schleip R: *Somatics* (website), http://www.somatics.de. This website contains a collection of relevant articles.
9. Schwind P: *Alles im lot—Eine einführung in die rolfing-methode*, München, 2001, Hugendubel.

MULTIPLE CHOICE TEST QUESTIONS

1) Structural Integration is
   a) a system of muscle stretches
   b) a sort of massage using oil
   c) a manual treatment of the connective tissue and movement education
   d) an Oriental form of bodywork

2) The main goal of Structural Integration is
   a) good alignment of the human body and well-coordinated movement
   b) to cure severe psychologic illness
   c) to reposition dislocated joints
   d) to cure neurologic disorders

3) Structural Integration was developed by
   a) Andrew Tailor Still
   b) Ida P. Rolf
   c) Moshe Feldenkrais
   d) Gerda Alexander

4) What kind of tissue is mainly treated in Structural Integration?
   a) the bones
   b) the muscle fibers
   c) the lymphatic system
   d) the fascia

5) The main function of connective tissue is
   a) to regulate blood pressure
   b) to connect and subdivide all components of the human body
   c) to produce blood cells
   d) to produce hormones

6) The connective tissue is present as
   a) a system of disconnected holes of the body
   b) an endless web
   c) a chemical substance inside the lymphatic system
   d) the magnetic field of the body

7) There is a force permanently acting on the human body. It is especially important for the theory and practice of Structural Integration. This force is called
   a) magnetic force
   b) force of acceleration
   c) gravity
   d) electromagnetic charge

8) The recipe of Structural Integration is
   a) an instruction about a sequence of medication
   b) a guide for muscle stretches
   c) a series of 10 manual treatment sessions
   d) a textbook of Oriental healers

9) Plasticity of the fascial system refers to the fact that
   a) this kind of tissue is soft and elastic
   b) this kind of tissue can be shaped by the hands of a practitioner
   c) this kind of tissue contains fluid elements
   d) this kind of tissue will never change

10) The dense part of the connective tissue is
    a) the ground substance
    b) the collagen fibers
    c) the blood cells
    d) the lymphatic fluid

11) When a practitioner of Structural Integration is doing visual analysis he/she is
    a) checking the client's eyesight
    b) checking whether the client shows rapid eye motion
    c) analyzing the client's physical structure as the client stands, sits, and moves
    d) diagnosing the client's psychologic state

12) The main goal of the first treatment of the standard sessions of Structural Integration is
    a) a free motion of breathing
    b) establishing good hinge functions in the legs
    c) balancing the head on top of the body
    d) reducing muscle tone in general

13) The main goal of the third treatment of the standard sessions of Structural Integration is
    a) to reduce tension within the client's back
    b) to reduce tension within the client's legs
    c) to allow better alignment along a lateral line
    d) to balance the client's cardiovascular system

14) There is a specific touch that is typical for Structural Integration. This kind of touch is characterized by
   a) using oil for intense sliding
   b) pushing very intensively onto the tissues all the time
   c) using a large variety of tactile contact from subtle to very intense
   d) being done from a distance within the client's electromagnetic field

15) When treating overly tense myofascial units of the musculoskeletal system, the practitioner of Structural Integration applies the following:
   a) He/she applies direct lengthening parallel to the muscle fibers and transverse to the primary fiber direction of fascia.
   b) He/she uses indirect technique.
   c) He/she massages the muscles.
   d) He/she manipulates the joint close to the most-strained place.

16) Working on the connective tissue system after a bone fracture will be beneficial
   a) immediately after the fracture has happened
   b) a few hours after the fracture has happened
   c) while the fractured part of the client's body has been put into a cast or splint
   d) after the cast or splint have been removed from the client's body

17) When working with elderly female clients, the practitioner has to be very careful in cases of
   a) a high-level muscle tension
   b) a low-level of muscle tension
   c) osteoporosis
   d) frequent activity in sports

18) During an acute phase of autoimmune diseases it is advisable
   a) to do shorter treatments
   b) not to do any treatment at all
   c) to do subtle work
   d) to add stretching to the manual work

19) When treating infants the practitioner has to make the sessions
   a) short and precise
   b) long and global
   c) only during morning hours
   d) later in the evening

20) On a psychologic level Structural Integration will help for
   a) curing psychosis
   b) curing bipolar disorder
   c) curing hysterical symptoms
   d) improvement of the balance of the autonomous nervous system

Traditional Thai Massage

Richard M. Gold

18

INTRODUCTION

Traditional Thai massage, also known as **Nuad Bo' Rarn,** is the physical medicine component of a complete indigenous system of traditional medicine, Traditional Thai medicine. The other components of traditional Thai medicine are herbal medicine, nutritional medicine, food cures, and spiritual practices, including meditation, yoga, incantations, and recitation of Buddhist **sutras.** Understanding the name Nuad Bo'Rarn can give us an insight into the nature of this form of healing body therapy. The word "Nuad" is from the Thai language and means to touch with the intention of imparting healing. The word "Bo'Rarn" is from the **Sanskrit** language of ancient India. It means something that is ancient and revered. So to the Thai people this work is held in the highest esteem and is understood to have specific healing attributes. The application of this work as a traditional medical modality is wide ranging. This includes the treatment of a wide range of medical problems such as myofascial, neurologic, orthopedic, internal medical, urogenital, gynecologic, and respiratory conditions and care during gestation and postpartum. In addition, Thai massage is used to treat psychologic problems. These techniques are utilized in pediatrics through gerontology and currently are being applied in situations of palliative care.[1]

HISTORY

Historically, Thai massage was not specifically what we in the West consider massage. It was considered and utilized as the hands-on practice of traditional medicine. Thai massage techniques were applied in the treatment of the varied ailments that afflict humanity, including mental and emotional illness. The historical founder of Thai Medicine is known as **Jivaka Kumar Bhaccha** (the Father Doctor). He is

To better understand concepts in this chapter, watch *Traditional Thai Massage* video on the **DVD** found at the back of this book.

351

identified by scholars as a close personal associate of the historical Buddha and was the head physician of the original **Sangha,** the community of followers that gathered around the Buddha. This would place him as living in India approximately 2500 years ago. As Buddhist monks and followers made their way from India to what is now modern Thailand in approximately the second century BC, traditional medicine came along with them. For centuries, the traditional medical knowledge was transmitted orally from teacher to student. Over the centuries, a distinct tradition evolved that was primarily influenced by the Ayurvedic traditions from India, but also began to incorporate theories and practices from ancient China. In addition, healing practices of the indigenous tribal peoples of the area also became part of the local medical practices. By the time **Theravada Buddhism** was declared the official religion of the kingdom in approximately 1292 AD, the traditional medicine was well established in the Buddhist monasteries, known as **Wats.** Traditionally, the Buddhist monks and to a lesser extent Buddhist nuns administered the healing work to the people.

Besides the specific hands-on techniques, herbs, and foods utilized in healing, Buddhist philosophy pervades the practice of medicine in Thailand. The practice of healing work is understood to be the practical application of "**Metta,**" loving kindness. Metta is understood to be a core component of daily life for each individual seeking awareness and fulfillment on the path taught by the Buddha. Teachers describe Metta as the "foundation of the world," essential for the peace and happiness of oneself and others.

In Thai Theravada Buddhism, significant emphasis is placed on the practical application of spiritual philosophy: that higher ideals be brought into everyday life and decisions. Accordingly, the practice of Thai massage demonstrates the practical application of the Four Divine States of Mind:

1. Metta, Loving Kindness
2. Compassion
3. Vicarious joy
4. Mental equanimity (brought to fruition through meditative practice)[1]

KEY DISTINCTIONS

Thai massage combines elements of yoga, meditation, acupressure, and assisted stretching to provide a unique and wonderful bodywork experience. Thai massage does differ in key aspects from Western massage.

Key distinctions:

1. Thai massage is practiced with the client fully clothed in loose-fitting clothing.
2. No oils or lubricants are used in Thai massage.
3. Thai massage is practiced very, very slowly.
4. Thai massage is a core component of an entire traditional medical practice: traditional Thai medicine.
5. Thai massage practice emphasizes pressing, compression, and stretching techniques. The stroking and rubbing techniques of Western massage (effleurage and petrissage) are mostly absent.
6. Thai massage practitioners utilize their feet, knees, elbows, body weight, and forearms in addition to their hands and fingers extensively during treatment.
7. Treatment sessions take place on a cotton pad or mat that is placed on the floor or on a low platform.
8. Thai massage practitioners are encouraged to work in a concentrated and meditative state of mind, unencumbered by thought or fantasy, and to transmit this quality of mind through their touch to the client.
9. Although it is the physical body of the client that is being addressed, the primary focus and intention of treatment are to bring balance and harmony to the "energetic" body and mind of the recipient.
10. Historically, very little emphasis was placed on precise anatomic landmarks.[1]

BENEFITS

Traditionally, Thai massage was utilized by doctors to treat the varied ailments that afflict humanity. These would include what are currently identified as internal medical issues, neurologic and orthopedic complaints, gynecologic issues, pediatrics, and psychoemotional challenges. Special benefit is also available for geriatric and palliative care concerns. As Thai massage is embraced in the West, the specific benefits of stress relief, mental quieting, and therapeutic stretching are achieved. The application of Thai massage as a type of assisted yoga brings the additional benefits associated with yoga into focus. These benefits include the apparent increase in flexibility but also the more subtle beneficial effects on the glands of the human endocrine system.

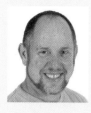

The synergistic combination of attributes offered by Thai massage consistently astounds me: even after 20 years of involvement! Both as a provider and as a recipient, I love and respect this style of work. The therapeutic benefits of Thai massage are available on multiple levels:

1. Physically: Thai massage is a great bodywork treatment. The diverse procedures that are applied with a client in four possible positions lead to an excellent physical bodywork experience.
2. Energetically: As a system of treatment based upon an energetic paradigm of human "beingness," Thai massage stimulates and balances the bioenergy in a calming and noninvasive manner.
3. Physiologically: As a system of peripheral stimulation, whereby points on the surface of the body are stimulated and cause specific physiologic effect on the internal organs, glands, and nervous system, Thai massage is extremely effective.
4. Spiritually: A clear intent of the practice of Thai massage is to create a meditative mindfulness for both the recipient and practitioner. This quality of mindfulness and mental equanimity is not necessarily specific to any one religion or spiritual path. The key issue here is that the practice of Thai massage induces and allows for an experience of mental quieting and calmness that allows both recipient and practitioner to experience a sense of unity and clarity of thought and purpose.

Thai massage has specific effects on the muscles and structures of the body. The primary therapeutic effects are accomplished with pressing and stretching techniques. Tense muscles become shorter. The ability of a muscle to produce movement at a joint is determined by the difference between the muscle's length when it is relaxed compared with when it is contracted. When muscles shorten and become persistently tense, they become hardened and oxygen depleted. Additionally, from an energetic perspective, a tense muscle further inhibits the smooth flow of bioenergy through the energetic pathways, designated as Sen.

This results in diminished flexibility, increased spasms, and sensations of pain and stiffness. Muscle shortening impacts the surrounding fascia. As the muscle tissue shortens, the fascia also shortens and loses elasticity. This contributes to increased tissue fibrosis and diminished flexibility. A further dynamic that occurs in the musculature is a weakening of the antagonistic muscles and the loss of tone due to the persistent contraction of the paired muscles. This weakening eventually contributes to postural imbalance. These interrelated phenomena ultimately result in decreased flexibility, increased susceptibility to injury, and pain and stiffness. Additionally, the blockage of bioenergy can actually contribute to a lessened physiologic functionality of the internal organs and blood stagnation that lead to disease and aging.

Pressing Techniques

The deep presses in Thai massage literally squash the muscles, stretching the myofascial tissues laterally. This pressing action helps to break down fibrotic tissues and helps stimulate the production of more elastic fibers. The blood flow through the entire affected musculature is enhanced. This brings increased nutrients and oxygen into the area and helps to flush out toxins, carbon dioxide, and other metabolic byproducts by enhancing the movement of the lymphatics and venous blood.

Stretching Techniques

The numerous sustained stretches in a Thai massage session are applied in a number of varied directions. The practitioner strives to alter the vectors of approach to the stretches thereby delivering a diversity of signals to the brain. The stretching takes the muscles just beyond what their normal relaxed length would be. The **muscle spindle organs** actively respond to this stimulation. (The muscle spindle organs are the sense organs in the muscles that provide a constant flow of information to the brain about the state of muscle contraction and any change in this state of contraction. Additionally, the tendons also contain sensory fibers, the Golgi tendon organs, that communicate with the brain on how much pull they are being subjected to as the attached muscles contract.) During the stretching, the muscle spindle organs signal the brain that the muscle is relaxed. This allows the inhibitory nerve impulses to the antagonistic muscles to stop and allow them to begin to regain their normal tone. This dynamic action helps to restore balance within and between functional muscle groups. This promotes increased flexibility, postural improvement, and diminished pain and suffering.[1]

BODY MECHANICS

Although Thai massage is traditionally practiced on a mat on the floor or on a low platform rather than upon a massage treatment table, the body mechanics of the practitioner remain of utmost importance. It is difficult to overstate the importance of proper body mechanics for the safety of the recipient and the health and longevity of the practitioner. Practitioners must always be highly aware of both their own body posture and that of the recipients in order to maintain a safe and therapeutic environment. As aspects of Thai massage are often a form of partner yoga, practitioners must always remain mindful of how they are using their body. Practitioners seek to be aware of the flow of gravity through their own body and into and through the body of their recipient. This attention to the routing of gravity is an essential component of safe and effective practice.

There are specific body positions or stances that the practitioner must learn to work in comfortably and with proper mechanics to allow for a fluidity of movement, an optimization of their strength, and the safety of both themselves and the recipient. The working postures of Thai massage are:

- Diamond stance: The practitioner kneels on the treatment mat with the knees together, buttocks resting on the heels, tops of the feet flat on the mat, spine straight, and head erect.
- Open diamond stance: The practitioner kneels on the treatment mat with the knees spread apart, buttocks resting on the heels of the feet, tops of the feet flat on the mat, spine straight, and head erect.
- Kneeling diamond stance: The practitioner stands erect from the knees, establishing a vertical line from the knees to the crown of the head. The knees can be close together or opened up.
- Cat stance: The practitioner kneels on the treatment mat with knees together or spread apart, buttocks resting on the heels, tops of the feet on the mat (same as in the diamond or open diamond stances). Keeping the spine straight, the practitioner leans forward from the hips and places the palms of the hands flat onto the mat with straight arms. An alternative to this is for the practitioner to come up on the toes, lifting the buttocks off the heels of the feet. This allows the practitioner to lean forward further without losing the straight line of the spine.
- Raised cat stance: The practitioner is positioned on the knees and flat palms of the hands. The spine is parallel to the floor. There is a vertical line running through the hips to the knees.
- Warrior stance: the lunge: The practitioner moves from the kneeling diamond stance rising up onto one knee, bringing 50% of his/her weight forward onto the foot. The weight can be easily shifted from front to back. The knee of the raised leg should not extend forward past a vertical line drawn down through the foot. The spine remains straight even as the weight is shifted forward.
- Archer stance: The practitioner is in a squatting position with the toes curled under. One knee is then placed down onto the treatment mat. The spine and head remain erect.
- T'ai chi bow stance: The practitioner stands maintaining soft knees and with the feet spread to shoulder width. The practitioner steps forward with one leg but only so far forward as to be able to keep the knee over the toes. The front foot points straight ahead, and the back foot turns slightly outward at a 45-degree angle. The spine remains erect even as the weight shifts back and forth from the back to the front leg.[2]

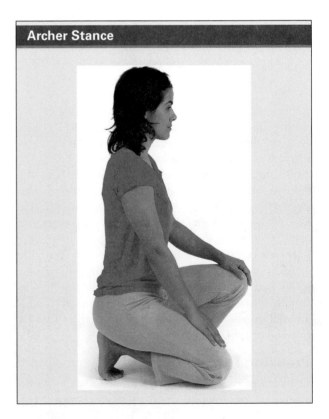

Archer Stance

T'ai Chi Bow Stance

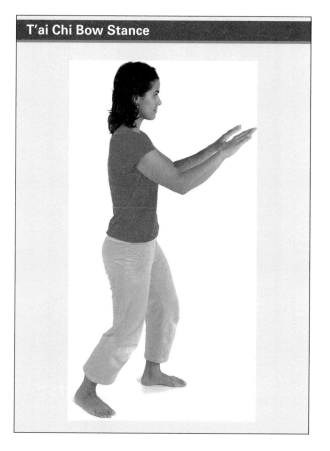

BASIC THEORY

The theories underlying the traditional medicine of Thailand represent an interweaving of the theories, philosophies, and practices primarily of ancient India's Ayurvedic medical tradition combined with some additional influences from ancient China. In addition, Thai medicine has evolved over the centuries in the context of indigenous Thai culture and Theravada Buddhist influences, giving this healing tradition a uniquely Thai expression. (In this chapter in the context of the entire text, I can only touch briefly on this theory. Please see the suggested readings if you wish to pursue the theory in more detail.)

In Thai philosophy, everything in our known world is composed of four elements: earth, water, wind, and fire. In healthy states, the four elements exist in a dynamic, interactive balance. When there is disease, the elements are out of balance and the individual suffers. A further aspect of Thai medical theory describes the three **doshas.** The doshas are the (Ayurvedic) dynamic principles of the body and are only assigned to living matter. The three doshas are:

- **Pitta**: Bile
- **Kapha**: Phlegm
- **Vata**: Wind

Human beings are influenced by all three of the doshas. For each individual, one of the three doshas will have a dominant influence. The dynamic interplay of the doshas is a key aspect of health and longevity. Imbalance in the doshas is a causative factor of disease.[3]

In addition, Thai medicine embraces an energetic view of the human body. This means that bioenergy flows through the body on specific pathways, known as **sen**. Ten main sen are identified. All the sen have their origins deep in the abdominal region in the vicinity of the navel and connect the core of the body to the sensory orifices, the excretory orifices, and the extremities. In Western terms, Thai massage is classified as a system of peripheral stimulation. This means that by stimulating specific points on the surface of the body that lie on the sen pathways, the internal functioning of the body's organs, glands, and nervous system can be affected.

In consideration of the basic theories of Thai medicine, the aspect that most clearly relates to the practice of Thai massage is the theory of vata, the wind. Quoting an old French text, "All functions of the body were discharged by a mysterious agency called the 'wind.'" It caused the blood to flow—you could feel it in the beating pulse—the digestion to act, the bowels to move, the skin to perspire. Indigestion was from excess wind. Headaches were caused be the wind from below blowing upwards. Pains in the legs were caused by the wind from above blowing downwards. The wind was the cause of most of the complaints from which the body suffered.[4]

According to Thai medical theory, wind (vata) is the only aspect that is identified as one of the elements and one of the three doshas. Wind is considered the most important of the three doshas because it sets the other two in motion and assists in the regulation of the functions of pitta and kapha.

In the practical application of the techniques of Thai massage, the slow, rhythmic presses and deep compressions are designed to affect the wind that is present in the body. The Thai massage practitioner seeks to facilitate the correct movement and placement of wind in the body and to release the wind from places where it has become stagnant. The numerous stretches that are a critical component of Thai massage are deigned to move wind that has accumulated and become stuck in the joints of the body structure.

THE IMPORTANCE OF ABDOMINAL THAI MASSAGE

According to the theory of Thai medicine, the abdominal region is of the utmost importance. The abdominal region is the place where vata (the wind) originates.

In addition, all the main sen energy pathways have their origins deep in the abdominal region in the vicinity of the navel. In order to have a healthy, functioning human being, the abdominal region must function normally. Therapeutic applications of Thai massage will always incorporate abdominal work. The practitioner will work with the client to establish an awareness of deep breathing into the abdominal region. All of the techniques that are applied to the abdomen are designed to invigorate the functioning of the internal organs and to eliminate energetic blockages and stagnation of blood and lymph. Improved functioning of the abdominal region will be reflected in the positive overall health and vitality of the client/recipient (Box 18-1).

TECHNIQUES

The application of the techniques of Thai massage utilizes the practitioner's fingers, palms, closed fists, forearms, elbows, feet, knees, upper thighs, and gluteals. The most basic and most frequently used technique is the palm press (Figure 18-1).

The entire palmar surface of the hand is evenly used, creating a direct downward vector into the client's body. The practitioner works with straight arms and uses

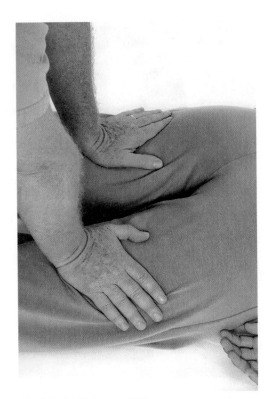

FIGURE 18-1 Palm press (PP).

shifting body weight to direct the pressure. Care must be made neither to emphasize the heel of the hand nor to knead with the fingers. The palm press procedure is designated as the integration technique that is utilized after detailed thumb and finger work has been applied. Palm presses are done with both hands working simultaneously or alternatively. Walking-palm presses, i.e., working from the feet up and down the legs or from the upper back to the sacrum, is an application of the technique that is frequently utilized.

The sole of the foot is utilized to deliver a firm compression to the client's body (Figure 18-2). The technique begins with the practitioner's leg bent and foot in direct contact with the client's body (e.g., the medial thigh muscles). As the practitioner's leg straightens, the foot applies the thrust of the pressure. A counterforce of pulling with the hand at the ankle usually accompanies the foot press. Care must be taken neither to use the heel of the foot nor to apply excessive pressure.

The ball of the thumb is utilized to exert a direct downward vector. The point or tip of the thumb is not used. Thumb presses are used to treat along the sen energy lines and into muscles (Figure 18-3). The thumbs deliver pressure that is generated from the abdominal

---

BOX 18-1 The Nine Zones on the Abdomen

The practitioner visualizes the abdominal region divided into nine equal zones, with the navel being in the center. The navel serves as the hub of the "wheel" and the lines that define the nine zones can be seen as the "spokes" of the wheel. The entire abdominal region is defined by the lowest ribs as the upper border, the pubic bone as the lower border, and the midaxillary lines establishing the lateral borders. All of the deep palm presses applied by the practitioner are directed (vectored) toward the navel. In Thai medical theory, all of the primary sen (energy) lines have their origins in the vicinity of the navel. These sen connect the physiologic center of the body with the sensory and excretory orifices. The deep work in the abdominal region helps remove stagnation in the abdominal viscera, invigorates proper functioning of the organs, and harmonizes the flow of bioenergy on the sen energy pathways.

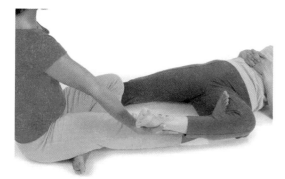

FIGURE 18-2 Foot press (FP).

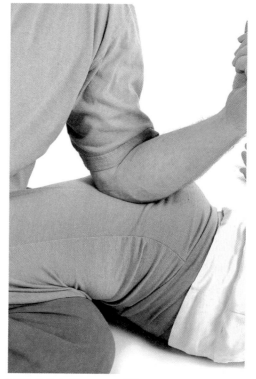

FIGURE 18-4 Elbow press (EP).

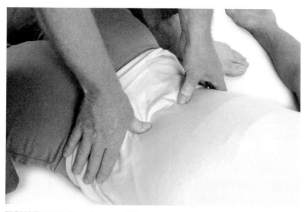

FIGURE 18-3 Thumb press (TP).

core of the practitioner and travels down the straight arms into the hands. Use of the thumbs by exerting force in the arms and hands can quickly lead to fatigue and discomfort. Often the thumbs work in a pattern/ sequence of "thumb-chasing-thumb but never catching." In this pattern, one thumb moves into the body as the other thumb lifts out, in a piston-like movement.

The elbow is used to treat points on the bottom of the feet and hip region (Figure 18-4). The elbow is placed on the point, and the practitioner's weight is pressed down into the elbow. The elbow pressure is released by bringing the forearm forward. The practitioner never lifts the elbow off the point.

The ulnar surface of the forearm is utilized to provide compression and stretch. The practitioner places the forearm(s) onto the body area to be worked (Figure 18-5). By rotating the radial (thumb) side of the arm forward, it deepens the compression and provides a stretch along the underlying muscles. This technique is utilized along the upper shoulders, back of the legs, low back, and the bottom of the feet.

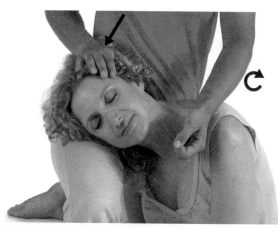

FIGURE 18-5 Forearm rolling pin.

Circular movements of the thumbs are used on the face, head, hands, and feet. Thumb circles are utilized over bones because the practitioner never presses directly down onto bones (Figure 18-6).

The tips of the finger(s), usually the three middle fingers, are utilized together in a circular motion (Figure 18-7). This technique is used over the sternum,

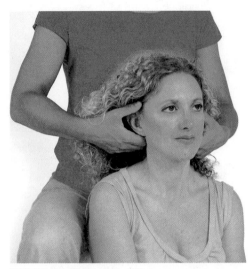

FIGURE 18-6 Thumb circle (TC).

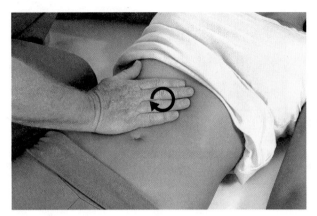

FIGURE 18-8 Palm circles.

A critical component of Thai massage is stretching of the limbs, torso, and neck. The stretching procedures are made by creating a force/counterforce in various locations of the body (Figure 18-9). The stretches create elongation and expansion and open up the joint spaces. The practitioner seeks to give the client an expanded sense of his or her body. With the application of the stretches, the goal of working very slowly is of the utmost importance. The practitioner must sense the holding patterns in the client's body and never forcibly stretch the client beyond what is comfortable.

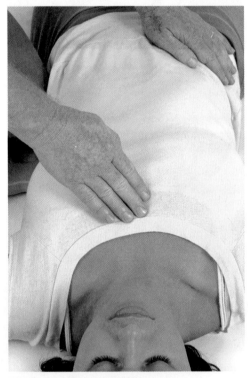

FIGURE 18-7 Finger circle (FC).

below the clavicle, in the intercostal spaces, along the edges of the scapula, and on the face.

Slow, circular movements are made with the entire palmar surface, including the heel of the hand and fingers. Palm circles are used extensively as an integrative procedure with deep abdominal treatment (Figure 18-8).

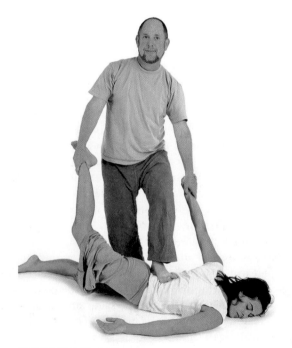

FIGURE 18-9 Stretching.

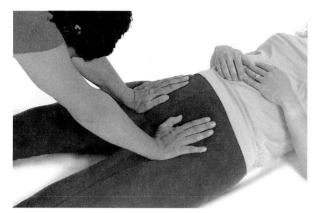

FIGURE 18-10 Stopping the blood flow.

On the femoral artery in the inguinal groove and on the axillary artery in the axilla, the practitioner locates the pulse by palpation and then exerts a deep downward compression with the heel of the hand in order to obstruct the superficial flow of blood. The compression can be retained for up to 30 seconds. The technique is never used on clients with a history of circulatory problems or cardiac problems or clients taking medication for the heart, circulation, or blood thinning. The purpose of this technique is to force the blood flow into deeper circulatory patterns and to help flush toxins and stagnation (Figure 18-10).

PRECAUTIONS AND CONTRAINDICATIONS

"Above all else, do no harm"

The techniques presented in this chapter comprise the physical medicine of traditional Thai medical practice. Throughout the history of Thailand, these techniques have been utilized to treat the wide array of complaints that afflict mankind, including problems of internal medicine as well as structural and neurologic complaints. Additionally, for many centuries Thai medicine has addressed problems of a psychologic and spiritual nature. As with any medical practice, traditional or modern, there are certain basic criteria that must be met before practical application commences. The practitioner must have a clear understanding of the problem(s) to be addressed. The practitioner must learn of any previous surgeries, current usage of medications, and any precautions advised by the client's medical doctor. The practitioner must have a treatment plan and specific goals that he or she seeks to accomplish in treatment. In addition, care and caution must always be exercised in treatment.

The nature of Thai massage demands that the practitioner be especially attentive to precautions in treatment and be very clear as to any preexisting problems the client might have that would require that certain procedures be eliminated from the treatment protocol. The following guidelines should be followed:

- Thai massage treatment is conventionally contraindicated in the treatment of cancer.
- Clients who are very ill and in a weakened state should not be treated.
- If there is high fever, treatment should not be given.
- Clients who suffer from osteoporosis should be treated with great caution with the stretching procedures and only with very light pressure.
- Clients who bruise quite easily and who are taking blood-thinning medication should be treated with only a very light pressure.
- Clients who are experiencing acute pain along the spine should not receive any procedures that worsen the pain and the stretches with the client in a prone position should be eliminated.
- If the client has previously had surgery on the spine (such as a laminectomy), all stretches in a prone position where the legs are raised are eliminated.
- Clients who are pregnant should be treated with caution. There should be neither abdominal work nor pressure on the low back. In addition, stretches need to be performed gently. All leg massage must be light, and ischemic compressions strokes must be avoided. The best approach for treatment of a pregnant woman is to work with the client in a lateral recumbent position.
- In Thailand, women are not treated during menses. This is a cultural taboo and not a medical precaution.
- The procedures known as "stopping the blood flow" are eliminated in treating clients with a history of heart problems, diabetes, and vascular problems.

> ### BOX 18-2 Localized Precautions
>
> There are specific localized problems that need to be noted and avoided during treatment. These include:
> - Fractures
> - Varicose veins
> - Wounds and bruises
> - Inflammation of joints and/or skin lesions
> - Abdominal area less than 1 hour after a meal[1]

OVERVIEW OF A TREATMENT

Practitioners are instructed to always interview all clients prior to beginning a session. With new clients, this is essential. Taking a thorough client history is vital. In addition to gaining a better understanding of the client and his or her medical history, the client will feel more confident and at ease. Positive rapport and open communication are invaluable in a therapeutic relationship.

Practitioners are seeking to learn as much as is relevant in order to provide a safe and therapeutic session. Be especially cognizant of any medical problems, prescription medications, and any previous surgeries or serious illnesses.

It is important to learn what the client's expectations are and their understanding of Thai massage. Find out if they prefer a light or deeper touch. For first-time clients, make certain that they understand that you will be working not just with your hands but with other body parts as well. Instruct the client to speak up if they feel a need to communicate a concern with you during the session.

In Thailand, sessions are approximately 2 hours or more. Standard sessions in the West will be 80 to 90 minutes. Hour sessions can be done but will feel rather incomplete. Sessions most often begin with the client in a supine position. The client remains clothed, preferably in loose-fitted clothes of natural fibers. No lubricants are used. The practitioner kneels at the client's feet and takes a moment to focus and become centered and offers a prayer that good will come from this work. The first procedure is to palm press the feet multiple times and then to palm press up and down the legs. This can also be repeated many times.

With clients who cannot lie comfortably supine, sessions can begin with the client prone, lateral, recumbent, or even seated. Directing the initial procedures to the feet and legs is designed to pull awareness out of the client's head, quiet thoughts, and to begin the process of deep relaxation. Depending on the client's needs and desires, the session can evolve in numerous ways. More or less time can be spent on the legs, arms, abdomen, head and neck, or back. If lying supine becomes uncomfortable, the client can shift to a lateral recumbent or prone position. Since so many of the procedures of Thai massage can be applied with the client in varied positions, the practitioner can be flexible about where and how to begin. Depending on the scheduled length of a session, the practitioner makes choices of what procedures are to be included. There is no set "recipe" of procedures that must be followed with each session. For specific treatment of particular problems, a more defined approach of therapy is recommended.

CERTIFICATION REQUIREMENTS

At this time, there is no national certification in Thai massage as a stand alone modality. Thai massage is an approved modality of the national organization, the American Organization of Body Therapies of Asia (AOBTA). Students who complete an AOBTA-approved curriculum of at least 500 hours, which can include Thai massage, are eligible to take a national certification examination administered by the NCCAOM (National Commission for Certification of Acupuncture and Oriental Medicine). In addition, students who complete an approved massage curriculum of at least 500 hours, which can include Thai massage, are eligible to take the national certification exam given by the National Certification Board for Therapeutic Massage and Bodywork (NCBTMB).

In 2005, an international not-for-profit, nonpartisan, professional organization, the Thai Healing Alliance International, was established to promote, unite, and establish academic requirements in the field of Thai healing arts, especially Thai massage.

CASE HISTORY

The client is a 45-year-old high school teacher who presented with radiating sciatic pain down the back and outside of her right leg. This condition had been problematic for 6 weeks. Her moderate pain is a constant with intermittent phases of intense pain. The pain is worse while standing. This is the first incident of sciatic pain she has experienced. The pain had a gradual onset and worsened during a period of overwork and personal stress. She has been seen by her private physician and by a neurologist. Her blood work showed a slightly elevated SED (sedimentation rate) rate and lymphocyte count. All x-rays and MRI scans showed no disk involvement. There were no indications of nerve damage or impaired reflexes. The physician prescribed pain mediations and NSAIDs (nonsteroidal antiinflammatory drugs). The medications provided some relief, but the pain reduction was short-lived and the patient felt dizzy from the pain medications and gastric irritability from the NSAID drugs. She no longer wanted to take mediations and therefore was seeking a natural approach to treat her sciatica.

After taking the client's history and reviewing her medical reports, we discussed the practice of Thai massage and the therapeutic benefit she could expect. We discussed in detail that she would remain clothed during the sessions, that I would be working with my feet, elbows, knees, and forearms, as well as with my hands, and that much of the time she would be lying in a lateral recumbent position. Also, I explained the importance of deep abdominal work and the energetic as well as physiologic correlations to her sciatic condition. I recommended that we do two sessions the first week, then one a week for 2 weeks and then reevaluate her condition. Each session was scheduled for 90 minutes and took place after her workday was completed.

Her sessions followed a specific protocol that began with palm presses on the feet and legs (Figure 18-11).

Next, abdominal work was applied. The abdominal work included palm circles in a clockwise pattern over the entire abdominal region, deep palm presses in nine zones, palm circles over the entire abdomen, deep thumb presses into points lateral to the navel, lateral and superior to the navel, and lateral and inferior to the navel, and finally an integration with gentle palm circles on the entire abdomen (Figure 18-11).

At the conclusion of the abdominal work, the client was placed into a lateral recumbent position with the right hip up. A pillow was placed between her knees for support and comfort. The sessions then proceeded with palm presses and thumb presses into the sen lines on the outer leg. Next, a series of leg stretches were applied with the practitioner's feet (Figure 18-13). Direct work on the hips and low back followed. The techniques included palm presses, deep elbow presses (Figure 18-14), forearm rolling, and more palm presses for integration. The final part of the session was composed of therapeutic stretching while the client remained in a lateral recumbent position (Figures 18-15 and 18-16).

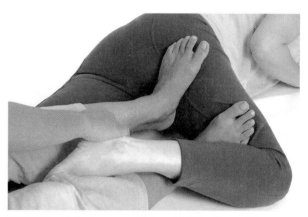

FIGURE 18-13 Foot presses with the client lateral recumbent.

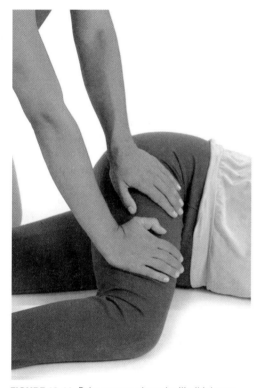

FIGURE 18-11 Palm presses along the iliotibial tract.

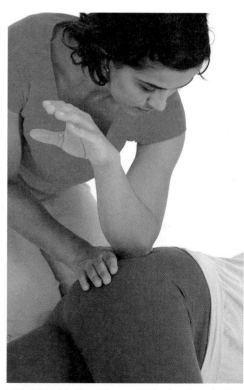

FIGURE 18-14 Deep elbow compressions into the hip to help relieve sciatic pain.

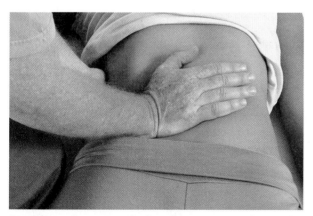

FIGURE 18-12 Deep compressions into nine zones on the abdomen.

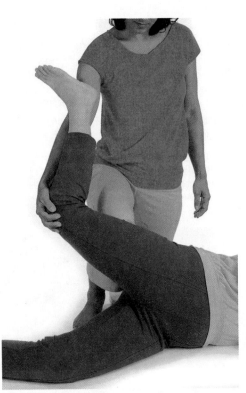

FIGURE 18-15 The leg is pulled back into the practitioner's knee. The knee compressions help alleviate pain in the hamstring region and along the posterior branch of the sciatic nerve.

During the first sessions, the client was only able to tolerate a light touch and minimal stretching. The abdominal region was particularly sensitive, especially in the lower right quadrant. After the first four sessions, the client reported a significant improvement in pain and a willingness to have deeper work and more thorough

stretching. She was able to stand for long periods without pain and had begun light exercise. We agreed to continue with weekly treatments and then, as needed, both for continued improvement in the sciatica condition and also because she appreciated the deep relaxation she experienced while receiving Thai massage.

After a total of nine sessions, she reported herself as free of all pain and able to exercise as she pleased. She continued to receive sessions on an average of once a month with the goals of remaining flexible, pain free, and reducing stress.

CHAPTER SUMMARY

In this chapter, the reader has been introduced to the hands on healing tradition of Thailand (ancient Siam). Known in Thailand as Nuad Bo'Rarn and in the West as Thai massage, this ancient system of healing bodywork dates back approximately 2500 years.

In the Thai culture, this healing work is used to treat the varied maladies that afflict humanity, including internal medical problems, psychoemotional issues, as well as musculoskeletal complaints. The techniques and application of Thai massage differ in many ways from Western massage therapy. Although Thai massage has only recently become known in the West, the acceptance of this style of work has grown rapidly. Currently, Thai massage courses are being taught at many schools and retreat centers in the Western world and there is a great demand for practitioners at spas and clinics worldwide. The learning, practicing, and receiving of Thai massage can be a wonderful and life-enriching experience.

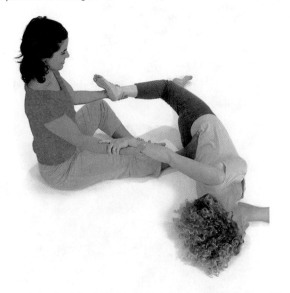

FIGURE 18-16 Leg extension with foot press into low back and hip.

SUGGESTED READINGS

Apfelbaum A: *Thai massage*, New York, 2004, Avery.
Asokananda: *The art of traditional Thai massage*, Bangkok, Thailand, 1990, DK Publishers.
Balaskas K: *Thai yoga massage*, London, 2002, Thorsons.
Bechert H, Gombrich R, eds: *The world of Buddhism*, London, 1984, Thames and Hudson.
Chopra D: *Perfect health*, New York, 1991, Harmony Books.
Chow KT: *Thai yoga massage*, Rochester, Vt, 2002, Healing Arts Press.
Frawley D: *Ayurvedic healing: a comprehensive guide*, Twin Lakes, Wis, 2000, Lotus Press.
Gold R: *Thai massage: a traditional medical technique*, St. Louis, 2007, Mosby.
Golomb L: *An anthropology of curing in multiethnic Thailand*, Chicago, 1985, University of Illinois Press.
Heyn B: *Ayurvedic medicine*, New Delhi, 1992, Harper Collins.
Lad V: *Textbook of Ayurvedic*, Albuquerque, 2001, Ayurvedic Press.
Mann N, McKenzie E: *Thai bodywork*, London, 2002, Hamlyn.

Mercati M: *Thai massage manual*, New York, 1998, Sterling Publishing.

Mulholland J: *Thai traditional medicine: a preliminary investigation*, Canberra, 1977, Australian National University Press.

Mulholland J: *Thai book of genesis: herbal medicine in pediatrics*, Canberra, UK, 1989, Faculty of Asian Studies Monograph, Australian National University.

Pierce SC: *Encyclopedia of Thai massage*, Forres, Scotland, 2004, Findhorn Press.

Riley JN, Mitchell JR, Bensky D: Thai manipulative medicine as represented in the Wat Pho epigraphies, *Med Anthropol* 5: p. 155-196, 1981.

Setthakorn C: *Nuad Bo'Rarn workbook, Foundation of Shivago Komparaj*, Chiang Mai, 1989.

Smith N: *Thai massage*, London, 2004, Lorenz Books.

Svoboda R: *The hidden secret of Ayurveda*, Albuquerque, 1996, Ayurvedic Institute Press.

Xinnong C, ed: *Chinese acupuncture and moxibustion*, Beijing, 1996, Foreign Language Press.

RESOURCES

Acupuncture.com
http://www.acupuncture.com/

American Massage Therapy Association
http://www.amtamassage.org/

American Organization of Body Therapies of Asia (AOBTA)
http://www.aobta.org/

National Certification Commission for Acupuncture and Oriental Medicine
http://www.nccaom.org/

National Institutes of Health (NIH)
http://nccam.nih.gov/health/ayurveda/

Pacific College of Oriental Medicine
http://www.pacificcollege.edu/

Thai Healing Alliance
http://www.thaihealingalliance.com/

Traditional Thai Massage: Sacred Bodywork
http://www.traditionalthaimassage.com/

REFERENCES

1. Gold R: *Thai massage: a traditional medical technique*, St Louis, 2007, Mosby.
2. Chow KT: *Thai yoga massage*, Rochester, VT, 2002, Healing Arts Press.
3. Svoboda R: *The hidden secret of Ayurveda*, Albuquerque, 1996, Ayurvedic Institute Press.
4. Smith M: *A physician at the court of Siam*, Oxford, 1957, Oxford University Press.

MULTIPLE CHOICE TEST QUESTIONS

1) The word "Nuad" is from what language?
   a) French
   b) Chinese
   c) Thai
   d) Sanskrit

2) The word "Nuad" translates to mean
   a) loving kindness
   b) to touch with the intention of imparting healing
   c) lying still
   d) meditation

3) The word "Bo'Rarn" is from what language?
   a) Thai
   b) Chinese
   c) French
   d) Sanskrit

4) The word "Bo'Rarn" translates to mean
   a) place where animals are kept
   b) deep touch
   c) massage
   d) ancient and revered

5) The historical founder of Thai medicine is known as
   a) Ravi Shankar
   b) Father Doctor
   c) Siddhartha
   d) Dali Lama

6) Circle the correct statement
   a) Thai massage practitioners only use their thumbs
   b) Thai massage is practiced very slowly
   c) Thai massage is practiced only very deeply
   d) Thai massage is only used with young clients

7) Thai massage is practiced with the client in what position?
   a) lateral recumbent
   b) supine
   c) prone
   d) all of the above

8) Thai massage is never practiced when the client has
   a) high fever
   b) pregnant
   c) stress
   d) acne

9) Metta means
   a) type of analysis
   b) deep touch
   c) loving kindness
   d) style of deep breathing

10) The practice of Thai massage is an expression of
    a) greed
    b) Nuad
    c) independence
    d) Metta

11) The primary focus of intention in treatment with Thai massage is (are)
    a) the neck
    b) the lower back
    c) the mind
    d) the feet

12) Thai massage is an aspect of
    a) system of traditional medicine
    b) an oil massage
    c) dietary options
    d) tourist attraction

13) Proper body mechanics in the practice of Thai massage
    a) are not necessary
    b) can be ignored
    c) are essential
    d) are moderately important

14) Thai massage practitioners utilize
    a) only their hands
    b) only their hands and feet
    c) only their feet
    d) their hands, forearms, elbows, knees, and feet

15) When a deep elbow compression is utilized in practice, the elbow is released by:
    a) a slow lifting release
    b) a rapid lifting release
    c) slowly bringing the forearm forward
    d) lifting slowly while rotating the elbow

16) The three doshas of Thai medical theory are
    a) wood, fire, earth
    b) earth, wind, fire
    c) kapha, pitta, vata
    d) kapha, vata, curry

17) The pressing techniques work by
    a) breaking down fibrotic tissues
    b) stimulating production of more elastic fibers
    c) enhancing blood flow through the affected musculature
    d) all of the above

18) The stretching techniques
    a) actively stimulate the muscle spindle organs
    b) are usually left out of sessions
    c) only provide routine signals to the brain
    d) are never done on pregnant clients

19) Stopping the blood flow technique is contraindicated when the client
    a) has a history of heart problems
    b) is on blood thinning medications
    c) has circulatory problems
    d) all of the above

20) The origins of the sen energy pathways are located in the
    a) brain
    b) extremities
    c) abdominal region
    d) palms and soles

Trager® Psychophysical Integration

Jack Blackburn

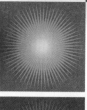

19

STUDENT OBJECTIVES

Upon completion of this chapter, students will be able to do the following:

- Understand the passive movements of tablework.
- Understand the active movements of Mentastics.®
- Recognize the importance of the practitioner's mental state during treatment.
- Anchor the client's awareness into feeling his/her body sensations.
- Recognize the perception that physical change depends upon a change of mind.

KEY TERMS

Drugless practitioner
Effortlessness
Gentleness
Hook-up
Listening hands
Mentastics®
Physical culturists
Presencing
Proprioception
Reinforce
Somatic awareness
Tensegrity
Trager® Psychophysical Integration
Weighing

OVERVIEW

Trager® Psychophysical Integration is a unique approach to manual therapy and movement reeducation that combines gentle touch, rhythmic motion, and client awareness in order to release tensions and limitations and to increase physical and mental expressiveness and articulation. Although the *Trager* approach is discussed in this book, the *Trager* approach is a form of movement education and not a form of massage, bodywork, or therapy. The main components of the approach are: sharing a state of presence with the client, tablework that involves passive client movement, and teaching active movements to clients that reinforce the benefits of the tablework. Milton Trager (Figure 19-1) influenced a number of bodywork and lay practitioners with his infectious presence and energetic role modeling. When he finally started teaching his work, which he called **Psychophysical Integration,** to others he was already in his late sixties. Most of his students were quite a bit younger than him and did not fully realize the connection he provided to an earlier time. His emphasis on physical movement and "agelessness" reflected the influences of the **physical culturists** of the early twentieth century. The real genius of his work was his realization that gentle, rhythmic movement, performed with great sensitivity, could effect positive and long-term changes in the client. The principles he discovered in refining his work seem almost zenlike in application. The stronger the resistance in the client, the less the amplitude of movement imposed by the practitioner. Soft hands supported by movement that is generated from the practitioner's whole body are more subtle and effective. The most powerful shifts often happen when the practitioner breaks physical contact giving the client space to integrate what has just been experienced.

HISTORY

In 1927 at the age of 19, without any formal training, Milton Trager started working on people's bodies to alleviate their pain and movement restrictions. Like many in those times, Trager was strongly influenced by Bernard McFadden, a strong proponent of physical

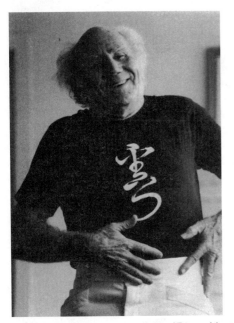

FIGURE 19-1 Milton Trager at age of 83. (*Trager:* Mentastics®: Movement as a way to agelessness, Barrytown, 1987, Station Hill Press.)

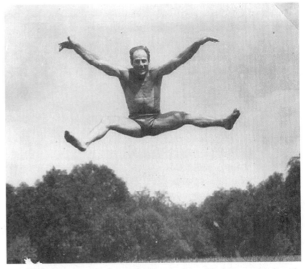

FIGURE 19-2 Trager as physical culturist-athletics on the beach, age 23. (*Trager:* Mentastics®: Movement as a way to agelessness, Barrytown, 1987, Station Hill Press.)

prowess, healthy living, and natural healing methods, and founder of the Physical Culture movement. Following the concepts and regimens of the physical culturists, Trager became a bodybuilder and developed himself as an athlete and dancer (Figure 19-2). Throughout the1930s and early 1940s, he worked with clients as a lay practitioner, experimenting and refining his methods, attempting to infuse his clients with his own experience of health and vitality. His way of working using the gentle, rhythmic, and painless movements that he was able to create in clients' bodies was unique. His intention was to instill feelings of physical freedom and well-being in them. The clients, though passive, would become aware of very pleasurable sensations in their bodies. It was as if Trager were giving them the feeling of dancing by dancing their bodies. He would then teach the clients to replicate these movements for themselves. His effectiveness in reducing pain and promoting movement was so dramatic that he confidently worked on clients with disabling illnesses such as cerebral palsy and polio-related paralysis.

During World War II, from 1943 to 1944, he served in the American Navy as a pharmacist's mate. On shipboard he tried out his techniques with his fellow sailors and army troops suffering from battle fatigue. Returning to civilian life after his discharge, he decided to become a professional health care provider. In 1944 he obtained a license in California as a **Drugless practitioner** (until repealed in 1949, this license covered chiropractors, naturopaths, osteopaths, midwives, and various manual therapies) and specialized in working with neuromuscular disorders. In 1950, in order to further validate his work, he decided to take advantage of the GI Bill and go to medical school to get an MD. Because of his age and limited educational background, he was not admitted into U.S. medical schools. He chose instead to study medicine in Guadalajara, Mexico. While in medical school he continued to work with clients when possible. He developed a reputation as a healer by helping ease the symptoms of children crippled with polio.

Trager completed his medical training in 1955 and did 2 years' residency in psychiatry while interning at the Territorial Hospital in Kaneohe, Oahu, Hawaii. In 1957, he opened a private practice in general medicine in Honolulu. Each day he would supplement his regular medical practice with one or two in-depth sessions in which he applied his techniques of manual practice. He eventually named his method *Psychophysical Integration* because of his strong belief, affirmed by years of experience, that profound changes in the body must be preceded or accompanied by profound shifts in the mind. He tried, over the years, to get this approach accepted by the medical community as a preferred treatment for patients with neuromuscular disorders. But, despite apparent success in treating the symptoms of difficult conditions such as muscular dystrophy, Parkinson's, and postpolio syndrome, he received a tepid response from his medical colleagues. They would refer patients to him for sessions and be surprised by the results. But, to Trager's dismay, none seemed to consider his drugless treatments as effective as surgery or medication. In 1977, at the age of 69, he retired from medical practice but continued to work with many patients considered "untreatable" by his medical colleagues.

In 1975, Trager demonstrated his approach at the Esalen Institute in Big Sur, California. One of the staff members, Betty Fuller, a teacher and sponsor of Moshe Feldenkrais's work, was so impressed that she became Trager's first pupil. She started arranging trainings for Milton with bodyworkers, other health care providers, and laypeople. Betty and other protégés founded the *Trager Institute* in 1980 in order to support the trainings and promote the work. From 1975 until his death in 1997 Trager continued to teach and refine his approach.[1]

▪▪▪ IN MY EXPERIENCE

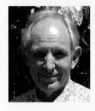

I was encouraged to become a *Trager* practitioner by my *vipassana* teacher in 1985. He said that he'd experienced many types of bodywork all over the world and that *Trager* came closest to the experience of insight meditation or *vipassana.* I have since become convinced that he was correct because so many of the principles of *Trager* emphasize presencing awareness through monitoring body sensations—the same is true of *vipassana.* I had no idea at the time what a gift he gave me with his suggestion. Studying with Milton Trager and joining a committed community of *Trager* practitioners has set the course of my whole life ever since. Every time I teach a class in a foreign land, or witness for a client who has a life-altering breakthrough, I am grateful to Milton Trager.

Another thing that I have realized over the years is that the principles that underlie what I do as a *Trager* practitioner have deeply affected how I experience life. I'm talking about principles like gentleness; patience; trust in the client and myself; curiosity; nonpushiness; effortlessness; and above all, presencing. I have followed those principles, and each has opened new doors of awareness and connected me to other teachers, philos-

ophers, and bodywork modalities. I have thus been able to set my own course based upon Milton Trager's example but not limiting myself to his understandings. Many times he had the humility to say to his protégés: "I have only scratched the surface—you will go much further." He taught that there is never an end to the awareness and body realizations that can happen.

Having been a bodyworker and *Trager* Practitioner for 21 years, I believe that as a profession, we are only scratching the surface of what is possible through the growth of somatic awareness. We all stand on the shoulders of the bodywork pioneers who taught us and then had the humility of Milton Trager to encourage us to go further. The same can be said for our humility and support of our clients—encouraging them to go even further than ourselves in self-discovery and presencing their own lives. We can also pass on the gift of our own playfulness and curiosity. Humankind is in need of a different way to appreciate the gift of life—to fully immerse ourselves in the joyousness and vitality that lay just beneath our willingness to listen into our bodies and humbly accept the fact that we have been wrong about our bodies. Descartes said "I think therefore I am." Milton Trager might say: "I Mind, through my body, and come closer to I AM."

TRAGER APPROACH: THREE COMPONENTS

Tablework

The *Trager* approach combines three main components for working with clients: tablework, **Mentastics®,** and **hook-up.** The tablework is the use of gentle rocking motions in combination with traction, compression, torqueing, and other forms of tissue engagement. The practitioner uses various methods of ongoing physical assessment during a session. At the beginning and end of a session the client's quality of movement and subjective experience of movement are explored. Throughout the session the client's structural relationship(s) to gravity and displacement is/are monitored, as are tissue

tonus, harmonic resonance, reflexive and autonomic responses, and quality of proprioceptive awareness. Range of motion, end feel, motility, and **tensegrity*** are assessed and iterated, nuancing the client's proprioceptive

---

*Tensegrity (tension-integrity) is a concept originally coined by Buckminster Fuller (inventor of geodesic domes) to describe the dynamic ability of living systems to maintain structural integrity in spite of perturbations and distortions. Based on his observations he designed light structures that depended upon a combination of solid beams and elastic trusses—held in place by their relationship of tension and compression. Deane Juhan, author of *Job's Body,* described the same relationship between bones and connective tissue. The body's shape and structural relationships are maintained through tensegrity. This is particularly important when we are distorting the passive body with rocking motion.

experience in numbers of different ways, while the body is in motion and at rest.

The practitioner's hands are used to isolate different joints, muscles, fascia, and other connective tissue. These portions of the client's body are supported and put into motion so that the momentum of the movement, while distributed throughout the client's body, can be anchored and vectored precisely. The practitioner focuses the client's awareness on the sensations being felt. These sensations are unique because most clients have not been supported and rocked in this way since they were cradled as infants. The movements are highly pleasurable and comforting and impose no painful stimuli. One physical therapist describes her experience using the tablework portion of Psychophysical Integration with patients (Figure 19-3).

> The movement done during the session is a subtle suggestion to the nervous system of what motion is possible. None of the movements done in a *Trager* session are forced. With gentle rocking, the body itself is never put into positions that are stressful to it. With the active participation of the subject removed, the body itself is learning in a proprioceptive way so that positions and movements are easily possible. Potential learned patterns resulting from previous pain avoidance can be overcome in this way. . . . The practitioner helps facilitate and restore normal movement to the ankle through repetitive, painless stimulation, and also increases "available" movement patterns to the hip, ankle, and cervical region. The joint mobilizaw-

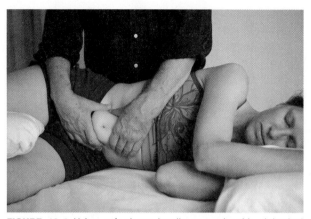

FIGURE 19-4 Using soft tissue handle to work with abdominal muscles and viscera. (Photo by Jennifer Richard.)

tion aspect of the *Trager* approach involves accessory and physiological motions that do not just mobilize the specific extremity part that the therapist is working on, but that affect the whole body simultaneously[2] (Figure 19-4).

Tablework Principles

Presence/Witnessing. Throughout a session the *Trager* practitioner tries to maintain a mental-physical state of continual presence, what Trager called "hook-up." This **presencing** state is not just concentration on what is occurring in the client's tissue from moment to moment, it is a sharing of feeling experience with the client. This state of awareness is essential for successful application of tablework in *Trager*. Maintaining presence is so important that, regardless of how skilled a practitioner is in the mechanics, technique, and even understanding of the work, without hook-up it can only be a superficial representation of what *Trager* has to offer.[3]

Gentleness. The second principle is **gentleness.** Gentleness, like presence, is a primary way of connecting with the client during the tablework. Gentleness does not mean a lack of strength or intention in the practitioner. Gentleness in *Trager* is like the "principle of gentleness" called *ju-no-ri* in judo. It is a way of working with resistance both in oneself and the client. Underlying this principle is the wisdom of not opposing resistance, but meeting it with pliancy, patience, and understanding. One must be peaceful and present

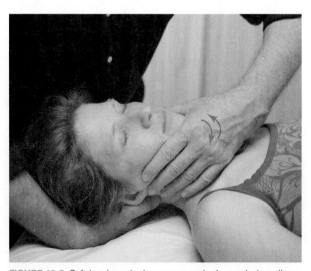

FIGURE 19-3 Soft hands anchoring movement in the cervical vertibrae. (Photo by Jennifer Richard.)

at the core. Gentleness rests upon qualities of patience, attention or listening, acceptance, and curiosity. These qualities inform the interaction during the tablework by the kind of contact and body movements that are created (Box 19-1).

No Pain: A Paradox

Trager would say: **"When you're creating pain you are not doing *Trager*."** He wasn't talking about preexisting discomfort; he was referring to anything the practitioner would attempt that increased pain in the client. All of the movement and positioning and hand contact in *Trager* tablework is designed to stay within a zone that does not trigger defensive reactions in the client. Even "good pain," the kind of pain that is welcomed by the client as a sign that relief is coming, seems to interfere with the unconscious mind's ability to trust and let go. There is a paradox here because many of the things a *Trager* practitioner does in a session might not take the client out of pain but do reduce the client's fear of pain as well as increase the client's **somatic awareness** and willingness to move. Whereas the pain of deep

---

BOX 19-1   Excerpt on Gentleness from a *Trager* Introductory Class, Seattle, 2002

Those hands that you had during the hook-up exercise were gentle hands. When I walked around and felt your hands, it felt like your hands were puffy, as if you were wearing soft mittens . . . these soft, listening hands. In *Trager* you learn to relax your hands into the contact and then bring the movement. What you are doing now is giving the person on the table some of *your* weight. You are still working with gravity, but now the person on the table has become a moving surface as she is feeling some of the weight of your upper body through your hands. Notice that your hands are still soft while you are doing this, making sure that you are just giving your weight, rather than "muscling in" to his/her resistance. The results feel very different to the person on the table. If you can bring in those hands that could feel the weight of the feather, then you can gather much more information from your client. If you meet resistance, lighten up. When you do less, it's an invitation for the client's mind to do more. There is no gain with pain in *Trager*. That doesn't mean that *Trager* practitioners don't do things that sometimes cause pain for their clients, but when we do, we are slipping out of *Trager*. Milton Trager believed that small increments of pleasure are much more effective than large increments of pain, when it comes to releasing patterns and producing actual change.[4]

---

compressions, trigger point releases, shiatsu, or spinal adjustments may take someone out of pain immediately but not necessarily increase somatic awareness or ease of motion.

Doing Less Is More

Another unique feature of Trager's approach to his clients was his emphasis upon **"effortlessness."** This concept applies to the tablework as well as the *Mentastics,* active movements the client is taught to initiate. Like the principle of "no pain," this concept can be misinterpreted to mean that there is a superficial and vapid quality to the work. Nothing could be further from the truth. The practitioner is continually asking him/herself: "How much effort is this requiring?" Trager believed that the more you "efforted," the more out of touch you are; the more out of touch, the less effective.

Soft Hands

Underlying all the work between practitioner and client is soft, full-handed contact. Trager was noted for this kind of contact: "His hands feel as if they are covered with chalk." The irony here is that chalk on the hands of athletes makes for more complete connection with the surfaces they encounter. Soft hands are better equipped to adapt to different kinds of tissue and surface contours. As with "empty hands" in *tai chi*, soft hands are not conditioned by preset muscular or movement patterns. They can then be fully responsive to what they encounter. Sometimes called **"listening hands"** in *Trager,* they are able to receive and send very subtle information from and to the client (Figure 19-5).

Addressing the Intrinsic Wholeness Within

It could be argued that in body-centered work practitioners are interacting with two contrasting facets of their client's body-mind. The first is the preset reactive conditioning. The second is an *intrinsic potential for therapeutic change*. The intrinsic potential for therapeutic change could be called an "inner healer." The preset conditioning could be called the "inner defender." Trager maintained that patterns of resistance accumulate in the client's unconscious mind. He concluded that positive change only happens when the client's mind has been changed through new experience. The author argues that an intrinsic potential for therapeutic change has shifted into conscious awareness. Trager would agree although he described this potential as the sharing of universal life force.

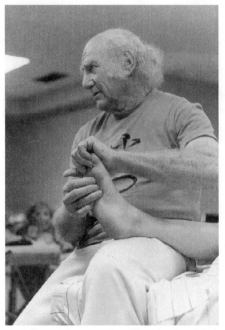

FIGURE 19-5 Trager demonstrating "listening hands" feeling for "what needs to happen." (Courtesy of US *Trager* Association.)

Reinforcement and Recall

One of the most important aspects of *Trager* tablework is the attention paid to any changes that occur. At the beginning of a session, before the client gets on the table, the practitioner will ask the client to perform a series of ordinary, simple movements, such as walking. Through such movements the practitioner can observe patterns of compensation and restriction. Even more significant for the session is to have the client become aware of and report how these movements feel from the inside.

The practitioner has now established the beginnings of somatic awareness in the client. This awareness is reinforced during the tablework so that the client becomes a willing partner to the changes that are occurring. After the tablework is completed, the learning of *Mentastics* movements further reinforces the client's somatic awareness.

Improvisation

Trager used to say that you have to "fool the mind" of the client. It's as if the client's unconscious mind gets used to certain movements and is able to adapt his/her resistance to those movements. But when the practitioner varies the movements, even very subtly by decreasing the amplitude or changing the direction,

this unconscious defensive adaptation-pattern protection begins to release. The practitioner that can continually improvise is thus able to challenge or coax the client's conditioned mind in an ever-changing variety of ways.

Curiosity

Curiosity would seem to subtend all of the characteristics that guide the tablework in *Trager*. When we are curious we are not imposing our preconceived ideas on a situation. When we are curious we ask questions that have an open-ended aspect to them. We want to find out how something IS—we are asking basic ontological questions such as "What is it like to be living life in this body?" Curiosity is interactive and relational. "What happens when I do this?" Guided by gentleness, curiosity wants to know more about this person, this body, this life (Figure 19-6).

Mentastics®

The second component of the work is called *Mentastics,* a word Milton Trager coined, which combines "mental and gymnastics." *Mentastics* are the movements combined with subjective internal monitoring. Trager said that he developed them so that he could experience, in his own body, what was happening for clients in the tablework (Figure 19-7). These movements are taught to clients so that they can re-create on their own the feeling of their sessions and thus recall and reinforce the changes that occurred during the tablework. These movements are gentle and very pleasurable. They are ways of using the gravitational field and momentum to

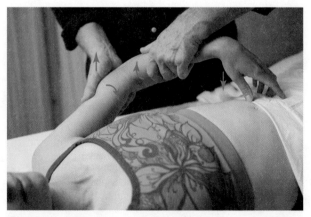

FIGURE 19-6 Various movement possibilities guided by practitioner's curiosity and responses in client's body. (Photo by Jennifer Richard.)

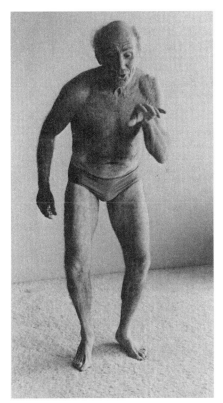

FIGURE 19-7 Trager demonstrating lightness and playfulness of *mentastics*. (Courtesy of Cathy Hammond and *Trager* International.)

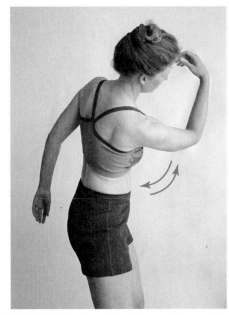

FIGURE 19-8 Releasing the weight of the arm into pendular momentum as torso rotates. (Photo by Jennifer Richard.)

stretch, open, and effortlessly move the joint or tissue in question. For this reason, many of the movements are carefully designed so that the muscles and joints to be addressed are passively affected, just as in the tablework. Also, as in the tablework, the client is encouraged to feel the range of sensations produced by the movement. This feeling awareness in the client can produce long-term changes in the client's holding patterns. Phil Witt has given a good description of *Mentastics* in application.

> *Mentastics* are best described as gentle, free flowing, dance-like movements whose main goal is to increase and provide the patient tools to increase his/her ability to move and control the pain... the unique feature of *Mentastics*... is that instead of requiring the patient to control the movements as in regular exercises, the patient is encouraged to "let go." In practice, this means the patient is instructed to initiate a movement and then let go of the muscle tension and allow the weight of the body part to carry the motion to completion. The better the patient becomes at this, the larger, freer and more effective the movement becomes[6] (Figure 19-8).

Principles of *Mentastics*: Movement for the Body

A Different Feeling Experience. Clients often lack words that can adequately describe their inner sensations. Two very important parts of the practitioner's role can be teaching the client to feel inside and help the client develop a feeling vocabulary. This is especially useful with *Mentastics* because the client is not aware of the many pleasurable sensations that are occurring that can aid the movement rather than restrict it. For instance a client who feels pain while moving her arm, who starts to become aware of the gentle pull of gravity lengthening her arm and the momentum that is keeping her arm in motion, discovers that these other signals, though less intense, can actually become more compelling.

Move Within Range of Comfort. Another important aspect of *Mentastics* is teaching the client to limit his/her movement, using minimal effort and maximal perception. Clients will often attempt to expand their range of movement beyond the range of no-resistance, trying to reach a certain goal rather than feeling for ease. The practitioner who is observant can spot the signs of restriction in the client's body language and confirm his/her hunch by palpating the tissue adjacent to the body part in motion. Then the practitioner can ask the

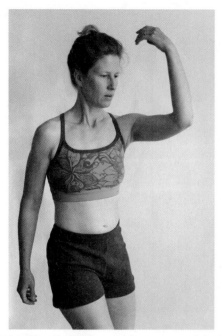

FIGURE 19-9 Client feeling for ease of movement, refining her input by asking. "What would be easier?" (Photo by Jennifer Richard.)

client, "What are you feeling?" If this does not produce a refinement in the movement, the practitioner can use words that tie up the intellect like: "What would be half of that?" The words lack specificity and take the client into a feeling state that bypasses thought. The client then makes an adjustment that comes from visceral searching. These enigmatic words can help the client to stop trying. Then all the practitioner needs to do is anchor that experience of least-efforting for the client by asking: "And what do you feel now?" (Figure 19-9).

Shifting from Watching to Feeling. The principles that underlie *Trager Mentastics* are dynamic and kinesthetic, based upon inner anatomy, somatic awareness, or felt-sense. Inner anatomy could be described as the client's awareness of the patterns of sensation produced by: **proprioception,** five-sense data, expenditure of effort or work, signals of restriction and limitation (such as tightness and pain), emotional states, mental states, degree of association or disassociation, and the degree of presence or hook-up. As such, *Mentastics* may be described as a dynamic yoga that allows the subject to monitor and interact with all the body's sensorial reflections in each moment. One of the difficulties in teaching *Mentastics* to groups is convincing the students to

remain **somatically aware.** Most are self-conscious and, as a result, compare themselves with others. The goal is to help them to shift their point of reference from external comparison to internal somatic awareness.

Moving with Presence. The unique feature about *Mentastics*, as compared with other movement systems like Feldenkrais, is the emphasis upon presence or hook-up. As elaborated in the second article of a series on *Trager*[7] Milton Trager found very ingenious, body-centered ways to teach continual presence. By far, the most difficult time to remain present is when the body is moving, when most of our sensory awareness becomes outwardly referenced through five-sense data. Trager's genius, whether native or trained, was to discover foolproof ways to keep the mind actively involved in maintaining presence during movement.

Practitioner Self-Awareness. When teaching *Mentastics* to a client the practitioner is aware of the feeling of weight, free movement, shimmering, rebound, and inner felt-shifts in his/her own body. This self-awareness allows the practitioner to show movements and give verbal suggestions that bring a similar awareness to the client. For instance, the practitioner is aware of a feeling of lightness or ease when demonstrating a repetitive movement. This feeling is transmitted to the client by visual and tactile cues and by open-ended questions that accompany the movements like: "How free can it be?" or "What could be lighter than that?" As stated before, these open-ended questions bypass the intellect and initiate a somatic inquiry that leads directly to presence.

The Importance of Recall and Reinforcement

Mentastics are an attempt to enhance the client's own movement and awareness and to re-create the effects of the tablework. It was Trager's intent to give the client some techniques that he/she could practice in order to **reinforce** the changes that had occurred in the session. By recalling the feeling that he/she had had, the client could then start from that felt-sense when practicing the movements. Trager was a master at the tablework and in his hopeful and positive encouragement of the client's own capabilities. But he would have considered himself a failure if he were not able to pass on his own key for self-renewal: *Mentastics*. He would often get the client up during the tablework and teach *Mentastics* to confirm that he/she could re-create the effects. Clients recall sessions in which he spent only a short time working on their body and spent most of the session teaching them *Mentastics*.

An Application of *Mentastics*: Playing with Balance

A good beginning *Mentastics* is finding the vertical center line of balance in any direction, becoming aware of that center line, noticing how the awareness of that center line affects our movement, learning to adjust our posture in order to keep that feeling of the center line alive as we make different movements, noticing the fine adjustments our body is making in order to maintain a sense of balance. The same thing applies to awareness of the horizon. The eyes and inner ear and our muscle memories give us a sense of where the horizon is located and help us to maintain our sense of balance in relation to both vertical and horizontal directions. All of our movements center around these axes, but through trauma, emotional upsets (such as body shame), and other inhibitions we lose our sense of playfulness and expressiveness that stem from body-centered awareness (Box 19-2 and Figure 19-10).

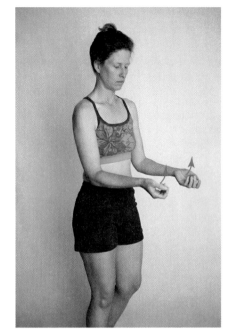

FIGURE 19-10 Weighing hands, wrists slack feeling the weight as interaction with gravity. (Photo by Jennifer Richard.)

> ### BOX 19-2 *Mentastic* Example: Playing with Balance
>
> Stand erect, feet shoulder width apart, knees soft. Close eyes and start to shift your weight from side to side. Feel the muscles of the legs engage and release as you shift back and forth. Notice that there is a place where the amount of muscle engagement in each leg is the same. Raise your forearms and feel the weight of your hands. Notice the tingly sensations of gravity as your hands pass through the lines of force of gravity. Now slow down and discover the thin vertical line of balance between right and left. When you feel that line, your inner awareness will light up—like the power signal on a radio tuner. Now rock forward and backward on your feet. Notice how your toes dig in as you rock forward and how they lift off as you lean back. Then slow down and discover the thin vertical line of balance between back and front . . . notice the feeling as you line up on the vertical. Check both directions: back-to-front and side-to-side until you feel perfect verticality. Store away that feeling. Take a deep breath and as you exhale softly open your eyes. As you look with your eyes remain aware of your inner somatic awareness. Now go for a walk and notice how your body remembers that feeling of vertical alignment. Notice what you feel in your extremities and how they move as you walk. Notice the relationship between your external senses and internal somatic experience.[8]

Hook-up

The third major component of the *Trager* approach is called *hook-up*. Trager used this phrase to describe the mental state of the practitioner as he/she works. This term literally means the practitioner is hooked-up or connected to what Trager called *universal mind* and thus to the client through the sharing of a common body-mind experience. One method for achieving this awareness is to keep the mind "present" by focusing on body sensations. This can become a very precise meditative tool for concentration. One might say that, when this concentration is achieved, the client and the practitioner are experiencing common sensations or sensory information packets from a shared perspective. In this way they are "hooked-up." These information packets can include the data of touch such as: texture, tonus, temperature, and signals of proprioception. It is the shared nature of this information that forms the basis of the approach. An example of what one experiences as *hook-up* would be dance couples that are so closely entrained that each can anticipate the movements from the thoughts and somatic experiencing of the other. While they are dancing, they seem to be of one mind, one body. Often in *Trager* sessions the practitioner feels a change in the tonus of the tissue under his/her hands just as the client becomes aware of very pleasant sensations in that part of his/her body. Milton Trager placed great emphasis on the *hook-up* portion of the work. Toward the end of his life he repeatedly said: "Hook-up is everything. It is the work."[4] Deane Juhan, author of *Job's Body*, in an article on hook-up, wrote:

> When a *Trager* Practitioner is in "Hook-up," specific molecular neuropeptide forms are operative that create this feeling state. Through the Practitioner's motor system this feeling state participates in the formation of movements. . . . the subtle cues embodied in these movements are taken in by the client who is then informed of the Practitioner's mental state [presence]. The client can then cultivate and receive this new feeling . . . and as it catches hold, this new feeling begins [in theory] to stimulate the production and release of reinforcing neuropeptides that mimic and perpetuate the particular chemistry of that particular feeling in the Practitioner. From this point on, the neurological substrates of a new memory are established, and any time the client actively [consciously] recalls that memory, the neuropeptide chemistry, associated with it can be reproduced[9] (Figure 19-11).

Hooking-up: Choosing To Be Present

One of the unique differences between the *Trager* approach and other forms of manual therapy is the emphasis Milton Trager put on the *choice* to maintain a

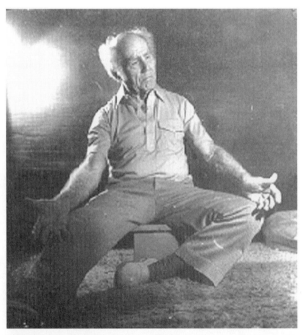

FIGURE 19-11 Trager in hook-up, staying present by attending to his bodily sensations continually. (*Trager:* Mentastics®: Movement as a way to agelessness, Barrytown, 1987, Station Hill Press.)

presencing state of mind by the practitioner. He discovered that this state of mind could dramatically influence the results of sessions. Trager taught practitioners simple but profound ways to attain and return to this state of awareness. He also stated that "hook-up" linked the practitioner with a "life regulating force" that also connected him/her with the client, mentally as well as physically. Trager had various ways of describing this state of mind: "deeper than relaxation," "It's like Zen," he would say, "it's like the feeling of . . . well . . . nothingness." "Recall how you feel when you are looking into the face of a baby, or when you are overwhelmed by a sunset."[10]

What is Hook-up?

What is this state of awareness that Trager lived for? What does it feel like? How does a practitioner learn to hook-up? What does the client experience when the practitioner is hooked-up? What are the results of a session where the practitioner is hooked-up? What physiologic and mental changes occur in the practitioner? Can hook-up be practiced no matter what technique is used? What about sessions in which both client and practitioner are hooked-up?

- Hook-up is a state of expanded mental, physical, and spiritual awareness. One becomes aware of a connection between inner and outer experiences, between one person and another, and a gnosis or inner knowing connection to universal being. Some might call it a state of communion.
- Hook-up feels deeply pleasurable and peaceful. One perceives dimensions that are usually in the background of our sensibilities, such as: timelessness, silence, stillness, emptiness, and unity. One feels spacious and loving, light and vibrant, awe-filled and expectant. Body and mind feel tingly or shimmery. These are called the "subtle sensations" in Buddhist meditation.
- One can hook-up by monitoring, moment to moment, the body's sensory responses from any phenomenon and then apprehend the effects of this process.
- When the practitioner is hooked-up the client feels gently held, respected, and guided into a state of deep peacefulness, trust, and nonpressured letting go.
- The results of such a session affirm the client's own inner resources: a fundamental participative process for self-healing that can continue long after the session is over.

- The practitioner becomes aware of heightened physical sensitivity that involves soft hands and a mental focus that is continuously listening, assessing, affirming, and adjusting to tissue change, rather than the removal symptoms.
- Since hook-up is primarily the apprehension of what is implicit in each moment; there is no reason why this state would not complement any modality. It is a matter of shifting other agendas like: fixing, mending, comparing, or protocol, into the background. Each session becomes unique and latent with possibility, as does each client.
- When practitioner and client are fully aware and conversant about what is occurring in the present moment, there is an interpersonal and reciprocal sharing of sensitivities; and change and transformation are multiplied.

What Does Hook-up Feel Like?

What does the state of hook-up or presence or mindfulness feel like to the practitioner? There is a deep sense of peace and assurance and connection with the client and the surrounding environment. The practitioner's hands become soft, warm, and spacious. Starting with the hands, the whole body feels like it's filled with a subtle effervescence. Movements produce pleasant shimmering sensations. The mind is clear and perceptive, able to discern very small increments of information. Like a rock climber in a dangerous ascent, all of the sensory channels both mental and physical are open, alert, and very receptive but with parasympathetic and liminal responses and no adrenaline rush. And there is also a strong sense of playfulness, expansiveness, and spontaneity. Trager described it as "swimming in a vast ocean of pleasantness."[11] Deane Juhan describes the feeling of hook-up as "a neuropeptide cocktail"[8] (Box 19-3).

Weighing: Relating to Gravity

Trager students learn to practice specific methods for remaining in hook-up. The first method is called "feeling the **weight**" (Box 19-4). The student is taught to weigh parts of his/her own body, with and without movement, and to experience the effects of hook-up. Then she/he learns to apply weighing and movement in producing and assessing responses in the client. As a *Trager* practitioner works with different parts of the client's body, he/she is always asking: "How much does it weigh?" "How does it move?" "How does it (the tissue) respond to my weight

---

> ### BOX 19-3 Exercise in Hook-up: Inside and Outside Are the Same
>
> Start by palpating or exploring an external object such as a flower or a sculpture or person's body. Notice the kinds of information you obtain through that experience. And notice what your mind does with that information. Continue the exploration until you feel satisfied that you have gathered as much information as you can . . . Then seat yourself. Get comfortable. Close your eyes. Take some time to recall what you just experienced and notice any visceral sensations still remaining in your body . . . Pause. Take some deep breaths down into your body. Notice the contact of your body parts that are being supported by other surfaces. Notice the downward pull of gravity in those places and sense the upward push of those supports. Notice how you assess the qualities of those supportive surfaces as experienced through your body. Next, feel the surface of your body; the weight, texture and constriction or looseness of your clothing. Then, feel the surfaces that are open to the surrounding air. Feel the temperature, the relative humidity, the movement of air around your body, and the ambience of the space. Next, go inside and focus into a part of your body that feels uncomfortable, pleasurable, or perhaps empty or numb. Carefully map out that area, notice the dimensions and layers of sensations or their lack . . . their intensity, rhythm, and direction. Notice how different types of sensation seem to arise and fade away. Notice that a part of your mind is able to keep track of any changes even as another part just monitors what is happening. Pause . . . Notice how you are now relating to this part of your body. What has changed? Take some time to feel any overall changes that have occurred in your body and mind. . . . Keeping your eyes closed, expand your attention to monitor what is happening outside your body: What do you hear, smell, or feel? Notice that what is occurring around you is mirrored by sensations you can feel inside. . . . Next open your eyes softly and notice what you feel inside as you observe spatial relationships and patterns and rest your eyes on the objects around you. . . . Then start to reexplore the object or person's body you were exploring before. Ask yourself some basic questions: What do I feel inside myself as I explore it? What can I feel from its surface? What kind of internal relationships can I feel in it? How is it affected by my exploration? After you have done this for sufficient time to feel complete, take a little time to sense inside your body and ask yourself, "How have I been affected by this experience?"[7]

---

and movement?" Passage through the linear rays of gravity triggers neurologic responses that contribute toward proprioception. This interactive device is deceptively simple . . . to apply it continually and with great specificity requires years of practice. What

BOX 19-4 **Exercise in Feeling the Weight**

Sit or stand comfortably and close your eyes. Now, keeping your upper arms comfortably close to your torso, raise your hands and forearms just enough so that you can feel the weight of your hands. Notice that as soon as you think of weight you will start to move your hands and forearms. That is because weight is a relationship between mass and gravity. You must move something through the lines of force of gravity in order to feel the weight. Notice the amount of "efforting" you are experiencing in your upper arms and shoulders. Notice also that as you focus into your palms and move them you feel a sense of warmth, tingling, and puffiness in your hands. If you don't feel these responses at first, try resting the weight of your hands and forearms on a comfortable surface like a pillow or massage table and then weigh your hands with the least possible effort. Next, weigh and explore three progressively smaller and lighter *imaginary* objects in your hands: a rock, a coin, and a small feather. Monitor the sensations your body-mind creates as you explore these imaginary objects and measure such things as weight, shape, texture, temperature, hardness, heft. Notice that as you explore these objects your hands and mind become more and more linked and that you become more acutely aware of fine sensations and the space around you. Next return your hands to your lap and notice how you feel inside. Bring your awareness into different parts of your body and notice that if you move that part slowly, you also become aware of the subtle sensations of gravity in that body part. Awareness of the subtle sensations directly affects your perception of other sensations. Notice that if you move very slowly it intensifies the subtle sensations from a feeling of effervescence to sparkles. Notice also that you are able to perceive sensation anywhere you put your attention including the space around you. Pause . . . take time to feel any changes in your body and overall awareness. Remind yourself that the potential for this shift in feeling and awareness exists in all persons at all times and that it is communicable. You can pass this same kind of feeling on to your clients . . . pause during the session, remove your hands, step back and weigh them, shift into hook-up, and then resume the session (Figure 19-12).

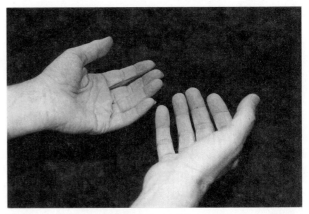

FIGURE 19-12 Soft "weighing hands" become warm, puffy, and highly sensitive. (*Trager:* Mentastics®: Movement as a way to agelessness, Barrytown, 1987, Station Hill Press.)

Hookup Summarized

Milton Trager opened a doorway in manual practices that can possibly alter the way we all work. His emphasis upon maintaining and sharing this state of awareness is the goal of the *Trager* approach and offering simple body-centered devices to achieve hook-up that were crucial contributions to his approach. The practice of hook-up or presence in the *Trager* approach can offer a wholly different way of perceiving our relationships with our clients. In presence everything is interrelated. There is no separation of phenomena from phenomena, distance from distance, or mind from mind. The end of separation is unity consciousness in which all time, all thought, all experiences, and all places are one interrelated continuum.

GENERAL PHILOSOPHY

Perhaps the most important three ingredients of the *Trager* approach are movement, awareness of feeling and sensation, and a focus on changing the mind of the client. The practitioner wants to create a new set of feeling experiences in the client through gentle, guided movement. There is an underlying assumption that everything that takes place in the body is reflected in the mind and vice versa. We can describe the mind as a continuum of awareness that is distributed throughout the body down to the cellular level, physically linked through neural, chemical, and electromagnetic transmitters. Although we often regard the body and mind as separate entities, they are one soma or functional unit.

Our conscious mind is only selectively aware of this two-directional communications link. For example, when we experience fear we can observe a cycle of sensations produced by the effects of the sympathetic response in our body. Through conscious monitoring,

is happening here? Measuring gravitational effects is a form of communion with this universal force of attraction and cohesiveness. The practitioner tracks the client's body response to increasing/decreasing weight and movement. Continuous weighing opens the door of presence because weight can only be felt in the moment. Opening the door of the *continuous now* gives us access to the gifts of presence mentioned above.

we can become aware of sensations related to processes controlled by the autonomic nervous system, such as the breath and heart rate. We also can monitor the amount of effort involved in voluntary and involuntary muscle movement. However, in most daily situations we pay little focused attention to these informational pathways.

What Trager proposed is that the body is replicated exactly in the unconscious mind that also contains stored memories. He further postulated that, in general, most clients are unaware of their pain-induced resistance patterns to movement as well as most of their bodily healing processes. For example: a person experiences an injury with accompanying trauma, pain, and other perceptions. In order to continue functioning without reinjury and in order to avoid feeling more pain, the mind automatically and unconsciously splints the region, emotionally through selective forgetting and physically through neuromuscular guarding. The mind buries the traumatic emotional material in obscure memory vaults. Both these responses are automatic and not consciously directed. We can think of these responses respectively as splinting or guarding, and numbing or avoiding the pain. The results often appear as deep-seated physical limitation and mental agitation. Trager recalled an incident that happened to him while he was interning in 1955.

It may be of interest that Trager's conjectures relating to tissue memory have also been observed and discussed by physiologists such as Speransky[11] and Selye[12] and by leading osteopathic researchers such as Korr[13] and Becker.[14]

Trager maintained that the unconscious mind holds a permanent record of *all* bodily transmitted experiences. Restimulation of this unconscious material can cause it to surface or become conscious again. The practitioner, through gentle, pleasurable movement, is introducing new information to the area of the unconscious mind associated with that part of the body. When the client feels these new pleasurable sensations in an area that has a stored record of trauma, his/her mind has the option of selecting this data over the old. This is a gentle and nurturing way of working with traumatic material, the obverse of using painful pressure to release emotionally based holding patterns. During the session the practitioner reinforces this selection by calling attention to the experience so that the client becomes consciously aware of the new sensations (Figure 19-13).

The enjoyable sensations in the body, imparted by the movement, become the medium for reaching or changing the mind of the client. The phrase *Psychophysical Integration* properly refers to the change of mind as the

EARLY *TRAGER* EXPERIENCE: ANESTHESIA

I was assigned to do a history and physical examination on a very stiff 75-year-old man who was to have surgery the next day. He was so rigid and tense that if he wanted to turn his head he would have to turn his whole body. I assisted in the surgery and when it was time to turn him on his side to do an additional small surgical procedure, it took seven of us to change his position. He didn't weigh that much, but he was so limp he would have fallen apart. Following surgery… I had to watch him while he recovered from the anesthetic. It was interesting to observe what went on as he slowly came to himself. By degrees his body returned to his original pattern of stiffness. Observing this I realized that the aging process is not just tissue involvement. What I had witnessed told me that we are the sum total of all the adverse happenings in our lives which cause these phenomena. . . . I am convinced that for every physical nonyielding condition there is a psychic counterpart in the unconscious mind to the degree of the physical manifestations.[10]

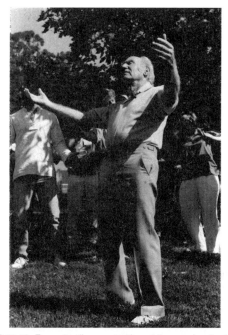

FIGURE 19-13 Trager leading mentastics while experiencing hook-up. (*Trager:* Mentastics®: Movement as a way to agelessness, Barrytown, 1987, Station Hill Press.)

objective in the therapeutic process in *Trager*. The client is intentionally guided to integrate the new information. Client example: "I thought this shoulder could not move in this way without pain. Now that I feel it moving and bringing me pleasurable sensations, I have another option." At this point the practitioner can reinforce this new awareness by teaching appropriate *Mentastics* to the client. Fine-tuning these gentle and pleasurable movements allows the client to reproduce the sensations he/she experienced on the table. Only this time the client initiates the movements rather than experiencing them passively. This completes the cycle of movement reeducation by affirming to the client that he/she can move with less pain and restriction. The more the client practices the movements the more freedom he/she develops. This is a similar process of reeducation to that used in Feldenkrais except that in *Trager* the emphasis is on using momentum and gravity in dancelike movements to create a feeling of effortlessness. Close monitoring of the ease of these movements is the motive force for change. In Feldenkrais the mind becomes more aware by carefully measuring the effort it takes to move the body. Positive change happens as a result of consciously refining movements based upon what produces more ease.[15]

CHAPTER SUMMARY

Physiologic and psychologic holding patterns are reactions to pain directed by the unconscious mind. Ordinarily these holding patterns are released as the body heals itself. Pathology can be thought of as an interruption or delay in this healing process. Body sensations provide a pathway into this unconscious holding. The *Trager* practitioner imparts new pleasurable sensations to reach and change the unconscious mind. Recall and reinforcement anchor these changes. During the table-work the practitioner does this verbally. After the table-work the practitioner teaches appropriate *Mentastics* movements to the client to further reinforce these changes.

The practitioner who is aware of the sensations in his/her own body in presence can induce the same kind of awareness in the client with the least amount of effort. Mental presence or "hook-up" in the practitioner imparts the same to the client.[16] The intent of the *Trager* approach is to enable the client to release unconscious physical and mental limitations or holding patterns. The work promotes deep relaxation and helps to increase physical mobility and mental clarity.

The principles that underlie the *Trager* approach are sometimes contradictory and paradoxical. The body is seen as a vehicle of communication in an exchange of information between practitioner and client. The practitioner asks questions through touch and movement. The client responds reflexively and those responses are mirrored and expanded to another set of questions by subtle changes or iterations in direction and pressure by the practitioner. As communication ensues, holding patterns or past conditioning, like tissue-stored memories, float to the surface similar to the way that rocks and boulders are buoyed to the surface by the lateral shifting of the earth. As these obstacles are gently coaxed to the surface, the pleasurable sensations of the movement are offered to replace the discomfort of the blocks. The general rule of thumb is that when resistance of any kind is felt, the practitioner responds by doing less. Doing less is a subtle beckoning for the client's unconscious to release more.

CASE HISTORY

In a session the author starts to explore the right arm of the client. "First I just hold the lower arm, feeling the weight and noticing the responses in the tissue as I weigh the arm in different positions. A change in weight signifies to me some kind of change in the connective tissue. I notice that as I pronate the forearm it feels lighter as I weigh it, and then drop-and-catch. Next I move my left hand so that it is supporting the arm under the elbow, and repeat the movements as described above, feeling the connective tissue responses in and around the elbow. I feel tautness in the thumb extensor and in the lower triceps. I palpate those attachments as I rotate the lower arm and elbow into different positions. I find a spot where there seems to be equal tautness in all directions; I gently hold that position and ask the client how that feels. She responds with a sigh. "I feel a big sense of relief." I immediately feel a release of the tautness in the connective tissue and proceed to more dropping and catching. All of a sudden there is a delightful freedom in the forearm, wrist, and hand, and the client can feel the change. I then proceed to do a similar kind of questioning of the upper arm, focusing on the freedom of movement, with and without support, under the shoulder joint. After freeing up the upper arm and shoulder joint, I proceed to the shoulder girdle, and its relation to the rib cage and sternoclavicular joint, combining movement, compression, distraction, and holding. When all segments have been explored in this way, I then create some complex movements that affirm, for the client and myself, the quality of movement available. Then finding that there is still some tautness in the thumb extensor, I check the thumb for movement and find some crepitus at its base. I support the forearm by holding the soft tissue of the flexors with my left hand, and then with my right hand holding the palm and back of her hand between my thumb and pads of fingers, I give her hand a rapid fluttering movement with my right hand, while palpating the extensors and flexors with my left. . . . The thumb flutters freely. . . . I continue until I feel a release in the thumb extensor. I then hold the thumb and wrist with both of my hands and then check the movement of the thumb. Once again there seems to be one position where there is a slight tautness in both directions. I hold the thumb and wrist in that position and ask the client to notice what she feels. She sighs again and says, "It feels so good. . . . It's hard to describe." I feel a slight reflexive tremor and then a release of all the tautness. I check the thumb for crepitus and find none. I ask the client to take some time to feel down into her arm and store away the feeling she has. After the tablework I teach her some Mentastics® movements so that she can replicate the feeling on her own." (Author session narrative, 2003)[5]

SUGGESTED READINGS

Calais-Germain B: *Anatomy of movement*, Seattle, 1993, Eastland Press.

Gendlin E: *Focusing oriented psychotherapy*, New York, 1996, Guilford Press.

Hanna T: *The body of life*, Rochester, VT, 1993, Healing Arts Press.

Hanna T: What is Somatics? In Johnson D, ed: *Bone breath and gesture*, Berkeley, Calif, 1995, North Atlantic Books.

Juhan D: *Job's body*, Barrytown, NY, 2003, Station Hill Press.

Liskin J: *Moving medicine: the life and work of Milton Trager*, Barrytown, NY, 1996, Station Hill Press.

Meyers T: *Anatomy trains*, New York, 2001, Churchill Livingstone.

Savage F: *Osteoarthritis: a step by step success story to show others they can help themselves*, Barrytown, NY, 1990, Station Hill Press.

Trager M, Guadagno C: *Trager Mentastics: movement as a way to agelessness*, Barrytown, NY, 1987, Station Hill Press.

RESOURCES

Trager International website
www.trager.com

United States *Trager* Association
Trainings, articles, requirements, membership
13801 W Center Street, Suite 3, PO Box 1009
Burton, Ohio 44021
440-834-0308, 440-834-0365 FAX
website:www.tragerus.org

REFERENCES

1. Liskin JH: *Moving medicine: the life and work of Milton Trager*, Barrytown, NY, 1996, Station Hill Press.
2. Waltrous I: The *Trager* approach: an effective tool for physical therapy, *Physical Therapy Forum* 72:22-25, 1992.
3. Blackburn J: Trager®—psychophysical integration—an overview, *Journal of Bodywork and Movement Therapies* 8:114-121, 2004.
4. Blackburn J: Trager® 2: hooking up: the power of presence in bodywork, *Journal of Bodywork and Movement Therapies* 8:114-121, 2004.
5. Blackburn J: *Trager*: at the table, *Journal of Bodywork and Movement Therapies*, 8:178-188, 2004.
6. Witt P: *Trager* psychophysical integration: an additional tool in the treatment of chronic spinal pain and dysfunction, *Whirlpool* 9:24-26, 1986.
7. Blackburn J: *Trager*: Mentastics®— presence in motion, *Journal of Bodywork and Movement Therapies* 8:265-277, 2004.
8. Juhan D: *The physiology of hook-up: how Trager® works*, Valley, Calif, 1993, The Trager Institute Mill.
9. Trager M, Guadagno C: *Trager Mentastics: movement as a way to agelessness*, Barrytown, NY, 1987, Station Hill Press.
10. Trager M: *Trager* psychophysical integration and Mentastics, *The Trager Journal* 1:5-9, 1982.
11. Speransky AD: *A basis for the theory of medicine*, New York, 1944, International Publishers.
12. Selye H: *The stress of life*, New York, 1976, McGraw-Hill.
13. Korr M: Somatic dysfunction osteopathic manipulative treatment and the nervous system: a few facts, some theories and many questions, *J Am Osteopath Assoc* 86:109-l14, 1986.
14. Becker A: Parameters of resistance, *J Am Osteopath Assoc* 73:38-51, 1973.
15. Feldenkrais M: *Awareness through movement*, New York, 1972, Harper and Row.
16. Blackburn J, Price C: Further implications of presence in the manual therapies, *Journal of Bodywork and Movement Therapies* 11:68-77, 2007.

1) What is hook-up?
   a) a hand position with tautness in both directions
   b) a state of presence that is shared with a client
   c) a way of connecting with the client's tissue so that there is no slipping
   d) client's way of noticing her postural position on the table

2) What is *Mentastics*?
   a) a series of mental puzzles to test body awareness
   b) a framework for assessing client body-mind connection
   c) a theory of homeostasis that originated in the twentieth century
   d) a series of movements involving mental and visceral awareness

3) Identify the principles that guide a *Trager* practitioner at the table:
   a) "When you meet resistance, do less."
   b) "No gain with pain."
   c) working with weight
   d) all of the above

4) What is the relationship of client pain to the *Trager* approach?
   a) Pain is a tool for working through the resistance.
   b) Pain should be released if possible before the session is over.
   c) The client's painful symptoms guide the practitioner through the session.
   d) The practitioner keeps the movements within the range that produces no added pain.

5) Which is not one of the three assessment tools used by *Trager* practitioners?
   a) tissue tonus
   b) quality of movement
   c) pain assessment on a scale of 1 to 10
   d) amount of client somatic awareness

6) At what age did Milton Trager start working with clients?
   a) 5 years
   b) 19 years
   c) 35 years
   d) 65 years

7) From Milton Trager's perspective, what role does the unconscious mind play in perpetuating symptoms?
   a) The client needs to become aware of unconscious psychological material before healing can be complete.
   b) The unconscious mind is a repository for traumatic situations that result in movement restrictions.
   c) The unconscious mind of the practitioner can block the awareness of certain solutions to the client's symptoms.
   d) The client and practitioner may have unconscious material in their relationship that must be resolved.

8) Reinforcement and recall apply to what portions of *Trager* sessions?
   a) intake
   b) tablework
   c) off of the table
   d) all of the above

9) What is meant by "psychophysical integration"?
   a) Various psychological theories current in the mid-twentieth century have proven the effects of the unconscious mind.
   b) The real change takes place in the mind of the client and therefore the practitioner addresses the session toward changing the client's mind.
   c) We must be very careful when working with clients so that we do not trigger unconscious emotional material.
   d) When a client has memories surface during the session, it is the practitioner's job to help the client address those issues in therapy.

10) Which is not a principle of *Mentastics*?
   a) Movement can be freeing if we push beyond our limits.
   b) The simplest movements when performed with awareness can produce the greatest results.
   c) What is half of that . . . and what is half of that?
   d) Pause and feel down into your body.

11) Which is not one of three forms of ongoing physical assessment used by *Trager* practitioners?
   a) client's quality of movement
   b) Swedish gymnastics
   c) tissue tonus
   d) client's subjective experience

12) Identify the *Trager* tablework principles:
   a) releasing trigger points and reassessing
   b) using hot packs before working painful areas
   c) listening hands
   d) isometric exercises to reinforce muscle adaptation

13) Which is not a benefit of working with hook-up (presencing)?
   a) practitioner can head off emotional releases of the client before they happen
   b) no separation of phenomena from phenomena, distance from distance, or mind from mind
   c) experience of unity consciousness
   d) a different way of perceiving our client relationships

14) Proprioceptive awareness includes all of the following except
   a) feeling the weight of your own body part
   b) feeling of pain in your shoulder
   c) feeling tightness in your hands and feet
   d) feeling movement along your spine as with pelvic motion

15) Which of these statements is true?
   a) Milton Trager strongly influenced twentieth century medicine.
   b) *Trager* works best when the client sleeps during the session.
   c) The *Trager* practitioner rarely speaks during a session.
   d) *Trager* sessions may include torqueing, traction, compression, weighing, and verbal interaction.

16) Which one of these quotes is false?
   a) "When you're creating pain you are not doing *Trager*."
   b) "The session is not over until the symptoms are gone."
   c) "When you find resistance do less."
   d) "It's like the feeling of . . . well . . . nothingness."

17) Why is pausing important?
   a) It allows the client to feel the changes that are happening.
   b) It gives the practitioner an opportunity to return to presence.
   c) The practitioner comes back in with less preconditioning.
   d) all of the above

18) Which statement about the use of soft hands in *Trager* is false?
   a) Preset hand muscular or movement patterns are not present in the practitioner's hands.
   b) Soft hands prevent the triggering of emotional responses in the client.
   c) Soft hands can be more responsive to the client's tissue.
   d) Soft hands can receive and send subtle information.

19) Milton Trager's conception of the unconscious mind includes all except
   a) holds a permanent record of *all* bodily transmitted experiences
   b) restimulation of unconscious material can cause it to surface or become conscious again
   c) gentle touch and movement are the obverse of using painful pressure to release emotionally based holding patterns
   d) a repository of repressed desires, childhood issues, guilt, and shame

20) Which statement does not reflect an experience of hook-up or presencing?
   a) The practitioner feels spacey, high, and free from any kind of body sensations.
   b) a deep sense of peace, assurance, and connection with the client and the surrounding environment
   c) The mind is clear and perceptive, able to discern very small increments of information.
   d) The practitioner's hands and the whole body can feel like they are filled with a subtle effervescence.

Trigger Point Release

Judith DeLany

20

Without question, pain is a driving force in the lives of many people. It negatively impacts the quality of life and the ability to work, concentrate, exercise, sleep, and to enjoy family and friends. Albert Schweitzer,[1] noted recipient in 1952 of the Nobel Peace Prize, aptly stated, "Pain is a more terrible lord of mankind than even death himself."

Regarding chronic pain, Kathryn Weiner, as director of the American Academy of Pain Management, shares some staggering figures[2]:

- Each year an estimated 50 million people in the United States alone suffer with chronic pain.
- In 1999, 4.9 million individuals saw a physician for chronic pain.[3]
- Four out of 10 people suffering moderate to severe pain were unable to find adequate pain relief.[4]

Efforts to diagnose the root cause of a person's chronic pain can be extensive since there are many sources of pain in the human body, including muscles, joints, and organs. There exists a multitude of standard medical tests, copious treatments, and numerous over-the-counter and prescription medications for chronic pain. One pervasive source of acute and chronic pain that is often overlooked in standard health care is a **myofascial trigger point,** a tender, hyperirritable spot within a muscle that, when provoked, refers pain and other sensations to a (fairly predictable) **target zone**[5]

(Figure 20-1). The associated target zone is usually peripheral to the **trigger point**, can sometimes be central to the trigger point, and is rarely in the same location as the trigger point. This chapter will consider trigger points, a variety of causes for their formation, and a number of treatment choices.

■ ■ ■ ■ IN MY EXPERIENCE

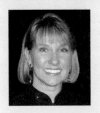

My personal and professional experience has taught me that it is valuable to consider the following:

- Many conditions masquerade as myofascial pain when a more serious, sometimes sinister condition is the primary cause. The most important skill a practitioner can have is to be able to recognize when and to whom to refer a person for further evaluation.
- A person can have more than one condition contributing to the symptom picture. For instance, it is entirely possible to find an abundance of hypertonic muscles and a number of trigger points that contribute to low back pain. A thorough search for additional trigger points that refer the same or similar patterns, as well as an evaluation of perpetuating factors, may yield a significant result. Additionally, there could also be zygapophyseal joint (articular process of a vertebra) involvement, a herniated or prolapsed disk, or kidney stones presenting alongside the myofascial syndrome.
- If the practitioner will ask the right questions and actively listen to the answers, the person will usually report more than enough clues to allow the practitioner to discern the cause of the problem. Rarely is chronic pain "all in the head," although there may certainly be central nervous system factors.
- The "thick file" chronic pain patient who has "been everywhere else" is one of the most exciting cases to see, although it is easy to be intimidated by cases that have already been reviewed by a number of "experts." In these cases, serious causes have usually been ruled out or treated, and trigger points have most likely been ignored. The practitioner with excellent trigger point treatment skills will often have success with those people where traditional medicine has failed to achieve satisfactory results.

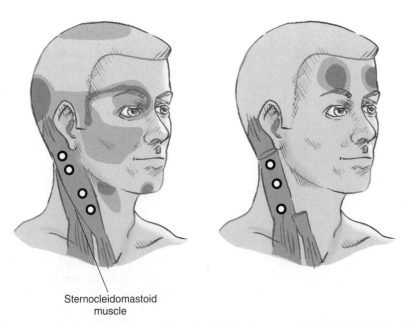

Sternocleidomastoid
muscle

FIGURE 20-1 Trigger points in sternocleidomastoid display a wide variety of referred symptoms, including facial and head pain as indicated, visual disturbances, ear pain, hearing loss, and disturbances in orientation. (From Chaitow L, DeLany J: *Clinical application of neuromuscular techniques,* vol 1, ed 2. *The upper body,* Edinburgh, 2008, Churchill Livingstone. Referred pattern is drawn after Simons et al, 1999.)

TRIGGER POINTS: A COMMON CAUSE OF PAIN

Trigger point release, as this chapter is titled, is not actually a modality. It is not a single or specific technique nor is it a particular application. Rather, it is a goal that many modalities and techniques strive to achieve. To release, or deactivate, a trigger point is to remove its ability to produce its referred sensation (often debilitating pain) and to improve the elements of soft tissue dysfunction that are associated with it.

In their original work, Travell and Simons[6] estimated that around 75% of pain clinic patients have a trigger point as the sole source of their pain. They note that trigger points often mimic carpal tunnel syndrome, tendonitis, bursitis, angina pectoris, sciatica, frozen shoulder, arthritis, and a plethora of other conditions.

The following research offers support in showing an all-too-common occurrence of trigger points.

- Two hundred asymptomatic Air Force recruits (ages 17 to 35) demonstrated trigger points in 54% of 100 females and 45% of 100 males tested.[7]
- They are often found in the upper trapezius (Figure 20-2) and quadratus lumborum[8] (Figure 20-3).
- A latent trigger point in the third finger extensor has been reported as possibly being more common.[5]

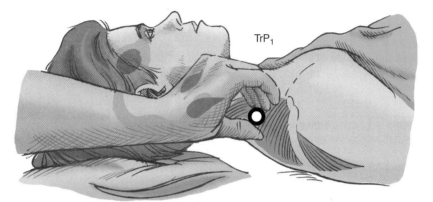

FIGURE 20-2 The outermost fibers of upper trapezius provoke intense referral patterns, particularly into the eye region. (From Chaitow L, DeLany J: *Clinical application of neuromuscular techniques,* vol 1, ed 2. *The upper body,* Edinburgh, 2008, Churchill Livingstone. Referred pattern is drawn after Simons et al, 1999.)

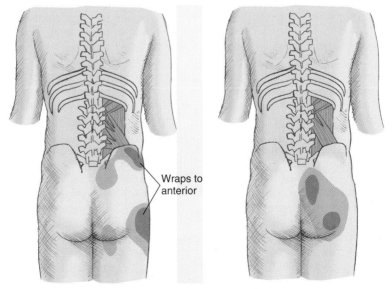

FIGURE 20-3 Quadratus lumborum trigger points refer into SI joint, lower buttocks, and wrap laterally along the iliac crest and hip region. A referral pattern into the lower abdominal region is not illustrated. (From Chaitow L, DeLany J: *Clinical application of neuromuscular techniques,* vol 1. *The lower body,* Edinburgh, 2002, Churchill Livingstone. Composite drawn after Travell and Simons, 1992, Fig 4.1 A-C. Williams & Wilkins.)

- Incidence of primary myofascial syndromes noted in 85% of 283 consecutive chronic pain patients[9] and 55% of 164 chronic head/neck pain patients.[10]

Practitioners who have the skill to successfully address trigger points and their associated soft tissue dysfunctions will not likely have a shortage of people to treat. The ability to explain these concepts to other health care practitioners and those people who may benefit from treatment will help to ensure a successful and rewarding clinical practice.

HISTORY OF TRIGGER POINT RELEASE

While most of the information currently considered as the foundational principles of trigger point formation and treatment has been developed in the last half century, referred pain from myofascial tissues, palpable myofascial nodules, and taut bands has been discussed in academic papers for much longer. Box 20-1 contains a historical summary of some of the most significant people whose work has influenced the modern concepts of trigger point therapies. Although this list is not comprehensive by any means and only covers the most prominent articles in the last 150 years, one can readily notice that the inquiry into the phenomenon of referred pain is multinational and multidisciplinary.

Although the list of all contributors to the current methods of trigger point treatment is far too great to contain in this chapter, two names are synonymous with trigger points in the United States and worldwide. American physicians Janet Travell and David Simons are responsible for the most detailed and definitive work[5,6,11] that built the current understanding of trigger points, thereby allowing a number of other pioneers to take diverse paths based on their foundational work.

BOX 20-1 Historical Discussions Regarding Chronic Referred Muscle Pain*

The following is a collection of some of the most prominent academic papers on what appears to be similar to if not the same condition as what is currently diagnosed as trigger points.

- F Valleix, 1841, in his *Treatise on Neuralgia* noted that when certain painful points were palpated they produced shooting pain to other regions *(neuralgia)*. He also reported that diet was a precipitating factor in the development of the painful aching symptoms of the back and cervical region.
- Johan Mezger, mid-19th century Dutch physician, developed massage techniques for treating "nodules" and taut cordlike bands associated with this condition.
- Uno Helleday, 1876 Swedish physician, described nodules as part of "chronic myitis."
- H Strauss, 1898 German physician, distinguished between palpable nodules and "bands."
- I Adler, 1900, identified clinical phenomena characteristic of MTrPs as muscular rheumatism.
- A Cornelius, 1903 German physician, demonstrated the pain-influencing features of tender points and nodules, insisting that the radiating pathway was not determined by the course of nerves, discussed it as possibly being due to *reflex mechanisms,* and showed that external influences (climatic, emotions, physical exertion) could exacerbate the already hyperreactive neural structures associated with these conditions.

- W Telling, 1911, called the condition *"nodular fibromyositis."*
- M Lange, 1931, wrote the first trigger point manual.
- J Edeiken, C Wolferth, 1936, showed that pressure applied to tender points in scapula region muscles could reproduce shoulder pain already being experienced. This work influenced Janet Travell (see below).
- Sir Thomas Lewis, 1938, a major researcher into the phenomenon of pain in general, charted several patterns of pain referral and suggested that Kellgren (see below), who assisted him in these studies, continue the research.
- J Kellgren, 1938, identified many of the features of our current understanding of the trigger point phenomenon, including consistent patterns of pain referral to distant muscles and other structures (teeth, bone, etc.) from pain points ("spots") in muscle, ligament, tendon, joint, and periosteal tissue—which could be obliterated by use of novocaine injections.
- A Reichart, 1938, physician who identified and charted patterns of distribution of *reflex pain* from tender points (nodules) in particular muscles.
- M Gutstein, 1938, refugee Polish physician working in Britain who identified that in treating *muscular rheumatism,* manual pressure applied to tender (later called "trigger") points produced both local and referred symptoms and that these referral patterns were consistent in everyone if the original point was in the same location. He deactivated these by means of injection.

*More extensive list and complete citations provided in Chaitow L, DeLany J: *Clinical application of neuromuscular techniques,* vol 1, ed 2. *The upper body,* Edinburgh, 2008, Elsevier.

BOX 20-1 Historical Discussions Regarding Chronic Referred Muscle Pain*—cont'd

- A Steindler, 1940, American orthopedic surgeon who demonstrated that novocaine injections into tender points located in the low back and gluteal regions could relieve sciatic pain. He called these points "trigger points." Janet Travell (see below) was influenced by his work and popularized the term *trigger points*.
- J Mennell, 1952, British physician described "sensitive areas" that referred pain and recommended treatment was a choice between manipulation, heat, pressure, and deep friction. He also emphasized the importance of diet, fluid intake, rest, the possible use of cold, and procaine injections as well as suggesting cupping, skin rolling, massage, and stretching to normalize "*fibrositic deposits.*"
- J Travell, S Rinzler, 1952, building on previous research and following their own detailed studies of the tissues involved, coined the word "myofascial," adding it to Steindler's term to produce "myofascial trigger points" and finally "*myofascial pain syndrome.*" This paper introduced referral patterns for 32 muscles.
- R Nimmo, 1957, following many years of research that paralleled chronologically that of Travell, this chiropractor, along with James Vannerson, described his concept of "receptor-tonus technique," involving virtually the same mechanisms as those eventually described by Travell and Simons in 1983 but with more emphasis on manual techniques.
- Janet Travell, David Simons, 1983, published *Myofascial pain and dysfunction: the trigger point manual,* volume 1, *the upper half of body,* which, along with its companion volume, became the definitive work on the subject of *myofascial pain syndrome* (MPS).
- K Lewit, D Simons, 1984, Czech neurologist Lewit described his simple manual treatment of MTrPs and later emphasized

joint dysfunction in MTrPs with suggestions as to joint mobilization and developed valuable concepts of chains of MTrPs.
- David Simons, 1986, American physician who collaborated with Travell in joint study of MPS also conducted his own studies into the connection between *myofascial pain syndrome* and *fibromyalgia syndrome,* finding a good deal of overlap.
- M Margoles, 1989, states that most patients with *fibromyalgia* demonstrate numerous active myofascial trigger points.
- R Bennett, 1990, suggests that many "tender points" in *fibromyalgia* are in reality latent trigger points. He believes that MPS and FMS are distinctive syndromes but are "closely related" and states that many people with MPS progress on to develop fibromyalgia.
- C-Z Hong, 1994, this physiatrist pioneered studies focusing on identifying taut bands of MTrPs.
- R Gerwin, S Shannon, C-Z Hong, D Hubbard, R Gevirtz, 1997, showed that interrater reliability of locating and identifying trigger points was improved with training, thereby establishing greater reliability of the physical examination for myofascial pain syndrome that is associated with trigger points.
- D Simons, J Travell, L Simons, 1999, published a second edition of volume 1 of their textbook, with emphasis on significant research conducted in the 15 years since the first edition, which altered the foundational platform of trigger point theories and treatment.
- J Shaw, T Phillips, J Danoff, L Gerber, 2003, revealed that higher concentrations of certain chemicals including substance P, calcitonin gene-related peptide (CGRP), bradykinin, norepinephrine, and others are present at the nidus of trigger points when compared with normal tissue.

Janet G. Travell, MD (1901-1997)

Dr. Janet G. Travell is usually recognized as the leading pioneer in the development of methods of diagnosis and treatment of myofascial trigger points. Although she did not single-handedly "create" this branch of medicine, her contributions through a half-century of life work were so enormous that many give her full credit. Although she used massage techniques and manual examination of the muscles as part of her work, the primary concepts for which she is remembered are dry needling and injection of trigger points as well as spray and stretch techniques.[5,6,11] Her dedicated effort to document her work and validate her theories was mirrored by her great passion to teach others, through her writings and lectures.

Travell's career as a physician was punctuated by many achievements. Among them was to serve as the first female Personal Physician to the President of the United States, which she did for President John F. Kennedy and for President Lyndon B. Johnson.[12] She published papers extensively between 1942 and 1990 while simultaneously co-authoring (with David Simons) the monumental textbooks, *Myofascial Pain and Dysfunction: The Trigger Point Manual,* Volume 1, *The Upper Body*[5,6] and its companion volume for the lower body.[11] The introduction of the term *myofascial pain syndrome*[13] pointed toward focal hyperirritable spots in muscles that strongly modulate central nervous system functions and the resultant collection of symptoms that these produce.

In addition to her medical career, this extraordinary woman was also a wife, mother, teacher, scientific investigator, author, and poet. Dr. Travell's own account of her inspiring life, as well as samples of her poetry and family letters, can be found in her autobiography, *Office Hours: Day and Night*.[12]

A number of teachers continue to train in the work developed by Travell, including Robert Gerwin, MD and Jan Dommerholt, PT, MPS, who together founded Myopain Seminars.[14] This postgraduate continuing education company has a distinct focus on myofascial pain syndromes and the treatment of trigger points with manual therapy and dry needling/injections.

David G. Simons, MD

Working alongside Dr. Travell for much of her life was another extraordinary person, Dr. David G. Simons. His life was equally fascinating, having started his medical career in aviation medicine after his completion of medical school in 1946. In 1957, then Air Force Major Simons set the world altitude record for a manned balloon flight. Featured on the cover of *Life* magazine[15] as the first man in the edge of outer space, his work demonstrated conclusive details regarding the threat of cosmic radiation as man ascended the atmosphere. Simons[16] subsequently wrote about his experiences in *Man High: A Space Scientist's Account of His Record Breaking Balloon Flight to 102,000 Feet*.

Dr. Simons was developing research programs in physical medicine and rehabilitation when he met Dr. Travell in 1963 as she lectured at the Air Force's School of Aerospace Medicine.[17] They soon united efforts to document trigger points, with the joint publication of their findings being enhanced by the synergistic relationship of these two dedicated doctors. It is certainly worth remembering that at the time their work was being compiled, the use of computers was "technology of the future," and the terms "cut and paste" still meant scissors and glue. The accumulation of data and the development of the manuscript for their textbooks was a laborious manual task that few today can even imagine.

In 2001, after 10 years of collaboration, Dr. Simons and co-author Professor Siegfried Mense published *Muscle Pain: Understanding its Nature, Diagnosis and Treatment*, ground-breaking for its integration of basic science neurophysiology principles with clinical practice.[18] With almost 200 publications to date and half of those concerning trigger points and chronic pain management, Simons most certainly has achieved international recognition as an authority in this field.

He currently serves as a clinical professor in the Rehabilitation Medicine department at Emory University and an adjunct professor at the University of St. Augustine for Health Sciences.

Bonnie Prudden

In the mid-1940s, noted rock climber and physical fitness expert Bonnie Prudden, using a fitness test devised by Drs. Hans Kraus and Sonja Weber, began testing children in Europe, Central America, and the United States. She noted a failure rate of 8% in Italy/Austria/Switzerland, 21% in Guatemala, and a substantially higher rate of 58% in the United States. Her report to President Eisenhower resulted in the development of the President's Council on Youth Fitness (now the President's Council on Physical Fitness and Sport), which made a significant impact on fitness awareness in the United States.[19]

Over the following years, Prudden wrote approximately two dozen books on physical fitness, produced a half dozen exercise albums, hosted the first regular exercise spots on national television as well as her own syndicated television show, and set up hundreds of exercise and fitness programs in a variety of settings including schools, hospitals, camps, factories, and prisons. Through these, she influenced exercise programs for babies, children, adults, and the elderly.

In 1980, Prudden published her book, *Pain Erasure: The Bonnie Prudden Way*, which detailed the use of manual pressure on trigger points to alleviate pain, based on the concepts of Travell's needling techniques.[20] The book offered self-help techniques for the person to use as well as treatment protocols for therapists. Although the book lacked detailed anatomy and gave little focus to perpetuating factors, it simplified trigger point treatment so that the nonprofessional could understand the concepts and helped trigger point therapy gain popularity with the public. Prudden taught her methods at her own School of Physical Fitness and Myotherapy. Today most of the students who attend her training typically seek employment in hospitals, doctors' and dentists' offices, or open their own pain clinics.

Nancy Shaw, a student of Prudden's as well as Travell's, encouraged myotherapists to form a myotherapy network. In 1995, at the request of Janet Travell,[21] the group adopted the name of "myofascial trigger point therapy" to denote their work, which, although showing roots in Prudden's myotherapy, also adopted Travell's perpetuating factors as a significant part of the treatment protocol. Today the National Association of Myofascial Trigger Point Therapists stands as a significant organization whose aim is to refine and promote manual treatment of TrPs.[22]

NMT: TRIGGER POINT APPLICATIONS FOR MASSAGE THERAPISTS

Between the mid-1930s and early 1940s, a European-style of neuromuscular techniques (NMT) first emerged in Great Britain, developed by the skillful hands of Stanley Lief and Boris Chaitow.[23] These cousins, trained in chiropractic and naturopathy, studied with teachers like Dewanchand Varma and Bernard Macfadden and integrated solid concepts of assessment and treatment steps for soft tissue dysfunction, with much of their focus on trigger points. Lief's world-famous health resort in Hertfordshire, England, presented them with a wide variety of conditions on which to test their theories and methods. Many osteopaths and naturopaths, including Peter Lief, Brian Youngs, Terry Moule, Leon Chaitow, and others, have taken part in the evolution and development of European neuromuscular techniques, which address trigger points as part of a soft tissue protocol.[23] Now taught widely in osteopathic and sports massage settings in Britain, NMT forms an elective module on the Bachelor of Science (BSc[Hons]) degree courses in Complementary Health Sciences at the University of Westminster, London, a program developed (in part) by Leon Chaitow, DO.

A few years later, across the ocean in America, Raymond Nimmo and James Vannerson first published their newsletter, *Receptor Tonus Techniques,* where they wrote of their experiences with what they termed "noxious nodules."[24] A step-by-step system incorporating **ischemic compression** (applied pressure to soft tissues) began to emerge. Eventually, several of Nimmo's students began teaching their own treatment protocols, based on Nimmo's work. Among these was Paul St. John, who developed his own system in the late 70s. In the mid-1980s, Judith DeLany (then Judith Walker) became St. John's first additional instructor of his method of neuromuscular therapy. She worked with St. John for 5 years (1984-89), where she assisted in the development of NMT techniques and protocols for massage therapy application. Their work together incorporated Nimmo's protocols and Travell and Simons' insights, with an emphasis on applied manual pressure as Prudden had discussed. In 1989, the two separated the work into two styles—NMT

St. John method and NMT American™ version. With both systems retaining a strong focus on Nimmo's original protocols and featuring significant focus on trigger points, both developers have significantly influenced his/her own particular method with unique insights and new techniques. A number of other teachers throughout the world have also developed their own systems of NMT based on the work of Chaitow, DeLany, and/or St. John.

In 1999, Clair Davies took a different route with Travell and Simons' extensive work and, through his book, *The Trigger Point Therapy Workbook: Your Self-Treatment Guide for Pain Relief,* simplified the concepts (even more so than Prudden) to make them accessible to the public.[25] His innovative methods of self-applied trigger point massage enable those in pain to help themselves and can be usefully incorporated by health care practitioners as an "easy to use" home care program.

In 2000, Leon Chaitow and Judith DeLany blended not only European and American NMT, but also osteopathic and massage principles, to produce the first set of comprehensive, anatomy-based, strongly referenced textbooks that use step-by-step massage-based protocols for the treatment of trigger points and myofascial pain. *Clinical Application of Neuromuscular Techniques,* Volume 1—*The Upper Body*[23,27] and its companion text for the lower body[26] integrate **trigger point pressure release** methods (precisely applied sustained pressure used to quiescent TrPs, formerly called ischemic compression) with other massage techniques. Alongside these, they offer positional release techniques, muscle energy techniques, regional anatomy, and substantial discussions regarding the physiology of the development of dysfunction in soft tissues. Additionally, over a decade of editorial services by each of them has made the peer-reviewed *Journal of Bodywork and Movement Therapies* (Elsevier) a showcase for manual technique applications in the treatment of trigger points.

While it is impossible to cover all of the advances that occurred during the last 60 years, one can readily see that many tools have emerged to contribute to the methodologies for assessing, treating, and preventing trigger points. Most treatment protocols are based on the practitioner's skill, anatomy knowledge, and precisely applied palpation. With a foothold planted in both traditional and complementary medicine, these techniques have long been commonplace in treatment rooms of massage therapy and are also now frequently used in occupational therapy, physical therapy, nursing, dentistry, chiropractic, osteopathic, and physical medicine clinics worldwide.

TRIGGER POINT RELEASE

To begin to understand trigger point release, the best place to start is by considering what constitutes a trigger point and how it forms. Many of the details regarding trigger points remain to be finitely defined by research. However, the current "integrated hypothesis of trigger point formation" as discussed by Simons et al[5] provides a plausible explanation of their formation, is the current most widely accepted model, and is the foundation for much of the following discussion (Figure 20-4).

A myofascial trigger point (MTrP) is a localized area within a muscle that, when sufficiently provoked (by pressure, needling, etc.), produces a referred **paresthesia** (sensation) to a particular, moderately predictable target zone associated with that muscle. Although the referral pattern is usually pain, it can also be tingling, numbness, burning, itching, or other sensations. The trigger point will usually cause the host muscle to test as weak, produce a loss of range of motion of the joint(s) served by the host muscle, cause pain and weakness when the muscle housing it contracts, and may affect the synergist and antagonists of the host muscle. The muscles in the target zone of referral may also be affected (become excited) and they may form **satellite trigger points** that then have referred patterns of their own.

The underlying physical mechanisms that cause trigger points to form and those which perpetuate them are not yet fully understood. How trigger points produce various referred phenomena, and which structures are involved (neural, fascial, etc.) are areas of current and potential research and, often, a focus of heated debate and academic discussion.[18] While several theories exist,[27] most point to changes in local biochemistry within the tissues that house the trigger point. The following summation follows the concepts presented by Simons et al[5] in their integrated trigger point hypothesis and overviewed by Chaitow and DeLany.[27]

It is important to differentiate between a **contraction** (voluntary, with motor potentials), a **spasm** (involuntary, with motor potentials), and a **contracture** (involuntary, without motor potentials). The primary difference is that while contractions and spasms are produced and maintained by action potentials (neural transmissions from the spinal cord), a contracture is apparently sustained by abnormal chemistry at the point where the muscle fibers are innervated by the motor neuron—the **myoneural junction** or **motor point** of the muscle fiber.

Muscle tissue is intricately organized in order to efficiently deal with the production and use of energy in an effort to provide gross and fine movements throughout daily life (Figure 20-5). In normal movement, a number of chemically induced signals take place from the brain to the muscle and then back to the brain. These signals are used to assess, recruit, and provide substantial information to and from a multitude of sites, tissues, and receptors. The motor point endplate is the site of significant biochemical activity that allows the neuron (nerve) to signal the muscle fibers to shorten. Following a strain, overuse, or trauma, endplate activity alters, resulting from the presence of excessive calcium ions, which produces excessive

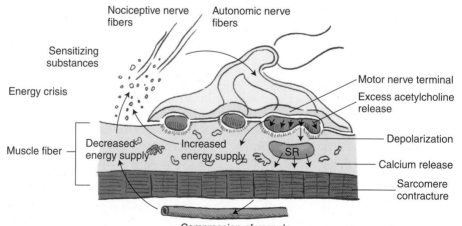

FIGURE 20-4 The integrated hypothesis of trigger point formation, as discussed by Simons et al, 1999, is based heavily on abnormal biochemistry associated with endplate dysfunction. SR - sacroplagmic reticulum. (From Chaitow L, DeLany J: *Clinical application of neuromuscular techniques, vol 1, ed 2. The upper body*, Edinburgh, 2008, Churchill Livingstone. Adapted from Simons et al, 1999.)

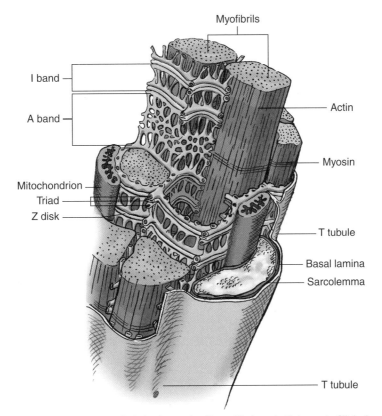

FIGURE 20-5 Details of the intricate organization of skeletal muscle. (From Chaitow L, DeLany J: *Clinical application of neuromuscular techniques,* vol 1, ed 2. *The upper body,* Edinburgh, 2008, Churchill Livingstone.)

release of a powerful neurotransmitter, **acetylcholine** (ACh). The continuous flow of ACh causes the actin and myosin filaments of the muscle fiber(s) to slide to a fully shortened position (a weakened state) in the immediate area around the motor endplate, which lies at the center of the fiber. Since the taut tissue compresses surrounding blood vessels, **ischemia** (lack of adequate blood) develops.

With reduced levels of blood arriving at the local tissues, cellular levels of oxygen and nutrient will also be reduced. Among the elements that are lacking are those that are used to produce adenosine triphosphate (ATP). ATP is the energy of the cell, and a lack of it produces a **local energy crisis.** That is, the body as a whole has adequate energy but the local tissues affected by the ischemia become deficient in ATP. Without available ATP, the local tissue is unable to remove the calcium ions that build up within the tissues, since this step requires **active transport,** a process that demands energy. The calcium-charged gates associated with ACh flow remain open, which allows continuous release

of ACh, thereby producing the contracture associated with the trigger point. Removing the superfluous calcium requires more energy than sustaining a contracture, so the contracture remains. The central sarcomeres shorten and form a contracture "knot." This knot is the "nodule" that is a palpable characteristic of a **central trigger point** (CTrP), one that has formed at the center of the fiber (Figure 20-6).

As the situation progresses, the remaining sarcomeres of that fiber (those that are not bunching) are being stretched. This produces the (usually palpable) taut band that is also a common trigger point characteristic. **Attachment trigger points** (ATrPs) may develop at the attachment sites (periosteal or myotendinous) of these shortened central sarcomeres. Persistent muscular tension provokes inflammation, fibrosis and, eventually, the deposition of calcium.

In addition to its location (central or attachment), a trigger point can be classified as to its state of activity (active or latent) as well as whether it is a primary, satellite, or key trigger point.

Trigger point complex

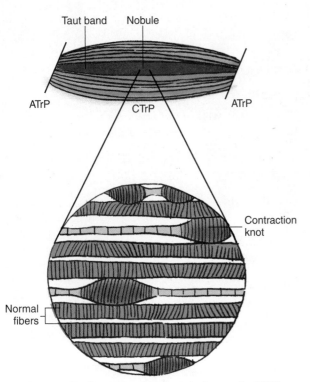

FIGURE 20-6 Tension produced by central trigger point (CTrP) can result in localized inflammatory response (attachment trigger point, ATrP). (From Chaitow L, DeLany J: *Clinical application of neuromuscular techniques,* vol 1, ed 2. *The upper body,* Edinburgh, 2008, Churchill Livingstone. Adapted from Simons et al, 1999.)

- An **active trigger point** refers a sensation to the target zone that the person recognizes as being (all or at least part of) the primary complaint. That is, when the trigger point is provoked the person experiences the pain, tingling, numbness, or other sensation(s) that have been aggravating him/her on a regular or constant basis.
- A **latent trigger point** has all of the same characteristics as an active trigger point, except that the person does not recognize the referral pattern as being a common complaint. The person will often be surprised when the sensation associated with a latent trigger point is provoked due to the fact that he/she has not ever, seldom, or at least for a long time, felt that sensation.
- A **primary trigger point** is an active trigger point that directly refers the sensation of which the person complains. In other words, it is primary to the person's paresthetic complaint. It should be borne in mind, however, that more than one trigger point could refer to the same region.

- A **satellite trigger point** is one that develops in the target zone of another trigger point. It is sustained by the referring trigger point. Satellite trigger points can also develop in the target zone of the satellite, thereby creating a "domino effect."
- A **key trigger point** is one that, when deactivated, also releases its associated satellite(s). In other words, it is the "key" to the chain and, until it is located and deactivated, attempts to eliminate the satellites will usually fail.

A latent trigger point can lie unnoticed and remain inactive for an indefinite period. Although activation usually occurs when the tissue is overused, strained by overload, or traumatized (as in a motor vehicle accident or a fall or blow), it can also be activated when the tissue housing it:

- is stretched or shortened (particularly abruptly)
- becomes overly chilled
- or when other perpetuating factors (poor nutrition, shallow breathing, hormonal imbalance, etc.) provide less than optimal conditions of health

TRP TREATMENT OPTIONS

It is important to note that there are two important steps to be taken in treatment of the trigger point—deactivation of the trigger point and elongation of the associated taut band. Deactivation can be achieved in a number of ways (discussed below). Elongation (stretching) of the tissues then follows in order to reset the appropriate relationship of the actin and myosin filaments. Prior to stretching, it is important to assess the condition of the attachment sites to avoid undue stress on any tissues that are already showing signs of inflammation. In other words, if attachment sites are moderately tender or if attachment trigger points exist, additional stress on these elements (through active or passive stretching) should be avoided. A more precise, manual elongation of the fibers housing the trigger point would be preferred (Figure 20-7).

A number of trigger point treatment options exist that can be used to deactivate the fibers housing a trigger point.[27] Among the most well known are:

- Trigger point pressure release (precisely applied sustained pressure)
- Chilling techniques (including spray and stretch technique, which uses a vapocoolant spray)
- Dry or wet needling (acupuncture, injection methods)
- Positional release methods
- Muscle energy techniques
- Myofascial release methods

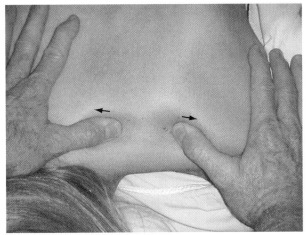

FIGURE 20-7 The thumbs, when gliding in opposite directions, provide precise traction of the central sarcomeres of the fibers and a local myofascial release. (From Chaitow L, DeLany J: *Clinical application of neuromuscular techniques,* vol 1, ed 2. *The upper body,* Edinburgh, 2008, Churchill Livingstone.)

It is also important to address additional factors that might include:

- Correction of associated osseous dysfunction, possibly involving high-velocity techniques (HVT) and/or other osteopathic/chiropractic mobilization methods
- Education to correct perpetuating factors (posture, hormonal, diet, stress, habits, etc.)
- Self-help strategies (stretching, hydrotherapies, changes in habits of use, etc.)

It is well beyond the scope of this text to describe each of the treatment options in detail. However, one technique has been shown by research to achieve greater results than other choices (Box 20-2). Trigger point pressure release uses sustained pressure directly applied to the CTrP to deactivate it. Elongation of the central sarcomeres accompanies the release in order to manually or actively separate the actin and myosin filaments and to lengthen the short fibers.

Palpating and Treating Trigger Points

Diagnostic criteria are commonly used in medicine to serve as the standards by which to judge if a particular condition is present. In order to determine that a central trigger point is present, a minimal criterion has been defined by Simons et al[5,18] as a nodule located in a taut band that, when properly provoked, produces a referral pattern. When provoked, these referred

---

BOX 20-2 Which Method Is Most Effective?

Researchers at the Department of Physical Medicine and Rehabilitation, University of California[28] used:

1. Ice spray and stretch (Travell and Simons approach)
2. Superficial heat applied by a hydrocolator pack (20 to 30 minutes)
3. Deep heat applied by ultrasound (1.2 to 1.5 watt/cm^2 for 5 minutes)
4. Dummy ultrasound (0.0 watt/cm^2)
5. Deep inhibitory pressure soft tissue massage (10 to 15 minutes of modified connective tissue massage and shiatsu/ischemic compression)

This study included 24 patients with active triggers in the upper trapezius that had been present for over 3 months.

- The pain threshold of the trigger point area was measured using a pressure algometer three times pretreatment and within 2 minutes posttreatment.
- The average was recorded on each occasion.
- Control group members were similarly measured twice (30 minutes apart) and received no treatment until after the second measurement.
- The results showed that all methods except the placebo ultrasound produced a significant increase in pain threshold following treatment. The greatest change was demonstrated by those receiving deep pressure treatment (which equates with trigger point pressure release).
- The spray and stretch method was the next most efficient in achieving reduction in pain threshold.

Research from Hong C-Z, Chen Y-C, Pon C, Yu J: Immediate effects of various physical medicine modalities on pain threshold of an active myofascial trigger point, *Journal of Musculoskeletal Pain* 1(2): 37-53, 1993.

---

patterns are (usually) painful and can present as patterns of tingling, numbness, itching, burning, and other sensations.

When palpating for central trigger points at approximately midfiber region, the practitioner will often encounter a dense, congestive thickening in the taut fiber. The more distinct "nodule" associated with the trigger point may not be obvious at first due to the sometimes extensive tissue congestion. However, the distinct characteristic of exquisite tenderness is usually felt by the person and pressure may need to be decreased when the person reports the discomfort level. The colloid-based matrix of the tissue can usually be softened by manipulation, gliding strokes, applications of heat (when appropriate), or by elongation of the tissue. These steps often result in a reduction in size of the taut band and a more distinct palpation of the nodules. Depending upon the tissue's availability to be grasped, compression and pincer palpation can then be precisely applied to capture the nodule between the thumb and finger (Box 20-3).

When the suspect tissue is located and found to meet the minimal criteria, other observable conditions may be present to help confirm that it houses a TrP. These include a local twitch response (LTR), pain upon contraction, host muscle testing as weak, or by altered cutaneous humidity, temperature, or texture (sweaty, hot/cold, or rough spots on skin).[27] Trigger points (whether central or attachment, active or latent) should be charted as to their location and referral patterns, and each should be reassessed after deactivation.

Additionally, they should be reexamined at future sessions.

Treating a Central Trigger Point

Trigger point pressure release is one of the most successful techniques used to deactivate central trigger points.[28] Trigger point pressure release is applied to central trigger points by compressing the nodule between the thumb and finger or against an underlying bone or tissue with just a little more pressure than that required to match the tension in the taut band (Figure 20-8). This amount of pressure should provoke the referred pattern of the trigger point if the digits are directly in contact with the central nodule (also called the active loci or nidus). The blanching effects of applied compression extrude the blood from the tissue

---

BOX 20-3 Trigger Point Palpation Exercise

The following is suggested as an exercise for developing palpation skills in locating and treating central trigger points as well as a general protocol for clinical application. This begins by addressing a central trigger point.[27]

- Place the tissue in a relaxed position by slightly (passively) approximating its ends (for example, for pectoralis major the arm would be passively supported in shoulder flexion and slight internal rotation of the humerus). The approximate center of the fibers should be located with a thumb or finger contact. In this example, the portion of the anterior axilla near the torso would be grasped between the thumb and finger.
- Tendon arrangement should be considered in order to determine the center of the fibers, which are also the endplate zones of most muscles and the usual location of central trigger points.
- Digital pressure (pincer compression in this case) should be applied to the center of the fibers where trigger point nodules are found while the muscle is slowly taken in to slight stretch, which may increase the palpability of the taut band and nodule.
- As the tension becomes palpable, pressure into the tissues should be increased by the practitioner into the tissues to meet and match the tension within the taut band.
- The fingers can then be slid along the taut band near midfiber region to assess for a palpable muscular nodule or thickening of the associated myofascial tissue.
- An exquisite degree of spot tenderness is usually reported near or at the trigger point sites.
- Sometimes a local twitch response may be felt, particularly when a transverse snapping palpation is used. When present, the local twitch response serves as a confirmation that a trigger point has been encountered.

- If pressure is increased into the core of the nodule (central trigger point), a referred sensation (usually pain) may be felt by the person, which he/she either recognizes (active trigger point) or does not (latent trigger point). Sensations can also include tingling, numbness, itching, or burning, although pain is the most common referral.
- The degree of pressure should be adjusted so that the person reports a midrange number between 5 and 7 on their discomfort scale, as the pressure is maintained.
- Alternative protocols for application of pressure to trigger points include sustaining pressure for longer durations or applying short duration pressure repetitiously, "pumping" the tissue with 3 to 4 seconds of pressure, followed by 3 to 4 seconds without pressure.
- The tenderness of the tissue will vary from person to person and even from tissue to tissue within the same person. The pressure needed can vary from less than an ounce to several pounds. The appropriate degree of pressure should provoke between a 5 and 7 on the person's discomfort scale (of 1 to 10).
- The practitioner will usually feel the tissues "melting and softening" under the sustained pressure if the tissue is releasing, and the person may experience a similar sensation. As this occurs, the pressure can be mildly increased as tissue relaxes and tension releases, provided the discomfort scale is respected.
- The length of time pressure is maintained will vary; however, tension should ease within 15 seconds and discomfort level should drop. If it does not begin to respond within 8 to 12 seconds, the amount of pressure should be adjusted accordingly (usually lessened), as possibly should the angle of pressure or location of pressure.

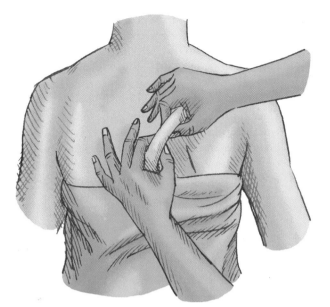

FIGURE 20-8 Trigger point pressure release can be applied precisely with fingertips, as shown here for lower trapezius. (From Chaitow L, DeLany J: *Clinical application of neuromuscular techniques*, vol 1. *The upper body*, ed 2, Edinburgh, 2008, Churchill Livingstone.)

and, when pressure is released, may enhance oxygen and nutrient availability as blood floods back into the localized area. Caution should be exercised however, as excessive restriction of blood can produce an ischemic state.

For best results, it is important to be directly on the central nodule, rather than near it. If the person keeps asking for more pressure, moving the point of pressure slightly one direction or another may reveal that the practitioner was close to, but not right on, the desired spot. It is also important to ask whether pain medication has been taken, which might be masking the sensations and requiring that excessive pressure be used to produce the expected sensation.

Tissue oxygenation, past trauma, previous therapies, general nutritional health, mineral imbalances, tissue toxicity, and dysfunctional postures all appear to influence the amount of pressure to use. The amount and duration of pressure appropriate for an individual or for individual muscles can vary greatly. In fact, if the tissue is extremely tender, the person may not tolerate any application of pressure. In such cases, lymphatic drainage or other light pressure techniques, such as positional release, would best be incorporated in the early stages of care.

Generally, when the correct pressure is precisely applied, the tissue should begin to soften within 12 to 15 seconds and the referred sensation(s) should decrease. Pressure can be maintained for longer; however, the practitioner should feel the tissues softening within 15 seconds. The person may feel a "melting" sensation in the tissues and may even suggest that the practitioner is decreasing the pressure. A reduction of discomfort may be achieved with pressure that lasts longer than suggested; however, clinical experience of this author suggests that increased pain and a decreased mobility often result posttreatment when overly sustained or heavy pressure is used. Pressure should be constant and may be mildly increased as the tissues begin to soften, but should be released within about 20 seconds from the onset of application.

In addition to matching the tension within the tissues, a 1 to 10 scale of the person's discomfort in the treated tissues may be used to help guide the practitioner.[27] With 1 representing a feeling of pressure only and 10 being extremely painful (which is to always be avoided!), a 5, 6, or 7 is ideal. Only enough pressure to elicit a mild to moderate state of discomfort (5, 6, 7) is used, with the higher end being reserved for the more robust person. The 9 or 10 level ("biting the bullet" or "digging it out") should always be avoided as this may result in tissue damage.

A more long-lasting effect may be gained when the practitioner returns to an area 3 to 4 times for a briefer period rather than sustaining pressure for an extended duration. In the time between briefer applications, the lymphatic and vascular systems will effectively enhance a fluid exchange, which usually results in a better outcome. The degree of pressure used may need to be periodically adjusted, particularly as the tissue improves.

Treating an Attachment Trigger Point

Once central trigger points have been assessed, the attachments should be examined (if palpable) as to general tenderness and inflammation. Attachment trigger points apparently form due to excessive, unrelenting tension on the musculotendinous or periosteal attachments (or both), which are often extremely sensitive and/or inflamed.[5] Palpation should be performed cautiously. If inflammation is suspected, the stretching components of the procedure should be delayed and a more precise manual myofascial release of the central sarcomeres substituted for the passive or active stretches until the attachment sites improve. Otherwise stretching techniques applied to tissues that house attachment trigger points may provoke or increase an inflammatory response.

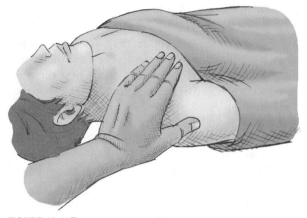

FIGURE 20-9 The upper trapezius fibers may be pressed against the underlying supraspinatus with gliding strokes applied in lateral or medial directions in order to elongate the central sarcomeres. (From Chaitow L, DeLany J: *Clinical application of neuromuscular techniques,* vol 1, ed 2. *The upper body,* Edinburgh, 2008, Churchill Livingstone.)

Gliding strokes may be applied from the center of the fiber toward the attachments (Figure 20-9), using one or both thumbs to lengthen the shortened fibers without placing undue stress on the attachments. These gliding strokes can begin at the center of the fibers and be directed toward one attachment and then repeated toward the other attachment or can be performed by using both thumbs and gliding from the center to both ends simultaneously.[27]

Once the associated central trigger point has been released, attachment trigger points usually respond without direct treatment. In the interim, cryotherapy (appropriately applied ice) can be used daily on the attachment trigger points until the central trigger points have been successfully deactivated.

A trigger point is more likely to be reactivated if the muscle in which it lies is not restored to its normal resting length following deactivating procedures. Therefore, muscle energy techniques and/or other appropriate stretching protocols (including manual elongation) should follow deactivation, if appropriate.

Trigger points ideally evidence their response to treatment by a reduction in referred phenomena and an increase in pain threshold. In other words, after successful treatment, more pressure is required in order to provoke the trigger point referral, and the referred sensations (including pain) are lessened or eliminated. It should be borne in mind that a TrP that is not responding to appropriate treatment could actually be a satellite trigger point, which will usually respond most favorably (and often spontaneously without direct treatment) when the associated key trigger point is located and deactivated.[5]

Other trigger point treatment considerations include the following:

- The taut fibers may sometimes be felt more distinctly by placing them in a slightly stretched position. However, if movement produces pain or if assessment of the attachment sites reveals excessive tenderness, the practitioner should exercise caution and suspect inflammation. Such conditions may be aggravated by applying additional tension, strumming of the taut fibers, or using frictional techniques.
- Trigger points frequently occur in "nests" and 3 to 4 repetitions (or more) of the TrP treatment may need to be applied to the same area, either within the same session or in subsequent sessions.
- The treatment of a trigger point is best followed by several passive elongations (stretches) of the tissue to that tissue's range of motion barrier. Unless contraindicated, passive stretching is then followed by at least 3 to 4 active repetitions of the stretch, which the person is encouraged to continue as "homework."
- It is important to avoid excessive treatment at any one session, as a degree of microtrauma is undoubtedly inherent in the processes described.
- While residual discomfort often accompanies this form of therapy, it may be reduced significantly by avoiding excessive treatment, by staying below 8 on the person's discomfort scale, and by using appropriate hydrotherapy applications during the session as well as at home.
- Since the elastic components of muscle and fascia are less pliable when they are cold,[29] myofascial tissues should be stretched when they are warm and while their ground substance is more solute. If prolonged application of cold (ice) has occurred, it is helpful to rewarm the area with a hot pack (unless contraindicated) or with mild movement before stretches are applied. Note: These precautions concern prolonged cold and do not apply for brief exposures to cold, such as spray and stretch or ice stripping techniques.

Based on the clinical experience, the following is suggested by the author of this chapter as a general guideline when addressing most myofascial tissue problems.[27]

- The most superficial tissue is usually treated before the deeper layers.

- The proximal portions of an extremity are treated ("softened") before the distal portions are addressed so that proximal restrictions of lymph flow are removed before distal lymph movement is increased.
- In a two-jointed muscle, both joints are assessed; in multijointed muscles, all involved joints are assessed. For instance, if biceps femoris is examined, both the hip joint and knee joint are assessed, and if extensor digitorum longus is treated, then ankle and all phalangeal joints being served by that muscle are checked.
- Most myofascial trigger points either lie in the endplate zone (midfiber) of a muscle or at the attachment sites.[5]
- Other types of trigger points may occur in the skin, fascia, periosteum, and joint surfaces.
- Knowledge of the anatomy of each muscle, including its innervations, fiber arrangement, nearby neurovascular structures, and overlying and underlying muscles, will greatly assist the practitioner in quickly locating and safely treating the muscle.[27]

COMMUNICATION DURING THERAPY

Clear communication is important for both the practitioner and the person being treated. The person can better assist and become involved in understanding his/her body when the practitioner understands what has brought on the condition and what helps to relieve it. A case history with full medical background of the condition will help guide the practitioner to use the appropriate protocols for treatment and to avoid those that are contraindicated. The following questions are frequently used to guide the session.

- *What is tender upon palpation?* Healthy, flexible tissues are not tender with appropriate pressure. Ischemic tissues and TrPs are usually tender. It is important to chart tender tissues and return to them for further inspection.
- *Are there referred sensations of pain, heat, tingling, cold, numbness, itching, or any other sensations to other body parts when the tissues are pressed?* Trigger points will refer sensations to other parts of the body. The location and target zones of referral as well as the type of referred sensations are important to know and to chart. These should be compared with the person's chronic pain patterns and should be reassessed at subsequent treatment sessions.
- *Is there a reduction of discomfort produced by applied trigger point pressure release?* This will help determine

if the desired results are being achieved. TrPs and ischemia may be reduced and, ultimately, normal tonus and tissue health restored to the area.

THE BENEFITS OF TRIGGER POINT RELEASE

Most chronic pain conditions have a trigger point element, either as the primary cause of pain or as a perpetuator. Treatment of trigger points may reduce or eliminate the pain, sometimes almost instantly. Additionally, in people who present with loss of range of motion, muscle weakness, joint imbalance, dental pain, abdominal visceral conditions, and structural misalignments, trigger points may be found to be the primary culprit or an adaptive mechanism that perpetuates the conditions.

Trigger points have been associated with headaches, hearing loss, vertigo, eye sight changes, TMJ syndrome, frozen shoulder, carpal tunnel syndrome, elbow pain, chest pain, sore throat, breathing difficulties, asthma, neck pain, low back pain, thyroid dysfunction, voice strain, various lower extremity conditions (from hip to toes), sciatica, and a host of other conditions. Each of these conditions may improve rapidly with appropriate trigger point release, despite the (often) associated failures in other fields of medicine. People in need of treatment may range in age from newborn infants to the most elderly, and, although not always, results from deactivation often appear to be miraculous, particularly in those who have already "been everywhere else."

CONTRAINDICATIONS

Trigger point release is safe in almost all conditions. However, when attachment trigger points display signs of inflammation, caution is suggested when lengthening the tissues, as previously discussed.

Additionally, release of taut tissue might be contraindicated in initial stages of some acute injuries. During the acute phase of tissue repair, the body often will produce swelling and splint the injured area,[30] which is a natural way to reduce hemorrhaging in torn tissues and to prevent movements that might further traumatize the fibers. Depending upon the degree of damage, treatments that might increase blood flow and allow increased mobility may not be appropriate on the recently injured tissues while they initiate the first phase of repair. Additionally, the person may need referral for qualified medical, osteopathic, or chiropractic assessment and care. Application of other techniques, such as lymphatic drainage[31] and certain movement therapies that are appropriate for acute injuries, may be used, if indicated.

Whether the tissues are in acute, subacute, or chronic stage of recovery, consultation with the attending physician is suggested if range of motion work is questionable (such as when a moderate or severe whiplash has occurred) to avoid further compromise to the structures (cervical disks, ligaments, vertebrae, etc.) that may have been damaged in the trauma. If symptoms of disk injury are present, regardless of length of time since the injury, diagnosis of the status of current disk health is suggested, as deterioration can be progressive.

When active or passive movements initiate a painful response, especially when that pain is elicited with little provocation, tissues associated with that movement need to be treated with particular care and caution. Gentle passive movement can safely accompany trigger point release, and mild active movements may be initiated with care. However, more comprehensive movements or exercises that involve weights should be left until the tissues respond to active and passive movement without pain.

As would be appropriate with all forms of massage applications, additional caution should be exercised for those people who present with open sores, postsurgical healing sites, herpes zoster (shingles), skin lesions, swelling, bruising, or other abnormal tissues until those conditions have been examined by a physician and approved for treatment. Special attention should be paid to enlarged (swollen) lymphatic nodes or lymphedema, and treatment of associated tissues should be avoided until the lymphatic condition has been fully assessed.

CERTIFICATION AND ADVANCED TRAINING

There are no legal requirements of training or certification in order to release trigger points. However, in those states that require a license to massage,[32] it would be necessary to complete the appropriate schooling, pass any required state boards, and acquire the appropriate license in order to treat trigger points and myofascial conditions. Additional licenses may be required in order to needle or inject trigger points, and in some states stretching the tissues, assigning exercise at home, working intraorally, or taking other steps to address perpetuating factors might also be regulated. For instance, some states allow intraoral protocols to be performed by a massage therapist while other states

restrict this treatment to the dental profession and its employees. Conversely, the practicing dentist may be confined to the area cephalad to the clavicles, even though the primary cause of TM joint dysfunction clearly may lie within a pelvic distortion. It is important that each practitioner understand his/her scope of practice and the legal boundaries that limit that practice, and to build a referral network with other qualified practitioners when proposed treatment lies outside the practitioner's scope of practice.

In order to be highly effective in locating and treating trigger points, the author of this chapter strongly suggests that a solid foundation of anatomy knowledge, palpation proficiency, an understanding of myofascial physiology, and skills in locating trigger points are valuable assets. Skill in assessing for and manually treating trigger points can be readily gained in seminars and other courses taught throughout the world. When learning certain techniques, tableside assistance with qualified instructors is imperative (such as work in the anterior neck or injection of trigger points). However, many of the manual protocols may be practiced by skilled therapists without supervision.

When designing and conducting clinical studies relating to soft tissue dysfunction, it is important that the examiners be experienced and well trained in those palpation skills and protocols required to accurately conduct the research. Those who are inexperienced (recent graduates or students, for example) or experienced practitioners with insufficient training in the specific techniques required may well fall short of the skills needed to apply technique-sensitive strategies. This is especially true for those applying manual techniques, since palpation skills take time and practice to perfect. Experienced practitioners who are trained to palpate for and identify specific characteristics that form part of research criteria will offer the most useful and valid findings.[5] Additionally, knowledge of fiber arrangement and the shortened and stretched positions for each section of each muscle will allow the practitioner to apply the techniques in such a way as to obtain accurate and reliable results. Knowledge of (or accessible charts showing) trigger point target zones is also of great benefit.

Both NMT American version™ and St. John method of NMT certification training have successfully been conducted in short course (seminar) events. Completion of four or five weekend courses is usually required, and it is usually suggested that adequate time be allowed between courses in order for the trainee to practice the techniques offered in the curriculum. Once all the required courses are completed, the trainee may take a certification examination that includes a written test as well as practical application of techniques and knowledge. There are no required continuing education courses to maintain the basic certification although advanced courses and seminars offering new developments within the field are often available.

Trigger point release has also been successfully taught in massage schools in a number of formats. NMT American version™ is an example where courses are conducted within the school's curriculum, taught by qualified instructors while using the same course manuals and protocols offered in the graduate-level short courses. The pace of the school curriculum is slower than the short course version, and the student has almost daily access to the instructors and assistants who can recheck the techniques learned previously. The graduating student receives NMT certification along with the massage school diploma and is ready to enter the job market as a certified NMT with well-trained skills in trigger point pressure release.

The European version of NMT is taught as a stand-alone module on undergraduate schemes, in the School of Integrative Health, University of Westminster, London. It is an elective module as part of a BS degree in *Therapeutic Bodywork* offered by the university. It is available as a stand-alone course to suitably qualified manual therapists who receive a certificate of proficiency on successfully completing the course and its knowledge and skills evaluation examinations.

The Pittsburgh School of Pain Management (formerly known as Academy for Myofascial Trigger Point Therapy) offers a 650-hour entry-level program for those interested in becoming myofascial trigger point therapists. Founded in 1995 in Pittsburgh, Pennsylvania, the program is recognized by the National Association of Myofascial Trigger Point Therapists (NAMTPT). Graduates are eligible to sit for the certification exam offered by the Certification Board for Myofascial Trigger Point Therapists, and many go on to receive recognition as Fellows or Clinical Associates with the American Academy of Pain Management.

Practitioners seeking training in trigger point pressure release are encouraged to contact the groups listed at the end of this chapter for the current standards of training and requirements for certification by each group. The information offered in these additional courses can be of substantial value, especially when built upon a foundation of comprehensive anatomy knowledge. Treatment of trigger points alone, however, is usually not sufficient to produce long-term results and is only one of many components addressed in comprehensive manual therapy practice setting.

CHAPTER SUMMARY

A thorough, whole-person approach to wellness has quickly come to the forefront in healthcare as complementary and integrative approaches are being incorporated into mainstream medicine. Even though it is not often practical, and at times not even legal, for each practitioner to address all aspects of wellness (illness), it is certainly relevant to bear in mind the interaction of biomechanical, biochemical, and psychosocial factors. Each or a combination of these factors may play a role in the formation and perpetuation of trigger points and associated myofascial pain syndromes. Integrative support by the practitioner and his/her referral network will offer the best possibility for a healthier outcome.

Trigger point release is a goal that can be accomplished by incorporating any one of a number of therapeutic interventions, such as trigger point pressure release, spray-and-stretch technique, dry needling, or injection. The most reliable trigger point release method is most likely to be the one that the practitioner has most fully mastered. Competency in any one of a number of techniques, coupled with anatomy knowledge and finely honed palpation skills, can dramatically increase the practitioner's ability to relieve chronic pain. There is no shortage of pain, and those who are prepared to address trigger points can easily have a very successful practice in a number of fields of medicine that incorporate trigger point release.

CASE HISTORIES

■ Case history 1

A 45-year-old female, mother of a 10-year-old child, presented with sporadic forearm pain and weakness in grip each time that she loaded the semisupinated forearm. Prior to the onset of her condition, she had no pain, weakness, or known injuries to the area in question.

When asked to recount what happened at the onset of this pain, she reported that one morning her daughter came running into the room waving a freshly extracted deciduous tooth. Joyfully the child ran into the bathroom to rinse it off and promptly dropped it down the drain. Acting quickly to turn off the running water to avoid washing the tooth down the pipes, the mother assessed the situation and decided to attempt to retrieve it by removing the drainpipe. Wielding her pipe wrench, she climbed under the sink and assumed a slightly strained, side-lying posture to reach the drain in the cramped space. Once the wrench was in place, she strained even further as she attempted to loosen the threads of the 80-year-old original plumbing. She recalls that while she was pulling on the wrench so hard that she thought she might break the pipe from the wall, it suddenly loosened and abruptly gave way. She felt a strain in her posterior and lateral forearm, yet was so focused on retrieving the tooth that she forgot about the incident until the following day when pain became the spontaneous reminder.

On the day following the strain, as she reached for a mug of coffee, she felt a "devastating pain" that incorporated the elbow, posterior forearm, and radial side of the wrist. She reports that the pain was so great that she almost dropped the mug and that she quickly reached over with her other hand to support the forearm. After she set the coffee mug down on the counter, the pain disappeared, only to reappear several more times that day and for several days thereafter whenever she lifted items that weighed approximately a half-pound or more.

She consulted a neuromuscular therapist a week after the incident. Passive and active range of motion tests (without resistance or loading with weight) failed to produce pain. Orthopedic and neurologic screening tests were negative. Examination of the right forearm muscles revealed trigger points in brachioradialis, supinator, and extensor digitorum. When provoked, the trigger point in brachioradialis precisely duplicated the reported symptoms, while the other two muscles referred patterns that were only similar to the reported symptoms. Trigger point pressure release successfully deactivated the trigger points, although the results were only temporary, with a slow return of symptoms to approximately 50% of the previous level within 3 days. A second treatment provided a similar result. On the third treatment, spray-and-stretch technique was added to the protocol, after which the condition was completely resolved.

■ Case history 2

A 36-year-old female teacher presented with a sore throat that had persisted off and on for approximately 4 months. Her physician had ruled out infection and inflammation and reported no apparent cause of her condition. She reported that the sore throat "comes and goes" but seems to be worse on days when she has to talk a lot.

Examination of her anterior throat area revealed tender and tight sternocleidomastoid, suprahyoid, and infrahyoid muscles bilaterally. While she did report that each of these referred into her throat, bringing on a feeling of tightness, none reproduced her symptom of throat pain. A further intraoral examination revealed very tender medial pterygoid muscles that did indeed feel to her like they were at least part of the problem. (It is suggested that practitioners be informed on state laws pertaining to intraoral work since scope of practice may vary from state to state.) When the practitioner's finger slid down onto the root of the tongue and pressed into hyoglossus muscle, the woman's eyes widened in surprise and she began a slight shaking of the head in a "yes" pattern to indicate apparent involvement of the tissue.

After the practitioner completed a treatment of short gliding strokes followed by sustained pressure on a portion of the right hyoglossus muscle and removed the finger to prepare for the other side, the person reported that the throat was completely relieved—but only on the right side! The left side was similarly relieved when that side of the tongue was treated.

The person was shown how to self-treat using static pressure on the hyoglossus muscles. She was also shown how to wrap the tongue in a cloth, pull the tongue forward and laterally in order to stretch some of the lingual muscles. On a subsequent appointment, she reported that she had been completely successful in eliminating this chronic condition although she still lectures the same amount as in the past.

SUGGESTED READINGS

Chaitow L, DeLany J: *Clinical application of neuromuscular techniques*, vol 1, ed 2. *The upper body*, Edinburgh, 2008, Churchill Livingstone.

Chaitow L, DeLany J: *Clinical application of neuromuscular techniques*, vol 2. *The lower body*, Edinburgh, 2002, Churchill Livingstone.

Davies C: *The trigger point therapy workbook: your self-treatment guide for pain relief*, Oakland, Calif, 1999, New Harbinger Pub.

Mense S, Simons D: *Muscle pain: understanding its nature, diagnosis, and treatment*, Philadelphia, 2001, Lippincott, Williams & Wilkins.

Simons D, Travell J, Simons L: *Myofascial pain and dysfunction: the trigger point manual*, vol 1, ed 2. *Upper half of body*, Baltimore, 1999, Williams & Wilkins.

Travell J, Simons D: *Myofascial pain and dysfunction: the trigger point manual*, vol 2. *The lower extremities*, Baltimore, 1992, Williams & Wilkins.

RESOURCES

Bonnie Prudden Myotherapy, Inc.
P.O. Box 65240
Tucson, AZ 85728-5240
(800) 221-4634
www.bonnieprudden.com

Myopain Seminars
Janet G. Travell, MD Seminar Series
7830 Old Georgetown Rd., Suite C-15
Bethesda, MD 20814
(301) 656-0220 E-mail *info@painpoints.com*
www.myopainseminars.com

NMT American Version™
NMT Center, Judith DeLany, Director
900 14th Avenue North
St. Petersburg, FL 33705
(727) 821-7167 E-mail: nmtcenter@aol.com
www.nmtcenter.com

St. John Seminars
6565 Park Blvd., Pinellas Park, FL 33781
1-888-NMT-HEAL E-mail: info@stjohnnmtseminars.com
www.stjohnseminars.com

Schools with Trigger Point Release Programs

Pittsburgh School of Pain Management
1312 E. Carson St.
Pittsburgh, PA 15203
(412) 481-2553
www.painschool.com

School of Integrative Health, University of Westminster
115 New Cavendish Street
London, W1M8JS, UK
44-7911-5000, ext. 3699

Organizations and Websites

International Myopain Society
www.myopain.org

National Association of Myofascial Trigger Point Therapists
www.myofascialtherapy.org

The International Myotherapy Association
www.myotherapy.org

REFERENCES

1. Schweitzer A: *On the edge of the primeval forest*, New York, 1931, Macmillan.
2. Weiner K: *Pain issues: pain is an epidemic, a special message from the director* (pdf online): http://www.aapain-manage.org/literature/Articles/PainAnEpidemic.pdf, American Academy of Pain Management. Accessed October 3, 2008.
3. *Pain management programs: a market analysis*, Tampa, Fla, 1999, Marketdata Enterprises.
4. Roper Starch Worldwide Inc: *Chronic pain in America: roadblocks to relief (online survey)*: http://www.ampainsoc.org/links/roadblocks/. 1999 Survey conducted for the American Pain Society, The American Academy of Pain Medicine, and Janssen Pharmaceutica. Accessed July 14, 2008.
5. Simons D, Travell J, Simons L: *Myofascial pain and dysfunction: the trigger point manual*, vol 1, ed 2. *Upper half of body*, Baltimore, 1999, Williams & Wilkins.
6. Travell J, Simons D: *Myofascial pain and dysfunction: the trigger point manual*, vol 1. *Upper half of body*, Baltimore, 1983, Williams & Wilkins.
7. Sola A, Rodenberger M, Gettys B: Incidence of hypersensitive areas in posterior shoulder muscles, *Am J Phys Med* 34:585-590, 1951.
8. Travell J, Simons D: Low back pain (pt 2), *Postgraduate Medicine* 73(2):81-92, 1983.
9. Fishbain D et al: Male and female chronic pain patients categorized by DSM-III psychiatric diagnostic criteria, *Pain* 26:181-197, 1986.
10. Fricton J et al: Myofascial pain syndrome of the head and neck: a review of clinical characteristics of 164 patients, *Oral Surgery* 6:615-663, 1985.
11. Travell J, Simons D: *Myofascial pain and dysfunction: the trigger point manual*, vol 2. *The lower extremities*, Baltimore, 1992, Williams & Wilkins.
12. Travell J: *Office hours: day and night. The autobiography of Janet Travell, MD*, Cleveland, 1968, New American Library.
13. Travell J, Rinzler S: The myofascial genesis of pain, *Postgraduate Medicine* 11:425-434, 1952.
14. www.myopainseminars.com
15. Simons D: From the edge of space—a pioneer's own story and photos, *Life* 43:19-26, 1957.
16. Simons D: *Man high: a space scientist's account of his record breaking balloon flight to 102,000 feet*, New York, 1960. Doubleday.
17. Simons D: Foreward. In Chaitow L, DeLany: *J Clinical application of neuromuscular techniques*, vol 2. *The lower body*, Edinburgh, 2002, Churchill Livingstone.
18. Mense S, Simons D: *Muscle pain: understanding its nature, diagnosis and treatment*, Philadelphia, 2001, Lippincott, Williams & Wilkins.
19. Lucey T: Catching up with Bonnie Prudden, fitness pioneer, *Sports Illustrated*, June 7, 1999.
20. Prudden B: *Pain erasure: the Bonnie Prudden way*, New York, 1980, Ballantine Books.
21. Goossen S: Personal communication with author, Jacksonville, FL, 2007.
22. National Association of Myofascial Trigger Point Therapists (website): http://www.myofascialtherapy.org. Accessed July 14, 2008.
23. Chaitow L, DeLany J: *Clinical application of neuromuscular techniques*, vol 1. *The upper body*, Edinburgh, 2000, Churchill Livingstone.
24. Nimmo RL, Vannerson JF: In Schneider M, Cohen J, Laws S, eds: *The collected writings of Nimmo & Vannerson, pioneers of chiropractic trigger point therapy*, Pittsburgh, Pa, 2001, self-published.

25. Davies C: *The trigger point therapy workbook: your self-treatment guide for pain relief*, Oakland, Calif, 1999, New Harbinger.

26. Chaitow L, DeLany J: *Clinical application of neuromuscular techniques*, vol 2. *The lower body*, Edinburgh, 2002, Churchill Livingstone.

27. Chaitow L, DeLany J: *Clinical application of neuromuscular techniques*, vol 1, ed 2. *The upper body*, Edinburgh, 2008, Churchill Livingstone.

28. Hong CZ et al: Immediate effects of various physical medicine modalities on pain threshold of an active myofascial trigger point, *Journal of Musculoskeletal Pain* 1(2): 37-53, 1993.

29. Lowe WW: *Orthopedic and sports massage reviews*, Bend, OR, 1995, Orthopedic Massage Education and Research Institute.

30. Cailliet R: *Soft tissue pain and disability*, ed 3, Philadelphia, 1996, FA Davis.

31. Chikly B: *Silent waves: theory and practice of lymph drainage therapy with applications for lymphedema, chronic pain and inflammation*, Scottsdale, AZ, 2001, IHH Publishing.

32. American massage therapy association: *States with massage therapy practice laws (website):* http://www.amtamassage.org/about/lawstate.html. Accessed July 14, 2008.

MULTIPLE CHOICE TEST QUESTIONS

1) Chronic pain
   a) is a rare occurrence
   b) does not present in people seeking massage
   c) occurs in approximately 50 million people in the United States annually
   d) is not a condition that a massage therapist will ever address

2) Which of the following is not part of the diagnostic criteria of a myofascial trigger point?
   a) a tender hyperirritable (usually) palpable nodule
   b) refers pain and other sensations when provoked
   c) taut band
   d) local twitch response (LTR)

3) Trigger point release is
   a) the application of a particular modality
   b) a goal that many modalities strive to achieve
   c) a specific technique performed by surgeons
   d) rarely accomplished

4) Travell and Simons estimate that around what percent of pain clinic patients have a trigger point as the sole source of their pain?
   a) 75%
   b) 99%
   c) 4% to 5%
   d) 50%

5) Trigger points can occur in any myofascial tissue but the most commonly identified TrPs are found in the
   a) lower trapezius and psoas major
   b) upper trapezius and quadratus lumborum
   c) sternocleidomastoid muscle
   d) abdomen

6) Practitioners who have skills in releasing trigger points
   a) can only work in a spa setting
   b) can work in a variety of practice settings
   c) must work in a doctor's office
   d) rarely meet people who need this skill

7) Academic papers regarding pain referred from myofascial tissues
   a) are rare
   b) have appeared in print for over 150 years
   c) are written only by American physicians
   d) are not reliable

8) Drs. Janet Travell and David Simons are
   a) credited with producing the most definitive written material on trigger points to date
   b) virtually unknown authors
   c) solely responsible for techniques and information pertinent to trigger points
   d) no longer considered significant figures in trigger point concepts

9) The first female Personal Physician to the President of the United States was
   a) Bonnie Prudden
   b) only the physician to one president
   c) Janet G. Travell, MD
   d) a single woman who was solely focused on her medical career

10) Dr. David Simons
    a) has almost 200 publications to his credit
    b) has achieved international recognition as an authority on trigger points
    c) was the first man to ascend to the edges of outer space
    d) all of the above

11) Bonnie Prudden
    a) made a significant impact on fitness awareness in the United States
    b) wrote *Erasing Pain with the Bonnie Prudden Method*
    c) denied that trigger points existed
    d) did very little to help the public understand trigger points

12) European-style NMT for trigger points first emerged in Great Britain, developed by the skillful hands of
   a) Leon Chaitow
   b) Stanley Lief and Boris Chaitow
   c) Bernard Macfadden
   d) a group of MDs who had read about Travell and Simons' work

13) In America, receptor-tonus technique was developed by
   a) Raymond Nimmo
   b) James Vannerson
   c) a and b
   d) none of the above

14) A localized area within a muscle that, when sufficiently provoked (by pressure, needling, etc.) produces a referred sensation to a particular target zone is called a
   a) satellite trigger point
   b) myofascial trigger point
   c) paresthesia point
   d) spasm

15) A contracture is apparently sustained by
   a) the central nervous system
   b) abnormal chemistry at the motor point of the affected muscle fibers
   c) the peripheral nervous system
   d) not enough ACh

16) A spasm is
   a) involuntary, with motor potentials involved
   b) another name for a contracture
   c) the same as a contraction
   d) none of the above

17) ATP is the energy of the cell, and a lack of it produces
   a) normal physiology
   b) no apparent change in muscle tissues
   c) a local energy crisis
   d) a need to use active transport

18) Attachment trigger points (ATrPs)
   a) can develop at the attachment sites of shortened tissues
   b) are almost the same as central trigger points
   c) are seldom present at the periosteal or myotendinous sites
   d) are not associated in any way with a CTrP

19) Deactivation of a TrP can be achieved by using
   a) dry or wet needling
   b) trigger point pressure release
   c) spray and stretch techniques
   d) all of the above

20) When treating a CTrP it is important to
   a) press as hard as possible
   b) lengthen the central sarcomeres after deactivation
   c) apply sustained pressure for as long as possible
   d) only treat it one time in order to avoid overtreatment

Tuina

Terry Norman

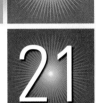

21

STUDENT OBJECTIVES

Upon completion of this chapter, students will be able to do the following:

- Understand the history and development of Chinese massage.
- Compare the schools of Tuina.
- Learn how Tuina differs from other forms of massage.
- Recognize the indications and contraindications of Tuina.
- Use Tuina techniques and procedures.

KEY TERMS

Acupoints
Acupressure
An Wu
Anmo
Bofa
Channels
Huangdi Neijing
Mofa
Na
Nafa
Qi
Reduction Method
Reinforcing Method
Roufa
TCM
Traumatology
Tui
Tuifa
Tuina
Yang
Yin
Yin and Yang Theory
Zang-fu

Tuina (pronounced "Tway Na-a") has been a medical therapeutic procedure in China for several thousands of years.[1] It can be translated as "Chinese Massage," but in reality it is much more. Tuina consists of spinal adjustments (as in chiropractic and osteopathic medicine), soft tissue manipulations (as in massage therapy), neuromuscular therapy (NMT), deep tissue therapy, myofascial release, physical therapy, acupressure (as in trigger point therapy), and energy balancing (as in meridian therapy). In fact, you could say that Tuina is the "Father" of all manual therapies, since components of Tuina can be found in all other therapies. If you travel to China and observe Tuina, you would find this statement to be true.

Tuina is a therapeutic system designed to deal directly with, and to prevent, the onset and development of sickness in a way suited to the natural healing process within the human body. It is based on an approach that will increase and strengthen the body's resistance to disease, illness, and fatigue, and actually speed up the healing of damaged areas due to injury or trauma by manipulating the body and points along the channels. The word "Tuina" is made up of two words, **"Tui"** meaning to push or stroke, and **"Na"** meaning to grasp or knead.[2] The Chinese characters are shown in Figure 21-1.

HISTORY OF CHINESE MASSAGE

It is important to note that when discussing procedures, techniques, events, and dates that go back several thousands of years, there will be some confusion and discrepancy as to the exact time in history these

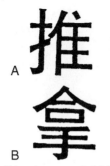

FIGURE 21-1 Chinese Tuina characters. **A,** Tui. **B,** Na.

events and names occurred. It is my intention to provide a picture that is as clear and accurate as possible based on information from several references, texts, and my own notes from the medical schools and hospitals in Shanghai and the National Olympic Training Center in Beijing.

ANMO

In ancient times, between 2700-770 BC, massage in China was referred to as **"An Wu."** Even then, massage was used to treat all types of medical conditions, although most of the techniques were for treating muscular injuries.[3] Later, by the Spring and Autumn Period (770-476 BC) and into the period of the Warring States (475-221 BC), massage was known as **"Anmo."** By this time, massage was being widely used in more medical situations.[4]

During the Sui and Tang Dynasties (581-907 AD), Anmo began to flourish. By the fifth century, Anmo had achieved the level of doctoral degree in the State Office of Imperial Physicians, showing that as a clinical subject of Chinese Medicine, it had developed to a higher level in its system of basic theory, diagnosis, and treatment. It was during this time that Anmo spread to other Asian countries such as Korea, Japan, and India.[3]

In the Song and Yuan Dynasties (960-1368 AD), Anmo became less popular and declined in use as a medical procedure. During this time, there was no Anmo department within the state medical institutions, but research continued to develop better Anmo techniques. For example, Anmo procedures to expedite childbirth were developed. Anmo was mainly used for treating osteotrauma, which laid the foundations for the medical system of bone setting called Tuina.[4]

During the Ming Dynasty (1368-1644 AD), Anmo began to flourish once again. In the Institute of Imperial Physicians, a specialty department of Anmo

was established. It was during this time that the term Tuina replaced Anmo. This is of profound importance in the developing history of Tuina, for it established a higher level of massage as a whole in China.[4]

Today, Anmo is referred to as "folk massage," while Tuina is considered "medical massage" and is performed in hospitals and clinics.

TUINA

Sui and Tang Dynasties were a flourishing age for Chinese massage. In the Office of the Imperial Physicians of the Sui Dynasty, a massage doctor was authorized to be in charge of daily medical treatment and teaching affairs. A massage specialty was set up in the Office of the Imperial Physicians of the Tang Dynasty and the massage practitioners were classified as massage doctors (massage practitioners with doctorates), practitioners, or workers, according to their training and responsibilities.[3]

During the Qing Dynasty (1644-1911 AD), Tuina fell out of favor with the government, although it was still used extensively by the people, especially in the area of infant Tuina. Remarkable development continued in this area, along with great achievements in the treatment of **traumatology,** treating traumatic injury patients, with Tuina. It was during this time that the school of Tuina traumatology was formed.[4]

Also during this period, the Portuguese opened up trade with China. With the Portuguese came the Jesuits, who established the first trade missions. The Jesuits were very organized and highly educated in science, mathematics, commerce, and politics, but especially in the craft of map making. They did not try to convert the Chinese to Christianity but attempted to learn all they could about the Chinese way of life, including their beliefs and forms of medicine. This included the study of Tuina.

Upon their return home, the Jesuits brought teaching manuals on Tuina back for study. These techniques and procedures spread throughout Europe, into France, making their way to Sweden, where a man by the name of Per Henrik Ling found and studied them. Combined with techniques he developed to treat injuries incurred by athletes, he developed what was later called Swedish massage. Unfortunately, most of the true nature of Tuina procedures and techniques, along with the unique diagnostic methods of Chinese medicine, were lost or misunderstood after several transcriptions and translations were done. We can only guess at what Per Ling saw and read in those texts on Chinese

Tuina. But it is fair to say that Swedish massage, along with all forms of massage and manual therapy, derived from Tuina.

After the foundation of the People's Republic of China in 1949, the government strongly endorsed the revitalization of **TCM,** Traditional Chinese Medicine, and began to look at Tuina with great interest. In 1956, the first training course in Tuina was established in Shanghai.[5] In 1958, the Shanghai Clinic of Tuina and Shanghai Technical Secondary School of Tuina were set up. By the 1960s, a professional contingent of Tuina clinics and courses had been formed in China. In 1974, the first section on Tuina appeared in the department of Acupuncture, Tuina, and Traumatology in the Shanghai College of TCM. Soon after, the same thing happened at the TCM colleges in Beijing, Nanjing, Fujian, and Anhui. And in 1987, the All-China Association of Tuina was established. Since then, academic exchanges of Tuina, both nationally and internationally, have been conducted.[4]

Over the years, there has been a great increase in the number of books written on Tuina, along with research into the essentials and clinical practice of Tuina. For example, the curative effects of Tuina in treating cervical spondylopathy, prolapse of lumbar intervertebral disk, infantile diarrhea, coronary heart disease, and cholecystitis have become known throughout the world.

Today, Tuina flourishes in China and plays a vital role in various medical fields such as prevention, traumatology, rehabilitation, sports medicine, and health care.[4] An increasing number of medical professionals in Western countries, such as Canada, United States, United Kingdom, Germany, and Italy, are beginning to look into the effectiveness of Tuina and how it can be incorporated with traditional Western therapies of physical therapy, massage, osteopathy, chiropractic, and sports medicine. Many Western countries even have Tuina clinics and schools that offer Tuina to the public and perspective students.

Schools of Tuina

Many schools of Tuina have been established throughout China. The reasoning for their establishment is influenced by different academic sources, lineages, targets of treatment, politics, economy, societies, culture, and geography. Even though these schools have many differences, they all share three common characteristics:

1. Long histories and popularity within a specific region

2. Respective theoretical guidance, medical experiences, specialized training methods

3. Specialized manipulations called "school manipulations" characteristic of that school

To introduce and discuss all the schools of Tuina would take quite a long time, so a few will be discussed at this time. Most of the schools in northern China are lucid and vigorous in their techniques, while those in southern China are exquisite and gentle. For example, Tuina practiced in Beijing tends to incorporate several techniques during a treatment with most of them being compression type, while Tuina practiced in Shanghai tends to use 1 to 5 techniques per treatment with the Rolling Method being the primary technique used during treatment.[3]

BASIC TUINA

Originally, along with treating soft tissue injuries, diseases, and general disorders, Tuina was used in areas of gynecology, neurology, and pediatrics. Today, the field of treatment also includes orthopedics, traumatology, cosmetology, rehabilitation, sports medicine, and general health care.

Tuina techniques used in orthopedics and traumatology are not only the fruit of clinical experience but also are an important part of Traditional Chinese Medical theory, which treats the whole body and all its symptoms together. There are different kinds of injuries, such as acute or chronic injuries to the soft tissues, bones, or joints, and therefore different methods of treatment are used depending on different clinical conditions. The pressure used in massage, whether heavy or light, skillful or unskillful, is very important in recovery from injuries. If done correctly, it is an important aid to healing; otherwise there are no good effects.[6]

Adult Tuina commonly deals with such conditions as cervical spondylosis, lumbar strain, herniation of intervertebral disk, arthritis, gastrointestinal disorders such as constipation or diarrhea, hypertension, diabetes, chronic coronary disorders, and stroke. Tuina has even been used to aid medicine in cases of internal infections. For infants, Tuina has been successful in controlling diarrhea, constipation, vomiting, abdominal pain, and intestinal obstructions.

Tuina has a "dual-direction" effect upon the body.[4] That means that Tuina has a **Reduction Method,** a reducing action on the flow of **Qi** and the condition, and a **Reinforcing Method,** an increasing action on the flow of qi and the condition. It can balance both hyperactivity and hypoactivity in the body, such as hypothyroidism or hyperthyroidism.

Research performed at major medical schools and hospitals in Shanghai and Beijing has shown that Tuina can improve the microcirculation of the blood and lymphatic systems, which will bring a faster recovery of sprains and contusions. Because Tuina can affect the nervous system, it may be used to bring about an anesthetic effect on the body such as reducing neuralgia or increasing endorphins. In addition, there are no harmful side effects with Tuina.

Tuina Differs from Other Manual Therapies

Tuina differs from other manual therapies mainly by the enormous scope of diseases and disorders it is able to effectively treat. Tuina is based upon the complex theories and principles of TCM. Among these theories is the Theory of Channels. This theory, and its applications, is what separates Tuina from all other manual therapies. It is also one of the oldest forms of bodywork, having evolved and developed over the last 5,000 years.[6]

Indications of Tuina

1. Disorders due to trauma—strains, sprains, contusions, subluxation of joints
2. Medical syndromes—asthma, headaches, insomnia, anemia, gastrointestinal dysfunctions, Bell's palsy, tinnitus and deafness, etc.
3. Surgical diseases—intestinal adhesions
4. Diseases of gynecology—dysmenorrhea, irregular menstruation, etc.
5. Diseases of pediatrics—cough, asthma, infantile diarrhea, constipation, vomiting, infantile myogenic torticollis, malnutrition, and food stagnation, etc.

Contraindications of Tuina

1. Acute and chronic communicable diseases—hepatitis, etc.
2. Infectious diseases—erysipelas (an acute superficial form of cellulitis caused by group A streptococci infection), medullitis (osteomyelitis), suppurative arthritis
3. Various hemorrhagic diseases—bleeding gastric ulcer, hematuria, etc.
4. Various malignant tumors—carcinomas, breast cancers, etc.
5. Inflamed and ulcerative dermatitis and dermatosis with pathologic changes and injuries, bruise, and scald

---

BOX 21-1 Scope of Practice

In China, the scope of practice for a Tuina doctor is quite different than for those in this country who incorporate Tuina as an adjunct modality to their profession as a manual therapist. Laws in this country do not allow massage therapists or physical therapists to perform spinal and joint manipulations. Only qualified and properly trained licensed professionals such as chiropractors and osteopaths are allowed to perform manipulations of this type. Still, there are many Tuina procedures and techniques that massage therapists, physical therapists, and rehabilitation therapists can perform and remain within the scope of their practices. Techniques that would be appropriate to perform are: pressing points along channels, stretching, soft tissue manipulations, and range-of-motion movements and exercises.

---

6. Bleeding due to trauma, fracture, and dislocation, a complete tear of a ligament, etc.
7. Lumbosacral and abdominal areas of a pregnant woman at any stage or during menses[4] (Box 21-1)

Rice Bag Training

Rice bag training is very important in the development of Tuina skills. Several Tuina techniques may require deep penetration into tissues or extended work on an area or acupoint. Therefore it becomes essential that you have the strength and endurance to perform the techniques and procedures correctly in order to achieve the proper results. This is where rice bag training comes in.

The rice bag simulates living tissue to a point and allows students to focus on their skills, build strength and endurance, and make mistakes without damaging anyone. As you practice, a skill base is formed from which more advanced and complex techniques can later be developed.

Bags are filled with rice, which gives both resistance and flexibility in the material, just as living tissue does (Figure 21-2). As your hands and fingers become stronger, you can substitute hard peas for the rice. And later, the peas can be replaced with sand or tiny stones.[6]

It is also important that you stay relaxed while practicing on the rice bag. This means that fingers, wrists, hands, arms, and shoulders must remain comfortably loose to minimize fatigue and prevent the chance of overstrain to the joints and muscles. Make sure to focus your attention on the technique you are practicing, and don't let your mind wander, for you may begin to practice incorrectly and develop an ineffective way of performing the technique. This can lead to injuring yourself and/or your client.

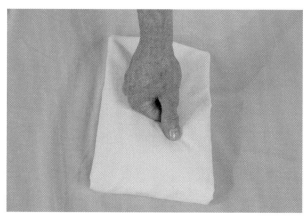

FIGURE 21-2 Rice bag training.

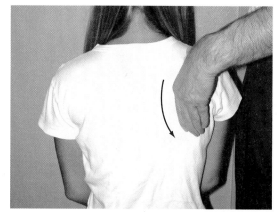

FIGURE 21-3 Tendon separating method (Bofa). (Courtesy of Terry Norman.)

There is an old Chinese saying often told to the student, "If you have done a thing a thousand times, you have only done it once." Try to remember this saying when practicing Tuina. Use all of your evaluating skills when practicing:

- Look at how your hand/fingers are performing the technique
- Listen to the sound your hand/fingers make on the rice bag
- Feel how your hand/fingers are feeling on the bag—is there any pain?

Tuina Techniques

In teaching and illustrating hand techniques used in Tuina, it is important to understand the scope of techniques used. Whereas there are 5 main techniques used in Swedish massage (effleurage, pétrissage, friction, vibration, and tapotement), Tuina uses over 1,000 hand techniques. All are designed to move qi (vital energy) and blood in a specific way to induce healing and bring about health as rapidly as possible. Some techniques are fairly easy to learn with only a minimal amount of practice, while others may take years to master.

Tendon Separating Method (Bofa)

Using the side of the index finger and pad of thumb, stroke down the medial side of the scapula, making a smooth, gentle penetrating movement, separating the tendons between the scapula and spine and the fascial sheaths (Figure 21-3). Repeat several times.

Kneading Method (Nafa)

Keeping wrist relaxed, gently knead with thenar eminence in a rubbing or kneading manner by moving the

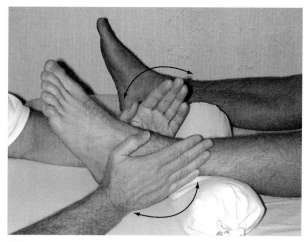

FIGURE 21-4 Kneading method (Nafa). (Courtesy of Terry Norman.)

hand in a circular motion, back and forth (Figure 21-4). Do not use friction. This should be done briskly at approximately 100 rpm, with hands moving in opposite directions.

Rubbing Method (Roufa)

Using the entire palm, with focus on the center of the palm, rub briskly in a semi-circular motion, keeping hands relaxed and moving in opposite directions (Figure 21-5). This should be done rapidly at approximately 100 rpm for 3 to 5 minutes.

Thumb Stroking (Tuifa)

Using the pad of the thumb, gently stroke across the area being worked (Figure 21-6). This technique is used in a smaller area like the forehead, face, neck, etc.

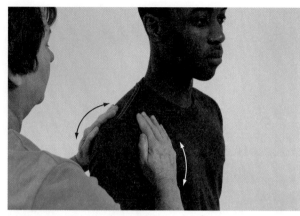

FIGURE 21-5 Rubbing method (Roufa).

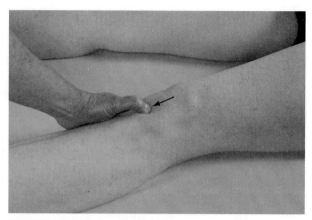

FIGURE 21-8 Scrape method (Cuofa).

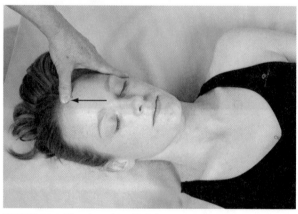

FIGURE 21-6 Thumb stroking (Tuifa).

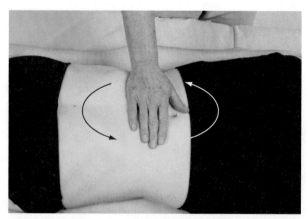

FIGURE 21-7 Palm rubbing method (Mofa).

Palm Rubbing Method (Mofa)

Gently rub with palm in circular fashion, keeping the wrist, arm, and shoulder relaxed (Figure 21-7).

Scrape Method (Cuofa)

Press deeply into affected area and scrape downward or back and forth within a very small distance, approximately one-fourth inch (Figure 21-8). This is similar to deep transverse friction but is not to be done rapidly.

TRADITIONAL CHINESE MEDICINE

There is a Chinese proverb that states, "The superior doctor prevents illness; the mediocre doctor cures imminent illness; the inferior doctor treats actual illness." Chinese medicine dates back to the late period of the New Stone Age about 5,000 years ago.[3] Ancient literature mentions the use of acupuncture, herbal medicine, and massage being performed during this time. It was during the Shang Dynasty, more than 3,000 years ago, that the philosophical thinking of **Yin** and **Yang** and the five elements were formed. This was when the basic theory of Chinese medicine began to spring forth.

The first book ever written on medicine, which included diagnosis of diseases, etiologies, treatment protocols, and treatment modalities, was the **Huangdi Neijing**, or the **Yellow Emperor's Classic of Internal Medicine**.[7] It was written several thousand years ago. Much of this book was devoted to the study and practice of Tuina, which in the early stages of development was known as "Anwu."

Traditional Chinese Medicine is based on a system of observing, listening, feeling, coordinating, and cataloging symptoms with pathology and etiology, along with an awareness of the balance of the human body in accordance with the rhythmic flow of nature and the universe.[8]

In TCM, each person is regarded as an integrated whole, without separation of mind, body, and spirit. Every part or function within the person can be seen primarily in terms of its contribution to the efficient functioning of the entire person. Therefore, it is said that "no one part can be understood except in its relationship to the whole." This makes the Chinese approach a holistic one.[9]

Acupressure

Acupressure is a therapeutic science that has been a major component of almost every form of massage and manipulative medicine for the last 5,000 years. Often referred to as "trigger point therapy" in the U.S. and other western countries, acupressure is actually a component of Tuina. Acupressure uses carefully administered pressure applied with the thumbs and fingers on specific points to relieve pain and tension and to bring about a state of health and wellness. Most of these specific points, or "acupoints," lie along channels running over the body. These channels, and the manipulation of such, are a key component of the theory of Traditional Chinese Medicine. Acupressure is still used today to deal with such medical conditions as neck tension and headaches, stroke, and cancer.[6]

Acupoints

Acupoints are points that are located along the channels of qi flowing throughout the body and are specific sites through which the qi of the organs and channels is transported to the body surface. They are not only the pathways for the circulation of qi and blood, but also the loci of response to disease and injury. In Tuina, proper techniques are applied on acupoints to regulate the functional activities of the body, speed the healing of injuries sustained in athletic competition, and strengthen the body's resistance to prevent and treat diseases.[8]

YIN AND YANG THEORY

The logic underlying Chinese medical theory assumes that a part can only be understood in its relationship to the whole. The entire universe and everything in it can be explained through the Yin and Yang Theory. There is a constant "give and take" process going on within all of nature as well as within our body. Simply stated, the **Yin and Yang Theory** is about relationships, patterns, and change.[9] If one can identify the patterns, see the inner relationships, and understand the changes taking place, or that will take place, it becomes easier to make adjustments to avoid imbalance that lead to illness and create or maintain a state of health. Therefore, the primary focus of the Tuina practitioner is to identify patterns of imbalance within the body and to reestablish patterns of balance.

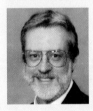
The Yin and Yang are not seen as forces or material entities but as complementary opposites. This is not some mythical concept that transcends rationality, but rather convenient labels used to describe how things function in relation to each other and to the universe. Yin is associated with such qualities as: cold, negative energy, passivity, darkness, the female, softness, inwardness (storing up), inactivity, and

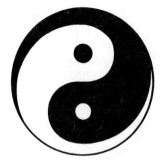

FIGURE 21-9 Yin and Yang symbol. (Courtesy of Terry Norman.)

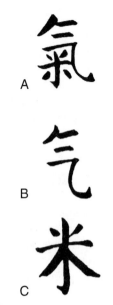

FIGURE 21-10 **A,** Qi. **B,** Vapor, steam, or gas. **C,** Uncooked rice. (Courtesy of Terry Norman.)

decrease. Yang implies qualities such as: heat, positive energy, the male, activity, vigor, stimulation, movement, light, firmness, excitement, outwardness (an outward flow), and increase. The Yin and Yang symbol is in Figure 21-9.

At the border between the two, there is a mutual and constant transformation of Yin to Yang and Yang to Yin taking place. When one reaches its maximum transformation, it begins to change into the other. This is not just a poetic metaphor but can be seen throughout nature with the changing of the seasons, or within the pathogenesis of a disease or chronic illness. There is no difference in the working mechanisms—they are all the same process (Box 21-2).

QI

Qi (pronounced "chee") is one of the fundamental substances that maintains the normal, vital activities of the human body and all of life.[9] Along with blood and body fluid, it is the material foundation for the physiologic functions of the zang-fu organs, tissues, and channels. Qi, while having an independent relationship with the

zang-fu organs, the tissues, and the channels, works together with the Yin and Yang Theory to explain the physiologic functions of the human body.[8] Since there is no "true" definition of Qi in the English language, the closest "functional" definition we can come up with is that Qi is known as "vital energy."

In Tuina, one of the most important goals is to rid the body of any blockages that might restrict the smooth flow of Qi, or to reduce it when it is overstimulated, thereby bringing the flow back into balance, or a state of Yin and Yang. By doing this, a state of balance or homeostasis can be produced within the body.

The character for Qi indicates that it is something both material and immaterial (Figure 21-10). An acceptable definition of Qi is "vital energy."

As the characters indicate, Qi can be as immaterial as vapor and as dense and material as rice. It is also a subtle substance, which makes it not so easy to see or feel, although its effects are often apparent.

THEORY OF CHANNELS

The function of the **channels** is to propel the circulation of Qi and blood in order to nourish Yin and Yang and facilitate the bones, tendons, and joints. The channels connect with visceral organs and the extremities along with the internal and external parts of the body. Any blockage in the channels will cause stagnant

---

BOX 21-2 Yin and Yang

Because Yin and Yang create each other in even the most stable situations, they are always subtly transforming into each other. This constant transformation is the source of all change. It is a give-and-take relationship that reflects the activity of life itself. Within the dynamics of the body, the natural transformational process can be illustrated by the manner in which inhalation is followed by exhalation. In life's normal state, such regular transformations occur smoothly, maintaining a proper, healthy balance of Yin and Yang within the body.

circulation of channel Qi and blood and many other diseases such as atrophy of muscles, tendons, channels and vessels, and joints due to the loss of nutrients. Malnutrition of the zang-fu organs may also occur.

Zang-fu relates to all the Yin and Yang organs. The Zang organs are the Yin organs, which are said to be "solid." They are as follows: Lung, Spleen, Heart, Kidney, Pericardium, and Liver. The Fu viscera are the Yang organs, which are said to be "hollow." They are as follows: Large Intestine, Stomach, Small Intestine, Bladder, Triple Warmer (San Jiao), and Gallbladder.[8]

Acupoints lie along these channels, and the Qi flowing in the channels can be affected by manipulating these points with Tuina and acupressure. Like small control buttons, Qi can be increased, decreased, or moved from one area to another and from organ to organ to bring about a balanced state of function within the body. Whether it is to calm an upset stomach, relieve a headache, or remove inflammation from a joint, balancing Qi along the channels is our main objective before a state of health and wellness can be reestablished.

By tracing the channels along their normal directional flow, you can increase the flow of Qi in the corresponding organ and channel (Box 21-3). This will cause a "reinforcing" effect, which is necessary if there is a deficiency. And by tracing the channels backwards of their normal flow, you will cause a "reduction" effect, which will reduce the flow of Qi along the channel and in the corresponding organ. This is one way to balance Qi within the body and to bring about a state of health.

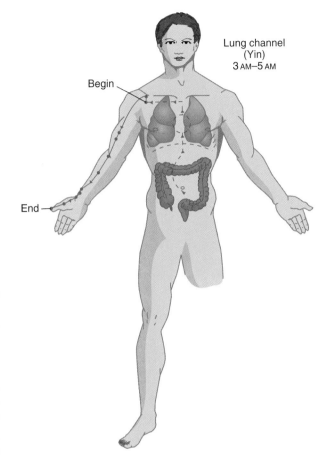

Begin

End

Lung channel
(Yin)
3 AM–5 AM

Figures in the next section illustrate the 14 major channels discussed above. I have provided the channel name, time of day it is most active, and whether it is Yin or Yang in nature. Remember, the first 12 channels are all bilateral (located on both sides of the body), while the last 2 are unilateral (one runs up the front and the other runs up the spine and over the head). The lines to be traced are shown in red. The blue lines indicate where the channel runs deep within the body.

Lung channel (Yin)
Large intestine channel (Yang)
Stomach channel (Yang)
Spleen channel (Yin)
Heart channel (Yin)
Small intestine channel (Yang)
Bladder channel (Yang)
Kidney channel (Yin)
Pericardium channel (Yin)
Triple warmer channel (Yang)
Gallbladder channel (Yang)
Liver channel (Yin)
Du channel (Governing vessel) (Yang) - unilateral
Ren channel (Conception vessel) (Yin) - unilateral

BOX 21-3 **Qi Channels**

The channels of Qi are named according to (1) the organ that is controlled by the energy flow, i.e., lungs, stomach, spleen, liver, etc., (2) the function of the energy, i.e., Governing Vessel (Du Channel), Conception Vessel (Ren Channel), Triple Warmer (San Jiao), and Pericardium, and (3) Yin or Yang quality. In the Yin channels, the Qi mainly flows upward—from ground to sky—and the channels are located on the anterior and medial sides of the body. In the Yang channels, the Qi mainly flows downward—from sky to ground—and the channels are located on the posterior and lateral sides of the body. The only exception is the Stomach Channel, which is located on the anterior of the body, but being Yang flows down the body.

There are 14 major channels that run throughout the body. Of the 14 major channels, 2 are unilateral and 12 are bilateral. And of the 12 bilateral channels, 10 correspond to organs and 2 correspond to functions.

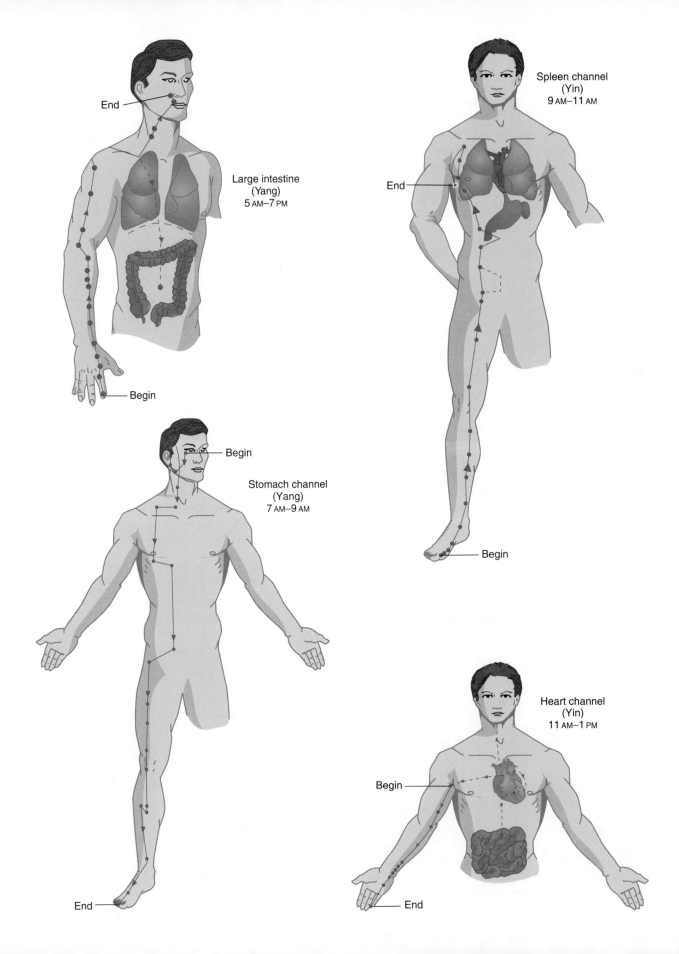

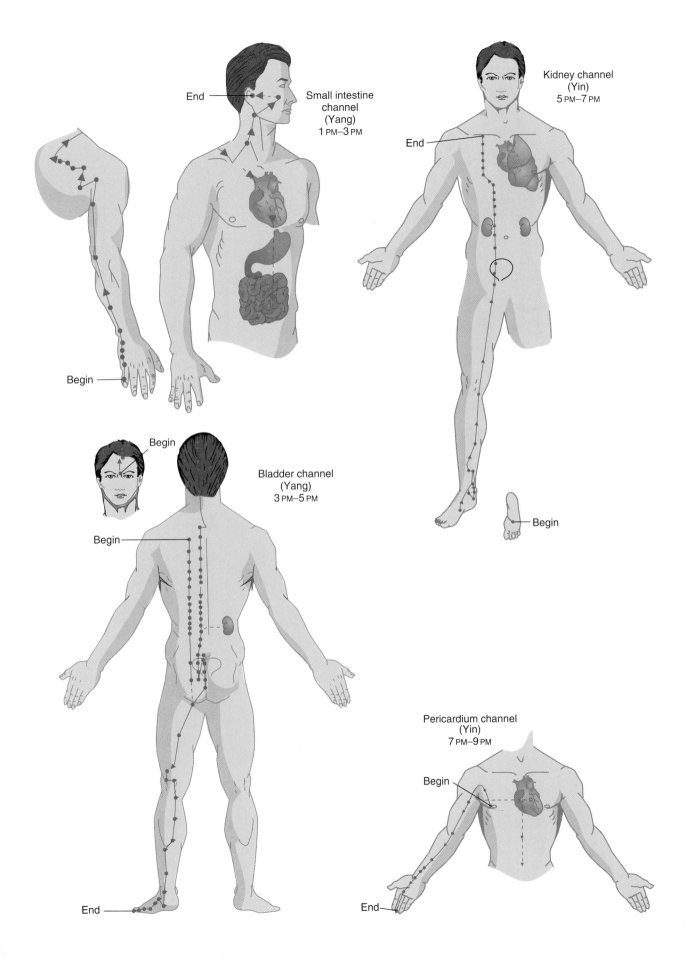

Small intestine
channel
(Yang)
1 PM–3 PM

End

Begin

Kidney channel
(Yin)
5 PM–7 PM

End

Begin

Begin

Bladder channel
(Yang)
3 PM–5 PM

Begin

End

Pericardium channel
(Yin)
7 PM–9 PM

Begin

End

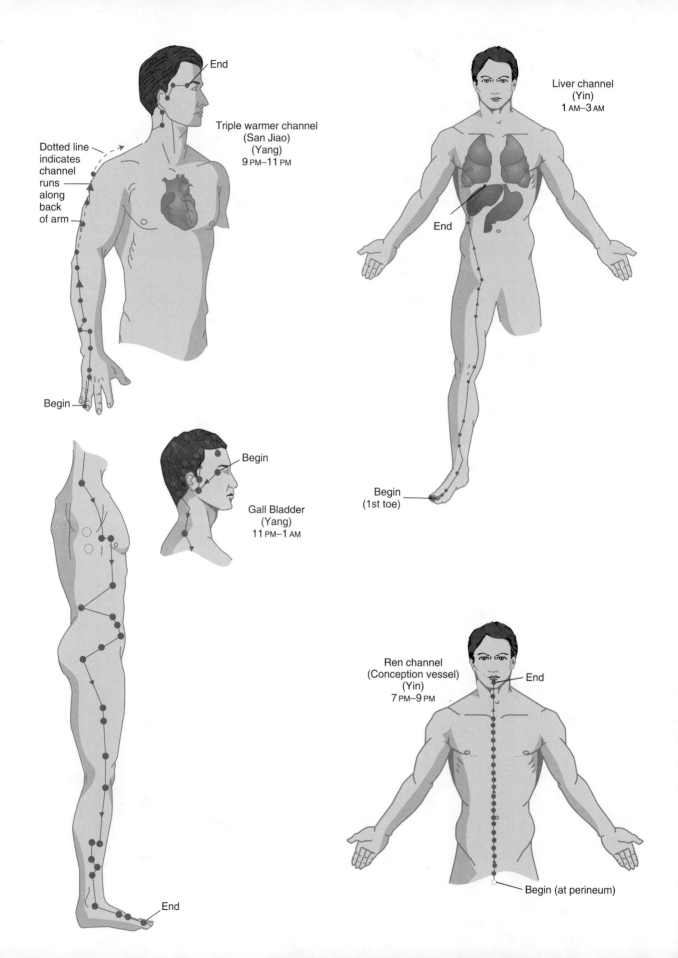

End

Triple warmer channel
(San Jiao)
(Yang)
9 PM–11 PM

Dotted line
indicates
channel
runs
along
back
of arm

Begin

Liver channel
(Yin)
1 AM–3 AM

End

Begin
(1st toe)

Begin

Gall Bladder
(Yang)
11 PM–1 AM

End

Ren channel
(Conception vessel)
(Yin)
7 PM–9 PM

End

Begin (at perineum)

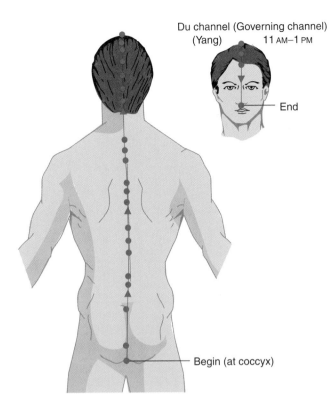

Du channel (Governing channel)
(Yang)   11 AM–1 PM

End

Begin (at coccyx)

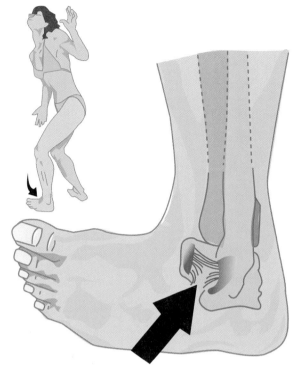

FIGURE 21-11 Lateral anterior talofibular ligament sprain.

TUINA THERAPEUTIC PROCEDURES

There are numerous therapeutic procedures in Tuina. I have chosen to address two of the more common injury sites that people suffer from: ankle sprains[1] and knee strains.[2] It's important to remember that in Tuina, the first thing you want to do is open up the channel. Then any manipulation of soft tissue that is applied to the area will produce a favorable effect. Otherwise any positive result produced will only be a partial one towards a total rehabilitation of the injury, resulting in a state of chronic weakness and/or tenderness of the area. Each procedure will be presented with the etiology and pathology of the injured area, along with the acupoints to work to open the channel, and lastly the Tuina techniques to treat the area.

Ankle Sprain

Etiology and Pathology

Figure 21-11 illustrates a common ankle sprain, which is usually caused by an inversion of the foot that tears the ligament. The ligament most often damaged is the anterior talofibular (ATF), as shown in the figure.

Acupoints to Treat Ankle Sprain.

1. Open up the channel that runs through the affected area: in this case the stomach and gall bladder channels. The first point is Zusanli (St-36) (Figure 21-12A). This begins to open up Qi flow into the leg and foot.

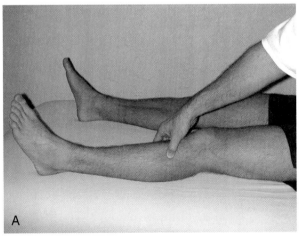

A

FIGURE 21-12A

2. Next, work Fuyang (Bl-59) (Figure 21-12B). Press and as the pain subsides, increase pressure and rub gently. Work approximately. 3 to 5 minutes, or until the pain stops.
3. Then work Kunlun (Bl-60) (Figure 21-12C) as in step #2.
4. Follow this with Pucan (Bl-61) in the same manner (Figure 21-12D). These points may be very tender if the Qi is stagnant at these locations.
5. Press and then rub Tongziliao (GB-1) located at the corner of the eye (Figure 21-12E).
6. Press Xiaxi (GB-43) for 3 to 5 minutes and increase pressure as the pain decreases (Figure 21-12F).

All of the above acupoints are to be worked on the affected side only.

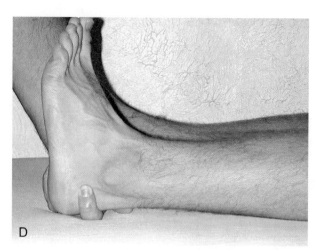

D

FIGURE 21-12D

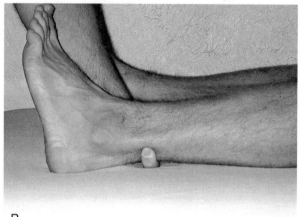

B

FIGURE 21-12B

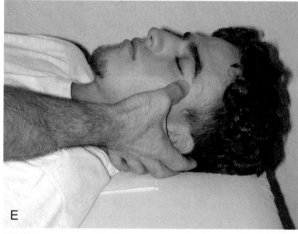

E

FIGURE 21-12E

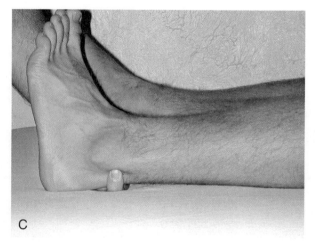

C

FIGURE 21-12C

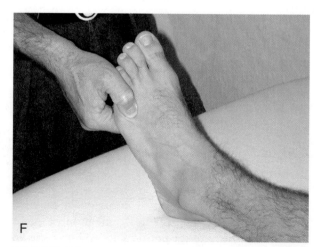

F

FIGURE 21-12F

Tuina Techniques

1. Laterally circumduct ankle 3 to 5 times.
2. Then, medially circumduct ankle 3 to 5 times.
3. Strongly dorsiflex the foot 2 to 3 times.
4. Plantarflex the foot 2 to 3 times.
5. Laterally rotate the ankle 2 to 3 times.
6. Medially rotate the ankle 2 to 3 times.
7. Scrape method to the talofibula ligament for about 30 to 90 seconds (Figure 21-12G).

If these ligaments are not pain free after applying the technique, don't repeat the technique. Continue to the next technique.

8. Kneading method to the ankle with the thenar eminences placed on both the medial and lateral malleolus. Kneading is performed rapidly and smoothly (Figure 21-12H).

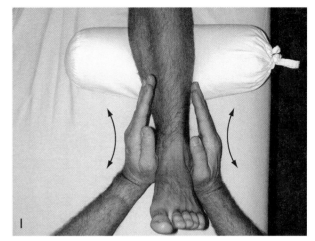

FIGURE 21-12I

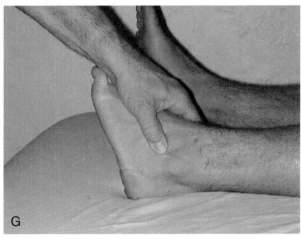

FIGURE 21-12G

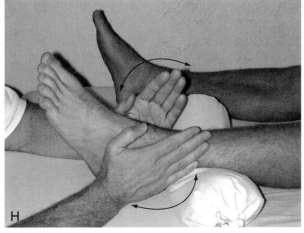

FIGURE 21-12H

9. Here is a top view showing the placement of the palms with only the thenor eminence on the malleoli and no palms. When done properly, the foot will mobilize automatically by moving side to side (Figure 21-12I).

This is not a friction type of movement, but one of kneading and rubbing the tissues under the thenar eminence. Pressure should be kept moderate, not heavy. And above all, your hands, shoulders, and wrist should be kept relaxed.

Knee Sprain

Etiology and Pathology

The knee is particularly vulnerable at full extension and in full weight-bearing position when the cruciate and collateral ligaments are taut and the anterior aspects of both menisci are secured between the condyles of tibia and fibula. Lateral impact to the knee can tear the meniscus or the cruciate ligaments. These are often caused from a blow to the lateral aspect of the knee, running, jumping, twisting of the joint, or falling on the knee (Figure 21-13A and B).

Acupoints

1. Begin every knee treatment with Futu (St-32). Hold the pressure for up to 3 minutes, and increase it as the pain subsides (Figure 21-14A).
2. Press Dubi (St-35), gradually increasing pressure as the pain subsides (Figure 21-14B).
3. Apply pressure to Zuzanli (St-36) as in steps 1 and 2 (Figure 21-14C).
4. Repeat procedure with Weizhong (Bl-40), being careful to press directly in the center of the back of

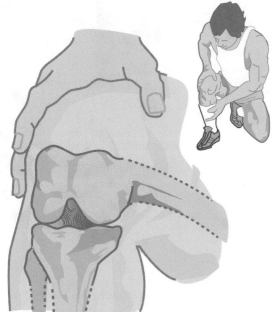

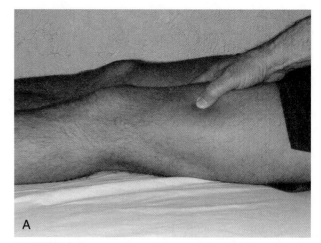

FIGURE 21-14A

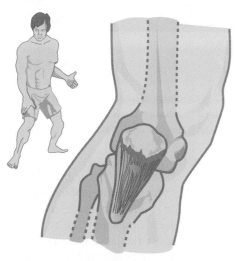

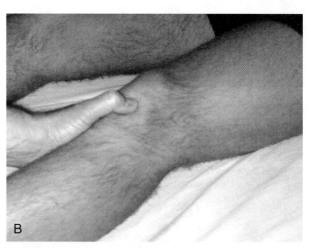

B

FIGURE 21-14B

A

B

FIGURE 21-13 A AND B Anterior cruciate ligament sprain.

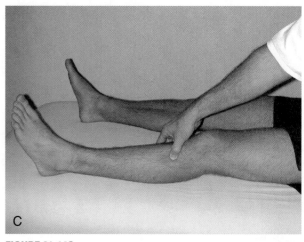

the knee. Avoid pressing the popliteal artery and nerve (Figure 21-14D). (NOTE: Some older systems of numbering the acupoints show Weizhong as Bl-54. The International System of numbering the points shows it to be listed as Bl-40. This system is more up to date and taught in most TCM schools around the world.)

Scrape method (Cuofa) to patella tendon until the pain decreases. Not to exceed 90 seconds of application (Figure 21-14E).

C

FIGURE 21-14C

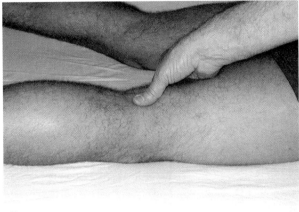

FIGURE 21-14D

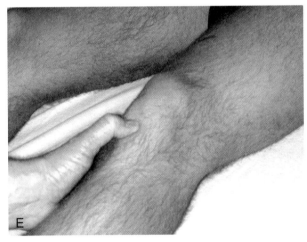

FIGURE 21-14E

CHAPTER SUMMARY

Chinese massage dates back some 5,000 years to around 2700 BC. It was originally known as "An Wu." Later, as it became more medical in its application, it was called "Anmo." Between 1368-1644 AD, a specialty department within Anmo was developed that was more scientifically medical in its application. This new form of massage was called "Tuina." Tuina is used in areas of gynecology, neurology, pediatrics, orthopedics, traumatology, cosmetology, rehabilitation, sports medicine, and general health care.

Tuina differs from other manual therapies mainly by the enormous scope of diseases and disorders it is able to effectively treat and the use and application of the channels. By using many of the 1,000 hand techniques available in Tuina, including Acupressure, the therapist can apply either the Reduction or Reinforcing Methods to rid the body of pain and disease, and reestablish a state of Yin and Yang, or health and balance.

Traditional Chinese Medicine (TCM), like Tuina, dates back more than 5,000 years. The first medical book ever written in the world was the *Huangdi Neijing*, or the *Yellow Emperor's Classic of Internal Medicine*. In this book, they discussed the Yin and Yang Theory, which covers the concept of relationships, patterns, and change within nature, the universe, and the human body. Also discussed was the concept of Qi, vital energy, how everything is made up of Qi, and how this Qi flows along pathways running throughout the body called channels. Qi can be manipulated by pressing or rubbing the acupoints that lie along the channels. Keeping this Qi flowing properly is what ensures a balance of Yin and Yang within the body. The result is a state of health and wellness.

CASE HISTORIES

▪ Case history 1

A 26-year-old female presents herself with a clinical diagnosis of polycythemia vera, a rare condition where the body makes too much blood. There is no clear diagnosis as to the cause in Western medicine, and patients that get the disorder find it is usually fatal, dying within 2 to 3 years from initial diagnosis. She had to have 2 to 3 pints of blood drawn off twice a week or her vessels would rupture from the pressure.

Using TCM, I discovered that the Liver was unstable, overcontrolling the Spleen, causing a deficiency of Yang within the Spleen and an increase of Damp to occur. By working Spleen points to increase Yang and Qi, dispel Damp, and improve the free flow of Qi by working Taichong (Liver-3), a state of normalcy in both blood volume and production was achieved in only 2 treatments. This was discovered after going to her doctor for her weekly examination.

▪ Case history 2

A 32-year-old male bodybuilder presents himself with mild atrophy of the left pectoralis major muscle and left triceps muscle, due to a herniated C-4/5 disk. Tuina was performed to the neck, left upper trapezius muscle, left pectoralis major, and left triceps muscles, along with opening up the Large Intestine channel, Gallbladder channel, Bladder channel, Small Intestines channel, and Triple Warmer channel, along the affected side. Stretching and ROM of the head, neck, and left shoulder, plus neuroreactivation of the radial nerve on the left side was performed. A normal state of muscle size and strength, along with replacement of the cervical disk, was achieved after six treatments.

SUGGESTED READINGS

Anhui Medical School Hospital of China: *Chinese massage: a handbook of therapeutic and preventive massage*, Vancouver, BC, 1983, Hartley & Marks.

Berk WR: *Chinese healing arts: internal Kung-Fu*, Burbank, Calif, 1986, Unique Publications.

Cao XI: *The massotherapy of traditional Chinese medicine*, Hong Kong, 1985 Hai Feng Publishing.

Gascoigne S: *The Chinese way to health: a self-help guide to traditional Chinese medicine*, Boston, 1997, Tuttle Publications.

Legge D: *Close to the 'Bone: the treatment of musculo-skeletal disorder with acupuncture and other traditional Chinese medicine*, Woy Woy, Australia, 1990, Sydney College Publications.

Luan C: *Concise Tuina therapy*, Jinan, China, 1997, Shandong Science and Technology Press.

Maciocia G: *The foundations of Chinese medicine: a comprehensive text for acupuncturists and herbalists*, New York, 1989, Churchill Livingstone.

Maoshing N: *The yellow emperor's classic of medicine*, Boston, 1995, Shambhala.

Mercati M: The *handbook of Chinese massage: Tui Na techniques to awaken body and mind*, Rochester, Vt, 1997, Healing Arts Press.

Nickel DJ: *Acupressure for athletes*, New York, 1984, Henry Holt.

Pritchard S:. *Chinese massage manual: the healing art of Tui Na*, New York, 1999, Sterling Publishing.

Reid D: *The complete book of Chinese health & healing*, New York, 1994, Barnes & Noble.

Schoenbart B:. *Chinese healing secrets*, Lincolnwood, 1997, LI. Publications International.

Sun C: *Chinese Massage Therapy*, Jinan, China, 1990, Shandong Science and Technology Press.

Sun S: *Atlas of therapeutic motion for treatment and health: a guide to traditional Chinese massage and exercise therapy*, Beijing, 1989, Foreign Language Press.

Wang F: *Chinese Tuina therapy*, Beijing, 1994, Foreign Languages Press.

Wang Z: *Acupressure therapy: point percussion treatment of cerebral birth injury, brain injury and stroke*, New York, 1991, Churchill Livingstone.

Xu M: *Manual treatment for traumatic injuries*, Beijing, 1997, Foreign Languages Press.

REFERENCES

1. Norman T: *Acupressure Course I* (course manual), Arlington, Tex, 1982.
2. Mercati M: *The handbook of Chinese Massage: Tui Na techniques to awaken body and mind*, Rochester, Vt, 1997, Healing Arts Press.
3. Zhang E: *Chinese massage, a practical English-Chinese library of traditional Chinese medicine*, Shanghai, 1988, Publishing House of Shanghai College of Traditional Chinese Medicine.
4. Xu Xi: *The English-Chinese encyclopedia of practical traditional Chinese medicine, Tuina therapeutics*, Beijing, 1994, Higher Education Press.
5. Pritchard S: *Chinese massage manual: the healing art of Tui Na*, New York, 1999, Sterling Publishing.
6. Norman T: *Asian Bodywork* (course manual), Arlington, Tx, 2001.
7. Veith I: *The yellow emperor's classic of internal medicine*, Berkeley, Calif, 1949, University of California Press.
8. Cheng X: *Chinese acupuncture and moxibustion*, Beijing, 1987, Foreign Language Press.
9. Kaptchuk TJ: *The web that has no weaver: understanding Chinese medicine*, Chicago, 1983, Congdon & Weed.

RESOURCES

www.aobta.com
www.tuina sports.com
Purchase Terry Norman's DVD on Sports Tuina contact Terry Norman at: tntll@earthlink.Net.

MULTIPLE CHOICE TEST QUESTIONS

1) The original form of massage done in China that dates back more than 5,000 years ago was called
   a) Anmo
   b) Shiatsu
   c) An Wu
   d) Tuina

2) Currently, in China today, the medical form of Chinese massage that is practiced by doctors in hospitals and clinics is called
   a) Anmo
   b) Amma
   c) An Wu
   d) Tuina

3) The term "Tuina" comes from the characters "Tui" and "Na," which mean
   a) stroke and knead
   b) beat and push
   c) pluck and pinch
   d) rub and press

4) One of the contraindications for doing Tuina is
   a) joint sprains
   b) asthma
   c) hepatitis
   d) intestinal adhesions

5) A technique that would be considered outside the scope of practice for someone performing Tuina in the United States would be
   a) stretching muscles and tendons
   b) pressing acupoints along channels
   c) soft tissue manipulations
   d) spinal manipulations

6) The fixed points that lie along the energy channels are called
   a) tsubo points
   b) acupoints
   c) ashi points
   d) primary points

7) The first book ever written on medicine was published in China thousands of years ago. The title of this book was the
   a) Ping T'sao
   b) Shang Hun Lun
   c) Huangdi Neijing
   d) Nei Chao T'u

8) Traditional Chinese Medicine began to decline in the nineteenth century due to
   a) the introduction of the x-ray machine
   b) political and foreign influences
   c) the death of a famous official
   d) Chinese doctors wanted a new approach to medicine

9) The revitalization of traditional Chinese medicine in the 1930s was largely due to
   a) Chinese rediscovering their roots
   b) foreign doctors had left China
   c) studies had proven its validity
   d) doctors were unable to get Western medications imported

10) The main difference between Western and Chinese medical approaches to illness and disease is that Western medicine attempts to eliminate the pathologic symptoms, where Chinese medicine focuses to reestablish
   a) a sense of euphoria
   b) a sense of balance
   c) a sense of awareness
   d) a sense of happiness

11) The main concept of the Yin and Yang Theory is
   a) negative and positive energies
   b) active, passive, and neutral energies
   c) relationships, patterns, and change
   d) expanding and contracting forces

12) The generally accepted definition of "Qi" is
    a) spiritual energy
    b) heat energy
    c) psychic energy
    d) vital energy

13) What is the number of major energy channels running through the body that Qi flows along, with acupoints located on them?
    a) 10
    b) 12
    c) 14
    d) 16

14) The root cause for the occurrence and development of all disease is imbalance between
    a) Yin and Yang
    b) Qi and blood
    c) channels and collaterals
    d) diet and exercise

15) In treating an injury or illness with Tuina, the first thing you want to do is
    a) increase blood flow
    b) make the person feel comfortable
    c) work on the most tender acupoints
    d) open up the channel

16) In treating an ankle sprain, the first acupoint you want to work is
    a) Zusanli (Stomach-36)
    b) Xiaxi (Gallbladder-43)
    c) Pucan (St-60)
    d) Tongziliao (GB-1)

17) In treating a torn anterior talofibular ligament of an ankle sprain, an effective Tuina technique to apply to the area is
    a) rubbing method
    b) thumb stroking method
    c) tendon separating method
    d) kneading method

18) In treating a knee sprain, the first acupoint you want to work is
    a) Futu (St-32)
    b) Dubi (St-35)
    c) Zusanli (St-36)
    d) Tongziliao (GB-1)

19) In treating any injury or illness, the primary goal is to reestablish
    a) the balance of Qi
    b) harmony of Yin and Yang
    c) the absence of pain
    d) peace of mind

20) Tuina is considered to be a manipulative art that is
    a) for relaxation only
    b) medically specific
    c) for soft tissue injuries only
    d) orthopedically specific

About the Contributors

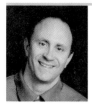

Dr. Joseph E. Muscolino, DC, a licensed Chiropractic Physician, is the author of *Kinesiology, the Skeletal System and Muscle Function; The Muscular System Manual, and the Skeletal Muscles of the Human Body, 2nd edition; The Musculoskeletal Anatomy Coloring Book.* The Muscle and Bone Palpation Manual with Trigger Points, Referral Patterns, and Stretching, all published by Mosby of Elsevier. He has a regular column entitled *Body Mechanics* in the *Massage Therapy Journal,* and often contributes articles to the *Journal of Bodywork and Movement Therapies.*

He has been an instructor of musculoskeletal and visceral anatomy and physiology, kinesiology, and pathology courses at the Connecticut Center for Massage Therapy (CCMT) for more than 20 years. He also runs numerous advanced study workshops, including deep tissue and joint mobilization workshops, kinesiology seminars, cadaver labs, and in-services for instructors of massage therapy.

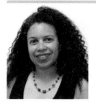

Sonia Elisa Masocco, MT, LDT, CAy, is an Ayurvedic instructor on the faculty of the Ayurvedic Institute in Albuquerque, NM. She has been in private practice for over 10 years. She is an ITEC qualified practitioner of aromatherapy, reflexology, and massage therapy. She completed her Ayurvedic training at the Ayurvedic Institute and the Ayurvedic Gurukula program in Pune, India.

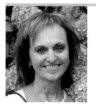

Beverly Byers, EdD, RN, LMT, MTI, is the founder and director of Oceans Massage Therapy Center, a school and spa in Lubbock, TX. Bev has been a registered nurse since 1981 and a professor of nursing at Lubbock Christian University since 1992. She is a licensed massage therapist and received her cancer massage training at the Scherer Institute in Santa Fe, NM and Memorial Sloan Kettering Cancer Center in New York City.

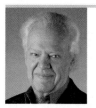

John E. Upledger, DO, OMM, is founder and president of The Upledger Institute and medical director of The Upledger Clinic, both headquartered in Palm Beach Gardens, FL. Dedicated to the natural enhancement of health, The Upledger Institute is recognized worldwide for its ground-breaking continuing-education programs, clinical research, and therapeutic services. The Upledger Clinic is world-renowned for its complementary care offered in both private sessions and intensive-therapy programs.

Throughout his career as an osteopathic physician and surgeon, Dr. Upledger has been recognized as an innovator and leading proponent in the investigation of new therapies. His development of CranioSacral Therapy has earned him an international reputation. *Time* magazine named him one of the world's next wave of innovators in 2001. His work has also been featured on Oprah, CNN, ESPN, Good Morning America, and in *USA Today* and many other national and international publications. In 2000 he testified before a U.S. Government Reform Committee meeting on the potential positive effects of CranioSacral Therapy on autism.

Dr. Upledger is a Certified Specialist of Osteopathic Manipulative Medicine, a Certified Fellow of the American Academy of Osteopathy, an Academic Fellow of the British Society of Osteopathy and a Doctor of Science. He has authored a wide range of books and research articles.

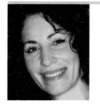

Sharon Desjarlais, CC, is a certified business coach and communications consultant for CranioSacral Therapists who want full and prosperous practices. She offers *CranioSacral Success*, a free e-mail newsletter full of unconventional tips for therapists to discover their blueprint for success and market their practices with joy.

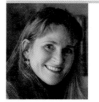

Susan G. Salvo, B Ed, LMT, NTS, CI, is a Nationally Certified, State Licensed Massage Therapist, and Natural Therapeutic Specialist. In 1982, she completed a 1000 hour program at New Mexico School of Natural Therapeutics. Ms. Salvo holds an associate degree in history and a baccalaureate degree in education from McNeese State University, where she is currently working on her Masters of Science degree in education. She owns and operates Bodyworks Massage Therapy by Susan Salvo and Associates which she founded in Lake Charles, Louisiana in 1983. In 1987, Ms. Salvo opened the Louisiana Institute of Massage Therapy in Lake Charles, which is a premier massage school. Ms. Salvo is a nationally known author, having written *Massage Therapy: Principles and Practice* and *Mosby's Guide to Pathology for the Massage Therapist,* both published by Elsevier. For the text *Teaching Massage,* produced by the Associated Bodywork Massage Professionals, she contributed the chapter entitled "Teaching Massage to Students with Special Needs" scheduled to be published by Lippincott, Williams, and Wilkins in 2008. Ms. Salvo co-authored a chapter entitled "The Atlas of Massage" for *Muscle and Bone Palpation Manual with Trigger Points, Referral Patterns, and Stretching* also scheduled to be published by Elsevier in 2008. Ms. Salvo is one of the featured experts interviewed in the documentary film, *History of Massage Therapy in the United States* released in 2007.

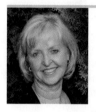

Diana Moore, MS, LMT, CIMI® is the founder and director of the International Loving Touch Foundation, Inc. (ILTF) in Portland, OR. She has been a licensed massage therapist since 1974 and a member of the American Massage Therapy Association for over 30 years. Her education includes a Master of Science in Management and Entrepreneurship from Marylhurst University with an undergraduate degree in Health Education and Sports Medicine from Portland State University. She received the Marylhurst Alumnus Award for Excellence in her field in 2002. In 2006, Diana received a Postgraduate Training Certificate in Infant Toddler Mental Health: A Relationship-Based Approach from Portland State University.

A pioneer in the global parenting tradition of infant massage, she began practicing and researching various methods in the mid seventies and subsequently developed the Loving Touch® Parent–Infant Massage Program. The International Loving Touch Foundation was incorporated in 1992. Diana teaches the Certified Infant Massage Instructor Program across the United States and internationally.

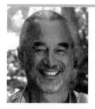

Dane Kaohelani Silva, DC, LMT, learned Hawaiian healing from his grandmother, Lily Kakani Nobriga, of Hāna, Maui, Uncle Harry Mitchell, and Papa Henry Auwae and was influenced by Auntie Margaret Machado. He earned his doctoral degree in chiropractic, is certified in acupuncture, is a licensed massage therapist, and is the founder of the Hawaiian Healing Center. Also one of the founders of the Hawaiian Lomilomi Association, he is an instructor for vocational, college, and graduate programs in Hawai'i, North America, Europe, New Zealand, and Japan. He is featured in the film, "Hawaiian Healing."

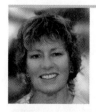

R. Makana Risser Chai, LMT, JD, first discovered her passion in life when she learned massage as a child from her grandmother. A licensed massage therapist, she studied with Auntie Margaret and Nerita Machado, authored the 2005 Bishop Museum book, *Nā Mo'olelo Lomilomi: The Traditions of Hawaiian Massage and Healing,* and with John Zak the 2007 pictorial, *Hawaiian Massage Lomilomi: Sacred Touch of Aloha.* In her past life she was a lawyer and CEO of a Silicon Valley training company. She founded Hawaiian Insights, Inc., to help perpetuate Hawaiian

traditions. She brings traditional practitioners to resorts and spas seeking to create authentic experiences, publishes the works of Native practitioners, and makes multi media presentations at meetings and conventions on Hawaiian ways to enrich life and work.

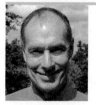

Robert Harris has a background in immunological research at the Max Plank Institute in Germany and holds a Higher National Diploma in Applied Biology from the U.K. He has been a Registered Massage Therapist in Ontario since 1980 and in British Columbia, Canada, since 1990 and has focused on Manual Lymph Drainage (MLD) and Combined Decongestive Therapy (CDT) since 1983.

Robert has dedicated his massage career to the Dr. Vodder method of MLD through clinical practice, lecturing, teaching, and as director and senior instructor at the Dr. Vodder School International training program, which he founded in 1994. His MLD training was completed at the Dr. Vodder School in Austria in 1984. Robert has translated and edited all of the Dr. Vodder School MLD textbooks and has authored many articles on the Dr. Vodder Method of Manual Lymph Drainage.

As the first teacher certified by the Dr. Vodder School in North America, Robert has taught and lectured on MLD throughout North America and has introduced the Vodder technique to New Zealand, Australia, Singapore, and Japan and in the UK. He has lectured extensively on the Dr. Vodder Method of Manual Lymph Drainage and Combined Decongestive Therapy.

Robert was elected as first president of the North American Vodder Association for Lymphatic Therapy (NAVALT) and served from 1992 to 1994. He has served on the Board of the Lymphology Association of North America (LANA). He is also a member of the AMTA, BCMTA, and International Society of Lymphology (ISL).

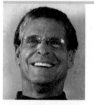

Art Riggs, CMT, is a Certified Advanced Rolfer® and massage therapist who practices in the San Francisco Bay area and has been teaching bodywork in the U.S. and internationally since 1988. His articles have appeared in several massage magazines and he is the author of *Deep Tissue Massage: A Visual Guide to Techniques* and the seven-volume accompanying DVD set, *Deep Tissue Massage and Myofascial Release: A Video Guide to Techniques.*

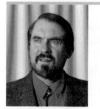

Keith Eric Grant, PhD, MS, BS, has been the senior instructor of sports and deep tissue massage at the McKinnon Institute, LLC in Oakland, CA since 1992. He is a computational physicist, an avid folk-dancer, and an advocate of teaching clinical massage techniques within the greater contexts of kinesthetic awareness and communication skills.

Dr. Grant has written the 'Ramblemuse' column for *Massage Today* since its inception in January 2001. He is currently a member of Massage Therapy Foundation's "Best Practices" Committee, working toward a system for creating evidence-based guidelines for application of massage to specific myofascial conditions. He is the author of two weblogs (blogs), The Massage Politics Sheet and Ramblemuse Touch Points, and the founding author of the Massage Medical Applications Project (MMAP).

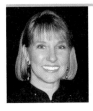

Judith DeLany, LMT, is founder and director of the International Academy of NeuroMuscular Therapies, a certifying body that sets standards for the training of healthcare practitioners in the use of NMT. She is the Director of the NMT Center, an educational/training organization that produces 80+ NMT events nationwide and internationally each year for the healthcare industry. She began teaching neuromuscular therapy (NMT) in 1984, emerging in a short time as a leading pioneer in the field of NMT. With many years as a clinician and educator, she refined and developed methods of teaching NMT American version™ and quickly excelled in curriculum development for continuing education for manual practitioners as well as curriculum development for basic manual training.

Ms. DeLany, together with Leon Chaitow, DO, ND, has co-authored two comprehensive textbooks on neuromuscular therapy titled *Clinical Application of Neuromuscular Techniques (volume 1 The Upper Body, volume 2 The Lower Body)* as well as the accompanying study guide, *Clinical Application of Neuromuscular Techniques—Case Study Exercises* (Elsevier). She has also contributed chapters on NMT to several books, including *Principles and Practices of Manual Therapeutics* (Pat Coughlin, MD, ed., Churchill Livingstone), *Modern Neuromuscular Techniques* (Leon Chaitow, DO, ND, 1st and 2nd eds., Churchill Livingstone), and *TouchAbilities: Essential Connections* (Iris Burman & Sandy Friedland, Delmar Learning). She has received recognition for outstanding instruction as well as legislative efforts and received "1999 Massage Therapist of the Year," awarded by the Florida Chiropractic Association.

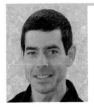

Whitney Lowe, LMT, is the author of the books *Orthopedic Assessment in Massage Therapy* and *Orthopedic Massage: Theory and Technique*, which are used in training programs and schools. He is currently a member of the editorial advisory board of the *Journal of Bodywork & Movement Therapies*. Lowe regularly authors works for publications such as *Massage Magazine, Massage Today, The Journal of Soft-Tissue Manipulation,* and *Journal of Bodywork & Movement Therapies*. Lowe directs the Orthopedic Massage Education & Research Institute (OMERI), through which he offers seminars and online training.

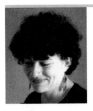

Leslie Korn, PhD, MPH, RPP, NCBTMB, has been in clinical practice since 1977. She specializes in natural approaches to mental health and the treatment of chronic illness and persistent health issues arising from posttraumatic stress. Dr. Korn has practiced therapeutic bodywork since 1977. She is a Registered Polarity Practitioner and Registered Polarity Educator. She is nationally board certified in therapeutic massage and bodywork and is a licensed mental health counselor. She has a PhD in Behavioral Medicine from

the Union Institute, an MA in cross-cultural health psychology from Lesley University, and an MPH from the Harvard School of Public Health where she carried out research in nutrition. She trained in psychotherapy and community mental health in the department of psychiatry at the Cambridge Hospital, Harvard Medical School where she was a Clinical Fellow in Psychology and Religion. She completed clinical internships at the Pain and Stress Clinic, Boston University and at the Trauma Clinic at the Massachusetts General Hospital.

She introduced polarity therapy and body-oriented psychotherapy for the treatment of PTSD in the department of psychiatry during her tenure at Harvard. Dr. Korn founded the Center for Traditional Medicine, a natural medicine public health center in rural Mexico serving a Mexican-Indian population and expatriates where she lived between 1973 and 1983 and again between 1997 and 2002. Dr. Korn has trained extensively in indigenous medical practices and has worked extensively with Hispanic and American Indian populations living in the Pacific Northwest and Canada.

She divides her clinical work with clients (assisted by Saba, the therapy dog) and writing between Olympia, WA and Puerto Vallarta, Mexico.

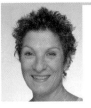

Elaine Stillerman, LMT, has been a New York State licensed massage therapist since 1978. She began her pioneering work in prenatal massage, labor support, and postpartum recovery in 1980. She is the developer and instructor of the professional certification workshop "MotherMassage®: massage during pregnancy" which she began teaching in 1990.

Elaine is the author of *MotherMassage: a Handbook for Relieving the Discomforts of Pregnancy* (Dell, 1992), *The Encyclopedia of Bodywork* (Facts On File, 1996), *Prenatal Massage: a Textbook of Pregnancy, Labor, and Postpartum Bodywork* (Mosby, 2008), and is the editor and contributing writer of *Modalities for Massage and Bodywork* (Mosby, 2009).

She writes the *Womankind* column for *Massage Today* and is an award-winning writer for the PBS-TV show "Real Moms, Real Stories, Real Savvy."

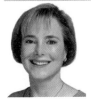

Laura Norman, MS, BS, LMT, began her career in reflexology in 1970—a time when complementary therapies were almost unheard of—and she has been on the leading edge of the holistic health movement ever since. Today, Laura is America's most celebrated practitioner of reflexology and a leading authority on reflexology, holistic healing, and wellness.

Through the Laura Norman Reflexology℠ Certification Program, Laura touches tens of thousands of people through her staff and her graduates. She also reaches out to millions more through her videos, DVDs, and other Laura Norman Reflexology℠ learning tools as well as through frequent local and national media appearances.

Feet First, A Guide to Foot Reflexology, Laura's international bestseller, is available in five languages. With over 500,000 copies in circulation, Laura has written what is considered to be an essential text on the fundamentals of reflexology and how it can improve the lives of people from birth through all the phases of life.

Laura is a nationally certified reflexologist and a licensed massage therapist and esthetician in the states of New York and Florida.

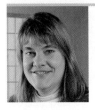

Sandra K. Anderson, BA, LMT, NCTMB, has been a licensed massage therapist since 1992, a certified shiatsu practitioner since 1999, and a certified Thai massage practitioner since 2002. She received all her training at the Desert Institute of the Healing Arts in Tucson, AZ. She taught at the Desert Institute for 12 years, in subjects ranging from anatomy and physiology to shiatsu, and was Chair of the Anatomy and Physiology Department for 5 years. Recently she was Director of Education for Cortiva-Desert Institute. She was Chair of the Examination Committee of the National Certification Board for Therapeutic Massage and Bodywork for 5 years and is currently Chair of the Awards Committee for the American Massage Therapy Association, Arizona Chapter. Sandra is co-owner of Tucson Touch Therapies, a treatment and continuing education center located in Tucson, AZ. She is Education Center Director for Tucson Touch Therapies and has presented numerous workshops on Asian bodywork techniques. Sandra is co-author of *Pathology for Massage Therapists* and author of *The Practice of Shiatsu*, 2007.

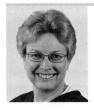

Sandy Fritz, MS, BS, NCTMB, is the Owner, Director, and Head Instructor of the Health Enrichment Center, Inc., School of Therapeutic Massage. Also in private practice for almost 30 years, Sandy works with a diverse clientele, dealing with everything from stress management massage to physician-referred rehabilitative care upon physician referral. She developed and supervises a student massage clinic with the Detroit Lions of the National Football League. She also provides professional sports massage and rehabilitation for individual athletes, primarily in golf, football, basketball, and baseball.

Sandy is the author of *Fundamentals of Therapeutic Massage, Mosby's Essential Sciences for Therapeutic Massage, Mosby's Massage Therapy Review Guide, A Massage Therapist's Guide to Lower Back and Pelvic Pain, Clinical Massage in the Healthcare Setting, Sports and Exercise Massage, A Massage Therapist Guide to Understanding, Locating, and Treating Myofascial Trigger Points,* and *Mosby's PDQ for Massage.*

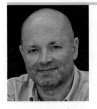

Peter Schwind, PhD, is a certified advanced Rolf practitioner. He has been a member of the Rolf Institute of Structural Integration since 1980 and has been teaching for the Rolf Institute in the U.S. and for the European Rolfing Association in Europe since 1985. He is the author of several books, including *Fascial and Membrane Technique: A Manual for Comprehensive Treatment of the Connective Tissue System* (Churchill Livingstone/Elsevier). He works in his practice in Munich and teaches Fascial and Membrane Technique for the Barral Institute and for the Munich Group.

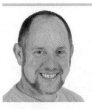

Richard Gold, PhD, LAc, graduated from Oberlin College in 1972 with a degree in Religious Studies. In 1978, he graduated from the New England School of Acupuncture. Since then, he has devoted himself to the study, practice, researching, and teaching of Asian Healing Arts. He participated in advanced studies in Chinese Medicine at Xinhua Hospital in Shanghai, PRC in 1980. In 1983, he earned a Doctorate in Psychology. He apprenticed to Seitai Shiatsu Master Kyoshi Kato in Osaka, Japan in 1986. Beginning in 1988, Dr. Gold began his studies of Traditional Thai Massage (Nuad Bo'Rarn) in Chiang Mai, Thailand at the Old Medicine Hospital, the Foundation of Shivago Komparaj. The first edition of his book, *Thai Massage: A Traditional Medical Technique* was published in 1998 by Churchill Livingstone with a second edition published by Mosby Press in 2007. Currently, Richard is the President and Chairman of the Board of the International Professional School of Bodywork (IPSB) in San Diego. He is also a senior faculty member at IPSB. In addition, he is on the Board of Directors of Pacific College of Oriental Medicine (PCOM).

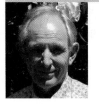

Jack Blackburn, LMP, Master's in Theological Studies, Certified Spiritual Director, Registered Counselor, specializes in body centered spiritual growth and healing. He has been a Trager® practitioner since 1986. He has been a Trager tutor since 1993, has taught Trager electives classes since 1996, and teaches a variety of classes to care giving professionals. He is a NCBTMB Approved Continuing Education Provider and AMTA National Presenter. He is a Focusing Trainer and teaches Bodywork Focusing classes for professionals. Jack is also a Reiki Master and teaches levels I, II, III and Advanced Reiki for Bodyworkers.

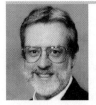

Terry Norman, BME, LMT has been performing Tuina for over 35 years. He has studied both in the U.S. and China and has over 6700 hours of study in a variety of fields within bodywork and Asian healing arts. Terry is nationally certified with the NCTMB, member of AOBTA, and serves on the Exam Development Committee of the NCBTMB.

He has studied Tuina at the University of Traditional Chinese Medicine in Shanghai, while doing clinical practice at the Yue Yang Hospital. Later, he was with the first group of foreign students to study Sports Tuina at the Olympic Training Center in Beijing. In 1996, Terry became the first foreign therapist to be allowed to work on Chinese Olympic athletes and to study at the Olympic Training Center as an individual therapist while performing internship studies at area hospitals and clinics in Beijing.

Terry has a practice in Texas and teaches classes in TCM, acupressure, Tuina, and sports Tuina at universities, colleges, massage schools, and physical therapy clinics in the Dallas/Ft. Worth area and nationwide.

ANSWERS TO MULTIPLE CHOICE TEST QUESTIONS

Chapter 1

1. c: Aaron Mattes began developing the AIS technique in 1972.

2. b: The primary purpose of every stretching technique is to increase the flexibility of the target tissues.

3. a: The "target" tissue is the tissue that we are targeting to stretch, hence the name.

4. d: A static stretch is so named because the client statically holds the position of the stretch.

5. a: By definition, a dynamic stretch involves more motion and less time in a statically held position. Therefore, dynamic stretches are usually held for only 1 to 3 seconds.

6. c: Because a dynamic stretch is primarily concerned with moving the target tissue, it is also known as a mobilization stretch.

7. c: The terms *active stretch* and *passive stretch* refer to the activity or passivity of the muscles of that joint. Therefore, an active stretch is one wherein the muscles of that joint bring the body to the position of the stretch.

8. d: It is often erroneously thought that a passive stretch requires the presence of a therapist. Although a therapist passively stretching the target tissues of the client is an example of a passive stretch, the presence of the therapist is not required. As long as the muscles of the client's joint where the stretch is occurring are relaxed, the stretch is passive. This means that a client can use another body part to create a passive stretch in his/her body.

9. d: Advanced stretching may be defined as a stretch that is facilitated by a neurologic reflex. PNF stretching is facilitated by the Golgi tendon organ reflex; AC stretching is facilitated by reciprocal inhibition. The Golgi tendon organ reflex and reciprocal inhibition are both neurologic reflexes.

10. b: The Golgi tendon organ reflex is used for CR stretching. Reciprocal inhibition is used for AC stretching. The muscle spindle reflex (also known as the stretch reflex) is never used to improve the efficacy of a stretch because it causes greater contraction of a muscle, thus greater tissue tension.

11. c: Reciprocal inhibition is used for AC stretching. The Golgi tendon organ reflex is used for CR stretching. The muscle spindle reflex (also known as the stretch reflex) is never used to improve the efficacy of a stretch because it causes greater contraction of a muscle, thus greater tissue tension.

12. c: The stretch phase of AIS technique involves the client actively moving into the position of stretch as well as the increased stretch done immediately thereafter, either by the client himself/herself or the therapist. The recovery phase involves the client returning to the initial starting position for the next repetition.

13. a: During AIS technique, the client exhales when actively moving the body part; think *exhale on exertion.*

14. c: One of the major factors for the increased flexibility gained by doing the AIS technique is the fact that multiple repetitions, usually 8 to10, are performed.

15. a: Given that multiple repetitions are performed, each repetition adds only a small amount of stretching force, usually 1 pound or less. It is important to not apply too much force when stretching a client's tissues or the muscle spindle reflex may be triggered, which would result in contraction of the muscle.

16. a: The muscle spindle reflex (also known as the stretch reflex) results in contraction of the muscle. It is a protective reflex, preventing the muscle from being overstretched and therefore torn.

17. c: Given that the AIS technique is based upon reciprocal inhibition, the muscles antagonistic to the target muscles must be actively contracted so that the target muscles are reciprocally inhibited from contracting, i.e., relaxed. The principle of reciprocal inhibition states that whenever a muscle is contracted, its antagonists will be reciprocally inhibited.

18. d: AIS technique results in increased flexibility of the target muscles because they are reciprocally inhibited and therefore relaxed so that they can be better stretched. The antagonist muscles to the target muscles are strengthened because they are actively contracted during the protocol. Due to the active movements involved, local circulation is increased; increased circulation also warms the area. And by contracting muscles, not only are they strengthened, but the neural pathways involved are facilitated as well. Hence, all choices are true.

19. c: Whenever a stretch is performed, it is crucially important that the line of tension of the stretch is focused upon the target tissue. This often requires the rest of the client's body to be stabilized. The hand of the therapist that does this is called the stabilization hand.

20. d: Marked osteoarthritis (also known as degenerative joint disease) and bulging or herniated disks may be contraindications to performing AIS technique if the positions attained during the protocol cause increased compressive force to the affected tissues.

Chapter 2

1. d: Ayurveda was developed in India and is a system of medicine that translates as "science of life."

2. d: Ayurveda was developed nearly 3,000 years ago.

3. c: The term *dosha* refers to bodily humor or bodily constitution. It is the conceptual union of predominance within the 5 elements. There are three doshas in Ayurveda: vata, pitta, and kapha, each with its own unique qualities.

4. a: Vata represents the union of ether and air and is responsible for space, movement, breathings, natural urges, and sensory functions. It is also the container for the superlative quality of prana.

5. b: Ayurveda holds that "like increases like."

6. c: Pitta is the time between 10 and 2 AM and PM, increasing in the summer and ripe for elimination in the fall. The ages of pitta are 14 to 50, or adulthood.

7. c: Toxicity shares some qualities with kapha.

8. d: Ayurveda respects the profound interrelationship between body, mind, and emotion in both health and disease, or toxicity.

9. c: Abhyanga is contraindicated with low agni and high ama.

10. a: Light, cool, and sweet oils are used with pitta predominance. Coconut or sunflower oils are examples of the types of oils used for pitta constitution.

11. c: Udvartana, or dry massage, is done roughly to help eliminate accumulated kapha or ama.

12. d: Udvartana is indicated for heavy, sluggish, congested symptoms.

13. d: Ayurveda does not recommend massage when a client has a fever.

14. b: Rubbing creates friction and can aggravate vata.

15. c: Pulling is used to release stress, suppressed emotions, and blocked energy.

16. d: It is best to avoid cold showers, a large meal, or wind after abhyanga or karna purana.

17. a: Pooling of warm oil in the lumbosacral area, or kati basti, relieves lower back pain and tension.

18. d: Lepana is the application of an herbal paste to the body and is beneficial in cases of localized swelling, inflammation, and generalized heat.

19. d: Pinda svedana, or poultice pounding therapy, helps eliminate toxins, encourages vitality, and rejuvenates the tissues.

20. b: During the period from 10 to 2 AM and PM pitta is at its highest.

Chapter 3

1. c: When normal cells become "out-of-control" and abnormally take over, they are considered cancers.

2. b: Massage for people living with cancer affects the immune system in a positive way.

3. a: Nausea, pain, anxiety, fatigue, and depression. Treatments for cancer cannot be isolated to

cancer cells, but rather affect normal cells as well, causing side effects of which the most common are nausea, pain, anxiety, fatigue, and depression.

4. d: All of the above. Research indicates massage reduces pain, improves appetite and quality of sleep, and strengthens the immune system.

5. b: Lymphedema. Lymph nodes act as filters and when those are nonfunctioning, lymph fluid becomes congested, causing swelling or edema in that particular part of the lymph system.

6. c: Radiation therapy. Radiation therapy uses radio waves in a controlled manner to deliver a beam of radiation to destroy cells; or in the case of internal implantation, the radioactive material acts as killers of cancer.

7. a: Lessened or dialed down. Because chemotherapy destroys normal cells along with cancer cells, the body is weakened and cannot tolerate deep pressure, nor can it dispose of the rapid release of toxins produce by deep or vigorous massage.

8. d: All of the above. Nausea increases the sensitivity of the senses, including movement and olfaction. Thus, increased movements and smells can be overstimulation for the person with nausea.

9. a: Deep vein thrombosis (DVT). Surgical interventions interrupt blood vessels and the normal flow of blood.

10. b: Complementary therapy. Massage is indicated for people with cancer, although is should not be used instead of conventional medicine, and it is not a cure for cancer. Rather, massage adds to (complements) the conventional treatments.

11. c: Metastasis. Rationale: When cancer cells acquire increased motility and invasiveness, the cells can move to an area in the body that is not directly connected.

12. d: Liquid tumors. Liquid tumors involve the cells that move in liquids such as blood and lymph.

13. a: Brain, colon, breast. Primary cancers frequently arise in these areas.

14. c: A port protects the blood vessels from the repeated entry of harsh chemicals. Because of the toxicity of chemicals, a port is implanted in a blood vessel to receive the drugs for

cancer, thus providing a barrier between the chemotherapy and the blood vessel.

15. b: Care given to ease a client's suffering. When treatment is no longer an option, comfort care (palliative) may help the person feel better.

16. b: Variables. The many types, severity, and side effects of cancer and cancer treatments place the client in different phases (of living with cancer) with unique circumstances and levels of pain, tolerance, and time.

17. d: All of the above. The variables of the disease phases, the treatments, and the side effects of the treatments influence the area(s) on the body to be massaged, the length of the massage, and the tolerance level of the person at any given time.

18. d: Both b and c. Deep tissue massage is contraindicated. Even the clients are not always aware of what their bodies are able to tolerate at the time. People with cancer often have blood values that are not in normal range and can easily bruise. In addition, their bodies may not be able to handle the release of toxins from deep tissue massage.

19. d: All of the above. The written health form and the communication between client and therapist should address questions related to pain, fatigue, and previous or current swelling related to cancer or the treatments for cancer.

20. a: Diagnosis. The diagnosis of cancer is the common ground for all people with cancer. After the diagnosis, individual phases, treatment choices, effects on the person, needs of the person, and successes of treatments make a unique case for the person with cancer.

Chapter 4

1. c: The craniosacral system creates the environment for the brain and spinal cord.

2. b: CST is based on the principle that the body is a self-correcting mechanism.

3. d: Fascia is a key vehicle that allows you to trace symptoms back to their source.

4. a: The Pressurestat Model is a semiclosed hydraulic system that forms the basis for the craniosacral rhythm.

5. c: Because the craniosacral system surrounds the brain and spinal cord, it directly affects the central nervous system (CNS) and indirectly affects all other body systems that are influenced by the CNS.

6. a: CST is designed to help you relieve the underlying source of problems so the client doesn't need to keep experiencing the symptoms.

7. d: When used gently with intention, the hands can become finely tuned devices for listening to the body and encouraging a response.

8. b: By identifying the rhythm's Symmetry, Quality, Amplitude, and Rate (SQAR), you can more easily pinpoint areas of the craniosacral system that are restricted or imbalanced.

9. c: Listening stations individually give you a quick read of the total body.

10. b: Active lesions may need to be resolved first before more subtle body restrictions can be identified and released.

11. a: The therapeutic nature of the Still Point has an overall calming and soothing effect on the body.

12. b: The motion or lack of motion is indicative of health or dysfunction.

13. d: By resisting the craniosacral rhythm at either the flexion or extension phase, you can bring about a momentary pause in the flow of the fluid and overall craniosacral motion.

14. c: By using body energy to store an energy cyst, less energy is available for other body functions.

15. b: Facilitated segments are areas of common pain and dysfunction.

16. d: Whether inspired on a subconscious level or by other means, a significance detector is one way the body communicates with the client and the therapist.

17. a: When the body can return to the original position it was in when it underwent a trauma, it can allow stored energy to be released along the same trajectory it came in through.

18. c: A tissue release can encompass any change; it can also vary from person to person, and from session to session.

19. b: Anything directly affected by the CNS can be influenced by CranioSacral Therapy.

20. c: When you have any questions as to whether changing a client's intracranial pressure will be detrimental, refer your client to their physician before proceeding.

Chapter 5

1. c: Population experts estimate that 53% of the population, will be 65 or older by 2020.

2. d: Geriatric massage is a form of massage designed to meet the specific needs of the elderly population.

3. b: Geriatrics is a branch of medicine concerned with the diagnosis and treatment of old age.

4. a: Dietrich Miesler founded the Day-Break Geriatric Institute in 1986. Essentially, this technique adapts traditional massage for the aging population, although there are a few unique techniques.

5. b: Comfort Touch was developed by Mary Kathleen Rose. She started teaching in 1991 and coined the phrase in 1993. This nurturing form of acupressure is consistent with hospice's philosophy of palliative care and avoids conventional massage in favor of broad perpendicular pressure.

6. d: Compassionate Touch was developed by Dawn Nelson in 1991 in California.

7. d: Use gentle stretching and joint movements as vigorous movements can be tiring for the client as well as bring harm in cases of increased bone porosity and osteoporosis.

8. a: The baby boomers are the people born between 1946 and 1964 and make up one third of today's population.

9. d: 90% of older persons reported to have at least one chronic condition and the majority had multiple conditions.

10. c: Life expectancy continues to get longer. Currently, the average life expectancy is around 77 years of age.

11. c: Senescence refers to the period of life from old age to death.

12. b: 65 is considered to be the beginning of old age in this country.

13. d: The branch of study concerned with normal aging is gerontology.

14. b: Orthostatic hypotension, also called postural hypotension, is the loss of balance brought on by a sudden drop in blood pressure when moving from a recumbent position to an upright position. To reduce the risk of falling, allow adequate time for the elderly to change positions. If needed, assist them in sitting or standing.

15. b: Senior citizens purchase 30% of all prescription drugs and 40% of over-the-counter medications.

16. c: 70% of the elderly population do not participate in activities on a regular basis and are considered to be sedentary. Geriatric massage should not replace appropriate exercise, however.

17. d: Prone positioning should be avoided when massaging the elderly population in favor of elevation of the client's upper body to promote proper breathing. Turning on the treatment table may also be problematic for some elderly.

18. b: Selective serotonin reuptake inhibitors, or SSRIs, are not commonly used medications by the elderly.

19. c: Hypertension is the leading chronic illness of the elderly.

20. a: Falling is the most common safety issue for people 65 and older. Medications can alter balance, coordination, and response time. Make sure your office is clear of any tripping hazards, such as loose rugs or furniture the elderly might not see.

Chapter 6

1. c: In India, Nigeria, and many other countries, mothers learn massage from *their* mothers and pass it along to the next generation. All over Nepal, writes Amelia Auckett, babies are massaged every day from just 2 to 3 hours old.

2. c: "With our babies more often in a container than in our arms, our infants are 'at odds' with their evolution, as anthropologist James McKenna put it," writes Heller.

3. b: In the past 30 years, the United States has begun to embrace the massaging of infants in the form of what is considered a parent-baby activity.

4. a: Much seminal work was done by Dr. Frederick Leboyer, whose highly popular 1976 book *Loving Hands* became the basis for most of today's infant massage training in the United States.

5. d: One of the first recorded mentions of infant massage in the United States dates from 1894, in a book *The Care and Feeding of Children* by Dr. Emmett Holt.

6. c: In general, infant massage should be performed in a smooth, rhythmic manner using moderate pressure and varying speeds.

7. b: The six behavioral states of the newborn can be used to help identify the best time to communicate with an infant.

8. a: In her classic study performed on premature babies, Tiffany Field was able to show that massage helped to facilitate weight gain, improve nervous system development, decrease levels of cortisol, increase muscle tone, and improve sleep and awake patterns.

9. d: The quiet alert state is the optimal time for communication and for infant massage activity to begin.

10. c: Leboyer noted that in South India, usual practice was to begin when the baby was 1 month old. Certainly, the abdomen should not be massaged until the umbilical cord stub has dropped off to allow time for proper healing.

11. a: Examples of engagement cues include smiling, cooing, and babbling. Disengagement cues include crying, gaze aversion, arching the body, and pushing away. Combined would be smiling and crying, for a cue of engagement and a cue of disengagement.

12. a: Premature infant. An infant born before the thirty-seventh week of gestation.

13. c: If allergies are suspected, it's wise to perform a simple patch test: place a small amount of the oil on the infant's wrist, leave for 20 to 30 minutes.

14. a: The formation of a close emotional tie between parent and infant is one of the defining purposes of infant massage. Bonding is defined as "a gradual, reciprocal process that begins with acquaintance. It is a unique and specific relationship between two people and endures across time."

15. d: Natural cold-pressed, or organic oils, such as sweet almond, apricot, sesame seed, or grape seed oil, will nourish the baby's skin and give a very smooth and pleasant feeling.

16. b: Both infant and parent will enjoy the bonding more if not distracted by too much excessive noise. Soothing music, nature sounds, or heartbeat sounds encourage relaxation.

17. b: Although mothers experience a sharp increase in bonding around the fifth month of pregnancy and have intensifying feelings throughout the pregnancy, the father's feelings usually tend to develop more slowly and become congruent after birth, when infant caretaking begins.

18. c: Floor time is an especially suitable occasion, in that it allows the baby to safely move around—not typically a concern with adult massage.

19. a: This varies according to the ability of the giver and the state of awareness of the infant.

20. c: Active toddlers often enjoy quick and vigorous movements accompanied with complementary activities such as singing and nursery rhymes to hold their attention.

Chapter 7

1. c: Although lomilomi was developed in Hawaii and came with the voyagers from the Marquesas, its roots are in China.

2. d: In addition to medical experts, children, servants of the chiefs, and martial arts masters practiced lomilomi in old Hawaii.

3. c: All of these techniques are part of lomilomi, but the two particularly important are stomach massage and back walking.

4. b: Physical aspects are the least important in determining if a particular style of lomilomi is authentic. What is important is the practitioner's mental, emotional, and spiritual approach.

5. d: Herbs are used as poultices, to create oil, and for aromatherapy.

6. a: Ti leaves are used for spiritual protection, medicinal properties, and as poultices, but not for their aroma, which is slight.

7. d: Sticks are used for all of these reasons: balance when back walking, compression, and self-massage.

8. b: Burning the skin is the safety concern when using hot rocks.

9. c: Every session of lomilomi begins with prayer. Although a prayer may be chanted, it also may be spoken or said silently.

10. a: Ho'oponopono is part of lomilomi because Hawaiians believe holding grudges causes illness.

11. b: The practitioner tells the client, "Observe the pain flow out on each breath like smoke."

12. d: Historically, Hawaiians created steam baths in all these ways, building huts over volcano vents and hot rocks, and covering themselves and a gourd of hot water with a blanket.

13. c: When creating a sacred space, although plants and candles may be used, what is required is prayer, intention, and a bowl of water for cleansing.

14. b: Telling the patient about similar cases you've seen is not important in making an assessment; visual observations of the patient's body, asking questions of patients and their families, and palpating with the hands are more useful.

15. d: The best place to start the physical strokes depends on the case; it could be at the head, the feet, away from the place of pain, or in another area.

16. d: All of these are reasons clients might experience different symptoms over time.

17. a: The most important factor in determining contraindications for lomilomi is the experience of the practitioner.

18. a: The "cutting the cord" ritual is performed to protect the practitioner from energies released by the patient.

19. d: A teacher learns lomilomi after years of study and practice.

20. c: Although the most fun way to find a teacher might be to move to Hawai'i, the best way is to check the Hawaiian Lomilomi Association web site.

Chapter 8

1. c: Only collector vessels have true valves, and the section from one valve to the next is called a lymphangion.

2. d: MLD is a light, gentle stroke that stretches the skin in a circular fashion.

3. a: Protein is a major component of lymph, pathogens are minor components, and red blood cells and carbohydrates are not usually found in lymph.

4. d: Sympatholytic effect is a lowered sympathetic nerve firing according to Professor Hutzschenreuter.

5. d: Colloid osmotic pressure is the water-attracting force of proteins.

6. c: MLD may affect other types of edemas, but the main use is in the treatment of lymphedema.

7. b: The innermost layer of lymph vessels (intima) is made of endothelial cells.

8. a: All of the answers are indications for MLD except acute infections.

9. b: MLD requires a specific stretching force to be exerted on the skin in order to stimulate contraction of lymph vessels.

10. c: Removal of proteins in the interstitium is considered to be the most important function of the lymph vessel system according to Professor Guyton.

11. a: Rotary technique can cover large surface areas most efficiently.

12. b: The Dr. Vodder method of MLD always begins in the most proximal parts (e.g., neck) and works toward the more distal parts, in relation to the lymph system.

13. b: There is a high protein level in the edema fluid of a lymphedema.

14. d: Compression therapy is one of the four key components of Combined Decongestive Therapy. The others are MLD, remedial exercise, and skin care.

15. c: Approximately 2 to 4 liters of lymph return to the heart every 24 hours.

16. c: Approximately 600 lymph nodes are found in the body.

17. d: The Dr. Vodder School was established in North America in 1994.

18. d: Efferent collectors take lymph away from the lymph nodes.

19. a: Lymphedema is a recognized complication of many dermatologic conditions including rosacea.

20. b: Venous disease does not cause lymphedema, but rather dynamic edema.

Chapter 9

1. c: For many, modern life has brought a more sedentary lifestyle that includes hours of sitting at desks or in front of computers with the back and hips flexed.

2. a: Myofascial release specifically addresses movement restrictions from adhesions.

3. b: By relaxing hypertonic muscles before doing direct techniques, postisometric relaxation provides an alternative to working directly against hypertonic muscles.

4. e: While MFR works by relieving movement restrictions and pain from soft tissue dysfunctions, important effects include benefits to posture and the sense of relaxed well-being.

5. a: Erik Dalton has described modern society as a society of flexion addicts.

6. b: MFR can include mechanical, neurologic, and movement-oriented approaches used in coordination to gain increased freedom from movement restrictions and pain.

7. a: Robert Ward, an osteopath, is credited with coining the name "myofascial release."

8. c: The orientation that our visual imagery ties in with neuromuscular patterns affecting our posture and body use is the core concept of "ideokinesis."

9. d: Ida Rolf's core focus was working along straight lines of fascial shortening to increase congruence with gravity.

10. d: Fascia supports the body at multiple levels, from wrapping individual fibers to broad sheets external to muscles.

11. a: Postural muscles are composed of more "slow twitch" fibers rather than more "fast twitch" fibers.

12. c: Direct MFR works in direct opposition to shortness and restriction.

13. c: Compression of the muscle localizes the stretch to specific areas of restriction. Compression of a lengthening muscle accentuates the lengthening. Compression of a shortening muscle accentuates the spreading and broadening.

14. b: Because it addresses deeper layers of tissue, MFR uses substantially less lubrication than more conventional massage.

15. d: In the upper body, a common postural dysfunction is upper crossed syndrome.

16. b: The direction of strokes should be dictated by the tissue-specific goals, such as lengthening a muscle against its pattern of shortness.

17. a: According to Wolff's law and Davis's law tissue is laid down along lines of stress.

18. c: Cellulitis is a serious and potentially life-threatening bacterial infection.

19. d: The authors of this chapter recommend learning the skills gradually and incorporating and practicing them as you gain expertise. This is a general technique for learning kinesthetic skills.

20. c: Dizziness, slurred speech, and/or a sharp headache can be signs of a stroke. While further assessment can be done, such as evaluating a history of such symptoms related to migraine headaches, awareness of the potential need for immediate medical care should be recognized as a first priority.

Chapter 10

1. b: NMT can be integrated into a variety of practice settings, including chiropractic, massage therapy, and medical offices, PT and OT clinics, spa settings, and sports arena.

2. d: NMT does not usually include bone density tests, which are diagnostic tests for evidence of osteoporosis.

3. d: Lief, Chaitow, and Nimmo all contributed techniques that became fundamental to American and European NMT.

4. c: Emotional stress is considered a psychosocial factor.

5. a: Biochemical factors include endocrine function, hydration, and mineral levels, along with many other elements that can influence chronic pain.

6. b: Biomechanical, biochemical, and psychosocial factors synergistically interface, with their interaction being quite astounding.

7. d: Colloids become more fluid when heated, shaken, or stirred and reset to a gel state when allowed to stand still.

8. b: Central trigger points develop at the midfiber region of muscle fibers and create what is usually felt as a nodule within a taut band.

9. d: Trigger point pressure release is a highly effective technique used to release central trigger points.

10. d: European and American versions of NMT share a common theoretical platform while having distinctly different application of techniques.

11. d: Hot and cold packs can be used, as appropriate, during NMT session or at home between sessions. Pressure bars have been used by NMT practitioners for many decades.

12. a: The thumbs, with their lateral surfaces touching, are the treatment tool when applying gliding strokes in NMT American version™. The fingers serve to steady the hand.

13. d: "Deep tissue massage" is an inaccurate label for NMT, which is only "deep tissue" when the source of the problem lies in the deeper tissues.

14. d: Gait assessment is most objectively performed with computerized equipment and other diagnostic tools. Visual methods, while offering some value, are much more subjective and leave a wide margin for error.

15. b: Central trigger points form at the center of muscle fibers and refer sensations to their associated target zones.

16. b: When the appropriate degree of pressure is precisely applied to a central trigger point and maintained for at least 8 to 12 seconds, the person usually reports that an associated referred sensation is fading away.

17. c: NMT protocols can be incorporated in any practice setting and provide a step-by-step examination process.

18. b: Pincer palpation and snapping palpation are both useful but dissimilar techniques that are used for different purposes.

19. d: Skin palpation has tremendous value in NMT application and can be used to assess the skin's freedom of movement from underlying tissues as well as to palpate the quality of the skin itself.

20. d: In two-jointed muscles both joints need to be assessed.

Chapter 11

1. c: A comprehensive rehabilitation approach in massage. Orthopedic massage is not a particular technique and is used only in certain applications.

2. a: They are the second most common reason for a patient to seek the care of a physician in the U.S. This statistic is presented early in the chapter in discussing the incidence of musculoskeletal disorders in our current health care system.

3. c: The primary reason for performing assessment is to determine if massage treatment is appropriate. There are a number of reasons to perform orthopedic assessment. However, the most important reason is to assure the practitioner that the client's condition has been accurately identified so appropriate treatment or referral can be offered. Assessment must be used to accurately identify the client's condition.

4. d: Normalize soft-tissue dysfunction. There are several steps listed as part of the rehabilitation protocol. Normalizing soft-tissue dysfunction is the first step in the protocol. The rehabilitation protocol is part of a comprehensive system of orthopedic massage.

5. b: Performing the same massage routine with each client. Orthopedic massage is a treatment approach that varies with each client depending on the specific needs for rehabilitation. Consequently, performing the same massage routine with each client is not a part of the orthopedic massage system.

6. c: Techniques vary based on the client's needs. The techniques of orthopedic massage are different depending on the needs of the client and the status of the client's condition. It is not necessarily painful, but it is adaptable with each client, so the treatment process would not always contain the same elements.

7. a: The practitioner uses the client's active muscle contraction to aid in the technique. In an active engagement technique, the client uses an active muscle contraction. The practitioner is performing some type of massage technique during the client's active muscle contraction. The muscle being treated in an active engagement technique is also the muscle that is being engaged in the contraction.

8. d: Deep longitudinal stripping. A pin and stretch technique is designed to encourage lengthening in a muscle. Deep longitudinal stripping is the most effective of these listed techniques to encourage lengthening of muscle tissue.

9. b: Massage of a client with a herniated lumbar intervertebral disk. A relative contraindication means there are certain circumstances under which this treatment could progress. Orthopedic massage methods could be used to treat a herniated intervertebral disk under certain circumstances. The other conditions described in this question would all be considered absolute contraindications, so this one is the only relative contraindication.

10. b: They are a pervasive health care issue in the U.S. This statement reflects the statistics given in the early part of the chapter related to the incidence of MSDs in the United States at the present time. They are a highly prevalent condition and one that massage therapists are likely to see.

11. a: Refer the client to another health care practitioner. If a client's condition is not within your ability or scope of practice, that client should be referred to another health care professional.

12. d: Matching the physiology of the tissue injury to the effects of treatment. A crucial component of orthopedic massage is to choose an appropriate form of treatment based on the nature of the client's condition. The question stem gives an example of this principle of matching the physiology of the injury to the effects of treatment.

13. c: Assessment is the same things as diagnosis. Assessment is the systematic process of gathering information. Diagnosis is the giving of a name or a label for a specific pathologic condition. Assessment is not the same as diagnosis.

14. d: It requires detailed knowledge of anatomy, kinesiology, and pathology. In order to perform orthopedic massage effectively, the individual must have detailed knowledge of these subject areas. Understanding of various pathologies, evaluation, and choice of appropriate treatment methods relies on fundamental knowledge from these fields.

15. a: First used in the early 1980s. The term *orthopedic massage* was first used extensively in the early 1980s by Tom Hendricson, DC.

16. b: First placed in a shortened position and then lengthened while a deep stripping technique is applied. This is a description of the technique applied to the target muscle in an active engagement lengthening technique (one attempting to lengthen the muscle tissue while using the client's active muscle contraction).

17. d: Asks for a general stress reduction and relaxation massage session. If the client asks for a general stress reduction and relaxation massage, then s/he is not wanting to have any particular pathologic condition addressed. Consequently, orthopedic massage is not an approach that would be used with that client.

18. a: During a concentric contraction. During a concentric contraction a muscle will also broaden. That is why the broadening techniques are applied during the concentric phase of muscle contraction.

19. c: Deep friction applied to an ankle sprain followed by flexibility training and eventual strengthening and conditioning. The rehabilitation protocol should follow a particular order that is described in the chapter. This answer demonstrates normalizing the soft-tissue dysfunction, reestablishing proper movement patterns, and then using strengthening and conditioning. This reflects the proper order of the rehabilitation protocol.

20. a: To accurately identify the nature of the client's problem and determine if massage is appropriate. Assessment is necessary to determine the nature of the client's condition and choose the most appropriate treatment approach.

Chapter 12

1. d: Polarity therapy integrates several methods to balance the energy field including light, medium, and deep touch on pressure points, rocking, breathing, sound techniques, and nutrition.

2. c: Polarity therapy was heavily influenced by both Ayurvedic medicine and cranial osteopathy.

3. b: Research by Korn and Ryser (2007) showed statistically significant reduction in depression following 8 PT sessions with dementia caregivers.

4. c: PT is primarily a method for balancing the human energy field even though it also influences circulation and lymphatic flow.

5. c: The five elements are ether, air, fire, water, and earth.

6. b: The vagus nerve is near the surface of the ear concha.

7. a: The air element includes the shoulders, kidneys, and the ankles as reflexes.

8. a: The cradle is often the first hold in the session where the therapist "cradles" the cranium to help the client achieve a parasympathetic state.

9. b: In asthma only cold is applied to the upper thoracic vertebrae to drive blood deep into the spinal cord and relieve congestion at the surface.

10. b: Tuning forks are another mode of PT that balance the energy field and vibrational body.

11. a: PT nutrition derived from India and emphasizes vegetarianism for both health building and cleansing.

12. a: Stone delineated the regions of the buttocks and breasts and earlobes as vitality center reflexes that reflected innate or constitutional vitality of the individual.

13. d: PT is a system designed to balance and support physical, mental, emotional, and spiritual well-being.

14. c: Cleansing diet is a vegan diet and is followed short term for detoxification and consists of special teas and liver flushes; the health-building diet incorporates grains and fermented milk to build cell health.

15. b: The five senses are assigned to each element; taste is associated with water.

16. d: The vagus nerve governs parasympathetic dominance, which improves sleep quality, digestion (excess gas) pain, and pain perception.

17. c: The right hand is considered positive and warming and the hand that "sends" energy, and the left hand, the negative pole, is the cooling hand and receives energy.

18. b: All function is triune. It is based on the concept of the interaction among positive, neutral, and negative polarities. This suggests that in order to release energy blockages or pain each pole (body reflex) must be balanced with the other to achieve full effect.

19. a: The trapezius is positive pole; the lungs are neutral, and the diaphragm composes the negative.

20. b: The types and depth of touch include the satvic (light), the rajasic (moderate), and the tamasic (deep).

Chapter 13

1. b: Pregnancy-induced hypotension, a decrease in maternal blood pressure cutting off blood and oxygen to the fetus, can be brought on by positioning your client flat on her back. In the supine position, her upper torso must be elevated from her hips at an angle between 45 and 70 degrees and her legs should be elevated (ideally above the level of her heart).

2. d: 10 to 30 grams of light pressure is the appropriate amount to use during manual lymphatic drainage. Light pressure is always provided in the direction of the heart for maximum drainage. Use a small amount of lubrication to ensure a stretching of the underlying skin.

3. d: The placenta is a specialized organ involved with maternal-fetal gas and nutrient exchange, and manufactures, elaborates, and stores essential hormones vital to the continuation of the pregnancy.

4. d: The posterior pelvis elongates the lumbar spine and decreases the exaggerated lordotic curve of late pregnancy.

5. a: Her cervical spine protracts and often contributes to weakness, numbness, and/or tingling in her fingers and hands.

6. b: Estrogen and relaxin affect the composition of cartilage and ligamentous structures, particularly the pelvis, by allowing them to soften and loosen.

7. c: Since most of the muscles in the front of her body are overstretched, and most of the muscles in the back of her body are compressed, the treatment goal is to shorten the anterior muscles and elongate those found on the posterior aspect of her body.

8. c: Blood volume starts to increase as early as the sixth week and continues through the end, with an average of 30% to 50%.

9. c: The pressure in her veins increases and contributes to lower limb swelling.

10. d: The decrease in anticoagulants along with vasodilation contribute to a five- to six-fold increase in the risk of blood clots during pregnancy.

11. a: The pretreatment evaluations test for pitting edema, which is often symptomatic of preeclampsia, and the presence of blood clots.

12. d: The top of the uterus is called the fundus.

13. a: Braxton Hicks contractions occur throughout the pregnancy to circulate the blood through the placenta and to strengthen the uterus for labor.

14. b: Oxytocin is the hormone of mother love, calmness, and uterine contractions.

15. d: Maternal blood pressure is normalized during a massage.

16. c: Gestational glucose intolerance (formerly called gestational diabetes) is not a contraindication to massage. However, since glucose levels decrease after any massage treatment, practitioners must pay particular attention to their client's posttreatment reactions and make sure clients eat or drink sufficient amounts of nourishment to normalize blood sugar levels before leaving their office.

17. a: Spleen 3 is safe during pregnancy and can be stimulated to help balance hormones.

18. c: The gentle (posterior) pelvic tilt decompresses the lumbar spine and elongates the muscles of the lower back.

19. b: It is always safe to massage a pregnant woman's abdomen provided you ask her permission first. The massage will always be slow, done with an open hand, gentle, and follow a clockwise direction.

20. d: Using and strengthening the transverse abdominis are instrumental in maintaining core muscle integrity, lumbar stability, and minimizing the separation along the linea alba called the *diastasis recti*.

Chapter 14

1. b: Zones and reflex areas in the feet and hands that correspond to all the parts of the body. Zones are energy pathways and the reflex areas are points/areas on the feet and hands that, when stimulated with thumb and finger pressure, trigger a healing response in other parts of the body.

2. a: Stress reduction that causes a physiologic change in the body. Reflexology soothes nerves that innervate other parts of the body and dilates blood vessels, which improves nerve function and blood supply.

3. b: Linked to a corresponding area or point in the foot. Empirical and clinical research studies have established that there are reflex areas and points on the feet and hands that correspond to various parts of the body.

4. b: 1890 by Sir Henry Head. In 1890 Sir Henry Head determined the divisions of the 10 zones (energy pathways) that travel from the feet to the head.

5. c: Lord William T. Riley. Lord William T. Riley had no involvement with Reflexology.

6. d: All of the above. Reflexology acts on the nervous system (nearly 15,000 nerves are in the feet), which has a calming effect on the rest of the body's systems.

7. c: Stress. Stress constricts blood vessels and does not allow blood, lymph, and nerves to function at optimal levels.

8. a: Thailand. Thailand is very progressive in its thinking about healthcare. The government approves of and encourages Reflexology as a therapeutic approach to better health.

9. a: Adaptation. People often adapt to pain and tune it out of their conscious awareness and don't realize there may be help to improve their condition.

10. a: Guidelines. Four horizontal imaginary lines on the feet and hands that differentiate the five sections of the body—neck/shoulder line, diaphragm line, waist line, pelvic line.

11. c: Diagnosis of illnesses. Diagnosis is not an appropriate role for Reflexologists.

12. c: Obesity. Reflexology is beneficial for obesity. Performing Reflexology when one of the other conditions is present could exacerbate the condition.

13. b: Reflexologists can diagnose diseases through developing sensitive touch techniques. Only physicians are licensed to diagnose disease.

14. d: Interlymphatory. There is no such mechanism as "interlymphatory."

15. d: All of the above. Dorsal—top of the foot; lateral—side of the foot; plantar—bottom of the foot.

16. b: Synergistically. The combined action of two things, such as the immune system and other body processes, is greater than the sum of their effects individually.

17. a: Run the length of the body. That is, energy pathways that run from the feet to the head.

18. c: Hook-in and back-up. "Hook-in and back-up" is considered a Reflexology technique, not a relaxation technique.

19. d: Thumb walking. Thumb walking is the main Reflexology technique used on fleshy areas.

20. b: Through local and international certification. ARCB promotes Reflexology through national certification in the United States.

Chapter 15

1. c: A is incorrect because lubricant is not used; b is incorrect because clients remain fully clothed; d is incorrect because that describes massage and myofascial techniques; c is the only answer that characterizes a shiatsu treatment.

2. d: D is correct because the feet are not used in massage therapy but are used in shiatsu. The forearms, elbows, and hands are all used in both massage therapy and shiatsu.

3. a: A is correct because that is the foundational concept of shiatsu. The other choices are Western and allopathic medicine concepts.

4. c: Acupuncture and Anmo are modalities; a tsubo is a point on a channel. Ki is defined as the energy or force that gives and maintains life.

5. a: A client with a flare-up stage of lupus is the only condition of the four listed that massage therapy is contraindicated for but that shiatsu may not be. Both massage therapy and shiatsu can be performed on clients with osteoporosis, cancer, and chronic insomnia.

6. d: Varicose veins are the only condition of the ones listed that are a local contraindication. All the others are not contraindications for shiatsu.

7. a: A is the only correct answer; none of the others are true.

8. a: Namikoshi founded the Japan Shiatsu Institute in 1940.

9. b: Yin and Yang are pivotal to the traditional philosophy, science, and culture of China and Japan. The concepts of Yin and Yang are not fixed; they are in constant motion and always transforming each other.

10. c: The definition of a channel is an organized system that Ki flows through.

11. a: The answer is lung. All the rest are Yang organs.

12. b: Blue is the color associated with the water element. White is associated with the metal element; yellow is associated with the earth element; green is associated with the wood element.

13. d: Joy is associated with the fire element. Fear is associated with the water element; sadness is associated with the metal element; anger is associated with the wood element.

14. a: Singing is associated with the earth element. Shouting is associated with the wood element; laughing is associated with the fire element; crying is associated with the metal element.

15. c: The hara is the abdomen.

16. b: The wide stance is the most effective body mechanics for shiatsu.

17. a: Blurred vision may indicate a wood imbalance; high blood pressure may indicate a fire imbalance; acid reflux may indicate an earth imbalance.

18. c: Needing to spend a lot of time alone may indicate a water imbalance; being incapable of connecting with others may indicate a fire imbalance; constantly worrying may indicate an earth imbalance.

19. a: Taking a bath, especially with salt, is a self-care recommendation for a client with a water imbalance; having a long conversation with a good friend is a self-care recommendation for a client with a fire imbalance; doing something nice for yourself is a self-care recommendation for a client with an earth imbalance.

20. b: Doing something nice for yourself is a self-care recommendation for a client with an earth imbalance; going to a party is a self-care recommendation for a client with a fire imbalance; avoiding smoke and polluted air is a self-care recommendation for a client with a metal imbalance; taking a bath is a self-care recommendation for a client with a water imbalance.

Chapter 16

1. b: Athletes train for performance, which is an outcome, and they desire specific results.

2. c: Performance by definition requires more energy expenditure than maintaining fitness.

3. a: Traumatic events are unexpected.

4. c: When an athlete is performing at his or her peak, he or she can enjoy maximum achievement but also incur greater chances of injury.

5. a: Intercompetition massage is defined as massage between events.

6. d: Palliative care typically soothes and supports all outcomes.

7. a: Physical therapy is rehabilitation to regain normal function.

8. b: The normal inflammatory response is an important factor in tissue healing.

9. c: Deep transverse friction is not indicated during the acute healing phase.

10. b: Mental focus is most related to autonomic nervous system function.

11. c: A bruise is a compression injury so the depth of pressure has to be modified to avoid aggravating the injury.

12. a: Gliding creates a tension force if there is sufficient drag.

13. d: This is the definition of muscle tone.

14. c: The tissue formation at the subacute healing phase is still fragile, and stretching could disrupt the healing process.

15. d: Scar tissue is connective tissue, predominantly collagenous fibers.

16. a: There is evidently some nerve involvement, which should be addressed by the appropriate professional.

17. c: Deep vein thrombosis, or DVT, can be life threatening if it moves to the heart or lungs. If you suspect your client has a blood clot, all massage is contraindicated and a medical professional should be consulted immediately.

18. d: All individuals should be evaluated for a, b, and c, but the general population does not usually have a specific activity related to physical performance.

19. b: PRICE stands for *p*rotection, *r*est, *i*ce—the relationship to hydrotherapy—compression, and *e*levation.

20. a: Massage begins on the surface of the body and then progresses to the deeper tissue layers.

Chapter 17

1. c: A manual treatment of the connective tissue and movement education. The practitioner uses his/her hands to release strain from the various kinds of connective tissues, especially from the fascial envelopes of the muscles, and educates the person about proper movement.

2. a: Good alignment of the human body and well-coordinated movement. Good alignment helps us avoid unnecessary compression of our body and enables us to move with grace.

3. b: Ida P. Rolf, PhD. Ida P. Rolf studied several alternative approaches for healthcare and developed structural integration outside of her career as a scientist.

4. d: The fascia. The fascia is a kind of connective tissue that wraps around and subdivides the muscles.

5. b: To connect and subdivide all components of the human body. The connective tissue wraps around muscles, bones, and organs as well as the elements of the nervous system and builds bridges between these different systems of the body. At the same time, it subdivides these systems down to the cellular level.

6. b: An endless web. It connects all parts of the body with each other.

7. c: Gravity. Because gravity is permanently acting on the body, good alignment of all segments of the human organism is essential not only for good posture, but also for appropriate fluid exchange among the different parts of the organism.

8. c: A series of 10 manual treatment sessions. During this series all segments of the human body are treated, the trunk as well as the extremities.

9. b: That this kind of tissue can be shaped by the hands of a practitioner. Shaping in this sense means influencing the viscoelasticity of the tissues and it also means stimulation of the mechanoreceptors of the fascia.

10. b: The collagen fibers. These fibers are built of protein and play an important role in connecting and stabilizing the individual parts of the body.

11. c: Analyzing the client's physical structure as the client stands, sits, and moves. This kind of analysis gives information about the way the client has shaped his/her body in everyday life and leads the practitioner to the most restricted areas of the client's organism.

12. a: A free motion of breathing. Breathing happens more than 20,000 times a day and contributes to the shape of the trunk more than any other physical activity.

13. c: To allow better alignment along a lateral line. Alignment in this sense means that the shoulder girdle and the pelvis are in a balanced relationship and the curvatures of the back, lumbar, thoracic, and cervical, show smooth transitions at the segments where one curvature meets another.

14. c: Using a large variety of tactile contact from subtle to very intense. Different types of tissues require different modes of touch for efficient treatment.

15. a: He/she applies direct lengthening parallel to the muscle fibers and transverse to the primary fiber direction of fascia. The practitioner crosses the fibers of the fascia to arrive at a better balance of the flexor and extensor muscles around a joint.

16. d: After the cast or splint has been removed from the client's body. While using a cast or splint, motion is drastically reduced. This leads to thickening of collagen fibers and motion

restriction around the related joints. The goal of the treatment is to restore proper fluid exchange within the tissues and to reduce strain.

17. c: Osteoporosis. In this condition bones lack density and there is a danger of fractures.

18. b: Not to do any treatment at all. The manual treatment could contribute to the ongoing inflammatory processes.

19. a: Short and precise. Small infants may easily be overstimulated if a treatment takes too much time.

20. d: Improvement of the balance of the autonomous nervous system. Ideally the client's organism will go through several cycles of stimulation and release while being treated by the practitioner.

Chapter 18

1. c: Nuad is from the Thai language.

2. b: Nuad means "to touch with the intention of imparting healing."

3. d: Sanskrit language from ancient India.

4. d: Translates as "ancient and revered."

5. b: The Father Doctor of Medicine, Shivago Komparaj.

6. b: A key element of the meditative aspect of Thai massage is that it is practiced slowly.

7. d: In addition, Thai massage techniques are practiced with the client seated.

8. a: This is an important contraindication. In pregnancy, special precautions are taken, but pregnancy is not a contraindication.

9. c: Loving kindness is a very important ideal throughout all Thai culture.

10. d: See under #9.

11. c: The practice of Thai massage is at its core a contemplative practice designed to bring mental equanimity to the recipient as well as the practitioner.

12. a: Traditionally, this system of bodywork was utilized to treat the varied ailments that afflict mankind as a key component of a system of medicine.

13. c: To ensure a safe practice and the health and longevity of the practitioner, proper body mechanics are essential.

14. d: Practitioners of Thai massage learn to utilize numerous parts of their own bodies as massage tools.

15. a: The slow, rhythmic practice enhances the meditative aspects of the work and also supports the safe practice, especially when advanced stretching techniques are applied.

16. c: The concept of the doshas is a key theoretical construct of Thai medicine and traces back to the influence of Ayurvedic medicine on Thai medicine.

17. d: These are key physiologic benefits of this practice for the recipient.

18. a: The stretching techniques facilitate a diversity of signals to the brain resulting in increased flexibility, postural improvement, and lessened pain and suffering.

19. d: Practitioners always find out if there is any history of heart and circulatory problems prior to the application of stopping the blood flow techniques. If a client is on blood thinning medications, deep pressure is also contraindicated.

20. c: All the sen pathways have their origins in the abdominal region in the vicinity of the navel. This is an energetic reason why deep abdominal work is very important in the practice of Thai massage.

Chapter 19

1. b: Hook-up refers to the state of conscious awareness of practitioner and client.

2. d: Mentastics are easy movements that involve continual monitoring and refinement of body sensations by the mind.

3. d: These are principles that are different from most other bodywork modalities.

4. d: The practitioner keeps the movements within the range that produces no added pain.

5. c: The Trager practitioner would be very unlikely to use a subjective pain scale since he/she is not focused on symptomatic relief.

6. b: 19 years.

7. b: The unconscious mind is a repository for traumatic situations that result in movement restrictions. By creating pleasurable movements

where movement has been unconsciously restricted, guarding is released.

8. d: All of the above. The Trager practitioner reinforces the client's awareness of the release of restrictions at any time during the session, by asking the client to feel into what is happening now in the body and also by teaching the client *Mentastics.*

9. b: The real change takes place in the mind of the client, and therefore the practitioner addresses the session toward changing the client's mind. Milton Trager came to the conclusion that this is universal.

10. a: Unlike many forms of exercise, clients are discouraged from pushing through movement restrictions when doing *Mentastics.*

11. b: Trager practitioners would not move a body part beyond the subtle movement restrictions—this could create even more restriction.

12. c: Listening hands. The others would be considered direct-mechanical technique.

13. a: There is no necessity to avoid client emotional releases in Trager.

14. b: Pain would not be considered a proprioceptive signal whereas movement restriction would be.

15. d: Trager sessions can include all of the practices listed in d.

16. b: In general the Trager session is not directed toward the removal of symptoms.

17. d: All of the above. Pausing is restorative for the practitioner, reinforcing to the client, and can allow the practitioner to become more creative.

18. b: Soft hands may indeed help a client to let go emotionally because he/she feels safe.

19. d: Unlike Freud, Trager did not consider the unconscious mind a repository of negative experiences or feelings. He considered that one of the ways the unconscious functions is to limit movement and muscle use in body parts that have been traumatized.

20. a: Hook-up is actually a state of heightened mental acuity and awareness of body sensations.

Chapter 20

1. c: Kathryn Weiner, in a special message as director of the American Academy of Pain Management, shares this figure when alleging that pain in an epidemic in America.

2. d: Travell and Simons developed a diagnostic criteria for TrPs that includes a palpable nodule within a taut band that when provoked, refers a sensation to the target zone associated with that muscle.

3. b: Releasing a trigger point is a goal in many modalities, and a number of techniques (manual release, needling, spray and stretch, etc.) can be applied to achieve this.

4. a: Within their original textbook published in 1983 and based on their clinical experience, Travell and Simons documented that approximately 75% of chronic pain patients have a trigger point as the sole source of pain.

5. b: Although a latent trigger point in the third finger extensor occurs more often, Travell and Simons note that upper trapezius and quadratus lumborum trigger points are more commonly located than any TrPs.

6. b: Practitioners who have manual skills in releasing trigger points are known by this author to work in private practice, medical offices (including dental, chiropractic, general medical, oncology), hospitals, athletic settings, rehabilitation (physical and occupational therapy, chronic pain clinics), and in spas.

7. b: Box 20-1 offers a substantial list of academic papers that explore referred pain from myofascial tissues, spanning a 150-year period.

8. a: It is rare to find a discussion on trigger points that does not include reference to the work of Travell and Simons, who are both given credit for developing the foundational platform as well as therapeutic applications for trigger points.

9. c: Janet Travell served as the first female Personal Physician to the President of the United States to John F. Kennedy, whom she met and treated for back pain when he was a U.S. senator.

10. d: Dr. David Simons first achieved international recognition when he ascended to 102,000 feet in a hot air balloon in 1957. He later met Janet

Travell, with whom he researched trigger points and chronic pain, which resulted in extensive publication of academic material.

11. a: Bonnie Prudden made a significant impact on fitness awareness in the U.S. by documenting and bringing to the attention of President Eisenhower that the children of the U.S. were substantially physically unfit.

12. b: Stanley Lief and Boris Chaitow developed European NMT in their famous healing center in Hertfordshire, England.

13. c: Raymond Nimmo and James Vannerson began writing of their experiences with what they termed "noxious nodules" and published their findings in their newsletters as receptor tonus technique.

14. b: A myofascial trigger point is defined as a localized area within a muscle that, when sufficiently provoked (by pressure, needling, etc.), produces a referred sensation to a particular target zone.

15. b: A contracture is apparently sustained by an abnormal, sustained flow of acetylcholine at the neuromuscular junction of the affected muscle fibers.

16. a: Spasms are involuntary (cannot be voluntarily relaxed) and present with evidence of motor potentials (neurologic influence).

17. c: A local energy crisis results when ATP (the energy of the cell) is not available in sufficient quantities to carry needed biological processes, such as active transport.

18. a: When central TrPs produce unrelenting tension on musculotendinous or periosteal tissues, attachment trigger points (ATrPs) often develop and may also be associated with inflammation, fibrosis, and calcification of those tissues.

19. d: A number of techniques can be used to deactivate a myofascial TrP. Mastery of one or more of the techniques discussed within this chapter can be accomplished with adequate training and practice.

20. b: It is important to lengthen the central sarcomeres associated with a TrP after deactivation. This can be accomplished by applying manual traction to the shortened actin and myosin filaments or, if appropriate,

though passive or active stretching of the muscle fibers.

Chapter 21

1. c: An Wu was the original form of massage performed in China.

2. d: Tuina is the medical form of massage done in China today.

3. a: Tui means to push or stroke, and Na means to grasp or knead.

4. c: Hepatitis is one of the contraindications for performing Tuina.

5. d: A Tuina practitioner may not perform spinal adjustments in the U.S.

6. b: Acupoints are fixed points that lie along the energy channels.

7. c: The Huangdi Neijing was the first medical book written in China.

8. b: TCM declined in the nineteenth century due to political and foreign influences.

9. c: By the 1930s, studies had proven the validity of TCM.

10. b: TCM attempts to reestablish a sense of balance within the body.

11. c: Relationships, patterns, and change are the concept of Yin and Yang Theory.

12. d: Qi is generally defined as "vital energy."

13. c: There are 14 major energy channels running through the body.

14. a: Imbalance between Yin and Yang is the root cause of all disease.

15. d: In treating an injury with Tuina, you must first open up the channel.

16. a: Zusanli (St-36) is the first acupoint to work in treating an ankle sprain.

17. d: Kneading method applied to an ankle sprain is an effective Tuina technique.

18. a: Futu (St-32) is the first acupoint to work in treating a knee sprain.

19. b: Reestablishing the harmony of Yin and Yang is the first goal in treating an illness.

20. b: Tuina is considered a medically specific manipulative art.

INDEX

Note: Page numbers followed by "f" indicate figures, "t" indicate tables, and "b" indicate boxes.